Praise for

Managing and Treating Urinary Incontinence, Second Edition

"This book, written by two of the world's authorities on urinary disorders, is an excellent overview of the management of the disorders of the pelvic floor, using a collaborative, yet inclusive, approach. The authors have condensed a very broad field ⟨...⟩ comprehensive in its inclusion ⟨...⟩ dysfunctions. The unique mer⟨...⟩ d strategy will benefit patients ⟨...⟩ f interventions. This is a must fo⟨...⟩ art in its context."

— *Roger Dmo⟨...⟩*
  Vanderbilt ⟨...⟩

"This is an outst⟨...⟩ e new and experienced clin⟨...⟩ excellent overview of the ⟨...⟩ incontinence, bowel dysfuncti⟨...⟩ e primary emphasis on cor⟨...⟩ recommended for nurses, phys⟨...⟩ apists involved in establishing c⟨...⟩ m care facility and hospital."

— *Jean F. Wy⟨...⟩ofessor*
  and Cora ⟨...⟩, Minnesota
  Continence ⟨...⟩sing

"An outstanding ⟨...⟩ perts. This should form the ⟨...⟩ ulum' in incontinence fo⟨...⟩"

— *Matt T. R⟨...⟩ters*
  and Presid⟨...⟩

"This second e⟨...⟩ nd innovators in the field is extremely well written, and, not unexpectedly, quite thorough. . . . Upon completion of this text, not only will the reader have a command of the diagnosis and management of urinary incontinence, but she or he will have an appreciation of how these skills and knowledge can improve the suffering and quality of life of those who are afflicted with this condition. Overall, I highly recommend this text to anyone with an interest in, or who is involved in, the diagnosis and treatment of urinary incontinence, including students, nurses, residents-in-training and other practitioners, and allied health care personnel."

— *Eric S. Rovner, M.D., Professor of Urology, Medical University of South Carolina*

"This second edition is a much needed update and contains the many advances in the field of incontinence care. The authors address the subject with expertise and experience while providing a unique guideline for assessment, which can be applied to patients in any setting. . . . Treatment options from the most simple behavioral to complex surgical are all-inclusive and provide an excellent resource for providers, caregivers, and students. . . . A 'must have' reference for anyone caring for the millions of people affected by urinary incontinence!"

—*Cindy Monaghan, R.N.C., M.S., F.N.P., Director, Seton Health Incontinence and Wound Services, Troy, New York*

Managing and Treating Urinary INCONTINENCE

Second Edition

Managing and Treating *Urinary* INCONTINENCE

Second Edition

by

Diane Kaschak Newman,
R.N.C., M.S.N., C.R.N.P., F.A.A.N.

Alan J. Wein, M.D., Ph.D. (hon)

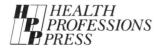

HEALTH
PROFESSIONS
PRESS

Baltimore • London • Sydney

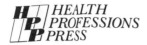

Health Professions Press, Inc.
Post Office Box 10624
Baltimore, Maryland 21285-0624

www.healthpropress.com

Typeset by Barton Matheson Willse & Worthington, Baltimore, Maryland.
Manufactured in the United States of America by Sheridan Books, Inc., Ann Arbor, Michigan.
Cover and interior design by Erin Geoghegan.

The cases described in this book are based on the authors' experience. In all instances, names and identifying details have been changed to protect confidentiality.

The information provided in this book is in no way meant to substitute for a medical practitioner's advice or expert opinion. Readers should consult a medical practitioner if they are interested in more information. This book is sold without warranties of any kind, express or implied, and the publisher and authors disclaim any liability, loss, or damage caused by the contents of this book.

Library of Congress Cataloging-in-Publication Data

Newman, Diane Kaschak.
    Managing and treating urinary incontinence / Diane Kaschak Newman, Alan Wein.—2nd ed.
        p. ; cm.
    Includes bibliographical references and index.
    ISBN 978-1-932529-21-0 (pbk.)
    1. Urinary incontinence. I. Wein, Alan J.   II. Title.
    [DNLM: 1. Urinary Incontinence. WJ 146 N5519m 2009]
    RC921.I5N488 2009
    616.6'2—dc22   2008037376

British Library Cataloguing in Publication data are available from the British Library.

Contents

About the Authors xi

Foreword   Diana J. Mason, Ph.D., R.N., F.A.A.N. xiii

Foreword   Joseph G. Ouslander, M.D. xv

Preface xix

Acknowledgments xxiii

1   Introduction 1

2   The Problem of Incontinence 13

3   Understanding Bladder and Pelvic Floor Function 61

4   Causes of Incontinence and Identification of Risk Factors 85

5   Bowel Dysfunction and Its Relationship to Urinary Incontinence . . 129

6   Clinical Assessment and Evaluation 175

7   Self-Care Practices and Lifestyle Changes to Reduce Urinary
    Symptoms 233

8   Behavioral Treatments: Implementing Toileting, Bladder Training,
    and Pelvic Floor Muscle Rehabilitation Programs 245

9   Drug Therapy for Incontinence and Overactive Bladder 307

10 Urinary Collection and Management Products 365

11 Evaluation and Management of Pelvic Organ Prolapse 485

12 Overview of Surgical Intervention for Incontinence 523

13 Continence Nurse Specialists and Service Models 565

Appendix A: Glossary 585

Appendix B: Resources 601

Index 615

Patient & Provider Tools & Forms CD-ROM

Care Plans

Care Plan #1 Nursing Diagnosis—Urinary Elimination: Altered Patterns Related to Transient/Acute Causes of Incontinence

Care Plan #2 Nursing Diagnosis—Urgency Urinary Incontinence and Overactive Bladder Symptoms of Urgency and Frequency That May Be Secondary to Detrusor Overactivity

Care Plan #3 Nursing Diagnosis—Stress Urinary Incontinence Related to Decreased Outlet Resistance from Weakened or Damaged Urinary Sphincter and/or Pelvic Floor Muscle

Care Plan #4 Nursing Diagnosis—Urinary Retention Related to Chronically Overfilled (Distended) Bladder with Loss of Sensation

Care Plan #5 Nursing Diagnosis—Functional (Urinary or Bowel) Incontinence Related to Decreased Physical or Cognitive Capability

Care Plan #6 Nursing Diagnosis—Impaired Skin Integrity Related to Urinary and/or Bowel Incontinence

Care Plan #7 Nursing Diagnosis—Urinary Tract Infection, Potential for, Related to Urinary and Bowel Incontinence

Care Plan #8 Nursing Diagnosis—Urinary Tract Infection, Potential for, Related to Use of Indwelling (Urethral or Suprapubic) Catheter

Care Plan #9 Nursing Diagnosis—Constipation, Colonic, Related to Lack of Dietary Fiber, Fluid Intake, and Exercise

Care Plan #10 Nursing Diagnosis—Constipation, Perceived, Related to Stool (Fecal) Impaction

Care Plan #11 Nursing Diagnosis—Bowel Incontinence Related to Decreased Rectal Tone

Care Plan #12 Nursing Diagnosis—Diarrhea Related to Laxative and Medication Use and Bacterial Infection

Patient Education Tools

What Is Urinary Incontinence?
Preventing Bladder Infections
What to Know About Your Bladder and Voiding
Caffeine Count
What You Eat and Drink Can Affect Your Bladder
Bladder Training—Controlling Urgency and Frequency
Exercising Your Pelvic Floor Muscles
Getting the "Knack" for Stopping Urine Leaks
Doing a Pad Test
Ways to Prevent Bladder Problems During the Night
Helping Your Bladder to Empty
How to Prevent Postvoid Dribble
The Side Effects of Treatment for Overactive Bladder
Using a Catheter—Men
Using a Catheter—Women

Care and Use of an Indwelling (Foley) Urinary Catheter
How to Use an External "Condom" Catheter
How to Care for Your Catheter Drainage Bag
Using a Pessary for Pelvic Organ Prolapse
Using Topical Estrogen
Tips for Keeping Your Bowels Moving
Self-care for "Painful Bladder Syndrome" (Interstitial Cystitis)

Assessment Forms

Incontinence Patient Profile
Past Medical History
Pelvic Floor Muscle Strength Assessment
Daily Voiding and Incontinence Record
Voiding Frequency–Volume and Incontinence Chart
Bowel Disorders Profile
Daily Bowel Record
Treatment Findings and Recommendations
Pelvic Floor Muscle Exercise Prescription
Initial Consultation (Long-term Care)
Bladder and Bowel Diary—Assessment of Bladder Function
    (Long-term Care)

Information Boxes

2.2   Summary of criteria for facility compliance with Tag F315
        (Urinary Incontinence and Catheters)
5.1   Bowel Function Evaluation Checklist
5.2   Elements of a successful bowel program in long-term care
6.1   Evaluation checklist
6.2   Evaluation checklist in long-term care residents
6.3   Simple UI-related questions
6.4   Patient Perception of Bladder Condition (PPBC)
6.5   Q-Tip procedure
6.6   Examiner instructions on how to perform a pelvic floor muscle (PFM)
        contraction during digital pelvic examination of female patients
6.7   Applications of a portable ultrasound machine (the BladderScan) in
        long-term care
6.8   Urodynamics terminology
6.9   Procedure for bedside or "eyeball" cystometrogram
7.1   Key components of lifestyle changes
9.1   Assessment of drugs used in the treatment of voiding dysfunction
10.1   Product Classification and Approval in the United States
10.3   Indications (medical necessity) for indwelling catheter
10.5   Medicare medical necessity and documentation requirements for
        intermittent catheters
11.2   Pelvic Organ Prolapse Quantification (POPQ) Measurement

Perineal skin care
Step-by-step approach to indwelling catheter removal
Best practices for indwelling urinary catheters
Changing a suprapubic catheter
Steps of a prompted voiding program
International Consultation on Incontinence Questionnaire (ICI-Q)

Tables

4.1   Lower urinary tract symptoms (LUTS)
4.4   Medications that affect bladder function
4.6   Common diagnoses and definition of terms for bladder and urethral dysfunctions
5.2   Common medications used for chronic constipation
6.1   OAB-q
6.2   Description of specific urodynamic studies
8.1   Description of types of bladder programs
8.2   Possible contributions and solutions to UI in patients with dementia
9.3   Drug therapy for underactive bladder and incomplete bladder emptying
9.4   Drug therapy for stress urinary incontinence
9.5   Estrogen hormone preparations
10.2 Common perineal skin conditions

Appendix 9.1   Drug therapy for overactive bladder and urinary incontinence
Appendix 9.2   OAB drug efficacy
Appendix 9.3   OAB drug side effect profile
Appendix 10.1 Product (HCPC) billing codes (as of 2008)
Appendix 10.2 Review of current skin care products
Appendix 11.1 Review of pessary types

Figures

6.1   Diagnostic algorithm for evaluation of urinary incontinence (UI)
6.6   Female body map and a pain scale for patient to mark pelvic pain
6.9   Pelvic floor muscle strength assessment
6.10 Male body map and a pain scale for patient to mark pelvic pain
6.12 UI care pathway
8.4   Management pathway for urinary incontinence in a long-term care setting
8.5   Urgency suppression wave
10.1 Types of incontinence products according to absorbency
11.5 Pelvic organ prolapse quantification

About the Authors

Diane Kaschak Newman, R.N.C., M.S.N., C.R.N.P., F.A.A.N., B.C.I.A.-P.M.D.B.

Ms. Newman is an adult nurse practitioner and a recognized expert in the field of nonsurgical management and treatment of urinary incontinence and related disorders. She is Co-Director of the Penn Center for Continence and Pelvic Health in the Division of Urology, University of Pennsylvania Health System in Philadelphia and an Instructor in the School of Medicine at the University of Pennsylvania. Her clinical practice is dedicated to the evaluation, treatment, and management of urinary incontinence and related problems. She has experience in treating patients in long-term care, home care, and office practice environments. Ms. Newman has participated in several research projects on the effects of behavioral treatment for urinary incontinence, overactive bladder, and interstitial cystitis.

Ms. Newman received her Master of Science degree in nursing from the University of Pennsylvania. She is Chairperson of the Committee on Promotion, Education, and Organization for Continence for the World Health Organization's International Consultation on Incontinence. She is the Chair of the International Continence Society Continence Promotion Committee.

She was a member of the planning committee of the *State-of-the-Science Conference on Prevention of Fecal and Urinary Incontinence in Adults,* National Institute of Diabetes and Digestive and Kidney Diseases, Office of Medical Applications of Research of the National Institutes of Health and presented at the December 2007 meeting. She is a member of the Patient Education Council of the American Urological Association Foundation. Ms Newman was a member of the panel of experts of the Center for Medicare and Medicaid Service's Scope and Severity of Nursing Care Deficiencies in Long-term Care on "Guidance to Surveyors on Incontinence and Catheters-Tag F315." She served as a member on the Gastroenterology and Urology Devices Panel of the Federal Drug Administration from 1998 to 2002. In 2002, the National Association for Continence presented her with the Continence Care Champion Award.

Ms. Newman is an internationally known speaker on the topic of urinary incontinence and the use of devices and products for the management of incontinence. A prolific writer, Ms. Newman has written and presented more than 125 scientific papers, chapters, and articles in major journals on the subject of assessment, behavioral treatment, and management of incontinence with an emphasis on the nurse's role. Her *American Journal of Nursing* article "Stress Urinary Incontinence in Women" was cited by *The New York Times* Personal Health Column (September 2003). She was interviewed in the August 2007 issue of Oprah Winfrey's *O* magazine and for *USA Today* in June 2008. She is the author of the book *The Urinary Incontinence Sourcebook*. She is the co-author with Dr. Alan J. Wein of *Overcoming Overactive Bladder*.

Alan J. Wein, M.D., Ph.D. (hon)

Dr. Wein is professor and chair of the Division of Urology at the University of Pennsylvania School of Medicine and Chief of Urology at the Hospital of the University of Pennsylvania. He is a graduate of Princeton University and received his M.D. from the University of Pennsylvania School of Medicine. He received his surgical and urology training at the University of Pennsylvania.

Dr. Wein has been recognized nationally and internationally through his many affiliations and professional memberships, which include the American Association of Genitourinary Surgeons, Clinical Society of Genitourinary Surgeons, American Surgical Association, Society of Surgical Oncology, Society of Urologic Oncology, Society of Pelvic Surgeons, Society for Urodynamics and Female Urology, Société Internationale d'Urologie, American Urological Association and the Royal Society of Medicine. He is a recipient of the Urodynamics Society Lifetime Achievement Award, the F. Brantley Scott Award of the American Foundation for Urologic Diseases, the Hugh Hampton Young Award of the American Urological Association, and both the Distinguished Service Award and the Distinguished Contribution Award of the American Urological Association.

Dr. Wein has authored or co-authored more than 830 articles and chapters, edited or co-edited 24 books, and has multiple multimedia presentations to his credit. He has been an editor of the gold standard text in the field, *Campbell's Urology*, since 1992 and is currently the editor-in-chief. He is a prodigious lecturer with over 600 invited academic activities over the course of his career, including the co-chairmanship of the 1st, 2nd, 3rd, and 4th International Consultations on Incontinence.

His fields of interest lie in urologic oncology, the physiology and pharmacology of the lower urinary tract, the evaluation and management of voiding function, and dysfunction and urinary incontinence.

Foreword

In 2002, I wrote the foreword to the first edition to *Managing and Treating Urinary Incontinence*. Noting my experience moderating a radio program on health, I pointed out that the public wants opportunities to talk about "bladder health" and incontinence—what many consider to be an embarrassment that should remain unspoken. Listeners will call in with questions and problems, finding courage to speak about their "loss of control" under the blanket of anonymity. In that earlier edition, I challenged readers to deepen their knowledge about urinary incontinence by using this rich resource by Diane Kaschak Newman, one of the world's leading experts on the topic.

Foolishly, I had hoped this book would be a panacea. Here, in one place, is a superb guide to the best practices and tools for managing and treating urinary incontinence. I believe this book has helped, but much more needs to be done. For example, we still do not have a famous champion or poster child for incontinence. Bob Dole made erectile dysfunction and Viagra household words. Katie Couric has created an unprecedented demand for colonoscopies following the death of her husband Jay Monahan from colon cancer. Lance Armstrong and testicular cancer; Nancy Reagan and breast cancer—where is the champion for openly discussing the prevention and management of incontinence?

Diane Newman has been that champion for the nursing and medical professions. She has nudged, cajoled, educated, and challenged nurses and physicians to pay attention to this hidden problem that is clinically and financially costly. But she is not a household name—only one that is trusted within urology, nursing, and policy-making circles. She has been a prime motivator behind getting the federal government to develop policies that will encourage clinicians and health care systems to be more responsive to the prevalent problem of incontinence.

Diane's efforts are undoubtedly part of the reason why this second edition of *Managing and Treating Urinary Incontinence* will turn into a best seller among nurses and other care providers. The Centers for Medicare and Medicaid Services (CMS) will no longer pay for the care needed to treat hospital-acquired urinary tract infections. The reflexive "Let's cath her" will no longer be a wise choice for the patient who has become incontinent. Readers will use this second edition to explore best practices for preventing and managing incontinence. The addition of a CD-ROM with care plans, education tools, and medical forms for monitoring incontinence could not be more timely.

At this writing, the CMS rules apply only to hospital care of individuals with UI. What about residents of long-term care facilities and those receiving home care? Do we need a CMS "rule" threatening no coverage to encourage everyone to provide appropriate interventions to ensure that our patients are continent?

I once experienced transient incontinence. I have to admit that I was hesitant to discuss it with Diane and my other nurse colleagues who know about this condition. But I did. I learned Kegel exercises and reminded myself of the added benefit I would have if I undertook a weight-loss program. If I, a nurse, have difficulty speaking the unspoken, what hope do your patients have of finding a clinician who will assess bladder health, talk openly about incontinence, and work with individuals on self-care management and other treatment options that can restore a feeling of "control"?

None of us wants to "lose control" of any bodily function. We want healthy lives. We also want clinicians who will engage us in authentic, caring conversations about our well-being. No clinician can have such conversations about urinary incontinence without the knowledge contained in this book. Keep it as a companion to your daily ventures in caregiving, share it with colleagues, explore which practices you are not doing but ought to, and use it to help the people who have entrusted you with their care.

Diana J. Mason, Ph.D., R.N., F.A.A.N.

Editor-in-Chief
American Journal of Nursing

Foreword

Rarely do you find a book or other educational resource that is authoritative, comprehensive, easy to read, and full of material useful in clinical practice. Rarer still do you have the opportunity to gain knowledge and insights from two of the world's leading experts on a topic representing two major health care disciplines. *Managing and Treating Urinary Incontinence, Second Edition,* is indeed one of those rare resources that come along too infrequently.

This book fulfills a major unmet need in the care of people with bothersome lower urinary tract symptoms. When I was in fellowship training in geriatric medicine in 1980, I asked the nurses what topics they would like to learn more about. The first one they mentioned was urinary incontinence. I diligently started my literature search (in the bowels of the UCLA medical library, not on the Internet), and came up pretty dry (pun intended). There was a dearth of literature, especially from the United States, to use in preparing a presentation. The best resources were written in geriatric medicine textbooks by some of the fathers of modern geriatrics in the United Kingdom (such as John Brocklehurst and Bernard Isaacs) and in *Incontinence in the Elderly* by Frederick Lane Willington in 1951. Thus began my almost 30-year journey of learning how to improve the quality of life and care of older people with incontinence and other bothersome urinary tract symptoms.

In 1989, I had an editorial titled "Incontinence—Out of the Closet" published in the *Journal of the American Medical Association* following the first National Institutes of Health Consensus Conference on Incontinence. Over the last 20 years, incontinence has certainly come out of the closet as a result of a plethora of research, advances in management and treatment, and the development of a variety of educational materials. Numerous national and international meetings, standards, guidelines, and publications have focused on the topic of incontinence. Indeed, Diane Newman and Alan Wein have been two of the major forces behind these efforts. Moreover, public awareness of the scope, severity, adverse consequences, and potential reversibility of incontinence and related urinary tract symptoms has increased substantially through the efforts of numerous organizations. More people now understand that incontinence is not just a hygienic problem or an inevitable consequence of aging. We still, however, have a long way to go. Data still suggest that a large proportion of people who experience the bothersome symptoms of incontinence and overactive bladder do not seek help from a health professional. Progress has been made, but much more work lies ahead.

One of the major barriers to improving incontinence care is a lack of education on the part of health professionals on screening for lower urinary tract symptoms and on the appropriate assessment and management of these symptoms. Health professionals cannot optimally manage a condition that they do not adequately understand. While the knowledge and tools to manage incontinence are now available, finding them in one place and in a usable format may be difficult in this age of information overload.

This is where *Managing and Treating Urinary Incontinence, Second Edition,* provides a timely solution. Building on a very successful first edition, Diane Newman, an acknowledged international authority in the field, had the foresight to include Alan Wein, arguably one of the top handful of urologists in the world for the last three decades, as a coauthor to enhance several areas of the text. Dr. Wein has provided outstanding additions to this second edition.

The text is easy to read and is complemented by useful tables and figures that are valuable for both learning and teaching. The references are comprehensive and up to date. I find every chapter extremely useful. The chapters on behavioral treatments (Chapter 8), drug therapy (Chapter 9), and urine collection and management products (Chapter 10) are most impressive, as would be expected given the expertise of the two authors. Two new chapters on pelvic organ prolapse (Chapter 11) and surgical intervention (Chapter 12) add great value for urologists, gynecologists, and nurses specializing in these areas. The additional resources provided on the CD-ROM are one of the most attractive features and should assist health professionals in translating research and knowledge into better practice for people with incontinence and related symptoms.

Health professionals from multiple disciplines, including nurses specializing in urology, gynecology, neurology, and geriatrics as well as urologists, gynecologists, geriatricians, neurologists, and primary care physicians will all benefit from learning from this book. I think the text should be required reading for advance practice nurses specializing in urology, gynecology, and geriatrics as well as fellows training in urogynecology and geriatric medicine. It will also be helpful for residents training in these fields.

Diane Newman and Alan Wein are not only international authorities in managing and treating incontinence and related lower urinary tract symptoms, they are also truly passionate advocates for the people who experience these conditions. *Managing and Treating Urinary Incontinence, Second Edition,* is a result of their passion and dedication, and will be a major resource for health professionals who are interested in and committed to improving the quality of life and care of their patients.

Joseph G. Ouslander, M.D.

Director, Institute for Quality Aging
Boca Raton Community Hospital

Professor of Medicine (Voluntary)
Assistant Dean for Geriatric Education
University of Miami Miller School of Medicine (UMMSM)
at Florida Atlantic University

Professor (Courtesy)
Christine E. Lynn College of Nursing
Florida Atlantic University

Preface

Urinary incontinence (UI) is a complex and costly medical condition. UI combined with overactive bladder (OAB) comprise two of the ten most chronic conditions in women in the United States, and they affect a higher percentage of individuals of all age groups than do hypertension, depression, or diabetes. UI and OAB affect the social, psychological, occupational, domestic, physical, and sexual lives of women and men of all ages and are increasingly adding to caregiver burden. The symptoms of UI and OAB are historically underreported because individuals perceive that current treatment is ineffective and that the symptoms are a normal consequence of aging or childbirth. People also feel embarrassment regarding these two conditions. The lack of knowledge on the part of clinicians about the causes and management options, and their assumption that UI and OAB are not true medical issues, hinder the detection and treatment of these insidious conditions. This book provides a comprehensive review of the problem of UI and OAB for health care providers of all disciplines (nurses, doctors, allied health professionals) who practice in primary care and who provide services to adults in acute care, rehabilitation centers, home care, and long-term care settings. This second edition of *Managing and Treating Urinary Incontinence* is unique in that it combines the expertise of a nurse practitioner (DKN) and a urologist (AJW), both of whom are authorities on UI and who blend their knowledge and perspective to present a thorough and practical review of the management and treatment of UI.

Since the first edition of this book, significant advances have been made in the management and treatment of UI. Professional organizations, government agencies, and consumer groups worldwide have developed practice guidelines on UI. In the United States, the 2008 National Institutes of Health State-of-the-Science Conference Statement on the Prevention of Fecal and Urinary Incontinence in Adults noted that preventive strategies need to be targeted to specific populations or clinical groups and should examine the impact of public health initiatives, increased public and provider awareness, changes in reimbursement mechanisms, and health delivery redesign. However, most health care providers are unaware of the existence of guidelines or consensus statements and thus have not incorporated them into their care practice.

Additionally, we continue to see an increase in research initiatives to determine the best treatment for UI so that providers can practice evidence-based care. Federal agencies have funded multiple research projects that look at the use of noninvasive behavioral treatments in ambulatory and long-term care settings. The National Institute of Diabetes and Digestive and Kidney Diseases has funded multisite networks that conduct research on UI, pelvic floor prolapse, and interstitial cystitis. The development of new drug therapy for OAB and innovative surgical approaches for incontinence and other pelvic floor problems have expanded the choices of treatments available to men and women. Research outlining the causes of UI and how to diagnose the condition has concluded that UI is treatable, even curable, and can always be managed to improve quality of life; however, the fact remains that men and women do not seek treatment.

In order to provide care for patients with UI, a few prerequisites must exist. First, a clinician must determine if incontinence or any lower urinary tract dysfunction exists and if the individual wants treatment. There is a stigma attached to UI and OAB, and people face social and personal barriers to admitting that they are "bothered" by these conditions. As health care providers, we must understand that individuals, especially women, despite their age, do not view UI as abnormal. Health care providers, doctors, and nurses must take the initiative and ask their patients the all-important questions, "Do you ever leak urine? Do you control your bladder or does your bladder control you?" We must begin to address the issues of UI and OAB because we will encounter the problems more frequently in our professional and personal lives as baby boomers age. Chances are that in the coming decades each of us will be in a position of caring for a family member who experiences incontinence. We must find the solutions and approaches to this problem now before it becomes an epidemic! Providers need to increase the dialogue about UI and OAB with their patients, colleagues, and friends because these conditions are costly, embarrassing, and distressing to society as a whole.

The second prerequisite is that clinicians must have a knowledge base from which to diagnose men and women with UI and OAB. This is one of the main objectives of the second edition of this book. Our colleagues tell us that they usually do not inquire about UI because, other than recommending an absorbent product, they are unsure of what else to tell people (they just "don't know"). This book provides readers with the basics to confidently discuss the most current and accurate information on UI with their patients and to initiate treatment. The book provides a comprehensive overview of UI, cites in detail the prevalence and risk factors (Chapter 2), and provides a thorough discussion of the anatomy and physiology of the lower urinary tract (Chapter 3). Chapters 4 and 6 are devoted to the causes of UI and the primary and secondary evaluation that should be done prior to initiation of treatment. Chapter 5 discusses the relationship between bowel function and UI. A major strength of this book is Chapters 7, 8, 9 and 12, which provide a very detailed review of the current treatments for UI and OAB. These chapters outline practical strategies for preventing UI; detail behavioral, drug, and surgical treatments; and provide the most current evidence-based outcomes research. This second edition also includes an expanded review of the use of catheters, including products and devices that can be used to manage UI as well as extensive illustrations and pictures of these products (Chapter 10). New to this edition is Chapter 11, which addresses pelvic organ prolapse in women and details the use of pessaries.

The third prerequisite is that clinicians must know where to go to find more information that will assist them in providing the most current care for UI. Appendix B (Resources) provides a list of companies that supply treatment products as well as a list of organizations that can offer support. For readers who are unfamiliar with terminology related to urinary and fecal function, incontinence, and the devices and strategies used to manage UI, an extensive glossary is provided (Appendix A). This edition also includes a CD-ROM that provides printable forms that can be used in the assessment of UI as well as helpful education tools that can be given to patients to enhance self-treatment and self-management of UI. Many of the chapter tables are also included on the CD-ROM so that clinicians can print them for reference and use them in clinical practice. In addition, several care protocols and forms are included on the CD-ROM that we have found to be useful in assessment, treatment, and management and that are often requested by colleagues and lecture/seminar attendees.

Our goal has been to make the second edition of *Managing and Treating Urinary Incontinence* a comprehensive, practical book that can be used in all care settings: acute care, primary care, home care, and long-term care. We hope that readers come away from this book better informed and inspired to approach the problems of UI and OAB with greater confidence, empathy, and energy.

Acknowledgments

Diane Kaschak Newman

A special and heartfelt thanks to my husband, Michael, who continues to support and encourage me through all my professional endeavors. To my lovely daughters, Carolyn Beth, Michelle Amelia, and Emily Joellis, who have assisted me with many of my writings through clerical and research work. To my co-author and colleague, Alan J. Wein, who selflessly offered his time and expertise to enrich this second edition of my book.

Alan J. Wein

To my lovely supportive wife, Noele, who puts up with me for unknown reasons. To our special girl, Nolan, who brightens our lives every day.

To the University of Pennsylvania Health System for encouraging and including education and research as a part of its mission statement.

A very special thank you to Robin Noel, Graphic Artist, Department of Surgery, University of Pennsylvania Medical Center, who tirelessly worked with us on developing and revising multiple illustrations.

We would like to thank all the many reviewers and contributors.

1

Introduction

Beth is 66 years old and has leaked urine, at least when she coughs or laughs, since her last child was born, over 25 years ago. In the past, this wasn't an inconvenience because it was only a few drops each time, occurring a couple of days a week when she played tennis. Neither her tennis partner nor her husband ever noticed she had a problem. About 10 years ago, when she began experiencing menopause, she noticed problems with urgency, the kind that she couldn't control, like the lady on the TV commercial who complains "Gotta go, gotta go!" She found herself anticipating the urgency, and, to prevent this, stopped at every bathroom she passed. But Beth does not feel this is a true problem, just an annoyance. Beth hasn't mentioned this problem to anyone.

Currently, Beth's world revolves around knowing the location of bathrooms everywhere. Her husband has begun noticing these frequent stops and is annoyed. Last week was very upsetting for Beth—she had two "accidents" trying to get to the bathroom. One happened when she was out with friends at a movie, and the urine leaked through her panties to her slacks. Thank goodness she was wearing black. Beth is contemplating seeing her physician but is unsure if she will "get up the nerve" to tell him about her problem. She may wait to see if it goes away because she is more secure since purchasing some thicker pads at the pharmacy and wearing those when she goes out or plays tennis. Beth has a memory of her mother having a "bladder" problem, but it was never discussed. Thinking back, she remembers things about her mother that make her think her mother may have had this same problem.

A MISUNDERSTOOD PROBLEM

Even though Beth does not think so, it sounds as though she has symptoms of urinary incontinence (UI) and overactive bladder (OAB), bladder control disorders that are both very common. These conditions are grouped under the heading of pelvic floor disorders (PFDs) and include pelvic organ prolapse (POP) and fecal or anal incontinence (AI). PFDs, such as UI and AI, affect between 12% and 42% of adult women (Fornell, Wingren, & Kjolhede, 2004; Melville, Newton, Fan, & Katon, 2006). They have been referred to as the "last real taboo of the 20th century" (Resnick, 1998). The World Health Organization has estimated that these conditions affect nearly 200 million people worldwide, and estimates of prevalence in the United States range from as low as 15 million (Fantl et al., 1996) to as high as 33 million people (Stewart et al., 2003).

These disorders affect more than twice as many women as men and are believed to be a significant health issue for aging women (Holroyd-Leduc & Strauss, 2004). UI and OAB are 2 of the 10 most common chronic conditions in women in the United States, and they affect a higher percentage of people of all age groups than does hypertension, depression, or diabetes. These conditions affect the social, psychological, occupational, domestic, physical, and sexual lives of adult men and women (Melville, Katon, Delaney, & Newton, 2005). Both sexes share similar misconceptions (e.g., incontinence is a normal part of aging, it is a result of a personal failing [obesity, sedentary lifestyle, diet], surgery is the only treatment option) and the belief that these "bladder control conditions" are comparatively minor problems (Diokno, Sand, Macdiarmid, Shah, & Armstrong, 2006; Newman & Wein, 2004). The lack of knowledge about etiology and management options on the part of clinicians, as well as their assumption that these conditions are hygiene issues and not true medical issues, obstructs the detection and treatment of these insidious diseases.

Urine loss can range from small drops, as seen in younger women, to moderate or severe leakage, meaning urine soaks through outer clothing. Approximately 1 in every 10 people who have UI experiences urine loss in amounts that soak through underclothes or more! Urinary frequency can be devastating to working women (Palmer & Fitzgerald, 2002). Frequency occurring every 30 minutes or less can cause women who cannot access the bathroom "at will" (e.g., teachers) to seek early retirement during their peak productive years (Linder, 2003). UI and OAB are also expensive medical problems, requiring $19.5 billion per year (2000 dollars) in the United States for management and treatment (Hu et al., 2004, 2005). This makes UI one of the most costly kidney or urological diseases (Office of Science Policy Analysis, 2000).

UI should never be accepted as normal, not even in older adults, people with dementia, or people living in nursing facilities. Although UI is treatable, manageable, and even curable, most people with UI do not seek help for their problem. There are disturbing statistics on the number of people who seek professional help for PFDs, especially among women. It is estimated that at least 50% of women with UI do not ask for care (Boreham et al., 2005; Hannestad, Rortveit, & Hunskaar, 2002; Melville et al., 2006). There is little information on health care seeking for AI in the general population, but one study found that only 11% of affected women who were visiting a general gynecologist had sought care (Boreham et al., 2005). Data are not available on POP care seeking in the general population (Morrill et al., 2007). The most common reasons given for not seeking help were the belief that UI is a normal part of aging (62%), there was no treatment for it (38%), UI was normal after childbirth (27%), or treatment would not help (10%) (Goldstein, Hawthorne, Engberg, McDowell, & Burgio, 1992). The common myths surrounding UI are discussed in Chapter 2.

What is disturbing is that help-seeking behavior has not changed since the authors started their UI practices over 20 and 30 years ago. People with UI and OAB do not realize that there has been a great deal of medical research looking at the assessment and management of UI. This research has helped doctors and nurses understand the prevalence, cause, assessment, and treatment of UI. New medications are effective and have fewer side effects. Direct-to-consumer advertisement has helped people to become better informed about OAB and available medications, and about appropriate incontinence products. Treatments—particularly behavioral interventions, medications, and surgery—can be successful in 8 of 10 people (Fantl et al., 1996).

PROFESSIONAL EDUCATION ON INCONTINENCE

The problem, unfortunately, is not just one of consumer awareness. Despite a growing body of available information on UI, professional education on incontinence and related disorders (e.g., AI, OAB) remains only a small or nonexistent part of the basic training of doctors, nurses, and allied health professionals (Newman et al., 2005). Many times, a person who admits to having UI is told that the cause is simply old age or typical body changes. These myths or untruths are detailed in Chapter 2. Self-care practices such as regular toileting, fluid intake modification, reduced caffeine intake, exercise, and weight reduction are some basic ways to prevent or reduce UI, but they are not actively promoted (Johnson, Kincade, Bernard, Busby-Whitehead, & DeFriese, 2000).

Although UI is more prevalent than diabetes mellitus, most health care professionals have received little education about UI, fail to screen for it, and view the likelihood of successful treatment as low. UI usually comes to a health care provider's attention only when the patient complains of specific symptoms. However, this is not often. Research has reported that only 38% of surveyed women initiated a conversation with a physician about incontinence (Kinchen et al., 2003). A survey conducted by one of the authors (DKN) indicated that more than half of women who discussed OAB with a health care provider (56%) had waited longer than 1 year to seek treatment; many attempted to self-manage their symptoms (Dmochowski & Newman, 2007).

Federal agencies have funded multiple research projects looking at the use of noninvasive behavioral treatments in the ambulatory and long-term care settings. In a surge of increased federal funding of incontinence research in the mid-1980s, significant development in the understanding of the prevalence, causation, assessment, and treatment of UI took place. This research has demonstrated that, after childbirth, UI is never normal, not even in older adults with dementia living in residential facilities. It outlines the causes of the problem and how to diagnose UI, and concludes that UI is treatable, even curable, and can always be managed. However, the fact remains that women do not seek treatment. A survey by the National Association for Continence (2004) showed that, on average, women wait 6.5 years and men 4.2 years before seeking a professional diagnosis once they begin experiencing loss of bladder control symptoms. The shorter interval for men may be because they are not used to wearing perineal pads, whereas women are. Women complain that, when they did tell their doctor or nurse about the problem, many were told to "live with it." The most common reasons cited for failure to seek treatment are either that incontinence is not seen as abnormal or that there is a low expectation of benefit from treatment.

Those people who seek treatment tend to have more significant symptoms (Newman, 2004). Older people may think incontinence is part of the normal aging process, and health care providers may dismiss it as not worthy of investigation and treatment. Unless the issue is specifically addressed by clinicians, most people are too embarrassed by their symptoms of UI to seek medical help. Even patients presenting with associated symptoms such as urgency and frequency may still be too embarrassed to mention urinary leakage. Patients are often unaware that there are effective behavioral and pharmacological therapies that can significantly reduce and even eliminate their symptoms. Consequently, whereas patients with severe symptomatology inevitably seek treatment, the majority of patients with mild or moderate symptoms of UI are often overlooked and become stigmatized by their condition. This is a common phenomenon; medical conditions that have greater stigma (and often are less life threatening) tend to take a much longer time to be declared to a physician—and even longer to family, friends, and others (Fonda & Newman, 2006).

Another confounding problem is that providers lack basic understanding of bladder control conditions. Many health care professionals tend not to inquire about UI because, other than recommending an absorbent product, they are unsure what else to tell their patients. According to a 1993 survey reported in *MMWR: Morbidity and Mortality Weekly Report,* many primary care physicians (PCPs) in Massachusetts and Oklahoma felt unprepared either to evaluate or to treat UI (Centers for Disease Control and Prevention, 1995). The survey further showed that most clinicians do not routinely ask their elderly patients about UI, and they are even less likely to routinely elicit bladder health information from their younger patients. Instead, UI is perceived as a diagnosis necessitating immediate referral to a specialist.

In response to this problem, the World Health Organization's Third Consultation on Incontinence recommended "compulsory inclusion of incontinence in the basic curriculum (physicians, nurses, physiotherapists and allied health professionals)" (Newman et al., 2005, p. 50). This group of experts believed that incontinence must be identified and preferably taught as a separate topic, not fragmented between different modules of the educational curriculum (Newman et al., 2005).

In the past two decades, many U.S. government agencies and professional organizations have issued practice guidelines on UI. In 1992 and 1996, the Agency for Health Care Policy and Research (AHCPR), now known as the Agency for Healthcare Research and Quality (AHRQ), produced Clinical Practice Guidelines called "Urinary Incontinence in Adults" (AHCPR, 1992; Fantl et al., 1996). In 1996 and 2005, the American Medical Directors Association issued guidelines for care of the resident with UI who lives in a long-term care facility. In 2005, the Centers for Medicare & Medicaid Services (CMS) issued new surveyor guidance for long-term care on UI and catheters. All of these guidelines were aimed at health care professionals and were intended to help standardize the assessment and management of UI in adults in both community and long-term care settings, with an ultimate goal of improving the lives of people with UI through early screening and treatment.

Although these readily available publications are widely quoted, they have largely failed to change the practice of many medical providers or their trainees. Bland et al. (2003) used a multifaceted educational intervention based on the 1996 AHCPR guideline in 20 of 41 primary care practices and failed to show an effect in increasing screening or management of UI by PCPs. The concept of using bladder diaries or checking postvoid residual urine as part of basic assessment is still foreign to most gynecologists, family doctors, and advanced practice nurses (APNs) not specializing in incontinence care. Specialist education programs with relevant accreditation mechanisms (and planned periodic re-credentialing) to safeguard patient interests need to be developed for urologists, gynecologists, specialist nurses, physical therapists, and others.

Since the first edition of this book, the number of doctors, nurses, and allied health professionals who are developing expertise in caring for incontinent patients has increased, but what is lacking are academic or clinical proficiency requirements to be considered a "continence practitioner or specialist." The American Board of Obstetrics and Gynecology, in collaboration with the American Board of Urology, issues credentials to urogynecologists and urologists who have undergone a fellowship of specialized training in academic medical centers. These centers have, in most instances, an existing multidisciplinary team consisting of individuals from the specialties of urology, gynecology, gastroenterology, colon and rectal surgery, and nursing. This allows the team to treat men and women for all conditions of the pelvic floor: UI, AI, POP, and chronic pelvic pain syndromes. The fear with such credentialing programs, however, is that incontinence may be seen as the province of an elite group of "super-specialists" who get further and further away from their colleagues (Newman et al., 2005).

Changing the current patterns of medical care with respect to detection and management of incontinence through education is a difficult task (Cohen et al., 1999). Unless there are other incentives (e.g., financial) or the removal of disincentives, guidelines are unlikely to cause rapid changes in actual practice. Also, because of the large number of patients with UI and OAB, the entire medical community, generalists and specialists, will need to be involved in screening and treatment. As part of its overall quality improvement efforts, in 2006, the CMS launched the Physician Voluntary Reporting Program (PVRP) (CMS, 2007). The goal of this new program is to improve the quality of care delivered to Medicare patients. A secondary benefit may be that it increases detection of UI in the community. Under the PVRP, physicians who choose to participate will help capture data about the quality of care provided to Medicare beneficiaries in order to identify the most effective ways to use the quality measures in routine practice and to support physicians in their efforts to improve quality of care. These quality measures include evidence-based, clinically valid measures that have been part of UI guidelines. The three measure descriptors for potential 2007 PVRP quality measures that relate to UI for geriatric patients are

1. Assessment of presence or absence of urinary incontinence in women aged 65 years and older

    • Patient documented to have been assessed for presence or absence of urinary incontinence

    • Patient not documented to have been assessed for presence or absence of urinary incontinence

    • Clinician documented that patient was not an eligible candidate for an assessment of the presence or absence of urinary incontinence

2. Characterization of urinary incontinence in women aged 65 years and older

    • Patient documented to have received characterization of urinary incontinence

    • Patient not documented to have received characterization of urinary incontinence

3. Plan of care for urinary incontinence in women aged 65 years and older

    • Patient documented to have received a plan of care for urinary incontinence

    • Patient not documented to have received plan of care for urinary incontinence

    • Clinician has not provided care for the patient for the required time to develop plan of care for urinary incontinence

Nurses, especially nurse practitioners, have attempted to use the AHCPR recommendations and the more recent CMS UI guidance, incorporating them into curricula, evidence-based clinical practice, and care pathways (Button et al., 1998; Newman, 2006a, 2006b; Ryden et al., 2000; Sampselle et al., 2000;

Thompson, 2004; Viktrup & Møller, 2004; Watson, Brink, Zimmer, & Mayer, 2003). Nursing models for providing continence care services are explored in Chapter 13. The certification board of the Wound, Ostomy, and Continence Nurses Society has developed a certification examination for continence care nurses (Jirovec, Wyman, & Wells, 1998; Newman, 2006a). The Society of Urologic Nurses and Associates certification program for APNs tests knowledge on UI and related urological disorders. Fortunately, the number of nurses certified through these two organizations is steadily increasing. However, as in other heath care disciplines, nurses are not always positive toward continence education. In one study, 20% of nurses polled thought that nurses working in nursing facilities would be apathetic or resistant to a program on incontinence (Palmer, 1995). Specific knowledge about UI is being outlined for use in graduate programs (Rogalski, 2005), but needs to be part of the undergraduate nursing curriculum also.

Part of the problem with management of UI by nurses is that nursing care of UI is fragmented and is practiced by several levels of nurses, from nursing assistants or aides to APNs. Because of this fragmentation, nursing's approach to basic assessment, treatment, and management strategies is not consistent. In most institutional health care settings, nurses not only provide direct patient care, they are also responsible for the philosophy, standard, and policy of care while supervising the performance of other nursing staff members, particularly nursing assistants (Bowers, Esmond, & Jacobson, 2001). Although manufacturers have introduced more diverse UI products in the U.S. retail market, nursing strategy for management of UI has centered almost exclusively on containment of urine leakage (i.e., incontinence absorbent pads, catheters) (Newman, Fader, & Bliss, 2004). Although UI prevalence rates for people living in long-term care facilities and in their homes are over 50%, prevention techniques and rehabilitative treatments are not routinely initiated by nurses caring for these patients. This is a growing dilemma that will only worsen as the U.S. population ages.

One group of allied health professionals—physical therapists—has targeted women's health as an integral part of the educational curriculum. The American Physical Therapy Association, Section on Women's Health, provides an educational program geared to therapists who are interested in women's health, particularly pelvic floor muscle disorders such as UI and chronic pelvic pain.

Besides formal training, doctors, nurses, and health care organizations have also established web sites on UI for consumers and health care professionals who are Internet users (Boyington, Dougherty, & Yuan-Mei, 2003; Diering & Palmer, 2001; Sandvik, 1999) (see Appendix B, Resources). For many professionals, these web sites are a significant source of expanded information on this problem.

Incontinence and OAB are often complex and multifaceted problems, particularly in frail or dependent individuals (Engberg, Kincade, & Thompson, 2004). These conditions usually require input from a wide variety of providers to be addressed effectively. However, if people do voice their incontinence problems, professionals must be educated on solutions that are individualized and effective. There are many solutions to incontinence, and there are many products and devices that can assist people with managing their problem, so that they can live an active and more enjoyable lifestyle.

Relief for Beth

When Beth next visited her family doctor, she mentioned her too-frequent bathroom visits. A urine test was negative for infection. Her doctor thought that a new medication might decrease her urinary frequency, which he explained was probably being caused by involuntary bladder contractions. At first the medication decreased her urgency and frequency and stopped her urine leakage episodes. However, after 6 months Beth noticed that she was starting to have "accidents" again. Her doctor suggested she see a specialist at a continence treatment center. The doctor at the center, a urologist, discussed the use of a Bladder Diary and performed an ultrasound that showed she was completely emptying her bladder. He then asked Beth to complete the Bladder Diary for 3 days and return to see his pelvic floor nurse specialist. Beth met with the nurse specialist, who reviewed her Bladder Diary and diet and pointed out foods and liquids that might be irritating her bladder. She taught Beth simple techniques for decreasing urinary urgency, and told her to keep taking the medication because all of these treatments would work together to improve her symptoms. After a month, Beth believed she had more control of her bladder, especially her urgency, and thought she could even ask to cut back on the medication when she next saw the nurse.

With better information and resources, providers could help more people like Beth regain control and confidence over this critical area of their lives. Here, collected in a single book, is much of what any professional needs to know. This book provides extensive information on underlying causes of UI and identification of people who are "at risk," it outlines the components of a basic evaluation, and it details information on various treatments and management practices. It was written for primary care specialists, including family physicians, general internists, nurses, and others who manage adult patients. It is intended to provide information that can be used in everyday clinical practice.

REFERENCES

Agency for Health Care Policy and Research. (1992). *Urinary incontinence in adults: Clinical practice guideline* (AHCPR Publication No. 92-0038). Rockville, MD: Author.

American Medical Directors Association. (1996). *Urinary incontinence clinical practice guideline.* Columbia, MD: Author.

American Medical Directors Association. (2005). *Urinary incontinence clinical practice guideline.* Columbia, MD: Author.

Bland, D.R., Dugan, E., Cohen, S.J., Preisser, J., Davis, C.C., McGann, P.E., et al. (2003). The effects of implementation of the Agency for Health Care Policy and Research urinary incontinence guidelines in primary care practices. *Journal of the American Geriatrics Society, 51,* 979–984.

Boreham, M.K., Richter, H.E., Kenton, K.S., Nager, C.W., Gregory, W.T., Aronson, M.P., et al. (2005). Anal incontinence in women presenting for gynecologic care: Prevalence, risk factors, and impact upon quality of life. *American Journal of Obstetrics and Gynecology, 192,* 1637–1642.

Bowers, B., Esmond, S., & Jacobson, N. (2001). The relationship between staffing and quality in long-term care facilities: Exploring the views of nurse aides. *Journal of Nursing Care Quality, 14,* 55–64.

Boyington, A.R., Dougherty, M.C., & Yuan-Mei, L. (2003). Analysis of interactive continence health information on the web. *Journal of Wound, Ostomy, and Continence Nursing, 30,* 280–286.

Button, D., Roe, B., Webb, C., Frith, T., Colin-Thome, D., & Gardner, L. (1998). Consensus guidelines for the promotion and management of continence by primary health care teams: development, implementation and evaluation. *Journal of Advanced Nursing, 127,* 91–99.

Centers for Disease Control and Prevention. (1995). Knowledge, attitudes, and practices of physicians regarding urinary incontinence in persons aged ≥ 65 years—Massachusetts and Oklahoma. *MMWR: Morbidity and Mortality Weekly Report, 44,* 747, 753–754.

Centers for Medicare & Medicaid Services. (2005). *State Operations Manual, Appendix PP—Guidance to Surveyors for Long-Term Care Facilities, Tag F315, §483.25(d) Urinary Incontinence* (Rev. 8, Issued: 06-28-05, Effective: 06-28-05, Implementation: 06-28-05) (pp. 1–39). Retrieved November 11, 2007, from http://www.cms.hhs.gov/transmittals/downloads/R8SOM.pdf.

Centers for Medicare & Medicaid Services. (2007). *Manual system: Additional codes for Physician Voluntary Reporting Program (PVRP).* Transmittal 259, January 7. Atlanta: Author.

Cohen, S.J, Robinson, D., Dugan, E., Howard, G., Suggs, P.K., Pearce, K.F., et al. (1999). Communication between older adults and their physicians about urinary incontinence. *Journal of Gerontology, 54A,* M34–M37.

Diering, C.L., & Palmer, M.H. (2001). Professional information about urinary incontinence on the World Wide Web: Is it timely? Is it accurate? *Journal of Wound, Ostomy, and Continence Nursing, 28,* 55–62.

Diokno, A.C., Sand, P.K., Macdiarmid, S., Shah, R., & Armstrong, R.B. (2006). Perceptions and behaviors of women with bladder control problems. *Family Practice, 23,* 568–577.

Dmochowski, R.R., & Newman, D.K. (2007). Impact of overactive bladder on women in the United States: Results of a national survey. *Current Medical Research and Opinion, 23,* 65–76.

Engberg, S., Kincade, J., & Thompson, D. (2004). Future directions for incontinence with frail elders. *Nursing Research, 53*(6 Suppl.), S22–S29.

Fantl, J.A., Newman, D.K., Colling, J., DeLancey, J.O.L., Keys, C., Loughery, R., et al. for the Urinary Incontinence in Adults Guideline Update Panel. (1996). *Urinary incontinence in adults: Acute and chronic management. Clinical practice guideline no. 2: Update* (AHCPR Publication No. 96-0682). Rockville, MD: Agency for Health Care Policy and Research.

Fonda, D., & Newman, D.K. (2006). Tackling the stigma of incontinence—promoting continence worldwide. In L. Cardozo & D. Staskin (Eds.), *Textbook of female urology and urogynecology* (2nd ed., pp. 75–80). Abingdon, UK: Informa Healthcare.

Fornell, E.U., Wingren, G., & Kjolhede, P. (2004). Factors associated with pelvic floor dysfunction with emphasis on urinary and fecal incontinence and genital prolapse: An epidemiological study. *Acta Obstetricia et Gynecologica Scandinavica, 83,* 383–389.

Goldstein, M., Hawthorne, M.E., Engberg, S., McDowell, B.J., & Burgio, K.L. (1992). Urinary incontinence: Why people do not seek help. *Journal of Gerontological Nursing, 18,* 15–20.

Hannestad, Y.S., Rortveit, G., & Hunskaar, S. (2002). Help-seeking and associated factors in female urinary incontinence. *Scandinavian Journal of Primary Health Care, 20,* 102–107.

Holroyd-Leduc, J., & Strauss, S.E. (2004). Management of urinary incontinence in women. *JAMA, 291,* 986–995.

Hu, T., Wagner, T., Bentkover, J., LeBlanc, K., Zhou, S., & Hunt, T. (2004). Costs of urinary incontinence and overactive bladder in the United States: A comparative study. *Urology, 63,* 461–465.

Hu, T.W., Wagner, T.H., Hawthorne, G., Morre, K., Subak, L.L., & Versi, E. (2005). Economics of incontinence. In P.A. Abrams, L. Cardozo, S. Khoury, & A.J. Wein (Eds.), *Incontinence: Proceedings from the Third International Consultation on Incontinence* (pp. 75–95). Plymouth, UK: Health Publications, Ltd.

Jirovec, M.M., Wyman, J.F., & Wells, T.J. (1998). Addressing urinary incontinence with educational continence-care competencies. *Image: Journal of Nursing Scholarship, 30,* 375–378.

Johnson, T.M., Kincade, J.E., Bernard, S.L., Busby-Whitehead, J., & DeFriese, G.H. (2000). Self-care practices used by older men and women to manage urinary incontinence: Results from the National Follow-up Survey on Self-Care and Aging. *Journal of the American Geriatrics Society, 48,* 894–902.

Kinchen, K.S., Burgio, K., Diokno, A.C., Fultz, N.H., Bump, R., & Obenchain, R. (2003). Factors associated with women's decisions to seek treatment for urinary incontinence. *Journal of Women's Health, 12,* 687–698.

Linder, M. (2003). *Void where prohibited revisited.* Iowa City, IA: Fanpihua Press.

Melville, J., Katon, W., Delaney, K., & Newton, K. (2005). Urinary incontinence in US women. *Archives of Internal Medicine, 165,* 537–542.

Melville, J.L., Newton, K., Fan, M.-Y., & Katon, W. (2006). Health care discussion and treatment for urinary incontinence in US women. *American Journal of Obstetrics and Gynecology, 194,* 729–737.

Morrill, M., Lukacz, E.S., Lawrence, J.M., Nager, C.W., Contreras, R., & Luber, K.M. (2007). Seeking healthcare for pelvic floor disorders: A population-based study. *American Journal of Obstetrics and Gynecology, 197,* 86.e1–86.e6.

National Association for Continence. (2004). *National survey on diagnosis and management of bladder control loss.* Unpublished study. Charleston, SC: Author.

Newman, D.K. (2004). Report of a mail survey of women with bladder control disorders. *Urologic Nursing, 24,* 499–507.

Newman, D.K. (2006a). The role of the continence nurse specialists. In L. Cardozo & D. Staskin (Eds.), *Textbook of female urology and urogynecology* (2nd ed., pp. 91–98). Abingdon, UK: Informa Healthcare.

Newman, D.K. (2006b). Urinary incontinence, catheters and urinary tract infections: An overview of CMS Tag F 315. *Ostomy/Wound Management, 52*(12), 34–36, 38, 40–44.

Newman, D.K., Denis, L., Gruenwald, I., Ee, C.H., Millard, R., Roberts, R., et al. (2005). Promotion, education and organization for continence care. In P.A. Abrams, L. Cardozo, S. Khoury, & A.J. Wein (Eds.), *Incontinence: Proceedings from the Third International Consultation on Incontinence* (pp. 35–72). Plymouth, UK: Health Publications, Ltd.

Newman, D.K., Fader, M., & Bliss, D.Z. (2004). Managing incontinence using technology, devices and products. *Nursing Research, 53*(6 Suppl), S42–S48.

Newman, D.K., & Wein, A.J. (2004). *Overcoming overactive bladder.* Los Angeles: New Harbinger.

Office of Science Policy Analysis. (2000). *Costs of illness and NIH support for selected diseases and conditions.* Retrieved December 31, 2006, from http://ospp.od.nih.gov/pdf/table_1.pdf

Palmer, M., & Fitzgerald, S. (2002). Urinary incontinence in working women: A comparison study. *Journal of Women's Health, 11,* 879–888.

Palmer, M.H. (1995). Nurses' knowledge and beliefs about continence interventions in long-term care. *Journal of Advanced Nursing, 21,* 1065–1072.

Resnick, N.M. (1998). Improving treatment of urinary incontinence [Commentary letter]. *JAMA, 280,* 2034–2035.

Rogalski, N.M. (2005). A graduate nursing curriculum for the evaluation and management of urinary incontinence. *Educational Gerontology, 31,* 139–159.

Ryden, M.B., Snyder, M., Gross, C.R., Savik, K., Pearson, V., Krichbaum, K., et al. (2000). Value-added outcomes: The use of advanced practice nurses in long-term facilities. *The Gerontologist, 40,* 654–662.

Sampselle, C.M., Wyman, J.F., Thomas, K.K., Newman, D.K., Gray, M., Dougherty, M., et al. (2000). Continence for women: A test of AWHONN's evidence-based protocol in clinical practice. *Journal of Obstetric, Gynecologic, and Neonatal Nursing, 29,* 18–26.

Sandvik, H. (1999). Health information and interaction on the Internet: A survey of female urinary incontinence. *BMJ, 319,* 29–32.

Stewart, W.F., Van Rooyen, J.B., Cundiff, G.W., Abrams, P., Herzog, A.R., Corey, R., et al. (2003). Prevalence and impact of overactive bladder in the United States. *World Journal of Urology, 20,* 327–363.

Thompson, D.L. (2004). Geriatric incontinence: The long-term care challenge. *Urologic Nursing, 24,* 305–314.

Viktrup, L., & Møller, L.A. (2004). The handling of urinary incontinence in Danish general practices after distribution of guidelines and voiding diary reimbursement: An observational study. *BMC Family Practice, 5,* 13.

Watson, N.M., Brink, C.A., Zimmer, J.G., & Mayer, R.D. (2003). Use of the Agency for Health Care Policy and Research urinary incontinence guideline in nursing homes. *Journal of the American Geriatrics Society, 51,* 1779–1786.

2

The Problem of Incontinence

Urinary incontinence (UI), the involuntary and unwanted leakage of urine, is a significant health problem. There are two main types of UI, stress and urge. Stress UI (SUI) is involuntary urine leakage on effort or exertion or on sneezing or coughing, as a result of insufficient closure of the urethra (Abrams et al., 2002). It is the most common form of UI and accounts for 50%–60% of women with UI. Urge UI (now referred to as urgency UI; UUI) is involuntary leakage accompanied by or immediately preceded by urgency, a strong, sudden, and uncontrollable desire to urinate as a result of involuntary bladder contractions (Abrams, Artibani, Cardozo, Khoury, & Wein, 2005). Mixed UI (MUI), a combination of UUI and SUI, is involuntary leakage with both urgency and exertion, effort, sneezing, or coughing. An estimated 15 million Americans have UI. The related condition of overactive bladder (OAB)—urinary urgency, with or without UI and frequency and nocturia—affects as many as 33 million Americans, according to survey data. Prevalence of UI is greater in women than men and steadily increases with aging. Frail elders living in their homes or in institutional settings are more likely to experience UI. UI and OAB significantly impact a person's quality of life (QoL), limiting social interaction and isolating people from family and friends. UI and OAB are costly conditions. This chapter provides an in-depth review of the prevalence of UI in all care settings, as well as comorbidities, impact on QoL, costs, and prevention strategies for these conditions.

The prevalence of UI (probability of having UI within a defined population at a defined point in time) ranges from 3% to 55% depending on the definition of incontinence used and the age of the population studied. Aging also increases the risk of developing UI and OAB, with a prevalence of 30%–40% in people older than 75 years of age. To put this into perspective, UI and OAB are more common than diabetes and are similar in prevalence to asthma (Ouslander, 2004).

Prevalence of UI is high, especially in older adults who reside in nursing facilities and those who are homebound. During 1995, an estimated 6.3 million community-dwelling older adults and 1.2 million nursing facility residents were living with UI (T.H. Wagner & Hu, 1998). Although prevalence can vary among individual long-term care (LTC) facilities, UI affects approximately 55%–65% of nursing facility residents, and the prevalence has been increasing over the past decade (Sahyoun, Pratt, Lentzner, Dey, & Robinson, 2001). Depending on the case mix, rates can be 70% and higher in facilities housing frail adults with functional impairments.

The type of UI may differ depending on the age group and gender studied. UI in women is part of female pelvic floor dysfunction, which also encompasses clinical conditions such as pelvic organ prolapse and fecal or anal incontinence. More than one main type of UI may occur in the same individual, with co-occurrence of SUI and UUI, referred to as "mixed urinary incontinence." Across all age groups, SUI is the most common type of UI, affecting approximately half (49%) of women with UI. The second most common type is MUI (29%), which typically presents with a heavy component of SUI, and the least common type is UUI (22%) (Hunskaar et al., 2003). Figure 2.1 shows the different types of UI in women. Advancing age is associated with an increased prevalence of UUI and MUI. The prevalence of UUI is low in premenopausal women but appears to change in mid-life (Waetjen et al., 2007). In contrast, the prevalence of SUI alone appears to remain stable across age groups (J.S. Brown et al., 1999; Holroyd-Leduc & Straus, 2004; Sampselle, Harlow, Skurnick, Brubaker, & Bondarenko, 2002).

INCONTINENCE, GENDER, RACE, AND AGING

Women are disproportionately affected by UI, with a ratio of women to men of 2:1 (Moore & Gray, 2004). The prevalence has been reported to be 38% in

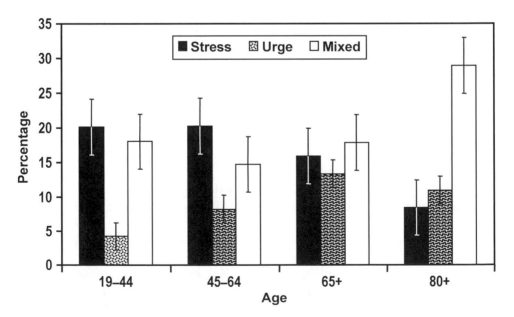

Figure 2.1.   Prevalence of urinary incontinence types in American women (37 studies). From Agency for Healthcare Research and Quality (2007).

women versus 19% in men, but increases in both genders with aging. Pooled analysis of epidemiological studies of UI prevalence in community-dwelling women suggested that the prevalence of ever having UI increased from 21% in 19- to 44-year-olds (17 studies) to 34% in 45- to 64-year-olds (45 studies), and to 39% among elderly women (11 studies) (Agency for Healthcare Research and Quality, 2007). Figure 2.2 shows the prevalence of UI in Norwegian women (Hannestad, Rortveit, Sandvik, & Hunskaar, 2000), and Figure 2.3 shows prevalence of UI in American men (Diokno, Estanol, Ibrahim, & Balasubramaniam, 2007). Anger, Saigal, Stothers, et al. (2006) noted that 17% of men 60 years and older experienced UI either daily (42%) or weekly (24%). Based on these prevalence rates, approximately 3.9 million men (2001 census) have UI (Stothers, Thom, & Calhoun, 2005). The prevalence of OAB has been estimated to be 16.9% for women (9.3% with urgency, frequency, and UI) and 16% for men (2.6% with urgency, frequency, and UI) (Stewart et al., 2003). Figure 2.4 shows the prevalence of OAB in men and women. More than 90% of all cases of UI occur in the community setting, affecting working and community-dwelling women from all age groups, with SUI the predominant type in younger adult women (Samuelsson, Victor, & Svardsudd, 2000; van der Vaart, de Leeuw, Roovers, & Heintz, 2002).

Ethnicity appears to have less of a role in prevalence in men than in women (Stothers et al., 2005), and increasing amounts of prevalence data are available on the types of UI in women of different races. In the Nurses Health Study of middle-aged nurses (mean age 44.8), self-reported prevalence of UI (leaking urine at least once a month) was 43% (Grodstein, Fretts, Lifford, Resnick, & Curhan, 2003). In a more recent publication on this ongoing study, the overall 2-year incidence (probability of developing or acquiring the condition during a defined period of time) of UI was 13.7%, which corresponds to an average incidence of 6.9% per year. Incidence generally increased across ages 36 through 50 years; however, after age 50 years (i.e., 51–55 years), there

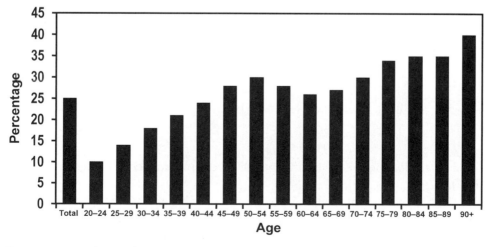

Figure 2.2. Prevalence of urinary incontinence in community-dwelling Norwegian women by age (N = 27,936). From Hannestad et al. (2000).

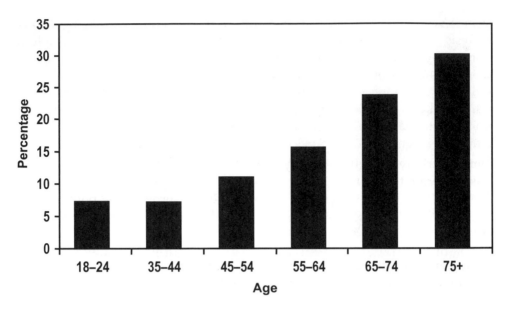

Figure 2.3. Prevalence of urinary incontinence in American men by age (*N* = 21,590). From Diokno et al. (2007).

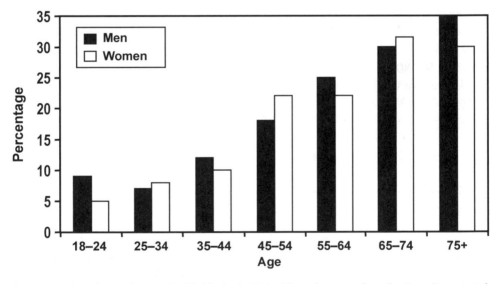

Figure 2.4. Prevalence of overactive bladder in the United States by age and gender. From Stewart et al. (2003).

was a small decline, most significant for severe incontinence (Townsend et al., 2007).

The type of UI may vary in women according to race. White women reported UI twice as often as black and Asian American women (Danforth et al., 2006). Lower rates of SUI have been reported by African American women when compared to white women. Hispanic and Asian American women have been shown to have rates of SUI equivalent to those of white women (J.S. Brown et al., 1999; Huang et al., 2006). African American and Asian American women have been shown to have higher rates of detrusor instability and UUI than women of other races (Duong & Korn, 2001; Thom et al., 2006). Espino et al. (2003) conducted the first community-based study of Mexican American older women (mean age 73 years) and found a prevalence of any UI in the past 12 months of 15%, which is lower than has been reported in other groups of women. Of those women who reported UI, 33% experienced symptoms of strictly UUI, 10% strictly SUI, and 42% MUI. Quantity of urine loss was moderate to severe.

Aging increases the prevalence of bladder disorders. The population of the United States is aging rapidly; the percentage of people over the age of 65 is expected to increase from 12.8% of the population in 1996 to close to 20.0% by 2030 (Bectel & Tucker, 1998). The most significant rise in the aging population is in the age group older than 85 years, often called the "old-old," whose numbers will more than double by 2030. This group tends to be frail, dependent in activities of daily living (ADLs) such as toileting, and increasingly in need of health care and custodial services. In women, the prevalence of SUI decreases with age, whereas the prevalence of UUI increases. Melville, Katon, Delaney, and Newton (2005) conducted a population-based, age-stratified postal survey of 6,000 women between 30 and 90 years of age who were enrolled in a large health maintenance organization in Washington State. Prevalence of UI increased with age, from 28% for 30- to 39-year-old women to 55% for 80- to 90-year-old women. Eighteen percent of respondents reported severe UI. The prevalence of severe UI also increased notably with age, from 8% for 30- to 39-year-old women to 33% for 80- to 90-year-old women. The rate of UI also rises in men as they get older (Anger, Saigal, Stothers, et al., 2006). OAB with UI increases substantially in men after the age of 40, and the incidence of UUI jumps nearly 15-fold for men and 6-fold for women when they reach 75 years or older (Milsom et al., 2001). Men have a more dramatic increase in incontinence as they age, compared with women (Parazzini, Lavezzari, & Artibani, 2002). Whereas the prevalence of UI doubles in women between the ages of 51 and 70+, it increases threefold for men.

One of the major differences between the manifestation of OAB in men and in women is that the majority of women with OAB symptoms do not have bladder outlet obstruction. In men, OAB symptoms often occur together with obstruction due to benign enlargement of the prostate, known as benign prostatic hyperplasia (BPH). The relationship between OAB and BPH is still unclear with regard to whether or not symptoms of OAB develop as a result of BPH (see Chapter 4). Approximately 50% of men with some type of prostatic obstruction also have detrusor overactivity. However, men younger than 60 who present with lower urinary tract symptoms tend not to have either an enlarged prostate or a history of BPH (Jaffe & Te, 2005).

Although age itself does not cause UI and OAB, factors that may lead to these conditions are more prevalent in older men and women (Irwin et al.,

2006). An increased risk of UI has been highly and independently correlated with several potentially reversible aging causes, including urinary tract infections (UTIs), depression, and physical restraints or environmental barriers that limit easy toilet access. Such barriers may increase the prevalence of UI in this population by as much as 50%. Interventions designed to address modifiable risk factors may help to prevent UI in this at-risk population of older men and women. Once UI occurs, it persists in the older adult, especially in someone who is frail and has multiple medical conditions. Importantly, because UI, OAB, and related pelvic floor disorders (Table 2.1) are multifactorial problems, they are difficult to distinctively diagnose and therefore treat in a straightforward fashion. Many men and women have overlapping lower urinary tract symptoms (Barry, Link, McNaughton-Collins, & McKinlay, 2008).

INCONTINENCE AND COMORBIDITY

Physician and nurse colleagues too often say that "incontinence never kills anyone," so it is not an "important medical problem." However, this was not the case for Janet:

> Janet, an 87-year-old woman with symptoms of OAB with UI, lived at home with minimal family assistance. One night, she was incontinent when trying to get to the toilet, slipped on her urine, fell, and sustained a hip fracture. After hip replacement surgery, she underwent rehabilitation in a nursing home. She never was able to ambulate on her own again and had to use a wheelchair. She died from complications due to a sacral pressure ulcer infection 8 months after sustaining her fall.

Although such scenarios are often seen in clinical practice, incontinence has not been directly linked with mortality, but instead is associated with adverse physical events in older patients. UI with associated urgency increases the risk of falls in elderly women and contributes to caregiver burden (J.S. Brown et al., 2000; Fantl et al., 1996). Older women who experience MUI (a combination of SUI and UUI) have been found to have an increased risk for falls and subsequent hip fractures when compared with continent women (J.S. Brown et al., 2000).

In addition to falling, comorbidities associated with UI and OAB include UTIs, disrupted sleep secondary to nocturia, and skin ulceration in incontinent patients (Darkow, Fontes, & Williamson, 2005). Moderate to severe UI is related to an increased risk of perineal dermatitis, particularly when urine leakage is managed by incontinence products, or occurs in a patient with diabetes mellitus or with deep skin folds resulting from obesity (Bliss, Zehrer, Savik, Thayer, & Smith, 2006). Incontinence has also been linked to an increased risk for hospital readmission, particularly in older adults with multiple chronic conditions (Thom, Haan, & van den Eeden, 1997). UI is associated

Table 2.1   Associated bladder and pelvic disorders

Condition	Description
Prostatitis	Prostatitis is an inflammation of the prostate gland caused either by a bacterial infection or by the backup of prostate secretions within the gland. Prostatitis may account for up to 25% of genital and urinary problems experienced by young and middle-aged men and approximately 2 million outpatient visits per year in the United States. The following classification system has been developed by the National Institutes of Health (NIH) (Krieger, Nyberg, & Nickel, 1999):

I.   Acute bacterial prostatitis—associated with severe symptoms of prostatitis, systemic infection, and acute bacterial urinary tract infection (UTI).

II.   Chronic bacterial prostatitis—caused by chronic bacterial infection of the prostate with or without symptoms of prostatitis and usually with recurrent UTI caused by the same bacterial strain.

III.   Chronic pelvic pain syndrome (CPPS)—characterized by symptoms of chronic pelvic pain (CPP) and possibly symptoms on voiding in the absence of UTI. This category is subdivided into inflammatory (category IIIA) and noninflammatory (category IIIB) prostatitis.

IV.   Asymptomatic inflammatory prostatitis—characterized by evidence of inflammation of the prostate in the absence of genitourinary tract symptoms; an incidental finding during evaluation for other conditions, such as infertility or elevated serum prostate-specific antigen (PSA) levels.

About 5%–10% of men with symptoms of prostatitis have acute or chronic bacterial prostatitis, which usually responds to antimicrobial therapy (Schaeffer, 2006). Symptoms include a small-volume watery urethral discharge, urgency, frequency, discomfort when urinating, and pain with ejaculation. Men with chronic bacterial prostatitis may be asymptomatic between acute episodes or have mild pelvic pain or irritative symptoms on voiding (frequency, urgency). History of recurrent UTIs indicates a diagnosis of chronic bacterial prostatitis. *Escherichia coli* causes approximately 75%–80% of episodes. Physical examination is not very helpful. To determine if the prostate is the source of the infection, obtaining a specimen through prostate massage is recommended (see Chapter 6).

Cases caused by a bacterial infection are the easiest to identify but are the least common, because acute and chronic bacterial prostatitis account for only 5% of patients presenting with this disorder. Chronic nonbacterial prostatitis is the most common form, and some of the symptoms, such as urinary frequency, urgency, and nocturia, can mimic overactive bladder (OAB). Asymptomatic inflammatory prostatitis, another common type, does not cause any urinary symptoms and is usually diagnosed only when the patient seeks medical care for another reason.

Treatment for chronic prostatitis involves the use of a prostate-penetrating antibiotic (e.g., a fluoroquinolone [Cipro, Levaquin, Proquin] 500 mg daily for 4 weeks or trimethoprim-sulfamethoxazole [Bactrim]160/800 mg twice daily for 4 weeks).

(continued)

Table 2.1   (continued)

Condition	Description
Chronic pelvic pain in men	This condition (NIH category III of prostatitis) is called CPPS and commonly manifests as pain in areas including the perineum, rectum, prostate, penis, testicles, and abdomen. It is often associated with symptoms of obstruction (e.g., hesitancy, weak stream) or irritative symptoms on voiding (Schaeffer, 2006). Men will complain of pain following orgasm/ejaculation. The symptoms usually remain stable or improve slightly over time, but some men have large fluctuations in the severity of symptoms. Most men with prostatitis present with pelvic pain without evidence of UTI.
	The NIH Chronic Prostatitis Symptom Index is a nine-item, self-administered tool that is reliable and valid and has been shown to be useful in assessing baseline status and responses to therapy (Litwin et al., 1999). Total scores range from 0 to 43 points, with higher scores indicating more severe symptoms. A reduction of 4 to 6 points is significant.
	History should determine if symptoms are associated with infection of the urinary tract, the prostate, or both. Both chronic bacterial prostatitis and CPPS have been associated with abnormalities in the semen and infertility.
	Initial treatment is a 12-week trial of alpha blocker therapy, which can be continued if pain relief occurs. Quercetin, a bioflavonoid with antioxidant properties that is available over the counter, has been reported to produce significantly greater improvement. Other therapies that have been only tested in small studies include gabapentin (neurontin), muscle relaxants, bee pollen extract, saw palmetto, corticosteroids, and allopurinol (Schaeffer, 2006). Acupuncture and physical therapies, including prostatic massage and sitz baths, have been recommended but have not been adequately studied.
Interstitial cystitis/ Painful bladder syndrome (IC/PBS)	IC/PBS is a chronic debilitating condition characterized by pelvic pain, urinary urgency, and urinary frequency (Hanno, 2007b). In the past IC was considered a bladder disease, but it is now considered a chronic pain syndrome that may begin as a pathological process in the bladder in most, but not all, patients. IC encompasses a major portion of the "painful bladder" disease complex, which includes a large group of patients with bladder, urethral, or pelvic pain or a combination of these; irritative voiding symptoms (urgency, frequency, nocturia, dysuria); and negative urine cultures (Hanno, 2007a). The true prevalence of IC has not been agreed on, but it occurs more frequently in women than men (ratio of 5:1) (Clemens, Joyce, Wise, & Payne, 2007).
	The exact cause of PBS is not universally understood, but includes a variety of factors such as chronic infection of the bladder, lymphatic disease, autoimmune (self-attacking disease—the body turns on itself) disorders, and even psychological and neurological conditions (Mayer, 2007). The quality of life of patients with IC/PBS is significantly degraded.
	The diagnosis of IC/PBS has been one of exclusion; as a result, IC/PBS is frequently misdiagnosed as urogenital infection, OAB, or endometriosis, among other conditions with similar symptomatology. A simple question will often suffice to differentiate between the two conditions: "Is your urgency to find a restroom because

Table 2.1   (continued)

Condition	Description
	you are afraid you will wet yourself or is it because you are in increasing pain and discomfort?" (Hanno, 2007a). People with IC/PBS have a bladder wall that is generally tender and easily irritated, leading to uncomfortable symptoms. Symptoms include pelvic pain, pressure, or discomfort related to the bladder that are usually associated with persistent urge to void *or* urinary frequency. These symptoms are in the absence of infection or other pathology. An associated symptom is painful sexual intercourse (dyspareunia). IC/PBS begins gradually and becomes progressively worse. Symptoms may go into remission but usually return (called flare-ups). Cystoscopy is usually performed to confirm a diagnosis.
	Treatment for IC/PBS includes pharmacological therapy (both oral and intravesical medications). Oral medication includes pentosan polysulfate sodium (elmiron) 100 mg 3 times a day, amitriptyline (elavil) 10–75 mg nightly, gabapentin (neurontin), and topiramate (topamax). Pentosan polysulfate sodium is the only FDA-approved oral medication for IC/PBS. Other treatments include myofascial release, bladder stretching, and biofeedback, and soft tissue massage, and other physical therapies such as trigger point release and pelvic floor muscle relaxation can alleviate pain and frequency. Bladder retraining with urge suppression (as described in Chapter 8) may be helpful, especially to decrease symptoms of urgency and frequency (Rosenberg, Newman, & Paige, 2007).
	Self-care practices are often recommended (see the companion CD under Patient Education Tools for "Self-Care for 'Painful Bladder Syndrome' " [Interstitial Cystitis]). Included are dietary modifications that may relieve and control symptoms and avoid flare-ups in the majority of IC/PBS cases (Mishell, 2006). Stress exacerbates IC/PBS symptoms or causes flare-ups. IC/PBS patients are advised to learn and practice basic relaxation techniques. Intravesical (in the bladder) therapy can be helpful in relieving symptoms. Dimethylsulfoxide (DMSO) is the only medication approved by the U.S. Food and Drug Administration for intravesical instillation for the treatment of IC/PBS (Hanno, 2007a).
Chronic pelvic pain in women	CPP in women is pelvic pain that continues for more than six months; it is seen more often in adult white women (Dutton, 2006). CPP accounts for 10% of gynecological visits. CPP can be identified clinically by six common characteristics: 1. Duration of six months or longer 2. Incomplete relief with most treatment 3. Significantly impaired function at home or work 4. Signs of depression (e.g., early morning awakenings, weight loss, anorexia) 5. Pain out of proportion to pathology 6. Altered family and social roles CPP originates in the region of the lower abdomen and pelvis (bladder), although the pain may extend downward to involve the lower extremities or upward to the thoracolumbar area. Changes associated with pain include physical and mental fatigue, cramp-

(continued)

Table 2.1   (continued)

Condition	Description
	ing, dysmenorrhea, premenstrual pain, depression and anxiety, dyspareunia causing decreased sexual activity, and interruptions in sleep (Hornick & Slocumb, 2008). Other typically reported symptoms include rectal itching, and burning on frequent bowel movements.
	Treatments are similar to those discussed for IC/PBS.
Vulvodynia	Vulvodynia is a broad umbrella group of conditions that cause vulvar pain. Of the different subtypes of vulvodynia, vulvar vestibulitis (VVS) is considered the most common. The main symptom of vulvodynia is vulvar pain. It is a chronic pain syndrome that affects up to 15%–20% of women (Arnold, Bachmann, Rosen, Kelly, & Rhoads, 2006; Bachmann et al., 2006), and is found in white and African American women but may be more common in Hispanic women. It is characterized by vulvar discomfort, most often described as burning or stabbing pain, occurring in the absence of other disorders. Women will have complaints of perineal burning, stinging, irritation, or rawness. The most common symptoms are dyspareunia, severe point tenderness on touch, perineal irritation, and vestibular erythema (ACOG Committee on Gynecologic Practice, 2006). It can be chronic or unremitting, intermittent, or episodic (often exacerbated premenstrually), or may occur in response to a stimulus (e.g., bicycle riding, tampon insertion, prolonged sitting, wearing tight clothes). Vulvodynia is not associated with sexually transmitted diseases (STDs) or STD risk factors, but affected women often have been treated repeatedly for candidal vulvovaginitis. *Candida,* a commensal microorganism known to cause the most common clinical infections of the vulva and vagina, may be a cause of vulvodynia. Pain of vulvodynia is not due to psychological issues, previous sexual abuse, or marital problems.
	Affected women are more likely to have altered contractile characteristics of the pelvic floor musculature; biofeedback therapy designed to address these alterations often results in improved muscle function and decreased vulvar pain. The pain can begin suddenly when provoked or triggered, and it tends to dissipate gradually. Women will report hours to days of discomfort after intercourse or a pelvic examination. Allodynia (i.e., pain elicited by a normally painful stimulus) and hyperpathia (i.e., when a stimulus causes greater pain than expected) suggest a neuropathic cause of the pain of vulvodynia.
	The diagnosis depends on a consistent history and lack of a documented infectious (e.g., negative yeast culture) or dermatological cause (e.g., normal pH). Women will report vulvar pain, dyspareunia, or pain with tampon insertion. Examination may review one or more focal inflammatory areas in the vestibule and tenderness when gentle pressure is applied by a cotton-tipped swab to the vulva, introitus, or hymenal areas (see Chapter 6). Many women with vulvodynia will also report urological symptoms such as urgency, frequency, and dysuria. These symptoms are similar to those seen with IC/PBS. Occasionally, the patient may not be aware that the sensitivity is in the area of the introitus, and she may describe the pain as deeper in the vagina or pelvis (Reed, 2006).

Table 2.1   (continued)

Condition	Description
	Medical therapies can be broadly categorized as medications that are being used to treat thinning of the vaginal tissues (estrogen), inflammation (corticosteroids), or pain (lidocaine [xylocaine], tricyclic antidepressants, gabapentin [neurontin]); depending on the drug, they can be given either topically or orally. Because the pain of vulvodynia seems to be neuropathic, many medications that have been used effectively in the treatment of other neuropathic disorders have been used in patients with vulvodynia (Goldstein, Marinoff, & Haefner, 2005). Tricyclic antidepressants (e.g., amitriptyline [elavil]) often are used as a first-line therapy; the antiepileptic drug gabapentin (Neurontin) has also been used.
	Prolonged treatment with oral fluconazole (Diflucan) has been recommended based on the supposition that chronic candidal infections may contribute to vulvodynia, but results have been inconsistent. This therapy should be reserved for patients with documented candidal infection. Biofeedback and physical therapy have been used to reverse changes in the pelvic floor musculature and to help women regain control of the muscles, including improving strength and relaxation (Glazer, 2000). Women should be counseled to avoid the use of harsh soaps and perfumed products in the vulvar region and to wear all-cotton underwear.
	Topical corticosteroids and estrogens generally have not been successful, and these treatments are used primarily in patients with specific indications (e.g., estrogen deficiency, lichen sclerosus). Similarly, the injection of steroids and interferon in women with localized symptoms has met with conflicting results and recommendations. Topical lidocaine (Xylocaine) has been used as needed (up to three or four vulvar applications per day) and recently has been used on a nightly basis in the introitus to minimize vulvar pain. Topical cromolyn sodium may be helpful in certain women.
	Surgery is indicated only in women with severe symptoms and in whom other treatments have not been effective.

with an increased risk for UTIs in perimenopausal and postmenopausal women (Foxman et al., 2001).

IMPACT ON QUALITY OF LIFE

Epidemiological and clinical studies of individuals with UI indicate that the condition has a considerable impact on overall QoL and well-being. The inability to control urine is one of the most unpleasant and distressing symptoms a person can experience, causing stigmatization and denial of the condition (Garcia, Crocker, & Wyman, 2005). It has been demonstrated that incontinent women have lower levels of emotional well-being than continent women (Wyman, Harkins, & Fantl, 1990). Both women and men with these conditions have significantly poorer QoL than age- and gender-matched populations. However, most QoL research has been conducted on community-dwelling white women, with little research on men and on people in LTC facilities.

The effect of UI on emotional well-being may differ between races, genders, and cultures (Bogner, 2004) and may have more of an impact on QoL when other comorbid medical conditions exist (Bogner et al., 2002; Ko, Lin, Salmon, & Bron, 2005). DuBeau, Simon, and Morris (2006) reported on 58,850 nursing home residents with UI and showed that new or worsening UI over six months was associated with worse QoL and was second only to cognitive and functional decline in predicting worse QoL. Therefore, QoL assessments are critical for conditions such as UI and OAB, which often go untreated and have consistently been shown to have a deleterious effect on health-related QoL in individuals of all ages and in all care settings.

UI can limit a person's social activities and interpersonal relationships. It can cause significant morbidity and affects the social, psychological, occupational, domestic, physical, and sexual lives of 15%–30% of women of all ages. UI is often the cause of social isolation and physiological problems. The emotional impact results from its effects in three areas: self-image, lifestyle, and relationships. Women who experience UI report anxiety and depression and feel that the abnormal symptoms associated with UI have rendered life intolerable. Women with SUI are more likely to report low levels of physical activity and to avoid participating in sports and other high-impact activities because of the fear of leaking urine (W.J. Brown & Miller, 2001). Although this strategy may reduce the frequency and severity of urinary leakage, it is harmful over the long term because it predisposes women to weight gain, which further increases the risk and severity of SUI (Subak et al., 2002; Sustersic & Kralj, 1998).

Some individuals may give up or restrict certain domestic routines and household chores, as well as outside activities such as shopping, traveling, and church attendance. Men and women will avoid or curtail activities in an attempt to prevent the possibility of an incontinence episode. Others will frequent only places where bathroom facilities are known and easily accessible. Women who are physically active and experience urine leakage during these activities will curtail and even stop such activities as exercising or dancing. Some will make adjustments in an activity or behavior that causes UI (e.g., change from high- to low-impact aerobics, avoid heavy lifting). UI and OAB negatively impact working women and cause them to work fewer hours (Fultz, Fisher, & Jenkins, 2004). Fultz et al. (2005) found that working women with UI reported an inability to concentrate on work, lower self-confidence, and an inability to complete tasks without interruptions (e.g., needing to go to the bathroom).

Women with UI tend to isolate themselves socially, increasing the risk for depression and removing themselves from social support systems needed to deal with this distressing condition. Melville, Delaney, Newton, and Katon (2005) conducted an age-stratified postal survey of 6,000 women ages 30–90 years. Subjects were randomly selected from enrollees in a large health maintenance organization in Washington State. Main outcome measures were prevalence of current major depression and adjusted odds ratios for factors associated with major depression in women with UI. The prevalence of UI was 42% ($n = 1,458$). The prevalence of major depression was 3.7% ($n = 129$), with 2.2% reported in those subjects without incontinence versus 6.1% in those with incontinence. Among women with incontinence, major depression prevalence rates differed by incontinence severity (2.1% in mild, 5.7% in moderate, and 8.3% in severe) and incontinence type (4.7% in SUI, 6.6% in UUI/MUI). Women with incontinence and major depression have a significantly increased incontinence symptom burden versus women with UI alone (Melville, Delaney, et al., 2005). The exact nature of the relationship among UI, depression, and recovery is not clear. In one study, the perception of the interference of incontinence with daily activities was the best predictor of depressive symptoms (Dugan et al., 2000). However, there are effective treatments for both UI and depressive symptoms in older adults.

The fear of incontinence during sexual intercourse severely affects intimate relationships. Both men and women may avoid sexual intimacy because of the fear of urine leakage during intercourse or of interrupting intercourse because of the need to urinate (Rogers, Villarreal, Kammerer-Doak, & Qualls, 2001). Among women, relationships with spouses and other family members may become constrained and the woman may feel rejected as she tries to conceal the condition, avoid possible embarrassment, and keep others from being repelled by the condition. This may lead to a decrease in sexual interest. In fact, UI is significantly associated with decreased libido, vaginal dryness, and dyspareunia (Handa, Harvey, Cundiff, Siddique, & Kjerulff, 2004). In an open-label prospective study of women treated with a transdermal antimuscarinic medication (oxybutynin [Oxytrol]), Sand, Goldberg, Dmochowski, McIlwain, and Dahl (2006) found that OAB affected the sex lives of 39% of women, and 24% reported that OAB affected relationships with partners. Embarrassment about bladder control issues causes many women to remain silent about the condition. Not only do they refrain from discussing the problem with family and friends, but many are too embarrassed to discuss it with their nurses and doctors—or they wait years before doing so. Men with erectile dysfunction and incontinence after radical prostatectomy surgery will limit sexual activity because of fear of urine leakage or because wives/partners fear urine contamination in the vagina. In general, UI and OAB can inhibit a sufferer's lifestyle, keeping him or her from receiving treatment in spite of the availability of several effective treatments.

The specific symptoms associated with UI and the severity of these symptoms are indicators of impact on QoL. Quantity of urine lost is an important measure because severe urine loss appears to have greater social and emotional consequences than does mild loss (Fultz & Herzog, 2001). OAB symptoms of urgency and frequency can be especially burdensome to a person who has difficulty with mobility or is recovering from an illness, or has conditions that may cause barriers to reaching the restroom (Newman & Giovanni, 2002). At night, urinary urgency may disrupt sleep.

As a result, individuals with these conditions gradually develop coping or self-care behaviors to manage their symptoms, instead of seeking treatment (Ricci et al., 2001). When UI becomes sufficiently so severe that it can no longer be easily hidden from others, QoL is significantly impaired. Emotional well-being is impaired, probably as a result of social isolation and feelings of stigmatization produced by the incontinence. For the elderly person, UI may provoke significant anxiety because it is a primary factor in the decision to enter an LTC facility (Coward, Horne, & Peek, 1995).

HELP-SEEKING BEHAVIOR AND SELF-CARE PRACTICES

Despite the considerable impact of bladder storage symptoms on QoL, many people never seek medical help and are thus uncounted (Kinchen et al., 2003). A European survey reported that patients wait from 2 to 11 or more years before seeking treatment (Sykes et al., 2005). Instead of seeking a solution for their UI, most patients will continue to alter their lifestyle and develop elaborate "self-care" practices (usually one or more) to hide or accommodate their symptoms (Huang et al., 2006; Koch, 2006). The use of self-care practices or self-management is a step-by-step process that involves the person making adjustments in activities and behaviors so that he or she can continue with daily life and stay in "control." If the self-management is successful, people become less troubled or bothered by their symptoms even if symptoms worsen (Bush, Castellucci, & Phillips, 2001). Self-care practices usually require little effort and are usually simple modifications (called behavior modifications) of normal daily activities. Reported self-care practices include restricting fluid intake, using absorbent pads, crossing the legs, carrying extra clothing, and wearing dark/loose-fitting clothing (see Chapter 7). Affected individuals may also avoid crowded places such as sports stadiums and movie theaters, where it may be difficult to get to a bathroom in time.

People with moderate to severe UI, urgency, and frequency may engage in a variety of behaviors to cope with unintentional urine loss. Some of these behaviors, such as defensive urination (urinating on a scheduled basis or prior to provocative events such as exercising), toilet mapping (searching out toilets in order to maximize access to toileting facilities), and, at the extreme, choosing to not leave the house, help people cope with bladder control disorders and do not compromise overall health. Although these measures help these individuals manage their symptoms, they can also be time consuming, require considerable planning, greatly impair social interaction, restrict movement, and diminish QoL. Management strategies in dealing with UI differ between genders. Men are more likely to limit fluids and decrease trips to the bathroom and are more likely to see a physician about their problem. Women more frequently limit fluid intake, increase trips to bathroom, and wear protective pads.

The fear of odor is a significant concern of women with UI, causing over-use of incontinence products, perineal perfumes and powders, and vaginal douches. Because of misconceptions surrounding UI, researchers have found that women typically resist acknowledging the disease as important, conceal or hide their condition from others, and seek help only when urine loss is so severe that it can no longer be hidden from family and friends (Fultz et al., 2003; Hägglund, Walker-Engstrom, Larsson, & Leppert, 2003; Shaw et al., 2006).

Current research in the area of help-seeking behavior (seeking help from a health care provider) in women with UI has determined that fewer than 38% sought help for their condition and they waited more than a year to do so (Koch, 2006). Huang et al. (2006) reported that fewer than 50% of women with clinically significant UI reported seeking treatment despite the fact that all women in this study were insured and had continuous access to a provider (Kaiser Permanente). Melville, Newton, Fan, and Katon (2006) surveyed pre-dominantly white, adult women in a nonprofit health maintenance organiza-tion in Washington State about incontinence symptoms, care-seeking behav-iors, and past and current treatments. Prevalence of UI (any leakage that occurs at least monthly) in this group was 41% and increased with age. Fifty percent of women had discussed their UI with a provider, but only 27% had made an appointment specifically to discuss their UI; only 8% had a history of surgery and only 16% reported current treatment of any kind (drugs, pelvic floor muscle exercises). Treatment for women who reported more severe UI was only slightly higher. Therefore, help-seeking behavior is poor.

The most common reasons that people with UI and OAB do not seek treatment are the (erroneous!) beliefs that 1) the symptoms are a normal con-sequence of aging, childbirth, or both; 2) it is too embarrassing; and 3) no treatment for these conditions is available (Diokno, Sand, Macdiarmid, Shah, & Armstrong, 2006). Women with SUI one year after childbirth had not sought help because they felt that their physician would not think UI was a serious problem (33%) and they themselves did not view it as serious (67%) (L. Mason, Glen, Walton, & Hughes, 2001). These and other myths or un-truths are detailed in Table 2.2. It is known that women who have more severe UI symptoms will seek treatment (Kinchen et al., 2003; Newman, 2004a). In addition, women who do seek professional help report higher levels of stress and suffering related to UI, and they tend to think it is a disease. A motivat-ing factor for seeking treatment in both men and women is the fear that symp-toms will worsen.

Most of the research on help-seeking behavior used questionnaires, so there was very little opportunity for respondents to explain in their own words the impact of the problem and why they had not sought treatment. To obtain this information, a mail survey was sent to customers of a mail-order incontinence product company (Newman, 2004a). Women surveyed described

Table 2.2 Common myths about urinary incontinence

Myth	Reality
UI is a normal part of aging.	Although UI is common, especially among older adults, it is not a normal part or consequence of aging. Possibly because of the prevalence and severity of UI seen among nursing home residents and homebound older adults, any UI is often erroneously perceived as an inevitable consequence of aging. Although the aging adult is more likely to experience bothersome LUTS, age-related changes do not inevitably lead to UI. This misconception is reflected in advertisements and greeting cards that link continence with younger, vibrant adults, while incontinence is seen as a sign of aging and loss of vigor and vitality. More significantly, women who see UI as inevitable report that this belief works against seeking assistance from health care providers, or causes them to postpone consultation until the condition has become so severe that they are no longer able to conceal its existence from family or close friends. Careful consideration of epidemiological statistics concerning UI, and a clear understanding of the pathophysiology of the lower urinary tract and the influence of normal aging on continence, can dispel this damaging myth.
UI is inevitable and not amenable to treatment.	One of the most significant obstacles in the diagnosis and management of UI is the pervasive perception among both patients and health care providers that it is inevitable and irreversible. The "stigma" surrounding bladder control problems, and the fact that people have many misconceptions about these conditions, prevent patients from seeking care. Townsend et al. (2007) found that only 13% of nurses in the Nurses Health Study reported receiving treatment for their incontinence.
If a patient has a UI problem, he or she will report it [belief of health care providers].	There is a disconnect between health care providers and their older patients: Only a minority (38%) mentioned leaking urine to their physician (Townsend et al., 2007). It has been reported that physicians "don't ask" and older adults "don't tell." The refrain "My patients would tell me if they had a problem with incontinence" is often heard from PCPs about patients of all ages.
	The reluctance to talk about UI and the lack of understanding of bladder control may contribute to miscommunication between providers and patients. One reason voiced by providers for women not discussing UI is that the women must not be "bothered" by it. However, Fultz et al. (2003) noted that, among women who were moderately to extremely bothered by their SUI symptoms, only 46.6% reported ever speaking with a physician about their problem, perhaps because of embarrassment. It may be that older adults are not asked because of time constraints and organizational barriers in providing comprehensive primary care to older adults. A U.K. study (Shaw et al., 2006) of women accessing primary care services indicated that women with SUI experienced their symptoms for 63 months prior to the study overall, and those with UUI for 42 months and with MUI for 69 months. A major reason given for this reluctance was the embarrassing nature of the condition. Many PCPs tell women to return if the problem "worsens" without knowing if the woman is seeking treatment or reassurance. Most women express a preference for having their health care provider initiate a discussion about incontinence rather than bringing it up themselves (L. Mason, Glen, Walton, & Hughes, 2001). The stigma associated with being unable to control bodily functions and the fear of other people's reactions, including those of health care providers, have led to people preferring to conceal their problem and manage it independently as

Table 2.2   (continued)

Myth	Reality
	long as they can (Horrocks, Somerset, Stoddart, & Peters, 2004). Physicians also tend to underestimate the degree to which patients are bothered by symptoms. Providers lack understanding regarding the problem, or their indifference may be a reflection of their lack of interest in a problem that is primarily a problem for women (Koch, 2006).
	Care processes are being developed. The ACOVE-2 intervention has been designed to improve primary care provided to older adults (≥ 75 years) who have UI through the use of a condition-specific intervention that includes collection of clinical data and medical records to prompt performance of essential care processes, and provide patient education material and physician education and support (Reuben, Roth, Kamberg, & Wenger 2003).
UI is a hygiene problem.	Perhaps the most significant impediment to optimal diagnosis and treatment of UI is the myth that it is a hygiene problem rather than a disorder. Individuals with UI commonly report a fear of odor and embarrassment. They feel unclean and become obsessed with personal hygiene. Women especially will prematurely turn to absorbent perineal pads to prevent the leakage from becoming noticeable and to avoid odor. Health care providers may unintentionally perpetuate this myth if they believe that the incontinence does not pose an immediate threat to life or act as a harbinger for malignancy or infection. Similarly, people with UI may unintentionally promote the misconception by denying their incontinence or assessing it as not sufficiently important to discuss with a health care provider. Defining UI as a hygiene problem rather than a medical condition is deleterious because it fails to recognize and confront the clinically relevant and often devastating adverse psychosocial consequences associated with UI, and it ignores the physical sequelae of incontinence, particularly in elderly patients.
UI is part of being "female."	Women tend to "accept" urinary symptoms such as UI more so than men (Fultz & Herzog, 2001). Some have thought that, because SUI may develop in relation to a normal life or natural event such as pregnancy and childbirth, women may see it as "normal" (Hägglund & Wadensten, 2007). Women's experience with managing menstrual bleeding (use of perineal pads) could be extended to managing urine loss, leading the woman to believe that UI is normal and having her adapt.
There is no effective treatment for UI.	Several factors contribute to the misconception that UI is unlikely to respond to treatment. If people believe that UI is an unavoidable consequence of aging, it logically follows that urinary leakage (like the aging process itself) cannot be alleviated or reversed, only postponed or covered up. A variety of effective treatments for UI exist, and novel treatments continue to be developed. Behavioral interventions, including pelvic floor muscle rehabilitation and bladder retraining, have proven effective for the management of UI and OAB. Alternative and effective treatments for SUI include surgery. A number of medications are available for OAB and UUI.

Key: LUTS = lower urinary tract symptoms; MUI = mixed urinary incontinence; OAB = overactive bladder; PCP = primary care provider; SUI = stress urinary incontinence; UI = urinary incontinence; UUI = urge urinary incontinence.

the initial loss of bladder control and noted things they would like providers to know (Box 2.1).

INCONTINENCE IN THE COMMUNITY

An estimated 15%–30% of community-dwelling older adults have UI. The prevalence rate among women 60 years and older, residing in the community, is 15%–35% (Fantl et al., 1996). UI affects up to 30% of the entire adult female population, and the prevalence increases among older age groups. From younger to middle-aged women, prevalence ranges from 16% to 31%, respectively, with a mean of 25% (Nygaard & Lemke, 1996; Thom, Nygaard, & Calhoun, 2005). Prevalence rates are 1.5%–5% for men ages 15–60 years and increase to 19% for men older than 60 years (Fantl et al., 1996). In pregnant women, incontinence affects between 32% and 64% for all UI and between 40% and 59% for SUI (including MUI) (Hunnskaar et al., 2005).

Several large epidemiological studies have reported on the prevalence of UI in community-residing women. A study of 3,273 adult women seeing primary care practices in a wide range of geographical and cultural settings in the United Kingdom indicated that 45.7% reported UI during the preceding month, with 25.5% having SUI, 3.5% UUI, and 20.7% MUI (Shaw et al., 2006). Women were asked to complete a questionnaire to determine if they had experienced a specific type of UI in the past month. Consistent with many other studies, 53% had not consulted a health care provider for their UI. Baseline data from the Heart and Estrogen/Progestin Replacement Study (HERS) in 2,763 older, community-dwelling women (mean age, 66.7 years) with coronary disease, who were not currently taking hormone replacement therapy, indicated that some type of frequent UI (≥ 1 episode in the prior week) occurred in more than half of the subjects (J.S. Brown et al., 1999). SUI and stress-predominant MUI occurred in 41.5% of the women reporting UI.

INCONTINENCE IN THE HOME CARE SETTING

UI is seen in 53% of homebound older adults and is a leading reason for caregivers to place a family member in a nursing facility. UI is a frequently seen diagnosis in patients requiring skilled nursing care in the home. Preliminary data from a survey of 8,400 home and hospice health agencies indicated that genitourinary conditions were among the 20 leading diagnoses for patients added to their caseloads (Strahan, 1994). UI is one of the 10 leading diagnoses for homebound individuals and first in total charges to Medicare for nursing services per person served (Ruther & Helbing, 1988). In a study of low-income, older individuals receiving publicly funded home care services, 23% were incontinent of urine and generated greater costs because of paraprofessional and other supportive care (Baker & Bice, 1995). UI tends to be severe among

Box 2.1   Women's statements about the impact of UI

Description of Initial Episode of Loss of Bladder Control

- Came home after church and wet pants before could enter bathroom.
- After having two children when I jumped around at an activity.
- Embarrassing; I was on a public bus.
- Annoying.
- Just couldn't control it.
- Wet in my pants and was not too happy about it. Embarrassed me so much.
- After riding a long way I can't get to a bathroom in time.
- On my way to the bathroom from bed.
- Stood up after sitting for a long while and drinking lots of fluids.
- After falling and breaking my hip.
- I was on a date and him and I were dancing. I was so embarrassed. He hung my panties on the radio antenna.
- Found my underwear wet.
- Shock.
- At my home; sudden urge, no control, therefore did not make it to bathroom.
- Disgusting.
- Laughed so hard at a joke, as a result lost control.
- I was in a grocery store, made a puddle on the floor, after that I started wearing pads 24 hours a day.
- Happened at home after awakening with bed wet. Have slept on plastic pads since.

Things They Would Like Professionals to Know

- Just let people know that it is a way of life and they aren't the only ones it happens to, so there is no reason to be ashamed.
- It's a real drag on my emotions.
- I am unable to tell anyone how to cope with this.
- It's hell.
- It's very inconvenient and embarrassing.
- I don't like people telling me that I have a wet pair of pants.
- Not being able to be myself.
- It's very inconvenient and bothersome.
- Constant worry.
- It has been a part of my life for so long I take it for granted.
- Limits ability to travel.
- I feel like I'm a prisoner in my own home because I'm afraid to stay out too long.
- Learn where all bathrooms are.
- I wish the products were packaged so they weren't so obvious and so I wouldn't be embarrassed to buy them. One cashier said when she saw the package "Oh you poor thing!" I was mortified and I've never gone to that grocery store again.
- I think the Dr. should ask about it during a checkup as we age.
- For Dr. to be more concerned and helpful.
- I find it degrading, disgusting, and very very uncomfortable.

homebound older adults in both frequency and volume. McDowell, Engberg, Rodriguez, Engberg, and Sereika (1996) examined the characteristics of frail homebound older adults with UI. Incontinence tended to be severe ($M = 3.8$ accidents/day), and almost all subjects reported having urge accidents (94.8%). Most subjects (80%) had functional limitations in ambulation, and levels of comorbidity were high ($M = 8.4$ medical problems).

Even though homebound older people tend to have multiple health and functional disabilities, they perceive UI to be a very disturbing problem that further restricts activities. The combination of decreased functional ability and UI is particularly challenging to both professional and nonprofessional caregivers. The magnitude of the problem of caring for incontinent homebound individuals will no doubt increase as the absolute number of older people increases and at-home care of dependent older people becomes more common. The effect of UI on vulnerable, frail, homebound elders is especially burdensome for them and also for families and caregivers. Home care providers will need to address this common and costly problem. The quality indicators that are used in LTC facilities could be applied when evaluating and treating vulnerable homebound elders for UI (Fung, Spencer, Eslami, & Crandall, 2007).

The psychosocial impact of UI imposes a significant burden on individuals and their families, caregivers, and health care clinicians. The proportion of older adults reporting impairments in ADLs (e.g., bathing, dressing, toileting, ambulation) increases sharply with age, with 73.6% of those over 79 years of age reporting at least one disability (Administration on Aging, 2002). Dependence on caregivers increases as incontinence worsens and as homebound older people use indwelling catheters and other supportive devices that increase the risk of infection, morbidity, and mortality. Most people with UI manage the condition using a combination of previous treatment strategies plus their own self-devised strategies. Most have little or no problem finding commercially available absorbent products. Sometimes, though, women refuse to participate in situations outside the home for fear of being incontinent, which can be especially frustrating for family members, particularly spouses (Baker & Bice, 1995; Mitterness, 1987). UI can predispose a woman to admission to an LTC facility. A study that examined reasons for placement in an LTC facility found that 44% of family members reported that UI was a significant factor in placing a relative in a nursing facility (M.J. Johnson & Werner, 1982). Thomas et al. (2004) found that incontinence was the most frequent caregiver complaint (68%) at the time of placement in an institution for a cohort of patients with dementia (75 females, 34 males).

Incontinence is a relentless source of weariness for caregivers, especially older caregivers. Caregiver burden, defined as the strain or load borne by an individual caring for an older, chronically ill or disabled family member or other person, increases day by day (Engberg, Kincade, & Thompson, 2004). People with functional impairment and UI need to be lifted and turned to prevent skin breakdown, their incontinence products and bed pads must be changed, and their soiled skin cleansed. In addition, incontinence is not only a daytime problem. During the night, a caregiver's sleep is disturbed to assist with toileting and transfers to commodes. In some situations the caregiver's burden is so great that he or she becomes ill. If older partners are frail themselves, they may even die before the incontinent person for whom they are caring.

Denial of incontinence by an older family member is a tricky dilemma for both family members and professionals who may be assisting the family with caregiving. Older people experience a loss of sensitivity to smell as they age. Also, some block out awareness of their incontinence to avoid its implications. If the family confronts the denial head on, they may provoke hostility and humiliation and cause an incontinent individual to further withdraw from acknowledgment of the problem.

The Centers for Medicare and Medicaid Services (CMS) Outcome and Assessment Information Set (OASIS; CMS, 2004) enables home health clinicians to address the problems of urinary and bowel incontinence in patients requiring home nursing care using the M0520 and the M0530 items to note when UI occurs. M0520 and M0530 are as follows:

M0520—Urinary Incontinence or Urinary Catheter Presence Levels

> 0—no incontinence or catheter (includes anuria or ostomy for urinary drainage) [if No go to M0520]
>
> 1—patient is incontinent
>
> 2—patient requires a urinary catheter (i.e., external, indwelling intermittent, suprapubic) [Go to M0540]

According to the OASIS User's Manual instructions:

- If the patient is incontinent AT ALL (i.e., "occasionally," "only once-in-a-while," "sometimes I leak a little bit," etc.), mark Response 1.

M0530: When Does Urinary Incontinence Occur?

> 0—timed voiding defers incontinence
>
> 1—during the night only
>
> 2—during the day and night

The OASIS User's Manual instructions note that:

- If patient is only "occasionally" incontinent, determine when the incontinence usually occurs.

- Any incontinence that occurs during the day should be marked with response 2.

The OASIS manual recommends that home health care nurses note the following:

- Review the urinary elimination pattern as you take the health history.

  - Does the client admit having difficulty controlling the urine, or is he/she embarrassed about needing to wear a pad so as not to wet on clothing?

- Do you have orders to change a catheter?

- Is your stroke patient using an external catheter?

- Be alert for an odor of urine, which might indicate there is a problem with bladder sphincter control.

- If the client receives aide services for bathing and/or dressing, ask for input from the aide (at follow-up assessment).

This information can then be discussed with the patient and caregiver.

INCONTINENCE IN LONG-TERM CARE FACILITIES

Over 65% of nursing home residents experience some type of UI, second only to dementia as a leading cause of placement in an LTC facility (Boyington et al., 2007; D. Mason, Newman, & Palmer, 2003). The prevalence of OAB is also high in the nursing home community—about 70% of residents have some difficulties with urgency and frequency in combination with incontinence. The relative risk of admission to a nursing home was 2.5 times greater for incontinent women and 3.7 times greater for incontinent men (Thom et al., 1997). Regional prevalence of UI has been reported as 65.4% at admission and 74.3% postadmission (Boyington et al., 2007). UI is the primary reason why many older adults are not accepted into the less expensive and less restrictive environment of assisted living facilities (Lekan-Rutledge & Colling, 2003; Newman, 2006).

Although very few medical records of newly admitted nursing home residents have an admitting or current diagnosis of UI, a large percentage of people admitted to LTC facilities "arrive" with UI (Anger, Saigal, Pace, et al., 2006). Few studies have investigated the incidence of incontinence. One study investigating newly admitted nursing facility residents reported that 24% of women residents who were continent at admission were incontinent one year after admission (Ouslander, Palmer, Rovner, & German, 1993). In that study, the development of UI was associated with cognitive impairment, the inability to transfer or walk independently, and poor adjustment to the nursing facility. In a study of 69 hip fracture patients, the incidence of UI in women was 24% (Palmer, Myers, & Fedenko, 1997). Immobility and dementia are the most critical factors contributing to the development of UI in nursing home residents (Schnelle & Leung, 2004). As with every other population studied, DuBeau et al. (2006) demonstrated that prevalent and new or worsening UI decreases QoL even in frail, nursing home residents with functional and cognitive impairments. These authors believe that improving continence care and quality in nursing homes by targeting interventions to those residents most likely to benefit will have an impact on resident QoL.

Incontinence itself is a strong predictor of nursing home placement. UI is a primary reason that brings on or contributes to a person's decision to enter a nursing facility or a family's decision to place an older family member into nursing facility care. Once UI occurs, it appears to persist throughout the resident's stay. Risk factors identified include presence of fecal incontinence, male gender, dementia, and impaired mobility, especially when the person is walking or being moved from one place to another (Palmer, German, & Ouslander, 1991).

Despite this highly prevalent condition, there is a lack of basic knowledge among nursing home staff about UI and its management. It is well known that staff are not performing assessments of residents with UI, but rather move forward with management or containment of urine leakage without determining the presence of confounding variables such as transient causes and without understanding the underlying causes (Newman, 2006; Watson, Brink, Zimmer, & Mayer, 2003). Watson et al. (2003) found that only 2% of incontinent women in the nursing homes studied had had a pelvic examination since admission, only 3% of residents received a specific treatment, and only 2% of residents or their families had their preferences for treatment recorded.

Causes of UI in Long-Term Care

There are many reasons for the occurrence of UI in nursing facilities. Restricted mobility is one of the main factors because residents who are placed in restraints or use assistive devices such as a walker, or who are in a wheelchair, are unable to toilet when needed. Social indifference and cognitive impairment also play a role in the prevalence of incontinence in nursing facilities. Many people enter a nursing facility continent but lose their ability to use the toilet soon afterward, usually because they are in a strange environment and the staff fail to take them to the bathroom as often as necessary (Holroyd-Leduc, Mehta, & Covinsky, 2004). Once in the nursing facility, most residents learn to live with UI. Residents will invest more time and effort in protecting themselves from the consequences of urine leakage by "managing" the problem themselves than in seeking treatment (Robinson, 2000).

In addition to UI, other bladder or incontinence-related disorders such as urinary retention and UTI are common in residents in nursing homes. Identified areas of concern include the use of indwelling catheters without medical necessity, poor perineal hygiene and care, inadequate indwelling urinary catheter care, repeated UTIs, lack of a toileting or bladder rehabilitation program, and the misuse of absorbent products (CMS, 2005; Newman, 2006).

It appears as though there is a discrepancy between the goals of residents and those of staff for UI treatment preferences in the LTC environment. Residents want treatment that allows them to remain dry but prevents dependence on staff. In a study that surveyed LTC residents, family members, and staff, residents perceived the staff as unwilling and unable to implement UI interventions such as toileting assistance (T.M. Johnson, Ouslander, Uman, & Schnelle, 2001). Residents expressed preference for medication and the use of absorbent products as treatments of choice. They viewed toileting or prompted voiding programs as fostering dependence. Families preferred medications to absorbent products. Staff in this study thought that prompted voiding was a more appropriate UI treatment than either absorbent products or more invasive treatments such as catheters; however, they very rarely implemented a prompted voiding program.

State and Federal Regulations

Incontinence poses risks to the LTC community and is demoralizing to staff, and there is a need for more structured guidance in dealing with bladder control problems in this environment. The prevalence of UI is considered an indicator of the quality of nursing facility care (Zimmerman et al., 1995). However, it is difficult to determine specific incontinence care processes despite attempts by government agencies. As part of the state certification survey that nursing facilities must submit annually to receive federal and state funding, surveyors look for a completed Minimum Data Set (MDS) and Resident Assessment Protocol (RAP) and appropriate and updated plans of care to address UI. The CMS Nursing Home Quality Initiative (NHQI) has made quality indicators for every nursing home available to consumers via the CMS web site (http://www.medicare.gov/).

The MDS has been found to be reliable when administered by nursing facility staff (N. M. Resnick, Brandeis, Baumann, & Morris, 1996). In recent years, use of the MDS has been expanded, and efforts are being made to compare nursing facilities on MDS-derived quality indicators and to track changes in quality of continence care over time. Quality indicator domains include (Schnelle & Smith, 2001) the following:

1. Prevalence of bladder or bowel incontinence: excludes residents who are comatose, or have an indwelling catheter or ostomy; includes either high-risk (severe cognitive impairment or *totally* dependent in ADLs having to do with mobility [bed mobility, transfer, and locomotion]) or low-risk (all other) residents

2. Prevalence of occasional or frequent bladder or bowel incontinence without a toileting plan and no bladder retraining program

3. Prevalence of indwelling catheters

4. Prevalence of fecal impaction

5. Prevalence of UTIs

These regulations have changed the atmosphere of LTC from a custodial to a rehabilitative environment.

The MDS gives a picture of continence (bladder function) over time and may not be objective or accurate, but will identify improvement or deterioration in bladder function. The MDS captures a 14-day window of time and can

THE PROBLEM OF INCONTINENCE

identify a transient episode of incontinence caused by acute illness that resolves before a continence evaluation can be initiated. The MDS 2.0 (Section H, 1b) criteria for levels of continence include the following:

0—Continent: complete bladder control (including control achieved by care that involves prompted voiding, habit training, reminders, etc.)

1—Usually continent: less than one bladder incontinence episode per week

2—Occasionally incontinent: more than two (but not daily) bladder incontinence episodes per week

3—Frequently incontinent: daily episodes of bladder incontinence, but some control is present (e.g., on day shift)

4—Incontinent: multiple daily episodes of bladder incontinence

The RAP on incontinence synthesizes a large amount of information into key points and recommendations (Dosa, Bowers, & Gifford, 2006). It provides a summary but very little information on overall guidance for assessment. However, when compared to the RAPs used for other conditions common in LTC, Dosa et al. (2006) found that the UI RAP best approximated the criteria of a guideline for clinical practice. However, most experts believe that the UI RAP needs to be updated to reflect current practice.

Assessment of residents is the responsibility of the staff as well as the practitioners, and supportive measures for UI and OAB should never be a substitute for proper assessment. Management strategies, drug therapies, and containment devices represent some of the treatment options available today that should be considered within the LTC community (CMS, 2005; Newman, 2003, 2004b). Because antimuscarinic medications have proven effective in clinical trials, their use along with toileting programs such as prompted voiding should be considered.

Since the 1980s, U.S. government agencies that have oversight for nursing home care have focused on the advances made in treating and managing this problem. Specifically, the National Institutes of Health (NIH) has funded multiple research projects investigating the effectiveness of toileting assistance programs in the LTC setting. Although the value of toileting programs, specifically prompted voiding, has been well documented in the research setting, other elements must be in place if these practices are to be transferred effectively to the clinical setting. Drug treatment is low (8.7%) and is reserved for residents having the most severe level of UI on the MDS (Level 4) (Jumadilova, Zyczynski, Paul, & Narayanan, 2005). Thus residents who may benefit from drug therapy are overlooked.

Clinical practice guidelines have been developed by both professional organizations (American Medical Directors Association, 1996, 2005) and government agencies (CMS, 2005; Fantl et al., 1996) to outline approaches to assessment, management, and care decisions. The most recent mandated government "Guidance" for meeting compliance in the evaluation and management of UI and urinary catheters in nursing home residents, known as the

F315 tag, was issued by the CMS Survey & Certification Group, Division of Nursing Homes (CMS, 2005). One of the authors (DKN) was a member of the panel of experts who developed this Guidance. F tags denote specific topic areas in the CMS manual used by state surveyors in conducting annual nursing home assessments (DuBeau, Ouslander, & Palmer, 2007). Deficiencies in care are identified by the relevant F tag in the Guidance and are available to consumers for every U.S. nursing home on the Nursing Home Compare web site (http://www.Medicare.gov/NHCompare).

In this new Guidance, Federal Tags 315 and 316 were combined in a single new F315 tag that addresses incontinence and urinary catheters; detailed criteria are presented in Box 2.2. This Guidance is intended to provide more information on assessment of UI and catheters and expand both the RAP and MDS in these areas. It is understood that each resident who is incontinent of urine will need to be identified, assessed, and provided appropriate treatment and services to achieve or maintain as much normal urinary function as possible. This intent is consistent with clinical practice guidelines. Key changes in the new Tag F315 from prior guidelines require LTC facilities to clearly diagnose the type of UI as well as delineate treatment options (Newman, 2006). LTC facilities will now consider incontinence as a void (such as wetness on the skin) along with little or no control. The Tag F315 Guidance has also been formulated to allow a facility to determine the type of UI once an assessment has been completed (Newman, 2006).

This new Guidance will most likely translate into a higher prevalence of UI in LTC facilities. With this emphasis on identifiable risk factors, accurate diagnosis, and individualized treatment of incontinence, LTC facilities are confronted with major clinical, financial, and regulatory burdens. It is the responsibility of the LTC facility to collaborate with the attending physician/ providers to develop a plan of care that includes several management options (behavioral programs, drug therapy, and other options). If these criteria are not met, LTC facilities can receive financial penalties up to $10,000/day. Understanding of the new Guidance is therefore important (Holroyd-Leduc, Lyder, & Tannenbaum, 2006).

However, what is lacking in the RAP, MDS, quality indicators, and Tag F315 are the clinical tools or algorithms to assist with the assessment process. Chapter 8 presents a treatment pathway for UI care in nursing homes (see Figure 8.4), and the companion CD has forms to use for bladder and bowel assessment in LTC facilities.

Barriers to Implementation of Incontinence Control Programs

Despite an established body of knowledge of effective treatment modalities for UI in LTC residents, a number of barriers impede optimal implementation (D. Mason et al., 2003). There is, for example, little evidence suggesting that clinicians have adopted and followed previous UI management guidelines, or

**Box 2.2   Summary of criteria for facility compliance with Tag F315
(Urinary Incontinence and Catheters)**

The urinary incontinence and catheters requirement has three aspects. The first aspect requires that a resident who does not have an indwelling urinary catheter does not have one reinserted unless the resident's clinical condition demonstrates that it is necessary. The second aspect requires the facility to provide appropriate treatment and services to prevent urinary tract infections, and the third is that the facility attempt to assist the resident to restore as much normal bladder function as possible.

For incontinent residents:

- Recognize/assess factors affecting the risk of symptomatic UTIs and impaired urinary function;

- Define and implement interventions to address correctable underlying causes of UI and minimize occurrence of symptomatic UTIs;

- Monitor and evaluate resident's response to preventive efforts and treatment interventions; and

- Revise approaches as appropriate.

For residents admitted with an indwelling urinary catheter or who had one placed after admission:

- Recognize/assess factors affecting urinary function and identify medical justification for indwelling urinary catheter;

- Define and implement interventions to minimize complications from an indwelling urinary catheter, and remove if clinically indicated;

- Monitor and evaluate the resident's response to interventions; and

- Revise approaches as appropriate.

For residents with a symptomatic UTI:

- Recognize/assess factors affecting risk of symptomatic UTIs and impaired urinary function;

- Define and implement interventions to minimize occurrence of symptomatic UTIs and address correctable underlying causes;

- Monitor and evaluate resident's response to preventive efforts and treatment interventions; and

- Revise approaches as appropriate.

Key: UI = urinary incontinence; UTI = urinary tract infection.
Adapted from Centers for Medicare and Medicaid Services. (2005). *State Operations Manual, Appendix PP—Guidance to Surveyors for Long-Term Care Facilities, Tag F315, §483.25(d) Urinary Incontinence* (Rev. 8, Issued: 06-28-05, Effective: 06-28-05, Implementation: 06-28-05) (pp. 1-39). Retrieved November 11, 2007, from http://www.cms.hhs.gov/transmittals/downloads/R8SOM.pdf

are aware of current research about the effectiveness of noninvasive programs in the LTC setting (Watson et al., 2003). In addition, many interventions are not implemented correctly and consistently because the success of the UI program relies heavily on the commitment and consistency of caregivers (Bowers, Esmond, & Jacobson, 2000; Kincade et al., 2003; Lekan-Rutledge & Colling, 2003). Berlowitz et al. (2001) surveyed staff at 36 Department of Veterans Affairs (VA) nursing homes to determine if employees were familiar with guidelines as well as whether five specific guidelines, including the Agency for Healthcare Policy and Research UI guideline (Fantl et al., 1996), had been read, were available, and had been adopted. Among 1,065 respondents (60% of those surveyed), 79% reported familiarity with guidelines. The proportion of staff at a facility reporting adoption of the guidelines was generally less than 50%. A similar study of nursing homes in New York found that only 31% of the guidelines standards were being met (Watson et al., 2003). Based on a survey of nursing home staff and state nursing home surveyors from a midwestern state conducted while attending two statewide workshops on the revised CMS Tag F315 Guidance, DuBeau et al. (2007) concluded that it will be unlikely to improve the quality of urinary continence care in nursing homes because of significant knowledge and attitudinal discrepancies between nursing home staff and state surveyors, facility staff's focus on documentation and staffing, and reliance on implementation strategies that have been shown to be ineffective. In this study, nurses voiced concerns that Tag F315 violates residents' rights.

Prior research has indicated that the two major issues/challenges that need to be overcome to improve urinary continence care in nursing homes are the establishment of appropriate infrastructure and of incentives (Ouslander & Johnson, 2004). Infrastructure includes such things as sufficient staff, agreed-on practice guidelines and quality indicators, dissemination of the guidelines, education on the use of the guidelines, and tools to facilitate guideline implementation. The infrastructure, however, is not anticipated to improve continence care without the establishment of incentives. Recommended external incentives include money, legal liability, and regulations. Suboptimal staff-to-resident ratios in some LTC facilities and inadequate and poorly supervised licensed staff further complicate UI management (Kincade et al., 2003).

These findings indicate that previous strategies and initiatives for UI management in the LTC environment are inadequate. To achieve the goals of UI management, both facility-level and individualized resident-level approaches to UI management are important (Kincade et al., 2003; Lekan-Rutledge, 2004; Lekan-Rutledge & Colling, 2003). Moreover, strategies must be realistic enough to be implemented in the complex care environment of the LTC facility (Thompson, 2004). Defining realistic strategies for success involves evaluating the facility, personnel, and resident limitations (Kincade et al., 2003; Lekan-Rutledge & Colling, 2003; D. Mason et al., 2003).

The Role of the Medical Director

The role of the medical director of an LTC facility in the implementation of a UI program is an important one. Many physicians are not familiar with the guidelines and processes that have been outlined by federal and state agencies. Also, many physicians believe that continence care is a responsibility of nurses. Therefore, it is the medical director's responsibility to ensure that the

UI policies of the LTC facility are developed and implemented. These policies will aid physicians in the care of the older adults residing in the facility. Implementing these guidelines will also improve the QoL and health of the residents and give the staff guidelines on how to handle one of the most common conditions found in LTC facilities (Prochoda, 2002).

The Role of the Advanced Practice Nurse

One study demonstrated significantly improved outcomes for three clinical problems—UI, depression, and pressure ulcers—when gerontological advanced practice nurses (APNs) worked with staff to implement scientifically based protocols (Bourbonniere & Evans, 2002; Maloney & Cafiero, 1999; Ryden et al., 2000; Zarowitz & Ouslander, 2006). This research indicates that, in addition to working with nursing facilities as "physician extenders" to provide resident evaluations, APNs can be an effective link between current research-based knowledge about clinical problems and nursing facility staff. Consistent educational efforts with staff and residents demonstrated that interventions can improve or stabilize the level of UI in many individuals. An expert panel outlined four models for APNs in nursing homes (Mezey et al., 2005). They concluded that APNs have the ability to influence positive changes in resident care. The most effective model appears to be when the APN is employed by the nursing home because he or she becomes embedded in the home's structure.

Staff Issues in Caring for Residents with UI

As noted, research clearly shows that implementation of toileting programs can improve the ability of residents to remain continent in LTC facilities. However, education alone is insufficient to change practice. Nursing staff in LTC facilities have stated that barriers to implementation of such programs include lack of time and resources, lack of authority to change practice, and little support from the administration, physicians, and other staff (Bowers et al., 2000; Lekan-Rutledge, Palmer, & Belyea, 1998). Another barrier is economic. It has been estimated that the additional cost of an effective incontinence management program is $9.09 per day per resident and that about 50% of this additional cost is due to labor (Frantz, Xakellis, Harvey, & Lewis, 2003). One study has shown that, although continence can be improved by an exercise and incontinence program, the costs incurred in treating acute conditions associated with incontinence and immobility are not affected (Schnelle et al., 2003). Thus, the primary argument for instituting an incontinence program must be improving QoL for residents and staff, as well as the considerable health benefits that occur when a patient is continent (DuBeau et al., 2006).

It takes support at all levels of the organization to successfully change the treatment of incontinence, but clearly the benefits are worth it. Problems associated with the delivery of continence care in LTC facilities have been identified (Lekan-Rutledge et al., 1998; Palmer, Bennett, Marks, McCormick, & Engel, 1994). They include the following:

- Inadequate initial staff education on UI and interventions appropriate for this population

- Lack of assessment or evidence of benefit before placing an incontinent resident on a toileting program

- Lack of individualized continence care; rather, care is at the convenience of the staff

- Inadequate staffing

- Poor communication and support from administrative staff regarding expectations

- Lack of financial incentives to keep residents dry

Current management practices in nursing facilities are not consistent with recommended guidelines. It is believed that remediable conditions exist in residents of nursing facilities that are not directly related to bladder dysfunction yet have an impact on continence (e.g., inability to transfer, inability to dress, inability to toilet, use of trunk restraints, inability to rise from chair, use of antianxiety/hypnotic medications) (Brandeis, Baumann, Hossain, Morris, & Resnick, 1997). However, staff are not actively addressing the problem.

Staff attitudes toward UI play a major role in the way incontinent residents are treated. Ninety percent of the actual care of residents—ADLs such as bathing, dressing, toileting, and feeding—is provided by certified nurse assistants (CNAs), who have limited training and education in the care of older adults. Staff may believe that incontinence is expected in nursing facility residents because they believe myths such as "UI is a natural part of aging," and they may convey their acceptance of incontinence directly to the resident (Yu, Kaltreider, & Brannon, 1991). Staff also may act out negative feelings toward these residents (Harke & Richgels, 1992; Lekan-Rutledge et al., 1998; Palmer, 1995; Smith, 1998). The resident with UI correctly perceives that the only way to get attention, although many times negative attention, is through incontinence. Staff also believe that it is quicker to change an absorbent incontinence pad than it is to toilet a resident. This leads to the usual routine seen in most nursing homes, which is to "check and change."

The hopeless acceptance of UI can make it into a "nonproblem." CNAs are not familiar with interventions such as prompted voiding and therefore are not supportive of treatment (B. Resnick et al., 2006). Identifying a continence nurse "champion" who has the knowledge, skills, and time to oversee a continence care program is one approach that can be successful. For interventions to be successful in nursing facilities, staff—particularly CNAs—must believe in the value of continence and be committed to achieving it (A. Wagner & Colling, 1993). Assessment of residents with incontinence is necessary to determine the pathophysiological causes and associated factors that can impede self-toileting. Nurses can perform this evaluation at the bed-side. Treatment techniques, specifically toileting assistance programs, can be readily incorporated into nursing practice. Most nursing facility staff can eas-ily adopt the use of interventions such as bowel and nighttime voiding man-agement and dietary modifications.

Research in nursing facilities has demonstrated the effectiveness of toi-leting assistance programs; however, very little of this research and few of the resulting documented techniques are being used by facility staff. A statewide assessment of Texas Medicaid nursing facilities (Cortes, Montgomery, Morrow, & Monroe, 2000) indicated that 63% of residents had UI but only 12% had appropriate inclusion of toileting assistance in their care plan. Among those residents for whom a toileting program would be desirable and likely benefi-cial, 80% did not receive it. The key to success is identifying which residents should be targeted for each specific program. Finally, staff education remains an ongoing issue. Staff must be aware of attitudes and beliefs about the aging process and its impact on the genitourinary system in order to provide effec-tive care (Palmer & Newman, 2004).

INCONTINENCE IN ACUTE CARE HOSPITALS AND REHABILITATION CENTERS

There are few recent prevalence estimates of incontinence in hospitalized pa-tients. In one report, approximately 24% of patients between 65 and 74 years of age and 48% of patients 75 years and older had at least one episode of in-continence during hospitalization (Palmer et al., 1997). Incontinence is often overlooked in hospitalized older patients, and few incontinent patients are identified. If nurses do not ask about bladder conditions such as incontinence during admission, these conditions are usually not identified. Schultz, Dicky, and Skoner (1997) found that 42% of 247 inpatients reported incontinence but only 10% had their incontinence documented on admission records. Re-searchers analyzing VA administrative data found that, although 43% of the patients were incontinent, only 3.4% of cases had incontinence as a discharge diagnosis (Armstrong & Ferguson, 1998). Although acute care hospital stays are generally short, UI is a significant health problem and should not be over-looked. In a geriatric rehabilitation unit, 21.9% of the patients had UI on ad-mission (Resnick, Slocum, Ra, & Moffett, 1996). During the course of rehabil-itation, there was a decrease in the incidence of UI to 16%. In this study, UI was highly correlated with limitations in ambulation.

As in other care settings, there appears to be a knowledge gap because acute care nurses do not appear to understand UI, do not know the causes, and therefore do not assess for the condition (Cooper & Watt, 2003). They also do not view it as a nursing care issue. Discharge nurses should design a plan that includes referral to a continence nurse or physician specialist (e.g., urologist) for further treatment. Protocols should be developed to direct acute care clinical practice (Bradway & Hernly, 1998). The NICHE project (Nurses Improving Care for Health System Elders) assists hospitals in implementing best practices for the care of older adults ("Geriatric models," 1994; Mezey et al., 2004). The Fulmer SPICES framework is helpful as a geriatric resource model of care. SPICES is an acronym that focuses nurses on six marker conditions in older adults: *s*leep disorders, *p*roblems with eating and feeding, *i*ncontinence, *c*onfusion, *e*vidence of falls, and *s*kin breakdown. These conditions are common and preventable and signal a need for further nursing assessment (Fulmer, 2007). The SPICES assessment tool can be found at http://www.hartfordign. org/publications/trythis/issue01.pdf

COSTS AND FINANCIAL ASPECTS

In the United States, society incurs a significant economic burden as a result of UI that has been increasing over the past decade (Thom et al., 2005). The cost (direct and indirect) of caring for incontinent people older than age 65 in the community and in nursing facilities was estimated to be $24 billion annually in 1995 (T.H. Wagner & Hu, 1998). This figure is the expenditure for 1995 Medicare Part A program costs and reflects the resources spent to treat UI and to mitigate its effects in people older than age 65. The direct costs were estimated as $16.3 billion, including $12.4 billion for women and $3.8 billion for men. This is more than the annual direct costs of breast, cervical, ovarian, and uterine cancers combined (Varmus, 1997). Costs for community-dwelling women older than 65 years ($8.6 billion) were greater than those for women living in LTC facilities ($3.8 billion) (Wilson, Brown, Shin, Luc, & Subak, 2001).

In the nursing home, UI accounts for 3%–8% of total costs, with the average nurse time spent managing a resident's UI being one hour per day. Costs are related directly to the need for increased nursing care from secondary problems such as UTIs, skin breakdown and infection, falls and subsequent injury, psychological distress, and withdrawal (Fantl et al., 1996; Hu et al., 2005). UI-related nursing home costs are only going to rise. Population projections from the Census Bureau suggest that there will be approximately 8.7 million nursing home residents by 2025, and the cost to treat incontinence in nursing home residents might surpass $25 billion by 2025 (in 2002 dollars).

OAB is also costly, especially because one third of patients have OAB with incontinence. A study by Hu et al. (2004) estimated that the direct cost of OAB in the United States was $12.6 billion during 2000. A disturbing part of these costs involves indirect costs, or costs associated with UI and OAB beyond the costs of the condition itself. These include the costs of related UTIs, falls, pressure ulcers, and depression, and they make up greater than 50% of the overall costs. Indirect costs such as these are not often seen in long-term chronic diseases. OAB-related costs also can be a burden to employers. Wu, Birnbaum,

Marynchenko, Williamson, and Mallett (2005) found that OAB was associated with work costs to employers resulting from increased employee sick days and increased risk of employee disability.

Currently, older adults account for more than two thirds of the cost of incontinence. These costs are predominantly for palliative (pads, protection, and laundry: 50%–75%) rather than rehabilitative services. In nursing homes, incremental labor costs (changing, turning, positioning, toileting) associated with caring for an incontinent patient (UI and fecal incontinence) are $4,957 per patient per year more than the cost for caring for a continent patient (Shih, Hartzema, & Tolleson-Rinehart, 2003). Wilson et al. (2001) calculated that, for women, the largest cost category was routine care (70%), followed by nursing facility admissions (14%), treatment (9%), complications (6%), and evaluation and diagnosis (1%). Coverage of treatment costs by third-party payers varies considerably. For example, because absorbent products are considered hygiene products, they are not reimbursed.

It is expected that overall costs for managing UI will increase as the aging population increases. Hu and Wagner (2005) believe that, because the health consequences of the costs of both UI and OAB are so significant, investing more health care resources to improve initial treatment may reduce costs of treating late-stage disease and its consequences. What is lacking in UI-related cost research is a cost-effectiveness analysis of current treatments. Only the data from such a trial will inform providers, payers, and patients as to whether the intervention is worth the extra cost and is the appropriate next step.

Langa, Fultz, Saint, Kabeto, and Herzog (2002) found that older individuals living in the community who had UI received a significantly greater quantity of informal (unpaid) care than those who were continent. In this study, the additional yearly cost of informal care associated with incontinence was $1,700 (did not use pads) and $4,000 (used pads) for incontinent men, whereas, for women in these groups, the additional yearly cost was $700 (did not use pads) and $2,000 (used pads). This increased "caregiver burden" is thought to be one of the main reasons why families seek nursing home care for a relative.

One study attempted to determine resource consumption within VA facilities for the treatment of UI (Armstrong & Ferguson, 1998). Facilities included those providing acute care and LTC and outpatient care. It was found that a large portion of resource consumption was due to nursing care for clients with UI. Ninety minutes per patient per day was required to clean patients after incontinent episodes ("check and change"), to apply skin products, and to change absorbent pads. An additional 90 minutes of nursing time per patient per day was used to assist patients to the bathroom. Based on these estimates, nursing time cost per incontinent patient per day was estimated to be $119.88. This study indicates that UI may have higher direct costs than was once believed. In 1997, LTC accounted for 35.8% of Medicaid spending, which itself accounted for one fifth of total spending (Lamphere, Brangan,

Bee, & Semansky, 1998). Whereas $10.5 billion of that went toward home- and community-based care, $32 billion went toward nursing homes (Bectel & Tucker, 1998).

The amount of "out-of-pocket" expense for routine care (e.g., absorbent pads, protection, and laundry) of UI has been measured in several studies and ranges from $50 to $900. Subak et al. (2006) found that women on average were spending about $900 per year out of pocket for managing urine leakage (purchase of absorbent products, laundry and dry cleaning). Subak and colleagues found that women were willing to pay almost $40 per month for a 50% improvement in UI and as much as $70 per month or more for cure of incontinence. Another study questioned community-dwelling, racially diverse women in the Kaiser Permanente Medical Care Program of Northern California. Of those who reported weekly UI, 69% reported incontinence-related costs, spending almost $200 per year out-of-pocket for routine incontinence, with African American women having higher routine care costs for incontinence than white women (Subak, van den Eeden, Thom, Creasman, & Brown, 2007).

PREVENTION OF INCONTINENCE

There is growing interest in the potential of preventing UI. It was one of the areas recently addressed by the NIH State of the Science Conference on "Prevention of Fecal and Urinary Incontinence" (NIH, 2007). Because UI and OAB are such prevalent public health problems, there is great potential for having an impact on these conditions through either primary (preventing the development of underlying bladder or sphincter dysfunction) or secondary (preventing a person with underlying bladder and sphincter dysfunction from developing UI) and tertiary (preventing UI from worsening or causing complications) prevention (Landefeld, 2008). Primary prevention strategies that address obesity, smoking, and poor mobility—all risk factors—could decrease UI prevalence (Sampselle, Palmer, Boyington, O'Dell, & Wooldridge, 2004). However, very little information relevant to incontinence prevention is available. Research has shown that there is incontinence prevention potential in community-dwelling older women (Association of Women's Health, Obstetric and Neonatal Nurses, 2000a, 2000b). It was estimated that, by increasing the number of women who discussed UI with their doctors from 41% to 71% and by assuming that they all performed effective bladder retraining, incontinence could be reduced by 50,000 cases annually (Fantl et al., 1996).

Because of their high prevalence and chronic but preventable nature, UI and OAB are reasonably framed as public health problems with an emphasis on primary prevention (Newman et al., 2005). Using this approach, key populations at risk of developing the condition will be identified, risk factors demonstrated, and public awareness strategies developed to help individuals alter modifiable risk factors (Sampselle et al., 2004). Risk factors are detailed in Chapter 4. Primary prevention should be the goal of all health care professionals because it means taking an active part in preventing the initial development of UI. The public is not aware that UI can often be cured (and may be prevented) with conservative, noninvasive, or minimally invasive techniques. Given that the process of storing and expelling urine is shaped by social rules for acceptable times and places for elimination, stigma is attached to incontinence. Programs to increase health promotion and education about UI may serve to deconstruct these barriers. A good example is one that promotes "bladder health" to seniors in the Philadelphia metropolitan area (Palmer & Newman, 2006). The goal of the program is to educate older adults about behaviors that may precipitate bladder symptoms, to outline self-care practices, and to decrease bladder symptoms.

The populations that have been researched concerning possible prevention of UI include (Lifford, Curhan, Hu, Barbieri, & Grodstein, 2005; Newman et al., 2005) the following:

1. *Women with childbirth-related incontinence*—Evidence exists that demonstrates that pelvic floor muscle training (PFMT) practiced during pregnancy results in a significantly lower incidence of UI in late pregnancy and during the postpartum period. Nulliparous women who received individual PFMT at 20 weeks of gestation were significantly less likely to experience UI at 6 weeks and 6 months postpartum (Sampselle et al., 1998). At 3 months postpartum, primigravid women who participated in supervised PFMT prenatally were 59% less likely to demonstrate UI, and those who practiced 28 or more contractions per day were more likely to remain continent than those who practiced a lower number (Reilly et al., 2002). Nulligravid women randomized to supervised PFMT, as compared to those who received routine care, were 39% less likely to report UI at 3 months postpartum (Morkved, Bo, Schei, & Salvesen, 2005).

PFMT initiated in the postpartum period has also demonstrated efficacy. At 3 months postpartum, prevalence of UI in a PFMT group was 31% as compared to 38% in a usual care group, with significantly fewer women classified with severe UI in the treatment group (Chiarelli & Cockburn, 2002). At 10 months postpartum, UI incidence decreased in 19% of women who received PFMT as compared to only 2% in the control group (Meyer, Hohlfield, Achtari, & De Grandi, 2001). An 8-week pelvic floor exercise (PFE) training program was effective in the prevention and treatment of SUI in the immediate postpartum period, and the benefits of the PFE program were still present 1 year after delivery (Morkved & Bo, 2000).

Elective cesarean delivery may be a UI prevention strategy because postpartum UI was found to be higher in primiparous women who gave birth vaginally as compared to those who had cesarean delivery. However, those in the cesarean group had significantly more UI than did nulliparous women (Rortveit, Daltveit, Hannestad, & Hunskaar, 2003).

2. *Men with postprostatectomy SUI*—Evidence is mixed about the value of PFMT pre- and postoperatively, with some studies finding a decrease in UI of at least 14% (Burgio et al., 2006; Sueppel, Kreder, & See, 2001; van Kampen et al., 2000) and others showing no effect (Bales et al., 2000; Porru et al., 2001).

3. *Older adults*—A randomized clinical trial provided evidence of the preventive effect of behavioral intervention (bladder training and PFMT), demonstrating the preventive capacity of these self-care strategies in older women (Diokno et al., 2004). Women ($N = 359$) from 55 to 80 years of age who were essentially continent were randomized to either a control group who received no treatment or a group who received treatment that included a 2-hour group session that presented information about UI and the role of bladder retraining and PFMT in bladder health. At 1 year postinstruction, women in the treatment group were more than twice as likely to remain or become absolutely continent as compared to their control group counterparts.

4. *Diabetics*—Nearly 50% of severe UI could be avoided by prevention of type 2 diabetes mellitus.

Based on this literature, the Third International Consultation on Incontinence recommended that 1) primary prevention studies should not be limited to individual interventions, but should also test the impact of population-based public health strategies; 2) PFMT should be a standard component of prenatal and postpartum care; 3) further randomized controlled trials should be conducted to test the preventive effect of PFMT for men after prostatectomy surgery; and 4) further investigation is warranted to assess the efficacy of PFMT and bladder retraining for primary prevention of UI in older adults (Newman et al., 2005).

CONCLUSION

Urinary incontinence is a considerable health problem affecting millions of Americans. In addition to UI, the related OAB is also prevalent. UI disproportionately affects women of all ages but is also seen in men, primarily as they age. Despite this high prevalence, professionals do not screen for UI, and the majority of patients do not seek help but rather suffer in silence. Quality of life of individuals with UI is significantly lowered, and the impact on caregivers is substantial. UI-related costs continue to increase as the population ages. Myths concerning the identification and treatment of UI persist, encouraging people to practice self-care as opposed to seeking professional care. Professional and federal agency guidelines have been developed for most clinical settings, but it is unclear if this will change the approach to the identification and treatment of this disease. There is new and promising evidence-based research in the area of prevention of UI.

REFERENCES

Abrams, P., Artibani, W., Cardozo, L., Khoury, S., & Wein, A. (2005). *Clinical manual of incontinence in women.* Plymouth, UK: Health Publications Ltd.

Abrams, P., Cardozo, L., Fall, M., Griffiths, D., Rosier, P., Ulmsten, U., et al. for the Standardisation Sub-committee of the International Continence Society. (2002). The standardization of terminology of lower urinary tract function: Report from the Standardisation Sub-committee of the International Continence Society. *Neurourology and Urodynamics, 21,* 167–178.

ACOG Committee on Gynecologic Practice. (2006). ACOG Committee Opinion: Number 345: Vulvodynia. *Obstetrics and Gynecology, 108,* 1049–1052.

Administration on Aging. (2002). *A profile of older Americans: 2002.* Retrieved January 25, 2007, from http://aoa.gov/prof/ Statistics/profile/profiles2002.asp

Agency for Healthcare Research and Quality. (2007, December). *Prevention of urinary and fecal incontinence in adults* (Evidence Report/Technology Assessment No. 161, Contract No. 290-02-0009). Rockville, MD: Author. Retrieved from http://www.ahrq.gov/downloads/pub/evidence/pdf/fuiad/fuiad.pdf

American Medical Directors Association. (1996). *Urinary incontinence clinical practice guideline.* Columbia, MD: Author.

American Medical Directors Association. (2005). *Urinary incontinence clinical practice guideline.* Columbia, MD: Author.

Anger, J.T., Saigal, C.S., Pace, J., Rodríguez, L.V., & Litwin, M.S., for the Urologic Diseases of America Project. (2006). True prevalence of urinary incontinence among female nursing home residents. *Urology, 67,* 281–287.

Anger, J.T., Saigal, C.S., Stothers, L., Thom, D.H., Rodríguez, L.V., Litwin, M.S., for the Urologic Diseases of America Project. (2006). The prevalence of urinary incontinence among community dwelling men: Results from the National Health and Nutrition Examination Survey. *Journal of Urology, 176,* 2103–2108.

Armstrong, E.P., & Ferguson, T.A. (1998, October). Urinary incontinence: Healthcare resource consumption in Veterans Affairs Medical Centers. *Veterans Health System Journal,* pp. 37–42.

Arnold, L.D., Bachmann, G.A., Rosen, R., Kelly, S., & Rhoads, G.G. (2006). Vulvodynia: Characteristics and associations with comorbidities and quality of life. *Obstetrics and Gynecology, 107,* 17–24.

Association of Women's Health, Obstetric and Neonatal Nurses. (2000a). *Evidence-based clinical practice guideline: Continence for women.* Washington, DC: Author.

Association of Women's Health, Obstetric and Neonatal Nurses. (2000b). *Quick care guide: Continence for women.* Washington, DC: Author.

Bachmann, G.A., Rosen, R., Pinn, V.W., Utian, W.H., Ayers, C., Basson, R., et al. (2006). Vulvodynia: A state-of-the-art consensus on definitions, diagnosis and management. *Journal of Reproductive Medicine, 51,* 447–456.

Baker, D.I., & Bice, T.W. (1995). The influence of urinary incontinence on publicly financed home care services to low-income elderly people. *The Gerontologist, 35,* 360–369.

Bales, G.T., Gerber, G.S., Minor, T.X., Mhoon, D.A., McFarland, J.M., Kim, H.L., et al. (2000). Effect of preoperative biofeedback/pelvic floor training on continence in men undergoing radical prostatectomy. *Urology, 56,* 627–630.

Barry, M.J., Link, C.L., McNaughton-Collins, M.F., & McKinlay, J.B., for the Boston Area Community Health (BACH) Investigators. (2008). Overlap of different urological symptom complexes in a racially and ethnically diverse, community-based population of men and women. *BJU International, 101,* 45–51.

Bectel, R.W., & Tucker, N.G. (Eds.). (1998). *Across the states 1998: Profiles of long-term care systems* (3rd ed.). Washington, DC: American Association of Retired Persons.

Berlowitz, D.R., Young, G.J., Hickey, E.C., Joseph, J., Anderson, J.J., Ash, A.S., et al. (2001). Clinical practice guidelines in the nursing home. *American Journal of Medical Quality, 16,* 189–195.

Bliss, D., Zehrer, C., Savik, K., Thayer, D., & Smith, G. (2006). Incontinence-associated skin damage in nursing home residents: A secondary analysis of a prospective, multi-center study. *Ostomy/Wound Management, 52*(12), 46–55.

Bogner, H.R. (2004). Urinary incontinence and psychological distress in community-dwelling older African Americans and whites. *Journal of the American Geriatrics Society, 52,* 1870–1874.

Bogner, H.R., Gallo, J.J., Sammel, M.D., Ford, D.E., Armenian, H.K., & Eaton, W.W. (2002). Urinary incontinence and psychological distress in community-dwelling older adults. *Journal of the American Geriatrics Society, 50,* 489–495.

Bourbonniere, M., & Evans, L.K. (2002). Advanced practice nursing in the care of frail older adults. *Journal of the American Geriatrics Society, 50,* 2062–2076.

Bowers, B., Esmond, S., & Jacobson, N. (2000). The relationship between staffing and quality in long-term care facilities: Exploring the views of nurse aides. *Journal of Nursing Care Quality, 14*(4), 55–64.

Boyington, J.E., Howard, D.L., Carter-Edwards, L., Gooden, K.M., Erdem, N., Jallah, Y., et al. (2007). Differences in resident characteristics and prevalence of urinary incontinence in nursing homes in the southeastern United States. *Nursing Research, 56,* 97–107.

Bradway, C., & Hernly, S. (1998). Urinary incontinence in older adults admitted to acute care. The NICHE Faculty. *Geriatric Nursing, 19,* 98–102.

Brandeis, G.H., Baumann, M.M., Hossain, M., Morris, J.N., & Resnick, N.M. (1997). The prevalence of potentially remediable urinary incontinence in frail older people: A study using the Minimum Data Set. *Journal of the American Geriatrics Society, 45,* 179–184.

Brown, J.S., Grady, D., Ouslander, J.G., Herzog, A.R., Varner, R.E., & Posner, S.F. (1999). Prevalence of urinary incontinence and associated risk factors in postmenopausal women. Heart & Estrogen/Progestin Replacement Study (HERS) Research Group. *Obstetrics and Gynecology, 94,* 66–70.

Brown, J.S., Vittinghoff, E., Wyman, J.F., Stone, K.L., Nevitt, M.C., Ensrud, K.E., et al. (2000). Urinary incontinence: Does it increase risk for falls and fractures? Study of Osteoporotic Fractures Research Group. *Journal of the American Geriatrics Society, 48,* 721–725.

Brown, W.J., & Miller, Y.D. (2001). Too wet to exercise? Leaking urine as a barrier to physical activity in women. *Journal of Science and Medicine in Sport, 4,* 373–378.

Burgio, K., Goode, P.S., Urban, D.A., Umlauf, M.G., Locher, J.L., Bueschen, A., et al. (2006). Preoperative biofeedback assisted behavioral training to decrease post-prostatectomy incontinence: A randomized, controlled trial. *Journal of Urology, 175,* 196–201.

Bush, T.A., Castellucci, D.T, & Phillips, C. (2001). Exploring women's beliefs regarding urinary incontinence. *Urologic Nursing, 21,* 211–218.

Centers for Medicare & Medicaid Services. (2004). *OASIS User's Manual, Revised Chapter 8* (pp. 78–79). Retrieved April 17, 2007, from http://www.cms.hhs.gov/HomeHealth QualityInits/14_HHQIOASISUserManual.asp

Centers for Medicare & Medicaid Services. (2005). *State Operations Manual, Appendix PP—Guidance to Surveyors for Long-Term Care Facilities, Tag F315, §483.25(d) Urinary Incontinence* (Rev. 8, Issued: 06-28-05, Effective: 06-28-05, Implementation: 06-28-05) (pp. 1–39). Retrieved November 11, 2007, from http://www.cms.hhs.gov/transmittals/downloads/R8SOM.pdf

Chiarelli, P., & Cockburn, J. (2002). Promoting urinary continence in women after delivery: Randomised controlled trial. *BMJ, 324,* 1241–1243.

Clemens, J.Q., Joyce, G.F., Wise, M., & Payne, C.K. (2007). Interstitial cystitis and painful bladder syndrome. In M.S. Litwin & C.S. Saigal (Eds.),*Urologic diseases in America* (pp. 123–156) (NIH Publication No. 07-5512). Washington, DC: National Institute of Diabetes and Digestive and Kidney Diseases. Retrieved June 11, 2008, from http://kidney.niddk.nih.gov/statistics/uda/Urologic_Diseases_in_America.pdf

Cooper, G., & Watt, E. (2003). An exploration of acute care nurses' approach to assessment and management of people with urinary incontinence. *Journal of Wound, Ostomy, and Continence Nursing, 30,* 305–313.

Cortes, L.L., Montgomery, E.W., Morrow, K.A., & Monroe, D.M. (2000). *A statewide assessment of quality of care, quality of life and consumer satisfaction in Texas Medicaid nursing facilities* (pp. 1–99). Austin: Texas Department of Human Services Long Term Care Office of Programs, Medical Quality Assurance.

Coward, R.T., Horne, C., & Peek, C.W. (1995). Predicting nursing home admissions among incontinent older adults: A comparison of residential differences across six years. *The Gerontologist, 35,* 732–743.

Danforth, K.N., Townsend, M.K., Lifford, K., Curhan, G.C., Resnick, N.M., & Grodstein, F. (2006). Risk factors for urinary incontinence among middle-aged women. *American Journal of Obstetrics and Gynecology, 194,* 339–345.

Darkow, T., Fontes, C.L., & Williamson, T.E. (2005). Costs associated with the management of overactive bladder and related comorbidities. *Pharmacotherapy, 25,* 511–519.

Diokno, A.C., Estanol, M.V., Ibrahim, I.A., & Balasubramaniam, M. (2007). Prevalence of urinary incontinence in community dwelling men: A cross sectional nationwide epidemiological survey. *International Urology and Nephrology, 39,* 129–136.

Diokno, A.C., Sampselle, C.M., Herzog, A.G., Raghunathan, T.E., Hines, S., Messer, K.L., et al. (2004). Prevention of urinary incontinence by behavioral modification program: A randomized controlled trial among older women in the community. *Journal of Urology, 171,* 1161–1164.

Diokno, A.C., Sand, P.K., Macdiarmid, S., Shah, R., & Armstrong, R.B. (2006). Perceptions and behaviours of women with bladder control problems. *Family Practice, 23,* 568–577.

Dosa, D., Bowers, B., & Gifford, D.R. (2006). Critical review of resident assessment protocols. *Journal of the American Geriatrics Society, 54,* 659–666.

DuBeau, C.E., Ouslander, JG., & Palmer, M.H. (2007). Knowledge and attitudes of nursing home staff and surveyors about the revised federal guidance for incontinence care. *The Gerontologist, 47,* 468–479.

DuBeau, C.E., Simon, S.E., & Morris, J.N. (2006). The effect of urinary incontinence on quality of life in older nursing home residents. *Journal of the American Geriatrics Society, 54,* 1325–1333.

Dugan, E., Cohen, S.J., Bland, D.R., Preisser, J.S., Davis, C.C., Suggs, P.K., et al. (2000). The association of depressive symptoms and urinary incontinence among older adults. *Journal of the American Geriatrics Society, 48,* 413–416.

Duong, T.H., & Korn, A.P. (2001). A comparison of urinary incontinence among African American, Asian, Hispanic, and white women. *American Journal of Obstetrics and Gynecology, 184,* 1083–1086.

Dutton, P. (2006). Factors predisposing women to chronic pelvic pain: Systematic review. *Journal of Family Planning and Reproductive Health Care, 3*(4), 244.

Engberg, S., Kincade, J., & Thompson, D. (2004). Future directions for incontinence research with frail elders. *Nursing Research, 53*(6 Suppl.), S22–S29.

Espino, D.V., Palmer, R.F., Miles, T.P., Mouton, C.P., Lichtenstein, M.J., & Markides, K.P. (2003). Prevalence and severity of urinary incontinence in elderly Mexican-American women. *Journal of the American Geriatrics Society, 51,* 1580–1586.

Fantl, J., Newman, D., Colling, J., DeLancey, J.O.L., Keeys, C., Loughery, R., et al. for the Urinary Incontinence in Adults Guideline Update Panel. (1996). Urinary incontinence in adults: Acute and chronic management. *Clinical practice guideline No. 2: Update* (AHCPR Publication No. 96-0692). Rockville, MD: Agency for Health Care and Policy Research.

Foxman, B., Somsel, P., Tallman, P., Gillespie, B., Raz, R., Colodner, R., et al. (2001). Urinary tract infection among women aged 40 to 65: Behavioral and sexual risk factors. *Journal of Clinical Epidemiology, 54,* 710–718.

Frantz, R.A., Xakellis, G.C., Jr., Harvey, P.C., & Lewis, A.R. (2003). Implementing an incontinence management protocol in long-term care: Clinical outcomes and costs. *Journal of Gerontologic Nursing, 29*(8), 46–53.

Fulmer, T. (2007). How to try this: Fulmer SPICES. *American Journal of Nursing, 107*(10), 40–48; quiz 48–49.

Fultz, N., Girts, T., Kinchen, K., Nygaard, I., Pohl, G., & Sternfeld, B. (2005). Prevalence, management and impact of urinary incontinence in the workplace. *Occupational Medicine, 55,* 552–557.

Fultz, N.H., Burgio, K., Diokno, A.C., Kinchen, K.S., Obenchain, R., & Bump, R.C. (2003). Burden of stress urinary incontinence for community-dwelling women. *American Journal of Obstetrics and Gynecology, 189,* 1275–1282.

Fultz, N.H., Fisher, C.G., & Jenkins, K.R. (2004). Does urinary incontinence affect middle-aged and older women's time use and activity patterns? *Obstetrics and Gynecology, 104,* 1327–1334.

Fultz, N.H., & Herzog, A.R. (2001). Self-reported social and emotional impact of urinary incontinence. *Journal of the American Geriatrics Society, 49,* 892–899.

Fung, C.H., Spencer, B., Eslami, M., & Crandall, C. (2007). Quality indicators for the screening and care of urinary incontinence in vulnerable elders. *Journal of the American Geriatrics Society, 55,* S443–S449.

Garcia, J.A., Crocker, J., & Wyman, J.F. (2005). Breaking the cycle of stigmatization. *Journal of Wound, Ostomy, and Continence Nursing, 32,* 38–52.

Geriatric models of care: which one's right for your institution? Nurses Improving Care to the Hospitalized Elderly (NICHE) Project. (1994). *American Journal of Nursing, 94*(7), 21–23.

Glazer, H.I. (2000). Dysesthetic vulvodynia: Long-term follow-up after treatment with surface electromyography-assisted pelvic floor muscle rehabilitation. *Journal of Reproductive Medicine, 45,* 798–802.

Goldstein, A.T., Marinoff, S.C., & Haefner, H.K. (2005). Vulvodynia: Strategies for treatment. *Clinical Obstetrics and Gynecology, 48,* 769–785.

Grodstein, F., Fretts, R., Lifford, K., Resnick, N., & Curhan, G. (2003). Association of age, race, and obstetric history with urinary symptoms among women in the Nurses' Health Study. *American Journal of Obstetrics and Gynecology, 189,* 428–434.

Hägglund, D., & Wadensten, B. (2007). Fear of humiliation inhibits women's care-seeking behaviour for long-term urinary incontinence. *Scandinavian Journal of Caring Science, 21,* 305–312.

Hägglund, D., Walker-Engstrom, M., Larsson, G., & Leppert, J. (2003). Reasons why women with long-term urinary incontinence do not seek professional help: A cross-sectional population-based cohort study. *International Urogynecology Journal and Pelvic Floor Dysfunction, 14,* 296–304.

Handa, V.L., Harvey, L., Cundiff, G.W., Siddique, S.A., & Kjerulff, K.H. (2004). Sexual function among women with urinary incontinence and pelvic organ prolapse. *American Journal of Obstetrics and Gynecology, 191,* 751–756.

Hannestad, Y.S., Rortveit, G., Sandvik, H., Hunskaar, S., for the Norwegian EPINCONT Study. (2000). A community-based epidemiological survey of female urinary incontinence: The Norwegian EPINCONT study. Epidemiology of Incontinence in the County of Nord-Trøndelag. *Journal of Clinical Epidemiology, 53,* 1150–1157.

Hanno, P.M. (2007a). Painful bladder syndrome (interstitial cystitis). In P.M. Hanno, A.J. Wein, & S.B. Malkowicz (Eds.), *Penn clinical manual of urology* (pp. 217–234). Philadelphia: Elsevier Saunders.

Hanno, P.M. (2007b). Painful bladder syndrome/interstitial cystitis and related disorders. In A.J. Wein (Ed.), *Campbell-Walsh urology* (9th ed., pp. 330–371). Philadelphia: Elsevier Saunders.

Harke, J.M., & Richgels, K. (1992). Barriers to implementing a continence program in nursing homes. *Clinical Nursing Research, 1*, 156–168.

Holroyd-Leduc, J.M., Lyder, C.H., & Tannenbaum, C. (2006). Practical management of urinary incontinence in the long term care setting. *Annals of Long Term Care, 14*(2), 30–37.

Holroyd-Leduc, J.M., Mehta, K.M., & Covinsky, K.E. (2004). Urinary incontinence and its association with death, nursing home admission, and functional decline. *Journal of the American Geriatrics Society, 52*, 712–718.

Holroyd-Leduc, J.M., & Straus, S.E. (2004). Management of urinary incontinence in women. *JAMA, 291*, 986–995.

Hornick, L., & Slocumb, J.C. (2008). Treating chronic pelvic pain. *ADVANCE for Nurse Practitioners, 16*(2), 44–54.

Horrocks, S., Somerset, M., Stoddart, H., & Peters, T.J. (2004). What prevents older people from seeking treatment for urinary incontinence? A qualitative exploration of barriers to the use of community continence services. *Family Practice, 21*, 689–696.

Hu, T.W., & Wagner, T.H. (2005). Health-related consequences of overactive bladder: An economic perspective. *BJU International, 96*(Suppl. 1), 43–45.

Hu, T.W., Wagner, T.H., Bentkover, J.D., Leblanc, K., Zhou, S.Z., & Hunt, T. (2004). Costs of urinary incontinence and overactive bladder in the United States: A comparative study. *Urology, 63*, 461–465.

Hu, T.W., Wagner, T.H., Hawthorne, G., Morre, K., Subak, L.L., & Versi, E. (2005). Economics of incontinence. In P. Abrams, L. Cardozo, S. Khoury, & A. Wein (Eds.), *Incontinence: Proceedings from the Third International Consultation on Incontinence* (pp. 75–95). Plymouth, UK: Health Publications, Ltd.

Huang, A.J., Brown, J.S., Kanaya, A.M., Creasman, J.M., Ragins, A.I., van den Eeden, S.K., et al. (2006). Quality-of-life impact and treatment of urinary incontinence in ethnically diverse older women. *Archives of Internal Medicine, 166*, 2000–2006.

Hunskaar, S., Burgio, K., Clark, A. Lapitan, M.C., Nelson, R., Sillen, U., et al. (2005). Epidemiology of urinary incontinence (UI) and faecal incontinence (FI) and pelvic organ prolaspe (POP). In P. Abrams, L. Cardozo, S. Khoury, & A.J. Wein (Eds.), *Incontinence: Proceedings from the Third International Consultation on Incontinence* (Vol. 1, pp. 255–312). Plymouth, UK: Health Publications, Ltd.

Hunskaar, S., Burgio, K., Diokno, A., Herzog, A.R., Hjalmas, K., & Lapitan, M.C. (2003). Epidemiology and natural history of urinary incontinence in women. *Urology, 62*(4 Suppl. 1), 16–23.

Irwin, D.E., Milsom, I., Hunskaar, S., Reilly, K., Kopp, Z., Herschorn, S., et al. (2006). Population-based survey of urinary incontinence, overactive bladder, and other lower urinary tract symptoms in five countries: Results of the EPIC study. *European Urology, 50*, 1306–1315.

Jaffe, W.I., & Te, A.E. (2005). Overactive bladder in the male patient: Epidemiology, etiology, evaluation, and treatment. *Current Urology Reports, 6*, 410–418.

Johnson, M.J., & Werner, C. (1982). We have no choice: A study of familial guilt feelings surrounding nursing home care. *Journal of Gerontological Nursing, 8*(11), 641–645, 654.

Johnson, T.M., Ouslander, J.G., Uman, G.C., & Schnelle, J.F. (2001). Urinary incontinence treatment preferences in long-term care. *Journal of the American Geriatrics Society, 49*, 710–718.

Jumadilova, Z., Zyczynski, T., Paul, B., & Narayanan, S. (2005). Urinary incontinence in the nursing home: Resident characteristics and prevalence of drug treatment. *American Journal of Managed Care, 11*(4 Suppl.), S112–S120.

Kincade, J.E., Boyington, A.R., Lekan-Rutledge, D., Ashford-Works, C., Dougherty, M.C., & Busby-Whitehead, J. (2003). Bladder management in adult care homes: Review of a program in North Carolina. *Journal of Gerontological Nursing, 29*(10), 30–36.

Kinchen, K.S., Burgio, K., Diokno, A.C., Fultz, N.H., Bump, R.C., & Obenchain, R. (2003). Factors associated with women's decisions to seek treatment for urinary incontinence. *Journal of Women's Health, 12,* 687–698.

Ko, Y., Lin, S.J., Salmon, J.W., & Bron, M.S. (2005). The impact of urinary incontinence on quality of life of the elderly. *American Journal of Managed Care, 11*(4 Suppl.), S103–S111.

Koch, L.H. (2006). Help-seeking behaviors of women with urinary incontinence: An integrative literature review. *Journal of Midwifery and Women's Health, 51*(6), e39–e44.

Krieger, J.N., Nyberg, L., & Nickel, J.C. (1999). NIH consensus definition and classification of prostatitis. *JAMA, 282,* 236–237.

Lamphere, J., Brangan, N., Bee, S., & Semansky, R. (1998). *Reforming the health care system: State profiles 1998.* Washington, DC: American Association of Retired Persons.

Landefeld, C.S., Bowers, B.J., Feld, A.D., Hartmann, K.E., Hoffman, E., Ingber, M.J., et al. (2008). National Institutes of Health state-of-the-art science conference statement: Prevention of fecal and urinary incontinence in adults. *Annals of Internal Medicine, 148*(6), 449–458.

Langa, K.M., Fultz, N.H., Saint, S., Kabeto, M.U., & Herzog, A.R. (2002). Informal caregiving time and costs for urinary incontinence in the United States. *Journal of the American Geriatrics Society, 50,* 733–737.

Lekan-Rutledge, D. (2004). Urinary incontinence strategies for frail elderly women. *Urologic Nursing, 24,* 281–283, 287–301.

Lekan-Rutledge, D., & Colling, J. (2003, March). Urinary incontinence in the frail elderly. *American Journal of Nursing,* (Suppl.), 36–46.

Lekan-Rutledge, D., Palmer, M.H., & Belyea, M. (1998). In their own words: Nursing assistants' perceptions of barriers to implementation of prompted voiding in long-term care. *The Gerontologist, 38,* 370–378.

Lifford, K.L., Curhan, G.C., Hu, F.B., Barbieri, R.L., & Grodstein, F. (2005). Type 2 diabetes mellitus and risk of developing urinary incontinence. *Journal of the American Geriatrics Society, 53,* 1851–1857.

Litwin, M.S., McNaughton-Collins, M., Fowler, F.J., Jr., Nickel, J.C., Calhoun, E.A., Pontari, M.A., et al. (1999). The National Institutes of Health Chronic Prostatitis Symptom Index: Development and validation of a new outcome measure. *Journal of Urology, 162,* 369–375.

Maloney, C., & Cafiero, M. (1999). Implementing an incontinence program in long-term care settings: A multidisciplinary approach. *Journal of Gerontological Nursing, 25*(6), 47–52.

Mason, D., Newman, D.K., & Palmer, M.H. (2003). Changing UI practice. *American Journal of Nursing, 103*(3 Suppl.), 2–3.

Mason, L., Glen, S., Walton, I., & Hughes, C. (2001). Women's reluctance to seek help for stress incontinence during pregnancy and following childbirth. *Midwifery, 17,* 212–221.

Mayer, R. (2007). Interstitial cystitis pathogenesis and treatment. *Current Opinion in Infectious Diseases, 20,* 77–82.

McDowell, B.J., Engberg, S., Rodriguez, E., Engberg, R., & Sereika, S. (1996). Characteristics of urinary incontinence in homebound older adults. *Journal of the American Geriatrics Society, 44,* 963–968.

Melville, J., Katon, W., Delaney, K., & Newton, K. (2005). Urinary incontinence in US women. *Archives of Internal Medicine, 165,* 537–542.

Melville, J.L., Delaney, K., Newton, K., & Katon, W. (2005). Incontinence severity and major depression in incontinent women. *Obstetrics and Gynecology, 106,* 585–592.

Melville, J.L., Newton, K., Fan, M.Y., & Katon, W. (2006). Health care discussions and treatment for urinary incontinence in U.S. women. *American Journal of Obstetrics and Gynecology, 194,* 729–737.

Meyer, S., Hohlfield, H., Achtari, C., & De Grandi, P. (2001). Pelvic floor education after vaginal delivery. *Obstetrics and Gynecology, 97,* 673–677.

Mezey, M., Burger, S.G., Bloom, H.G., Bonner, A., Bourbonniere, M., Bowers, B., et al. (2005). Experts recommend strategies for strengthening the use of advanced practice nurses in nursing homes. *Journal of the American Geriatrics Society, 53,* 1790–1797.

Mezey, M., Kobayashi, M., Grossman, S., Firpo, A., Fulmer, T., & Mitty, E. (2004). Nurses Improving Care to Health System Elders (NICHE): Implementation of best practice models. *Journal of Nursing Administration, 34,* 451–457.

Milsom, I., Abrams, P., Cardozo, L., Roberts, R.G., Thüroff, J., & Wein, A.J. (2001). How widespread are the symptoms of an overactive bladder and how are they managed? A population based prevalence study. *BJU International, 87,* 760–766.

Mishell, D.R. (2006). Chronic pelvic pain in women: Focus on painful bladder syndrome/interstitial cystitis. *Journal of Reproductive Medicine, 51*(3 Suppl.), 225–226.

Mitterness, L.S. (1987). The management of urinary incontinence by community-living elderly. *The Gerontologist, 27,* 185.

Moore, K.N., & Gray, M. (2004). Urinary incontinence in men: Current status and future directions. *Nursing Research, 53*(6 Suppl.), S36–S41.

Morkved, S., & Bo, K. (2000). Effect of postpartum pelvic floor muscle training in prevention and treatment of urinary incontinence: A one-year follow up. *BJOG, 107,* 1022–1028.

Morkved, S., Bo, K., Schei, B., & Salvesen, K.A. (2005). Pelvic floor muscle training during pregnancy to prevent urinary incontinence: A single blind randomized control trial. *Obstetrics and Gynecology, 101,* 313–319.

National Institutes of Health. (2007). *State of the Science Conference: Prevention of Fecal and Urinary Incontinence in Adults. Draft statement, December 12, 2007.* Retrieved February 11, 2008, from http://consensus.nih.gov/2007/IncontinenceStatementDRAFT 121207.pdf

Newman, D.K. (2003). Mentioning the unmentionables (Part 1). *ADVANCE for Providers of Post-Acute Care, 6*(5), 89–91, 100.

Newman, D.K. (2004a). Mentioning the unmentionables (Part 2). *ADVANCE for Providers of Post-Acute Care, 7*(1), 22, 24.

Newman, D.K. (2004b). Report of a mail survey of women with bladder control disorders. *Urologic Nursing, 24,* 499–507.

Newman, D.K. (2006). Urinary incontinence, catheters and urinary tract infections: An overview of CMS Tag F 315. *Ostomy/Wound Management, 52*(12), 34–36, 38, 40–44.

Newman, D.K., Denis, L., Gruenwald, I., Ee, C.H., Millard, R., Roberts, R., et al. (2005). Promotion, education and organization for continence care. In P. Abrams, L. Cardozo, S. Khoury, & A. Wein (Eds.), *Incontinence: Proceedings from the Third International Consultation on Incontinence* (pp. 35–72). Plymouth, UK: Health Publications, Ltd.

Newman, D.K., & Giovanni, D. (2002). Overactive bladder: A nursing perspective. *American Journal of Nursing, 102*(6), 36–46.

Nygaard, I.E., & Lemke, J.H. (1996). Urinary incontinence in rural older women: Prevalence, incidence and remission. *Journal of the American Geriatrics Society, 44,* 1049–1054.

Ouslander, J., & Johnson, T.M. (2004). Continence care for frail older adults: It is time to go beyond assessing quality. *Journal of the American Medical Directors Association, 5,* 213–216.

Ouslander, J.G. (2004). Management of overactive bladder. *New England Journal of Medicine, 350,* 786–799.

Ouslander, J.G., Palmer, M.H., Rovner, B.W., & German, P.S. (1993). Urinary incontinence in nursing homes: Incidence, remission and associated factors. *Journal of the American Geriatrics Society, 41,* 1083–1089.

Palmer, M.H. (1995). Nurses' knowledge and beliefs about continence interventions in long-term care. *Journal of Advanced Nursing, 21,* 1065–1072.

Palmer, M.H., Bennett, R.G., Marks, J., McCormick, K.A., & Engel, B.T. (1994). Urinary incontinence: A program that works. *Journal of Long Term Care Administration, 22*(2), 19–25.

Palmer, M.H., German, P., & Ouslander, J. (1991). Risk factors for urinary incontinence one year after nursing home admission. *Research in Nursing and Health, 14,* 405–412.

Palmer, M.H., Myers, A., & Fedenko, K. (1997). Urinary continence changes after hip fracture repair. *Clinical Nursing Research, 6,* 8–24.

Palmer, M.H., & Newman, D.K. (2004). Bladder matters: Urinary incontinence in nursing homes. *American Journal of Nursing, 104*(11), 57–59.

Palmer, M.H., & Newman, D.K. (2006). Bladder control educational needs of older adults. *Journal of Gerontological Nursing, 32*(1), 28–32.

Parazzini, F., Lavezzari, M., & Artibani, W. (2002). Prevalence of overactive bladder and urinary incontinence. *Journal of Family Practice, 51,* 1072–1074.

Porru, D., Campus, G., Caria, A., Madeddu, G., Cucchi, A., Roverto, B., et al. (2001). Impact of early pelvic floor rehabilitation after transurethral resection of the prostate. *Neurourology and Urodynamics, 20,* 53–59.

Prochoda, K.P. (2002). Medical director's review of urinary incontinence in long-term care. *Journal of the American Medical Directors Association, 3*(1 Suppl.), S11–S15.

Reed, B.D. (2006). Vulvodynia: Diagnosis and management. *American Family Physician, 73,* 1231–1238.

Reilly, E.T.C., Freeman, R.M., Waterfield, M.R., Waterfield, A.E., Steggles, P., & Pedlar, F. (2002). Prevention of postpartum stress incontinence in primigravidae with increased bladder neck mobility: A randomized controlled trial of antenatal pelvic floor exercise. *BJOG, 109,* 68–76.

Resnick, B., Simpson, M., Galik, E., Bercovitz, A., Gruber-Baldini, A., Zimmerman, S., et al. (2006). Making a difference: Nursing assistants' perspectives of restorative care nursing. *Rehabilitation Nursing, 31,* 78–83.

Resnick, B., Slocum, D., Ra, L., & Moffett, P. (1996). Geriatric rehabilitation: Nursing interventions and outcomes focusing on urinary function and knowledge of medications. *Rehabilitation Nursing, 21,* 142–147.

Resnick, N.M., Brandeis, G.H., Baumann, M.M., & Morris, J.N. (1996). Evaluating a national assessment strategy for urinary incontinence in nursing home residents. *Neurourology and Urodynamics, 15,* 583–598.

Reuben, B.D., Roth, C., Kamberg, C., & Wenger, N.S. (2003). Restructuring primary care practices to manage geriatric syndromes: The ACOVE-2 intervention. *Journal of the American Geriatrics Society, 51,* 1787–1793.

Ricci, J.A., Baggish, J.S., Hunt, T.L., Stewart, W.F., Wein, A., Herzog, A.R., et al. (2001). Coping strategies and health care-seeking behavior in a US national sample of adults with symptoms suggestive of overactive bladder. *Clinical Therapeutics, 23,* 1245–1259.

Robinson, J.P. (2000). Managing urinary incontinence in the nursing home: Residents' perspectives. *Journal of Advanced Nursing, 31,* 68–77.

Rogers, G.R., Villarreal, A., Kammerer-Doak, D., & Qualls, C. (2001). Sexual function in women with and without urinary incontinence and/or pelvic organ prolapse. *International Urogynecology Journal and Pelvic Floor Dysfunction, 12,* 361–365.

Rortveit, G., Daltveit, A.K., Hannestad, Y.S., & Hunskaar, S. (2003). Urinary incontinence after vaginal delivery or cesarean section. *New England Journal of Medicine, 348,* 900–907.

Rosenberg, M.T., Newman, D., & Paige, S. (2007). Interstitial cystitis/painful bladder syndrome: Symptom recognition is key to early identification, treatment. *Cleveland Clinic Journal of Medicine, 74*(Suppl. 3), S54–S62.

Ruther, M., & Helbing, C. (1988). Health care financing trends: Use and cost of home health services under Medicare. *Health Care Financing Review, 10,* 105–108.

Ryden, M.B., Snyder, M., Gross, C.R., Savik, K., Pearson, V., Krichbaum, K., et al. (2000). Value-added outcomes: The use of advanced practice nurses in long-term facilities. *The Gerontologist, 40,* 654–662.

Sahyoun, N.R., Pratt, L.A, Lentzner, H., Dey, A., & Robinson, K.N. (2001). *The changing profile of nursing home residents: 1985–1997.* Aging Trends No. 4. Hyattsville, MD: National Center for Health Statistics. Retrieved January 14, 2007, from http://www.cdc.gov/nchs/data/ahcd/agingtrends/04nursin.pdf

Sampselle, C.M., Harlow, S.D., Skurnick, J., Brubaker, L., & Bondarenko, I. (2002). Urinary incontinence predictors and life impact in ethnically diverse perimenopausal women. *Obstetrics and Gynecology, 100,* 1230–1238.

Sampselle, C.M., Miller, J.M., Mims, B.M., DeLancey, J.O.L., Ashton-Miller, J.A., & Antonakos, C.L. (1998). Effect of pelvic muscle exercise on transient incontinence during pregnancy and after birth. *Obstetrics and Gynecology, 91,* 406–412.

Sampselle, C.M., Palmer, M.H., Boyington, A.R., O'Dell, K.K., & Wooldridge, L. (2004). Prevention of urinary incontinence in adults: Population-based strategies. *Nursing Research, 53*(6 Suppl.), S61–S67.

Samuelsson, E., Victor, A., & Svardsudd, K. (2000). Determinants of urinary incontinence in a population of young and middle-aged women. *Acta Obstetrica et Gynecologica Scandinavica, 79,* 208–215.

Sand, P.K., Goldberg, R.P., Dmochowski, R.R., McIlwain, M., & Dahl, N.V. (2006). The impact of the overactive bladder syndrome on sexual function: A preliminary report from the Multicenter Assessment of Transdermal Therapy in Overactive Bladder with Oxybutynin trial. *American Journal of Obstetrics and Gynecology, 195,* 1730–1735.

Schaeffer, A.J. (2006). Chronic prostatitis and the chronic pelvic pain syndrome. *New England Journal of Medicine, 355,* 1690-1698.

Schnelle, J.F., Kapur, K., Alessi, C., Osterweil, D., Beck, J.G., Al-Samarrai, N.R., et al. (2003). Does an exercise and incontinence intervention save healthcare costs in a nursing home population? *Journal of the American Geriatrics Society, 51,* 161–168.

Schnelle, J.F., & Leung, F.W. (2004). Urinary and fecal incontinence in nursing homes. *Gastroenterology, 126*(Suppl. 1), S41–S47.

Schnelle, J.F., & Smith, R.L. (2001). Quality indicators for the management of urinary incontinence in vulnerable community dwelling elders. *Annals of Internal Medicine, 135,* 752–758.

Schultz, A., Dicky, G., & Skoner, M. (1997). Self-report of incontinence in an acute care setting. *Urologic Nursing, 17,* 23–26.

Shaw, C., Gupta, R.D., Bushnell, D.M., Assassa, R.P., Abrams, P., Wagg, A., et al. (2006). The extent and severity of urinary incontinence amongst women in UK GP waiting rooms. *Family Practice, 23,* 497–506.

Shih, Y.C., Hartzema, A.G., & Tolleson-Rinehart, S. (2003). Labor costs associated with incontinence in long-term care facilities. *Urology, 62,* 442–446.

Smith, D.B. (1998). A continence care approach for long-term care facilities. *Geriatric Nursing, 19,* 81–86.

Stewart, W.F., Van Rooyen, J.B., Cundiff, G.W., Abrams, P., Herzog, A.R., Corey, R., et al. (2003). Prevalence and burden of overactive bladder in the United States. *World Journal of Urology, 20,* 327–336.

Stothers, L., Thom, D., & Calhoun, E. (2005). Urologic Diseases in America Project: Urinary incontinence in males—demographics and economic burden. *Journal of Urology, 173,* 1302–1308.

Strahan, G.W. (1994, July 22). An overview of home health and hospice care patients: Preliminary data from the 1993 National Home and Hospice Care Survey. *Advance Data,* (256), 1–12.

Subak, L., Van Den Eeden, S., Thom, D., Creasman, J.M., & Brown, J.S., for the Reproductive Risks for Incontinence Study at Kaiser Research Group. (2007). Urinary incontinence in women: direct costs of routine care. *American Journal of Obstetrics and Gynecology, 197,* 596:e1–596:e9.

Subak, L.L., Brown, J.S., Kraus, S.R., Brubaker, L., Lin, F., Richter, H.E., et al. (2006). The "costs" of urinary incontinence for women. *Obstetrics and Gynecology, 107,* 908–916.

Subak, L.L., Johnson, C., Whitcomb, E., Boban, D., Saxton, J., & Brown, J.S. (2002). Does weight loss improve incontinence in moderately obese women? *International Urogynecology Journal and Pelvic Floor Dysfunction, 13,* 40–43.

Sueppel, C., Kreder, K., & See, W. (2001). Improved continence outcomes with preoperative pelvic floor muscle strengthening exercises. *Urologic Nursing, 21,* 201–209.

Sustersic, O., & Kralj, B. (1998). The influence of obesity, constitution and physical work on the phenomenon of urinary incontinence in women. *International Urogynecology Journal and Pelvic Floor Dysfunction, 9,* 140–144.

Sykes, D., Castro, R., Pons, M.E., Hampel, C., Hunskaar, S., Papanicolaoi, S., et al. (2005). Characteristics of female outpatients with urinary incontinence participating in a 6-month observational study in 14 European countries. *Maturitas, 52*(Suppl. 2), S13–S23.

Thom, D.H., Haan, M.N., & van den Eeden, S.K. (1997). Medically recognized urinary incontinence and risks of hospitalization, nursing home admission and mortality. *Age and Ageing, 26,* 367–374.

Thom, D.H., Nygaard, I.E., & Calhoun, E.A. (2005). Urologic Diseases in America Project: Urinary incontinence in women—national trends in hospitalizations, office visits, treatment and economic impact. *Journal of Urology, 173,* 1295–1301.

Thom, D.H., van den Eeden, S.K., Ragins, A.I., Wassel-Fyr, C., Vittinghof, E., Subak, L.L., et al. (2006). Differences in prevalence of urinary incontinence by race/ethnicity. *Journal of Urology, 175,* 259–264.

Thomas, P., Ingrand, P., Lalloue, F., Hazif-Thomas, C., Billon, R., Vieban, F., et al. (2004). Reasons of informal caregivers for institutionalising dementia patients previously living at home: The Pixel study. *International Journal of Geriatric Psychiatry, 19,* 127–135.

Thompson, D.L. (2004). Geriatric incontinence: The long-term care challenge. *Urologic Nursing, 24,* 305–313, 356.

Townsend, M.K., Danforth, K.N., Lifford, K.L., Rosner, B., Curhan, G.C., Resnick, N.M., et al. (2007). Incidence and remission of urinary incontinence in middle aged women. *American Journal of Obstetrics and Gynecology, 197,* 167.e1–167.e5.

Van der Vaart, C.H., de Leeuw, J.R., Roovers, J.P., & Heintz, A.P. (2002). The effect of urinary incontinence and overactive bladder symptoms on quality of life in young women. *BJU International, 90,* 544–549.

Van Kampen, M., DeWeerdt, H., VanPoppel, H., DeRidder, D., Feys, H., & Baert, L. (2000). Effect of pelvic floor re-education on duration and degree of incontinence after radical prostatectomy: A randomized controlled trial. *Lancet, 355,* 98–102.

Varmus, H. (1997). *Disease-specific estimates of direct and indirect costs of illness and NIH support.* Bethesda, MD: National Institutes of Health.

Waetjen, L.E., Liao, S., Johnson, W.O., Sampselle, C.M., Sternfield, B., Harlow, S.D., et al. (2007). Factors associated with prevalent and incident urinary incontinence in a cohort of midlife women: A longitudinal analysis of data. Study of Women's Health Across the Nation. *American Journal of Epidemiology, 165,* 309–318.

Wagner, A., & Colling, J. (1993). Resistance to change: Understanding the aides' point of view. *Journal of Long-Term Care Administration, 21*(2), 27–30.

Wagner, T.H., & Hu, T.W. (1998). Economic costs of urinary incontinence in 1995. *Urology, 51,* 355–361.

Watson, N.M., Brink, C.A., Zimmer, J.G., & Mayer, R.D. (2003). Use of the Agency for Health Care Policy and Research Urinary Incontinence Guideline in nursing homes. *Journal of the American Geriatrics Society, 51,* 1779–1786.

Wilson, L., Brown, J.S., Shin, G.P., Luc, K.O., & Subak, L.L. (2001). Annual direct cost of urinary incontinence. *Obstetrics and Gynecology, 98,* 398–405.

Wu, E.Q., Birnbaum, H., Marynchenko, M., Williamson, T., & Mallett, D. (2005). Employees with overactive bladder: Work loss burden. *Journal of Occupational and Environmental Medicine, 47,* 439–446.

Wyman, J.F., Harkins, S.W., & Fantl, A. (1990). Psychosocial impact of urinary incontinence in the community dwelling population. *Journal of the American Geriatrics Society, 38,* 282–288.

Yu, L.C., Kaltreider, D.L., & Brannon, D. (1991). Urinary incontinence: Nursing home staff reaction toward residents. *Journal of Gerontological Nursing, 17*(11), 34–41.

Zarowitz, B.J., & Ouslander, J.G. (2006). Management of urinary incontinence in older persons. *Geriatric Nursing, 27,* 265–270.

Zimmerman, D.R., Karon, S.L., Arling, G., Clark, B.R., Collins, T., Ross, R., et al. (1995). Development and testing of nursing home quality indicators. *Health Care Financing Review, 16,* 107–127.

3

Understanding Bladder and Pelvic Floor Function

The urinary tract, composed of the upper and lower urinary tracts, is a highly efficient system for removing waste products from the blood and excreting them from the body. The *upper urinary tract* includes the two kidneys and two ureters (Figure 3.1). The paired, fist-sized kidneys filter impurities from the blood and excrete them in the urine. They also regulate the chemical makeup of the blood and preserve the correct balance between salt and water in the body. Urine is transported from the kidneys through the ureters down to the bladder. In relation to bladder disorders, conditions such as unresolved urinary retention, high urinary storage pressure, and untreated urinary tract infections can cause upper urinary tract damage.

The *lower urinary tract* is composed of the bladder, prostate (in men only), urethra, internal and external sphincters, and urinary meatus (Figure 3.2A and B and 3.3). The lower urinary tract is located in the pelvic cavity, anterior to the sacrum. The urinary bladder lies posterior and slightly superior to the pubic bone and superior to the pelvic floor. The bladder fills and expands passively with urine, which is passed out of the body via the urethra. In relation to bladder disorders, conditions such as urinary incontinence (UI) and overactive bladder (OAB) usually affect only the lower urinary tract.

ORGANS AND STRUCTURES OF THE URINARY TRACT AND ASSOCIATED ORGANS

Bladder

The bladder is a hollow, distensible, muscular organ whose size, shape, and position vary in relation to the amount of urine it contains. It is divided into two parts, the detrusor and the trigone, but the entire structure often is (erroneously) referred to as the "detrusor." The bladder lies behind the pubic sym-

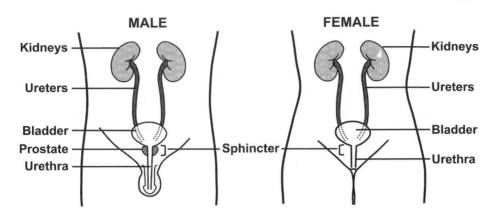

Figure 3.1.   Frontal view of the male and female urinary tract system. (Courtesy of Robin Noel.)

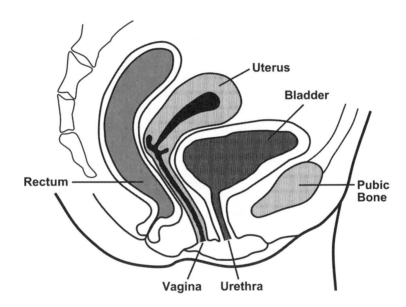

Figure 3.2A.   Lateral view of the female urinary system. (Courtesy of Robin Noel.)

physis (the center front portion of the pelvic bone) when empty and may rise above the level of the symphysis when full, sometimes making it palpable (Newman, 2002). It is freely moveable except at the base, where it is continuous with the urethra. The posterior base of the bladder, or *trigone,* is a triangle of smooth urothelium between the two ureteral orifices and the beginning of the urethra (Brooks, 2007) (Figure 3.4). At the interior angle of the trigone is the bladder neck, where the bladder muscle and the urethra meet. The bladder neck is normally closed at rest.

The detrusor is composed of several layers of smooth muscle bundles that crisscross and interlace with each other. The central muscle layer is made up

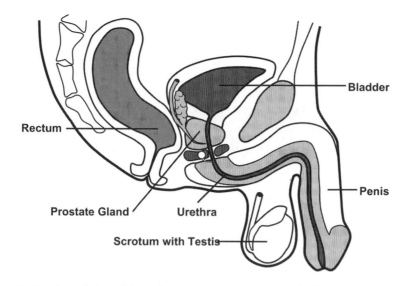

Figure 3.2B. Lateral view of the male urinary system. (Courtesy of Robin Noel.)

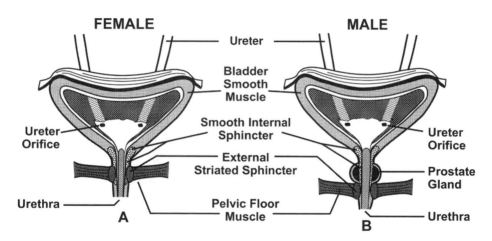

Figure 3.3. The lower urinary tract. (A) The female pelvis. (B) The male pelvis. (Courtesy of Robin Noel.)

of smooth muscle fibers and elastic connective tissue. This muscle layer expands as the bladder fills with urine and then contracts to expel it. The internal surface of the detrusor is the *urothelium,* which consists of three to seven layers of cells and appears smooth when the bladder is full. The urothelium has several receptors for neurotransmitters, primarily acetylcholine, adenosine triphosphate (ATP), and substance P. The urothelium lies on a thick layer of elastic connective tissue that allows the bladder to distend and expand as it fills with urine (Brooks, 2007). It has substantial sensory processes.

The superficial and deep trigonal detrusor musculature comprises the *trigone,* a small muscular triangular area that is continuous with the urethra at

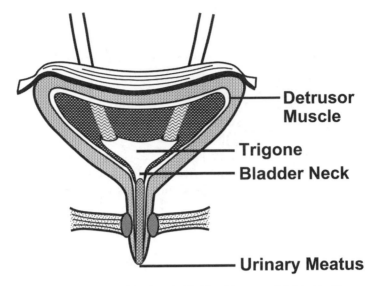

Figure 3.4. Trigone of the female bladder. (Courtesy of Robin Noel.)

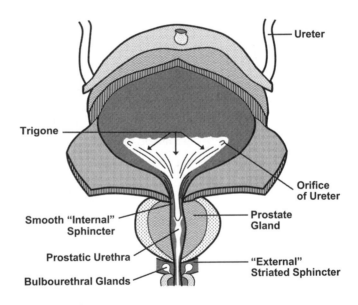

Figure 3.5. Anatomy of the male bladder and urethra. (Courtesy of Robin Noel.)

the bladder neck (see Figure 3.5). A functional sphincter mechanism exists at the bladder neck–proximal urethral area. This consists of smooth muscle, is not under voluntary control, and is often referred to as the internal sphincter or "smooth sphincter" mechanism. The bladder smooth muscle contains a variety of receptor sites (primarily cholinergic, alpha and beta adrenergic, and purinergic) that affect both bladder filling/storage and bladder emptying (Wein & Moy, 2007).

The bladder's function is to fill with, store, and then empty urine through the urethra (voiding or urination). It operates as a low-pressure, high-volume system (Wein & Moy, 2007). In order to fill and store urine normally, the bladder must exhibit normal (high) compliance (tonic change in pressure/volume), must not exhibit any involuntary phasic increases in pressure, and must be capable of transmitting normal sensory information. During the filling phase, the bladder wall expands to allow accommodation of increasing volumes without significant increases in bladder pressure. Normally, the bladder has a capacity of 500 mL (about 16 ounces) of urine, which is called the *functional capacity* of the bladder. The bladder increases to about the size of a softball when full. When empty, the bladder is a compact structure of folded tissue.

Urethra

The urethra is a thin, muscular tube that exits the trigone or base (neck) of the bladder to the outside of the body. It is made up primarily of smooth muscle and, therefore, is not under voluntary control. The urethral orifice, or *urinary meatus,* is the opening of the urethra to the outside (see Figure 3.4). When not passing urine, the urethral tube is collapsed and held closed by various factors that include the tone of its smooth muscle and the striated muscle that surrounds a portion of the urethra in both men and women.

In females, the urethra is approximately 1.5 inches (3–4 cm) in length. It exits the bladder neck through the urogenital diaphragm to the external urethral orifice (*meatus urinarius*), anterior to the vagina. The lower third of the urethra is fused with the vagina (DeLancey, 2006). Inferior to the bladder, smooth muscle from the trigone of the bladder extends longitudinally into the urethral wall, forming a functional but not an anatomic sphincter. A circularly oriented sleeve of striated muscle covers an inner layer of smooth muscle (*rhabdosphincter* at the midpoint), which together form the urethral wall in that area. In addition, the urethra is surrounded by a striated muscle group commonly known as the "external" sphincter at approximately its midpoint. This periurethral striated muscle is what allows individuals to voluntarily interrupt the urinary stream during voiding. Interaction between the urogenital diaphragm and the pubococcygeus muscles in the adjacent pelvic floor assists urethral closure (Figure 3.6). Many small mucous glands open in the urethra and can lead to urethral diverticula (Brooks, 2007). These glands, which are found distally in the urethra, are called *Skene's glands*. The urinary meatus is located just between the clitoris and the vaginal opening. The mucosal lining of the urethra in women is different from the lining in men in that it contains stratified squamous epithelium, which is subject to effects of the hormone estrogen. After menopause, the lack of estrogen is reflected in poorer quality of collagen, muscle, and skin tone and is thought to contribute to urogenital atrophy, perhaps contributing to symptoms such as frequency and urgency.

In males, the urethra begins at the bladder neck, passes downward through the prostate gland and the urogenital diaphragm, and finally passes

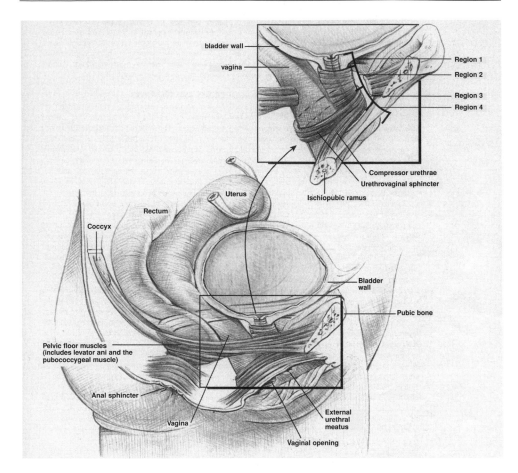

Figure 3.6.   Mechanism of urethral control in women. The urethra is 3 to 4 cm in length and can be considered to consist of four unequal regions (textbooks vary in their interpretations). Region 1 contains the internal urethral sphincter. The lumen is surrounded by smooth muscle and the bladder neck. In region 2, the middle portion, the lumen is surrounded by the striated sphincter urethra muscle as well as smooth muscle. In region 3, the lumen is surrounded by the striated urethrovaginal sphincter, which also loops around the vagina, and the compressor urethrae muscle. The striated muscles in regions 2 and 3 are referred to collectively as the external urethral sphincter. The internal and external sphincters form the sphincter complex, which maintains tone and prevents involuntary voiding. In region 4, the smooth muscle that originates in region 1 terminates in the fibrous tissue surrounding the external urethral meatus. (From Newman, D.K. [2003]. Stress urinary incontinence in women. *American Journal of Nursing, 103*[8], 46–55; reprinted by permission.)

along the length of the penis until it ends at the urinary meatus at the tip of the penis (referred to as the *glans penis*). It is 8 inches (18–20 cm) in length. The upper-most portion (also called the *prostatic* or *sphincteric urethra*) is approximately 3 inches long. In the preprostatic region, immediately inferior to the bladder, a circular collar of nonstriated muscle extending from the trigone of the bladder surrounds the urethra, forming the "internal" urethral sphincter (*sphincter vesicae*). The internal, involuntary sphincter prevents the flow of semen into the bladder during ejaculation and plays a role in maintaining urinary continence. In the membranous region, a circularly oriented layer of skeletal muscle (a portion of the urogenital diaphragm) surrounds a thin layer of nonstriated muscle. This layer is continuous with the prostatic urethra and forms the "external" urethral sphincter (*sphincter urethrae*) (Brooks, 2007). The voluntary external urethral sphincter plays an active role in maintaining urinary continence.

Sphincters

When an individual is not urinating, the urethral tube is closed. Box 3.1 lists the functions of the external and internal urinary sphincters.

Traditionally, the sphincter has been described as two muscles: a smooth (internal or proximal) annular muscle and a striated (external) muscle, which surround the proximal and middle urethra, respectively. However, in both men and women, the internal sphincter is not an anatomic structure but a physiological junction of the bladder neck and proximal urethra. It responds to alpha adrenergic stimulation and blackade. Research in women has led to a new understanding of the urethral sphincter mechanism as a combination of compressive and muscular elements that act together to ensure continence, even in the presence of physical exertion (DeLancey, 2006). The compressive elements of the sphincter include a moist urethral mucosa and an underlying vascular cushion. Muscular elements of the sphincter mechanism in women are the striated (voluntary) muscle fibers both within the wall of the urethra

---

Box 3.1   Function of the urinary sphincters

Internal Sphincter (Proximal Smooth Muscle)

- Located at the level of the bladder neck and proximal urethra.

- Formed by a ring of involuntary smooth muscle from the bladder trigone and two "U"-shaped loops of smooth muscle derived from the detrusor muscle.

- Operates in concert with the pelvic support structures to keep the proximal urethra closed.

- Innervated by autonomic fibers (alpha adrenergic and cholinergic).

- Involuntary and cannot be trained with active exercise.

- In men, removed or damaged during prostate cancer surgery, causing dependence on the function of the skeletal muscles of the external sphincter and pelvic floor.

External Sphincter (Striated Muscle)

- Consists of three small striated skeletal muscles, largely made up of slow-twitch muscle fibers, which are well suited to maintaining constant tone.

- Formed by the muscle of the striated urogenital sphincter.

- Voluntarily relaxes to facilitate emptying of the bladder.

- Voluntarily contracts to prevent urine leakage when abdominal pressure is increased, such as during effort, coughing, laughing, or sneezing.

(called the rhabdosphincter-skeletal muscle) and in the extramural portion, which is in the adjacent pelvic floor and under voluntary control. The "striated" sphincter, or "external" sphincter, comprises the striated muscle, which surrounds the urethra at that point, a part of the urethra at the level of what is referred to as the "urogenital diaphragm" (Wein & Moy, 2007).

During bladder filling and storage, the internal sphincter is thought to progressively increase smooth muscle tone (resistance) to ensure that the soft, moist urethral mucosa forms a watertight seal, preventing urine loss from the bladder neck and urethra even during periods of physical exertion. These smooth muscle fibers extend submucousally down the urethra and lie above the external sphincter. The smooth muscle in this area has a large amount of sympathetic alpha receptors, which is hypothesized to cause closure when stimulated. Normally during bladder filling, the tension in the striated (external) sphincter in both men and women gradually increases (the so-called guarding reflex), mediated by impulses coming via the pudendal nerve. During urination, the muscular elements of both sphincter mechanisms relax, allowing efficient and unimpeded evacuation of urine from the bladder. Because striated and smooth muscle fibers are primarily responsible for maintaining sphincter closure, it is essential to understand the neurological control of these muscles and the effects of specific pharmacological agents on sphincter function.

The external sphincter has voluntary control and has somatic innervation from the sacral region (S_3–S_4) via the pudendal nerve, allowing the sphincter to be closed at will. In males, the external sphincter has the bulk of the fibers at the membranous urethra, but some fibers also run up to the bladder neck.

Prostate

The prostate gland in men is located at the base of the bladder and urethral junction (urethrovesical region) and its inferior extent is at the urogenital diaphragm. It is pierced through its vertical aspect by the prostatic urethra (see Figure 3.5). The prostate is composed of glandular and stromal (smooth muscle and connective tissue) elements. The glandular tissue can enlarge, causing benign prostatic hyperplasia (BPH), and can undergo malignant transformation. The main function of the prostate is the manufacture of secretions that become components of semen.

Vagina

The vagina is a hollow, muscular tube that extends from the introitus to the cervix. The normal length is approximately 10–12 cm, and the upper vagina has a greater diameter than the lower portion (see Figure 3.2A). Anteriorly, the vagina is in contact with the bladder base, from which it is separated by loose connective tissue, and with the urethra. The base of the bladder rests on the vaginal wall in front of the cervix. The vagina is in a near-horizontal position when a woman stands. The middle to lower vagina is supported by connections to the pelvic diaphragm and lower endopelvic fascia. The lower third is further attached to the perineal body. In women, the perineum lies between the pubis, thighs, and buttocks (Figure 3.7A).

Pelvic Floor Muscle Anatomy

The "pelvic floor" is a term that has been used to refer to the pelvic floor muscles (PFM), but it actually includes additional structures such as the pelvic viscera; the peritoneum overlying it; the endopelvic fascia; the levator ani, coccygeus, obturator internus, and piriformis muscles; and the perineal membrane (DeLancey, 2006). The bony pelvis offers support and protection to the organs and structures located within the pelvis. The bladder itself lies deep in the bony pelvis, as do the lower two thirds of the ureters. The major bones of the bony pelvis—the ilium, the ischium, the pubis, and the coccyx—provide a framework to contain the pelvic organs and to support the PFM.

The PFM extend from the inner surface of the pubic bone anteriorly to the pelvic surface of the ischial spine posteriorly. They form a sling that is often referred to as the *pelvic diaphragm* (Figure 3.7B). These are a group of muscles know collectively as the levator ani and coccygeus. The levator ani consists of the pubococcygeus, the iliococcygeus, and the puborectalis mus-

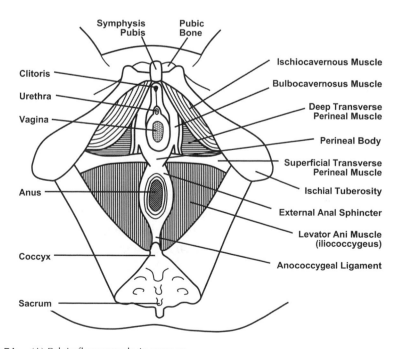

Figure 3.7A.   (A) Pelvic floor muscle in women.

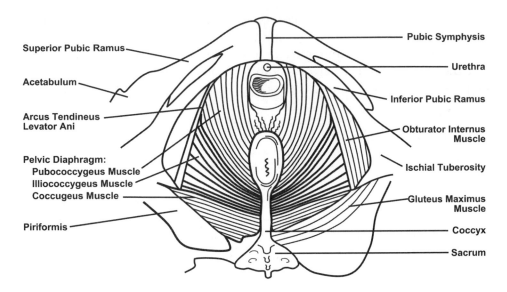

Figure 3.7B.   (B) View of the levator ani muscles in the pelvis. (Courtesy of Robin Noel.)

cles (Scarpero & Dmochowski, 2006). The PFM are entirely under voluntary control and play an important role in maintaining continence and preventing UI. They can become weakened with childbirth, lack of use, decrease in the hormone estrogen, aging, surgery, and injury.

The pelvic and urogenital diaphragms act together. In the resting position, they gently support the internal organs and structures. During physical activities or when there is a need to urinate and the toilet is not readily available, they tighten by pulling up and in, to prevent leakage.

Supportive Structures of the Pelvic Floor

The supportive structures of the pelvic floor include the endopelvic fascia, the pelvic and the fibrous urogenital diaphragms, and the levator ani and internal obturator muscles (Ashton-Miller & DeLancey, 2007; Newman, 2000, 2003).

Endopelvic Fascia   The endopelvic fascia, which is made up of collagen and smooth muscle, surrounds the vagina and attaches it laterally to the arcus tendineus fasciae pelvis. The arcus tendineus fasciae pelvis in turn is attached ventrally to the pubic bone and dorsally to the ischial spine. The arcus tendineus fasciae pelvis is located on either side of the urethra and vagina. It acts like a suspension bridge and provides the support needed to suspend the urethra on the anterior vaginal wall. It fuses with the endopelvic fascia, where it merges with the levator ani muscle.

Pelvic and Fibrous Urogenital Diaphragms   The pelvic diaphragm is a group of paired muscles (referred to as the pubococcygeus muscle) consisting of the levator ani and coccygeus muscles. The levator ani muscle is subdivided, from medial to lateral, into three muscles: the pubococcygeus, the puborectalis, and the iliococcygeus (Cundiff & Fenner, 2004). These muscles originate from the pubic rami on either side of the midline at the level of the arcus tendineus musculi levator ani.

The fibrous urogenital diaphragm, or perineal membrane, is located below the levator ani and spans the anterior portion of the pelvic outlet, connecting the perineal body to the pubic bone. It consists of superficial muscles that primarily assist the sexual and urethral sphincter muscles.

Levator Ani   The levator ani is a paired muscle that forms a hammock-like sheet of muscle anterior to the coccyx and posterior to the pubis. The muscles extend laterally from one pelvic wall to the other. The opening within the levator ani muscle through which the urethra and vagina pass (and through which pelvic organ prolapse occurs) is called the *urogenital hiatus* of the levator ani (Ashton-Miller & Delancey, 2007). The rectum also passes through this opening; however, because the levator ani muscles attach directly to the anus, it is not included in the name of the hiatus (DeLancey, 2006). The normal function or activity of the levator ani muscle is to keep the urogenital hiatus closed. It squeezes the vagina, urethra, and rectum closed by compressing them against the pubic bone. It also lifts the pelvic floor and pelvic organs in a cephalic (toward the head) direction.

The levator ani muscle is divided into three functional parts (Figure 3.8) (Aston-Miller & Delancey, 2007):

- The *pubococcygeus muscle,* the main part of the levator ani, arises from the pubis and inserts into the coccyx and anococcygeal ligaments. Muscle fibers extend from the main muscle mass and attach to the urethra, the external urethral sphincter (*sphincter urethrae* muscles), the prostate in men (*levator prostatae* muscles) or the middle of the vagina in women (*pubovaginalis* muscles), and the rectum. The majority of the fibers then merge with the perineal body. The muscle plays a role in sexual function because a pleasurable rhythmic contraction is felt during orgasm. It can also develop tension and spasm, causing pelvic pain disorders.

- The *iliococcygeus muscles* arise laterally from the tendinous arch of the obturator fascia and the ischial spine. The muscles attach to the last two segments of the coccyx and merge with the anococcygeal ligaments. The iliococcygeus muscles form a horizontal sheet or shelf that spans the opening of the posterior region of the pelvis.

- The *puborectalis muscles,* the medial portions of the pubococcygeus muscles, merge with the perineal body, forming a "U"-shaped sling that is situated posterior and lateral to the anorectal junction. The puborectalis muscles hold the anorectal junction anteriorly, preventing the passage of feces from the rectum to the anal canal and relieving pressure on the anal sphincter. Relaxation of the puborectalis muscles aids defecation.

The levator ani muscles have constant activity, like that of other postural muscles and like the external anal sphincter. They close the lumen of the vagina in a way similar to that by which the anal sphincter closes the anus. They form a horizontal sling on which the pelvic organs are supported, and their constant action prevents any opening within the pelvic floor through which a pelvic organ could prolapse. The constant resting tone of the puborectalis and pubococcygeus pulls the distal vagina and anorectal junction toward the pubic symphysis, creating a 90-degree angle between the anal and rectal canals, referred to as the *anorectal angle*. These muscles are composed mainly of two types of striated muscle fibers: type I and type II. Type I (slow-twitch) muscle fibers are approximately 80% of the muscle and, therefore, they maintain constant resting tone over time. They are recruited and fatigue slowly. Each muscle group also contains a smaller proportion of type II (fast-twitch) muscle fibers (approximately 20%). Type II muscle fibers can be recruited rapidly, permitting them to respond quickly during sudden increases in intra-abdominal pressure, but they tend to fatigue rapidly. It has been suggested that the successful treatment of stress UI by pelvic floor muscle exercises or electrical stimulation may be caused by the conversion of fast-twitch striated muscle fibers to slow-twitch fibers (Yoshimura & Chancellor, 2007).

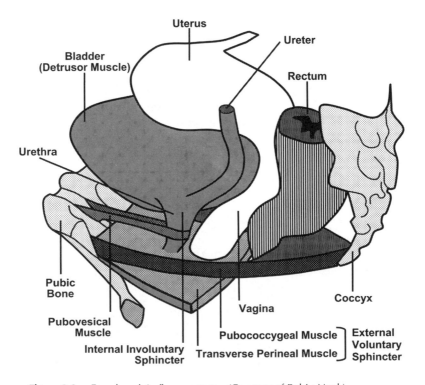

Figure 3.8.   Female pelvic floor anatomy. (Courtesy of Robin Noel.)

Internal Obturator   The internal obturator muscle is connected to the muscles of the pelvic floor and is another important muscle that lines the lower pelvis. It attaches to the obturator tendon within the pelvis and to the greater trochanter of the femur. As the obturator muscle contracts, it acts as a pulley, lifting the bladder and urethra into the optimum functional position. At rest, it maintains the bladder position in the pelvis.

Rectum and Anal Canal

The rectum is located posteriorly in the pelvis and is composed of a mucosa, a submucosa, and a circular and a longitudinal layer of smooth muscle. In women, the anterior wall of the rectum is located directly adjacent to the posterior vaginal wall. The rectum serves as both a storage area and a conduit from the colon to the anal canal. The anal canal is defined proximally by the levator ani muscles and includes the puborectalis muscle, which creates the anorectal angle (Figure 3.9). Two sphincters encircle the anal canal: the internal anal sphincter, which is a continuation of the circular smooth muscle of the rectum, and the external anal sphincter, which consists of striated muscle innervated by the pudendal nerves arising from sacral nerves S_2, S_3, and S_4. Extrinsic innervation of the internal anal sphincter is by the sympathetic and parasympathetic autonomic nerves (Wald, 2007).

    The internal and external anal sphincters form a complex system with the anal canal, having a pressure level to secure a waterproof closure, thus preventing unwanted leakage of feces. The inner-most layer is the lining of the anal sphincter complex. This mucosal lining is surrounded by the internal anal sphincter muscle, a thickened prolongation of the circular smooth muscle layer of the distal rectal wall that is under autonomic control. The internal sphinc-

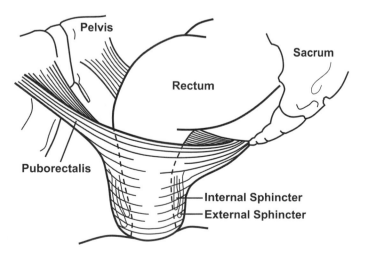

Figure 3.9.   Anal sphincters. (Courtesy of Robin Noel.)

ter is responsible for 80% of resting pressure of the anal sphincter system. The smooth muscle of the internal sphincter generates a constant tension or contraction over long periods of time. Between the internal and the external anal sphincters are the fused longitudinal fibers of the intestinal wall and levator ani muscles that continue into the superficial part of the external anal sphincter muscle.

The external anal sphincter is voluntary, striated muscle that has a predominance of slow-twitch, fatigue-resistant muscle fibers (Madoff, Parker, Varma, & Lowry, 2004). It provides 20% of the anal resting tone. It is mainly composed of two parts: a deep part and a superficial part, separated by a connective tissue layer. The superficial part forms a round structure at the edge of and below the caudal end of the internal sphincter. Both parts send connective tissue fibers to the tip of the coccyx. In the female, the external anal sphincter is shorter anteriorly than posteriorly.

The third part of the anal continence mechanism is the puborectalis muscle, which forms a sling around the rectum. The anal sphincter and the puborectalis muscle function as one unit to bring about voluntary sphincter contraction. Although the internal anal sphincter is responsible for the maintenance of resting pressure, both the external anal sphincter and the puborectalis muscle actively contract and thereby increase anal pressure in situations of fecal urgency and increases in intra-abdominal pressure, such as during coughing. Resting anal sphincter tone is associated with internal sphincter function and is known to be lower in women after vaginal birth complicated by a third-degree perineal tear.

ROLE OF THE NERVOUS SYSTEM

The functions of the lower urinary system are dependent on an intact, functioning brain and nervous system (NS) (Figure 3.10). The NS of the body is divided into a central nervous system (CNS) and a peripheral nervous system (PNS) portion. The CNS contains the brain and the spinal cord. The PNS contains the autonomic (both the sympathetic and parasympathetic NS) and somatic peripheral nerves. The lower urinary tract is innervated by three sets of peripheral nerves involving the sympathetic, parasympathetic, and somatic NS.

The *autonomic NS* includes the parasympathetic (cranial and sacral spinal cord origin) and sympathetic (thoracic and lumbar) nerve fibers and upper lumbar region (sympathetic nerve fibers). The autonomic NS regulates or influences many involuntary bodily functions (remember, though, that normal voiding in the adult is voluntary!). Fear or anxiety can therefore cause diarrhea, inability to void, nausea, cold sweaty hands, increased heart rate, and the like. Injuries to the nerves of the autonomic NS usually cause diffuse pain. Breathing exercises such as those used in bladder training can help calm down an autonomic NS in distress.

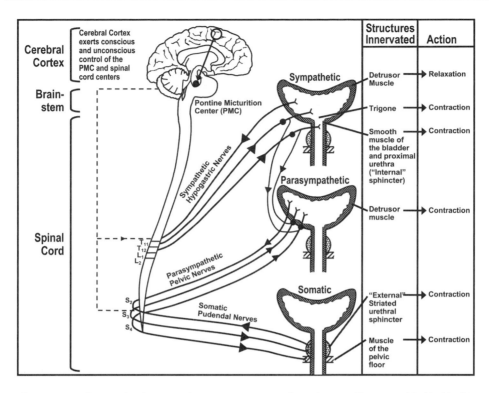

Figure 3.10.   Connection between the nervous system and continence. (Courtesy of Robin Noel.)

The *sympathetic NS* has efferent pathways that arise from the thoracic and lumbar segments of the spinal cord that are thought to contribute to urine storage. The sympathetic NS is thought to contribute to bladder storage by 1) inhibiting the parasympathetic pathway responsible for bladder contraction, and 2) contracting the smooth muscle of the bladder neck and proximal urethra (internal sphincter) via activation of alpha-adrenergic receptors.

The *parasympathetic NS* efferent pathways are located in the cranial and sacral spinal cord (S_2–S_4) and contain neurons responsible for micturition, defecation, and vaginal relaxation. The nerve terminals end on the urinary smooth muscle and epithelium. The fibers that are responsible for micturition reside in the pelvic nerve. The parasympathetic NS promotes bladder emptying by 1) stimulating the bladder smooth muscle to contract; and 2) relaxing the internal urethral sphincter, which allows urine to enter the urethra.

Fibers carrying sensation (afferent or sensory nerves) from the bladder and urethra and other pelvic structures travel along with other efferent nerves back to the spinal cord and connect with fibers ascending to the brain or with fibers that can elicit local reflexes.

The *somatic NS* is under voluntary control. The somatic NS sends a signal to the striated external urethral sphincter via the pudendal nerve either to contract, preventing urine leakage, or to relax, allowing the release of

Table 3.1   Nerve activation in normal bladder function

Nervous system	Nerve	Originates	Innervates	Function
Storage				
Involuntary (sympathetic)	Hypogastric	T_{10}–L_2	Detrusor muscle and smooth (internal or proximal) muscle	Allows detrusor to expand during filling/ storage and contracts smooth internal sphincter (maintains closure to prevent urine from entering the bladder)
Voluntary (somatic)	Pudendal	S_2–S_4	Pelvic floor muscles	Contracts external urethral sphincter (maintains closure) or relaxes smooth muscle at proximal urethra, allowing the release of urine
Emptying				
Voluntary and involuntary (parasympathetic)	Pelvic	S_2–S_4	Detrusor muscle	Stimulates the detrusor muscle to contract and relaxes the smooth muscle at the proximal urethra to allow urine to enter the urethra (causing emptying)

urine. The pudendal nerve is involved in innervation of the external urethral and anal sphincters and the clitoris, labial skin, and superficial perineal muscles. Because this nerve runs along the superior surface of the pelvic floor, it is susceptible to injury during vaginal delivery. The detrusor (bladder) muscle normally does not increase its activity as the bladder fills with urine. The PFM and urethral sphincter muscle remain contracted to prevent release of urine. Table 3.1 presents a summary of nerve activation of the bladder.

The NS functions on electrical impulses transmitted through the release of chemicals known as neurotransmitters. Neurotransmitters that relate to bladder and urethral function are primarily cholinergic and adrenergic (Wein & Moy, 2007). Control of the bladder is mediated primarily through the cholinergic fibers of the pelvic nerve. The pelvic nerve releases acetylcholine to effect contraction (to empty the bladder) of the detrusor muscle. Modulation of pelvic nerve activity by local reflex arcs and by the pontine micturition centers, and frontal cortex allows for accommodation of the bladder and storage of urine. The term *cholinergic* refers to those receptor sites where acetylcholine is a primary neurotransmitter. Acetylcholine stimulates muscarinic receptors in the bladder to contract. Neurotransmitters may have differing effects in different organs or anatomic locations. There are five differ-

Table 3.2 Possible peripheral neurotransmitters and modulators in the lower urinary tract

Transmitter (receptor)	Effect	Site of action
Acetylcholine (M_3)	Contraction	Bladder smooth muscle
Acetylcholine (M_3, M_2)	Excitation (?)	Peripheral afferents
Acetylcholine (M_2)	Contraction (?)	Bladder smooth muscle
Acetylcholine (M_1, M_3)	Contraction (?)	Prejunctional
Acetylcholine (M_2, M_4)	Relaxation	Prejunctional
Norepinephrine (β_3)	Relaxation	Bladder smooth muscle
Norepinephrine (α_1)	Contraction	Bladder smooth muscle
Adenosine triphosphate ($P2X_1$)	Contraction	Bladder smooth muscle
Adenosine triphosphate ($P2X_3$)	Excitation	Peripheral afferents
Nitric oxide (NO)	Relaxation	Bladder base smooth muscle
Nitric oxide (NO)	Inhibition	Peripheral afferents
Serotonin ($5\text{-}HT_1$, $5\text{-}HT_2$)	Contraction	Bladder smooth muscle
Prostanoids	Contraction	Bladder smooth muscle
Prostanoids	Excitation	Peripheral afferents
Leukotrienes (LTB_4)	Contraction	Bladder smooth muscle
Angiotensin (AT1)	Contraction	Bladder smooth muscle
Bradykinin (B_2)	Contraction	Bladder smooth muscle
Endothelin (ETa)	Contraction	Bladder smooth muscle
Tachykinins (NK2)	Contraction	Bladder smooth muscle

From Wein, A.J., & Moy, M.L. (2007). Voiding function, dysfunction and urinary incontinence. In P.M. Hanno, A.J. Wein, & S.B. Malkowicz (Eds.), *Penn Clinical Manual of Urology* (pp. 341–478). Philadelphia: Elsevier Saunders; reprinted by permission.

ent muscarinic receptor subtypes, M_1–M_5. The majority of those in the bladder smooth muscle are of the M_2 subtype, although bladder smooth muscle contraction is mediated primarily by the M_3 subtype.

The term *adrenergic* is applied to those receptor sites where a catecholamine is the neurotransmitter (Wein & Moy, 2007). Most postganglionic sympathetic fibers are adrenergic receptor sites, including those to lower urinary tract smooth muscle, where the catecholamine responsible for neurotransmission is norepinephrine. Adrenergic receptor sites are further classified as alpha (α) or beta (β) on the basis of the differential effects elicited by a series of catecholamines and their antagonists. Classically, the term *alpha-adrenergic effect* designates vasoconstriction or contraction of smooth musculature, or both, in response to norepinephrine. There are numerous other potential neurotransmitters in the periphery and in the CNS that may affect lower urinary tract function (Table 3.2 and Table 3.3).

Efferent innervation for the external urethral sphincter is classically thought to be somatic and to emanate from *Onuf's nucleus* in the sacral spinal cord (segments S_2–S_4), exiting the cord as the pudendal nerve. The peripheral neurotransmitter is acetylcholine, but the receptor type is different from that

Table 3.3   Potential CNS neurotransmitters other than opioids and their effects on the micturition reflex

Neurotransmitter (receptor)	Site	Predominant action*
Glutamate	Brain, spinal cord	+
Glycine	Brain, spinal cord	−
GABA (Á-aminobutyric acid)	Brain, spinal cord	−
Serotonin	Spinal cord	−
Acetycholine (M_2, M_4)	Brain	−, +
Dopamine (D-2)	Brain	+
Dopamine (D-1)	Brain	−
Norepinephrine (α_1, α_2)	Brain, spinal cord	+, −
Tachykinins (NK1, NK2)	Brain, spinal cord	+

From Wein, A.J., & Moy, M.L. (2007). Voiding function, dysfunction and urinary incontinence. In P.M. Hanno, A.J. Wein, & S.B. Malkowicz (Eds.), *Penn Clinical Manual of Urology* (pp. 341–478). Philadelphia: Elsevier Saunders; reprinted by permission.

*+ = enhances micturition reflex; − = inhibits micturition reflex.

in smooth muscle in the bladder (called "nicotinic" as opposed to "muscarinic"). Activation causes sphincter contraction. At the level of Onuf's nucleus, during filling and storage serotonin and norepinephrine stimulate the pudendal nerve and therefore striated urethral sphincter activity (Wein & Moy, 2007).

UNDERSTANDING MICTURITION

Under normal conditions, urine continuously and gradually accumulates as the normal bladder accommodates increasing volumes of urine with little or no increase in pressure within the bladder. In the absence of any pathological factors, the sense of bladder filling is not perceived until approximately 40%–50% of the functional bladder capacity is reached. In order to understand bladder disorders, it is important to understand how the bladder empties.

At a socially acceptable time and location, voluntary urination (*micturition*) is initiated by a complex set of reflexes organized and facilitated at the level of the brain stem. Various micturition centers in the brain, brain stem, and spinal cord are involved in emptying the bladder. These centers control the reflexes to empty the bladder and coordinate its filling. Information from the bladder is transmitted via afferent or sensory reflex pathways to the CNS. It first reaches the pontine micturition center in the brain stem. The micturition center of the brain stem conveys the information that the bladder is filling up to the brain (cortex) and to important areas within the brain such as the limbic system (center for motivation and memory) and the cerebellum (responsible for some muscle control). The connection to the cortex enables a

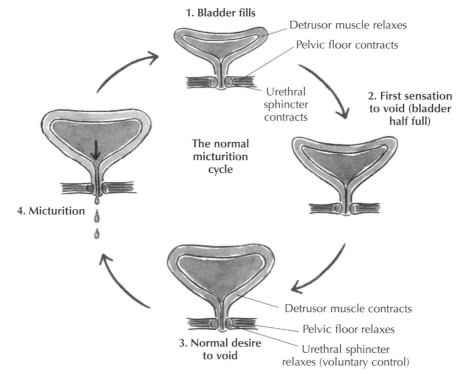

Figure 3.11. The steps of the normal urination cycle.

person to make a conscious decision to delay micturition or to empty the bladder early. Descending connections to the pontine micturition center convey information to activate or inhibit bladder emptying.

Interestingly, the bladder muscle is under voluntary control even though it consists of smooth muscles that cannot normally be controlled voluntarily. A special feature of the bladder is that emptying can be delayed or done early, even when the bladder is not full. Motor outflow to the bladder and urethra is via an efferent (as opposed to afferent) limb. A person usually empties the bladder when it is most convenient, normally every 4–5 hours during the daytime and less often at night.

Normal voiding is a coordinated event, and the steps of the micturition cycle are as follows (Figure 3.11):

1. The bladder expands as it fills with urine. The periurethral striated musculature and the urethral sphincter muscle remain contracted to prevent release of urine.

2. As the bladder fills to half its capacity, neurons from the bladder carry messages to the brain and the first sensation of the need to void occurs.

3. Because voiding is voluntary, the individual makes a conscious decision to void or to delay voiding. Voiding occurs by relaxation of the striated urethral sphincter and activation of the spinal reflex pathways, which is

> **Box 3.2   Micturition cycle or voiding**
>
> Bladder filling/urine storage requires the following:
>
> 1.   Accommodation of increasing volumes of urine at a low intravesical pressure (normal compliance) and with appropriate sensation.
>
> 2.   A bladder outlet that is closed at rest and remains so during increases in intra-abdominal pressure.
>
> 3.   Absence of involuntary bladder contractions (detrusor overactivity).
>
> Bladder emptying/voiding requires the following:
>
> 1.   A coordinated contraction of the bladder smooth musculature of adequate magnitude and duration.
>
> 2.   A concomitant lowering of resistance at the level of the smooth and striated sphincter.
>
> 3.   Absence of anatomic (as opposed to functional) obstruction.
>
> Adapted from Wein, A.J., & Moy, M.L. (2007). Voiding function, dysfunction and urinary incontinence. In P.M. Hanno, A.J. Wein, & S.B. Malkowicz (Eds.), *Penn clinical manual of urology* (pp. 341–478). Philadelphia: Elsevier Saunders.

coordinated in the pons. Increases in parasympathetic transmission to the bladder cause contraction and increase pressure in the bladder (detrusor). These same pathways act to inhibit sympathetic and pudendal outflow to the urethra, causing relaxation of the urethral sphincters and pelvic floor muscle.

4.   Voiding (*micturition*) occurs.

Voiding, or the micturition cycle, involves two relatively discrete processes: 1) bladder filling and urine storage and 2) bladder emptying or voiding, which are outlined in Box 3.2.

In order for the individual to maintain continence, the bladder pressure must be less than the pressure within the urethra. However, under certain conditions, an involuntary contraction of the detrusor muscle (erroneously referred to as "spasm") may spontaneously occur at any point during bladder filling. This phenomenon will raise the pressure within the bladder precipitously, and, if sensation is intact, will result in a perceived sensation of impending micturition and urinary urgency. This precipitous rise in bladder pressure may result in the unexpected involuntary expulsion of urine through the urethra (i.e., UI). Urinary frequency occurs as a result of reduced functional bladder capacity, or, rarely, as a result of structurally diminished bladder capacity. It can also be due, at least partly, to a coping mechanism adopted by the individual to avoid leakage of large volumes of urine by maintaining a relatively low volume in the bladder through frequent urination.

Men and women have different habits when they void. Men stand to void and often void in public (at urinals) next to other men. They often contract their abdominal muscles to aid in complete bladder emptying. Women tend to void in private and must relax to open the external sphincter. They will sit or squat over a toilet seat to void. This position is important because many women compress their abdomen to empty the bladder.

AGING AND CHANGES IN THE LOWER URINARY SYSTEM AND PELVIC FLOOR

The physiological, psychological, and environmental changes that accompany aging do not directly cause the bladder to malfunction, but they do predispose older adults to an increased risk or incidence of disorders (Palmer, 2004; Resnick & Yalla, 2007). One of the primary changes with age is a shift in the circadian rhythm of water excretion that leads to the greatest proportion of urine production occurring at rest, usually during the night (Pfisterer, Griffiths, Schaefer, & Resnick, 2006). Contributing to this is the blunting of the nocturnal phase of the release of the antidiuretic hormone, arginine vasopressin (AVP), which is released during the day and night. Also, during the day, fluid accumulation occurs in extracellular spaces; at night, there is a lower level of physical activity and the individual is lying flat, promoting the movement of body fluid from extracellular spaces to blood vessels. This increased renal perfusion, and excretion of excess renal fluid may cause an increase in the amount of urine in the bladder, called *nocturnal polyuria*.

Some older people may excrete 50% or more of their 24-hour urine output during the night (DuBeau, 2007). This is especially true in women who have delayed fluid excretion. Because of this larger volume of urine in the bladder, urine loss can occur during sleep (called *nocturnal enuresis* or *nighttime incontinence*). This is also why older adults experience *nocturia,* or the complaint that the person has to wake at night one or more times to void (Van Kerrebroeck et al., 2002). Nocturia should be recorded from the time the individual goes to bed with the intention of going to sleep, to the time the individual wakes with the intention of rising. Older adults with nocturia are usually troubled by sleep impairments to a greater degree than those individuals without nocturia. They have frequent awakenings, have difficulty returning to sleep after awakening, and may have nighttime symptoms such as muscle cramps in the legs. One of the most serious consequences of nocturia is falls and fractures (Asplund, 2007). An occurrence of two or more nocturnal voids is associated with a twofold increase in such falls (Stewart, Moore, May, Marks, & Hale, 1992).

A common cause of nocturia is the use of diuretics. If these drugs are taken in the morning, they can result in increased thirst and increased fluid intake in the daytime and increased nocturnal urine output. If a loop diuretic (e.g., furosemide [Lasix]) is taken 6 hours before going to bed, nocturnal diuresis and nocturia often can be reduced (Reynard, Cannon, Yang, & Abrams, 1998).

Another cause of nocturia in older adults is nocturnal polyuria (NP). NP is present when greater than 20% of the 24-hour urine production common in "young adults," and greater than 33% in those over 65 years, occurs at night (Abrams et al., 2002). Chronic medical conditions such as congestive heart failure, venous stasis with peripheral edema, hyperglycemia and excess urine output, obstructive sleep apnea, and use of diuretics, as well as evening and nighttime fluid consumption, are causes of NP (Colling, Owen, & McCreedy, 1994). NP can also be caused by low bladder capacity secondary to overactive bladder, BPH, urethral obstructions, atrophic vaginitis, low bladder compliance, and even bladder cancer. Treatment could be something as practical as fluid restriction, giving diuretics at 2:00 P.M. rather than 6:00 P.M. or 7:00 P.M., afternoon naps with elevation of the legs, compression stockings, or treatment with the vasopressin analogue desmopressin (DDAVP), which increases reabsorption of fluid in the kidneys. For low bladder capacity resulting from overactive bladder, antimuscarinic therapy and behavioral modification are generally the treatments of choice.

In addition to the shift in the circadian rhythm of water excretion, the following normal age-related changes occur in the urinary system:

- There is a 30%–40% loss of functional cells (nephrons) in the kidneys.

- There is a decrease in the kidney's ability to filter blood and concentrate urine.

- Ability to postpone urination is decreased because there is a delay in the time before a person perceives an urge sensation (Resnick & Yalla, 2007). Sensory nerve tracts from the bladder through the spinal cord and to the brain often "wear out," creating breaks in the neural pathway. There is "short-circuiting" of nerve firing, and messages may not completely reach the brain. In general, the nervous system takes longer to respond to sensory stimuli.

- Detrusor overactivity (involuntary bladder contractions) results in small, frequent contractions that create the urge to void before the bladder is full (Pfisterer, Griffiths, Schaefer, & Resnick, 2006). These bladder contractions, over which the person has no control, cause urine leakage (urge UI) on the way to the bathroom. Detrusor overactivity may affect bladder function parameters because it is associated with decreased bladder capacity and increased bladder sensation (Pfisterer, Griffiths, Roisenberg, Schaefer, & Resnick, 2006).

- Detrusor muscle becomes less contractile as muscle fibers stiffen and atrophy. This can prevent the bladder from emptying completely (called *urinary retention*). This may be why some elderly persons need to void more frequently in small amounts. The urine that remains in the bladder after the individual has voided (*postvoid residual*) also may become infected with bacteria, causing an increased incidence of urinary tract infections.

- Urethral length and closure pressure decrease significantly with age in women, and may be related to numbers of pregnancies and deliveries (Pfisterer, Griffiths, Schaefer, & Resnick, 2006). Aging also causes a deterioration of the urethral musculature as the total number of striated muscle fibers in the urethra decreases (Ashton-Miller & Delancey, 2007).

- Although bladder capacity does not change with age, there is an increased flow time and decreased flow rate.

- Hypoestrogenization of the perineal area occurs in women. Estrogen receptors are found in squamous epithelium of the urethra, vagina, and bladder trigone in women. The PFM are also estrogen sensitive. After menopause, the tissue lining the vagina and urethra becomes thin and less vascularized, leading to urogenital atrophy/atrophic vaginitis and possibly contributing to urinary symptoms such as urgency and frequency. Also, estrogen reduction in the genitourinary tract increases the risk of urinary tract infections by depletion of vaginal colonization of lactobacilli. These changes can appear immediately following menopause or several years after.

- The prostate gland in men enlarges with aging and can cause bladder outlet obstruction leading to BPH and lower urinary tract symptoms, especially urgency and frequency.

CONCLUSION

The structures of the lower urinary tract work in unison to store and empty urine. Any disruption in the function of the bladder, urethra, sphincters, or pelvic floor can impair lower urinary tract function. Any injury to the brain and CNS can adversely affect urinary function. An unavoidable cause of urinary tract dysfunction is aging, which can predispose a person to bladder dysfunction. Clinicians who manage people with UI and related pelvic dysfunction need to have a working knowledge of anatomy and physiology of the different structures of the lower urinary tract.

REFERENCES

Abrams, P., Cardozo, L., Fall, M., Griffiths, D., Rosier, P., Ulmsten, U., et al. (2002). The standardisation of terminology of lower urinary tract function: Report from the Standardisation Sub-committee of the International Continence Society. *American Journal of Obstetrics and Gynecology, 187,* 116–126.

Ashton-Miller, J.A., & DeLancey, J.O. (2007). Functional anatomy of the female pelvic floor. *Annals of the New York Academy of Sciences, 1101,* 266–296.

Asplund, R. (2007). Pharmacotherapy for nocturia in the elderly patient. *Drugs and Aging, 24,* 325–343.

Brooks, J.D. (2007). Anatomy of the lower urinary tract and male genitalia. In A.J. Wein, L.R. Kavoussi, A.C. Novick, A.W. Partin, & C.A. Peters (Eds.), *Campbell's urology* (9th ed., pp. 38–77). Philadelphia: Elsevier Saunders.

Colling, J., Owen, T., & McCreedy, M.R. (1994). Urine volumes and voiding: Patterns among incontinent nursing home residents. *Geriatric Nursing, 15,* 188–192.

Cundiff, G.W., & Fenner, D. (2004). Evaluation and treatment of women with rectocele: Focus on associated defecatory and sexual dysfunction. *Obstetrics and Gynecology, 104,* 1403–1421.

DeLancey, D.O. (2006). Anatomy. In L. Cardozo & D. Staskin (Eds.), *Textbook of female urology and urogynecology* (2nd ed., pp. 115–126). Abingdon, UK: Informa Healthcare.

DuBeau, C.E. (2007). Beyond the bladder: Management of urinary incontinence in older women. *Clinical Obstetrics and Gynecology, 50,* 720–734.

Madoff, R.D., Parker, S.C., Varma, M.G., & Lowry, A.C. (2004). Faecal incontinence in adults. *Lancet, 364,* 621–632.

Newman, D.K. (2000). *Continence for women: Research-based practice.* Washington, DC: Association of Women's Health, Obstetric and Neonatal Nurses.

Newman, D.K. (2002). *Managing and treating urinary incontinence* (pp. 19–28). Baltimore: Health Professions Press.

Newman, D.K. (2003). *Pelvic muscle rehabilitation: Clinical manual.* Dover, NH: The Prometheus Group.

Palmer, M.H. (2004). Physiologic and psychologic age-related changes that affect urologic clients. *Urologic Nursing, 24,* 247–252.

Pfisterer, M.H., Griffiths, D.J., Roisenberg, L., Schaefer, W., & Resnick, N.M. (2006). The impact of detrusor overactivity on bladder function in younger and older women. *Journal of Urology, 175,* 1777–1783.

Pfisterer, M.H., Griffiths, D.J., Schaefer, W., & Resnick, N.M. (2006). The effect of age on lower urinary tract function: A study in women. *Journal of the American Geriatrics Society, 54,* 405–412.

Resnick, N.M., & Yalla, S.V. (2007). Geriatric incontinence and voiding dysfunction. In A.J. Wein, L.R. Kavoussi, A.C. Novick, A.W. Partin, & C.A. Peters (Eds.), *Campbell's urology* (9th ed., pp. 2305–2321). Philadelphia: Elsevier Saunders.

Reynard, J.M., Cannon, A., Yang, Q., & Abrams, P. (1998). A novel therapy for nocturnal polyuria: A double-blind randomized trial of furosemide against placebo. *British Journal of Urology, 81,* 215–218.

Scarpero, H.M., & Dmochowski, R.R. (2006). Pelvic anatomy for the surgeon. In C.R. Chapple, P.E. Zimmern, L. Brubaker, A.R.B. Smith, & K. Bo (Eds.), *Multidisciplinary management of female disorders* (pp. 3–12). Philadelphia: Elsevier Saunders.

Stewart, R.B., Moore, M.T., May, F.E., Marks, R.G., & Hale, W.E. (1992). Nocturia: A risk factor for falls in the elderly. *Journal of the American Geriatrics Society, 40,* 1217–1220.

Van Kerrebroeck, P., Abrams, P., Chaikin, D., Donovan, J., Fonda, D., Jackson, S., et al., for the International Continence Society. (2002). The standardization of terminology in nocturia: Report from the standardization subcommittee of the International Continence Society. *BJU International, 90*(Suppl. 3), 11–15.

Wald, A. (2007). Clinical Practice: Fecal incontinence in adults. *New England Journal of Medicine, 356,* 1648–1655.

Wein, A.J., & Moy, M.L. (2007). Voiding function, dysfunction and urinary incontinence. In P.M. Hanno, A.J. Wein, & S.B. Malkowicz (Eds.), *Penn clinical manual of urology* (pp. 341–478). Philadelphia: Elsevier Saunders.

Yoshimura, N., & Chancellor, M.B. (2007). Physiology and pharmacology of the bladder and urethra. In A.J. Wein, L.R. Kavoussi, A.C. Novick, A.W. Partin, & C.A. Peters (Eds.), *Campbell's urology* (9th ed., pp. 1922–1972). Philadelphia: Elsevier Saunders.

4

Causes of Incontinence and Identification of Risk Factors

Urinary incontinence (UI) is defined as any involuntary loss or leakage of urine. In addition to UI, associated lower urinary tract symptoms (LUTS) consisting of storage or emptying symptoms may be present and include urgency, frequency, nocturia, postvoid dribbling, nocturnal enuresis, straining to void, hesitancy, and weak urinary stream (Table 4.1) (Rosenberg et al., 2007). The term *lower urinary tract symptoms* is now being used to describe urinary symptoms in men and women of all ages (Wein & Lee, 2007). In addition to the underlying physiological origins, in many patients UI is associated with psychological, functional, environmental, and social factors. Incontinence is also a symptom that, especially in older adults, can be caused by two or more interrelated factors.

Because UI is such a prevalent problem in adults, understanding its causes is imperative. The variety of causes and types of UI has led to a number of attempts at classifying the problem. Assessment of UI in all care settings is necessary and, in the case of nursing home facilities, is required by federal regulations. To perform a thorough assessment, the clinician must understand the underlying causes of UI, be able to differentiate between transient and persistent UI, and identify those patients at risk. This chapter discusses current definitions for the different types of UI (transient and persistent), its underlying pathophysiology, and related risk factors. Emphasis is on UI in older adults. This chapter reflects the nomenclature of the International Continence Society (ICS) for lower urinary tract dysfunction (Abrams et al., 2002). Terms such as "reflex incontinence," "detrusor hyperreflexia," and "overflow incontinence" are, according to the ICS, no longer valid.

TYPES OF INCONTINENCE

There are two classifications, or types, of UI: 1) transient (i.e., reversible or acute), and 2) persistent or chronic. The distinction between transient and persistent UI is clinically important. Persistent UI refers to incontinence that continues over time and is unrelated to an acute illness.

Table 4.1   Lower urinary tract symptoms (LUTS)

Symptom	Description	Causes
Storage/Filling Symptoms		
Dysuria	Painful or difficult urination, often described by patients as "burning when passing my urine."	Irritative symptom that could be caused by urinary tract infection or urethritis, and inflammation or presence of a foreign body such as stones, or tumor.
Frequency	Voiding more than 8 times in a 24-hour period.	Usually caused by overactive bladder, increased urine output (uncontrolled DM or diabetes insipidus), reduced bladder capacity, or painful bladder syndrome.
Incontinence	Involuntary loss or leakage of urine.	Depends on type of incontinence.
Nocturia	Wakening from sleep to void more than twice a night.	Use of diuretics. Nocturnal polyuria, overactive bladder. Sleep apnea, CHF, hyperglycemia, incomplete bladder emptying, hypnotics and sedatives.
Nocturnal enuresis	Urinary loss while asleep.	Abnormal circadian secretion of antidiuretic hormone, DO, abnormal control of the micturition reflex, use of sleeping aids and hypnotics.
Pressure (bladder, suprapubic)	Feeling that the bladder is full and the urge to void will occur shortly.	Causes include incomplete bladder emptying. Discomfort that is relieved by voiding may indicate IC/PBS (see Chapter 2).
Urgency	Sudden, compelling desire to urinate that is difficult to defer. In certain cases, it can lead to urge/urgency UI if the person does not void immediately. Should not be confused with "urge" or the normal desire or need to void.	Distinctive symptom that is usually caused by DO. Other causes include infection and inflammation or presence of a foreign body such as stones or tumor.
Urinary retention	The inability or failure to empty the bladder completely. Can occur as an acute event with complaints of severe suprapubic discomfort, or chronic event that causes large amounts of urine to be retained with minor symptoms.	Chronic retention may be secondary to progressive obstruction or bladder decompensation. Acute retention may be due to recent neurological injury or may occur after pelvic surgery.

Table 4.1 *(Continued)*

Symptom	Description	Causes
Emptying/Voiding Symptoms (Outlet Obstruction)		
Hesitancy	Difficulty in starting or initiating urine stream and delay in onset of voiding or in initiating urine stream when person wants to void.	Commonly seen in men with BOO. Other causes include 1) DSD, 2) the detrusor muscle is not contracting effectively during voiding, and 3) psychological inhibition of bladder contraction (e.g., patient unable to void in public restrooms; referred to as "shy bladder").
Incomplete emptying	The sensation that urine remains in the bladder after micturition.	Causes include fluid remaining in the bladder and abnormal bladder sensations; also occurs after contractions of the bladder. Seen in men and women with BOO, neurological diseases, and pelvic organ prolapse in women.
Intermittent stream	Stopping and starting of urine stream while voiding.	BOO.
Postvoid dribbling (sometimes called "terminal dribbling" or postmicturition voiding)	Intermittent urine loss immediately after voiding. Men will complain that this occurs as they leave the toilet and women complain that it happens when rising from the toilet.	Causes include urinary retention, urethral diverticulum in women.
Slow, weak, or "poor" stream	Decreased or reduced force of urine stream when compared to previous performance (rare in women).	Causes include: 1) reduced voided volumes; 2) in men, BOO; and 3) decreased bladder contractility.
	Patients may report that they have reduced and prolonged urine flow and may complain of not emptying their bladder.	May be a sign of urinary retention.
"Sprayed" or "split" stream	Symptoms of double stream or spraying of the urinary stream.	Secondary to urethral stricture or may occur without obvious pathology.
Straining to void	Need to use intra-abdominal or muscular effort to initiate, maintain, or improve the urinary stream. Intra-abdominal pressure is increased during a Valsalva maneuver, which increases the intravesical pressure, and this can improve bladder emptying. The urinary stream may be impaired and intermittent. If straining occurs over many years, pelvic organ prolapse may occur.	BOO, poor bladder contractility.

Key: BOO = bladder outlet obstruction; CHF = congestive heart failure; DO = detrusor overactivity; DM = diabetes mellitus; DSD = detrusor–sphincter dyssynergia; IC/PBS = interstitial cystitis/painful bladder syndrome; UI = urinary incontinence.

Potentially Reversible and Treatable Causes of Incontinence

Treatable and potentially reversible conditions that can contribute to UI have been referred to as "transient or acute" incontinence. Two mnemonics—DRIP and DIAPPERS (Table 4.2A and B)—have been described and used by clinicians for many years (Kane, Ouslander, & Abrass, 1994; Resnick & Yalla, 2007). Another, developed by one of the authors (DKN), is the mnemonic PRAISED, outlined in Table 4.2C. These mnemonics prompt the clinician to search for factors that, when addressed and treated, might resolve transient or transiently exacerbated UI. Once the underlying disorder is reversed or treated, the incontinence usually disappears. Table 4.3 highlights predisposing conditions and solutions for resolving acute UI. The causes of transient UI are outlined in more detail in the following text using the mnemonic PRAISED.

P—Pharmacological/Psychological

Pharmacological causes of UI may be the result of polypharmacy (the use of multiple drugs), which is frequent among many older adults. An adult older than age 65 takes an average of four to five drugs per day. Many of these medications have UI and related LUTS as possible side effects. Thus, the more drugs an individual takes, the greater the potential for UI and LUTS. The possibility that prescription drugs may cause UI among older adults is often overlooked by the clinician prescribing them. Table 4.4 outlines medications that can alter bladder function.

Psychological causes, including chronic anxiety and learned voiding dysfunction, can cause symptoms of overactive bladder (OAB). Major depression is more prevalent in women with both UI and fecal incontinence (Melville, Delaney, Newton, & Katon, 2005; Melville, Fan, Newton, & Fenner, 2005). Screening for depression in women with UI may lead to greater adherence to treatments and better outcomes.

R—Restricted Mobility/Retention

Restricted mobility—the impaired ability to use the legs, arms, or upper or lower body—and other physical disabilities are obstacles to using the toilet and can worsen urinary urgency and frequency, leading to urge UI. Especially for older people, physical limitations present difficulties when the person attempts to self-toilet. Recovery from surgery, serious illness, and bed rest also limit physical mobility and present additional toileting challenges. Inability to independently toilet can lead to UI during some stage of a person's incapacity (Coppola et al., 2002). Environmental factors often accentuate immobility and cause a sudden onset of UI. If toilet facilities are not easily reached and accessible, if a portable bedside commode or urinal is not at hand, or if no one is near to provide assistance in getting up and walking to a bathroom, sitting on a toilet, or using a bedpan, toileting may be impossible. Physically

Table 4.2 Mnemonics for causes of incontinence

A. Acute and potentially reversible incontinence[a]

D	Dehydration
	Delirium
	Diapers
R	Retention
	Restricted mobility
I	Infection (acute symptomatic UTI)
	Inflammation (atrophic vaginitis/urethritis)
	Impaction (fecal)
P	Polypharmacy
	Polyuria (hyperglycemia, hypercalcemia—rare)

B. Transient or reversible incontinence[b]

D	Delirium, confusion, or both
I	Infection—urinary (symptomatic)
A	Atrophic urethritis or vaginitis
P	Pharmaceuticals (causing urinary symptoms)
P	Psychological, especially depression
E	Excessive urine output (e.g., from diuretic use or metabolic disorders such as CHF, hyperglycemia, elevated blood sugar)
R	Restricted or decreased mobility (musculoskeletal disorders, fear of falling, poor eyesight)
S	Stool impaction

C. Potentially reversible causes of incontinence[c]

P	Pharmaceuticals
	Psychological, causing depression, grief, anxiety
R	Restricted mobility
	Retention
A	Atrophic urethritis or vaginitis
I	Infection—urinary (symptomatic)
S	Stool impaction
E	Excessive urine output, caused by endocrine and cardiovascular disorders, excessive fluid intake, and pedal edema
D	Dehydration
	Delirium and other confusional states

[a]Adapted from Kane, R., Ouslander, J., & Abrass, I. (1994). *Essentials of clinical geriatrics* (3rd ed., p. 194). New York: McGraw-Hill.

[b]Adapted from Resnick, N.M., & Yalla, S.V. (2007). Geriatric incontinence and voiding dysfunction. In A.J. Wein, L.R. Kavoussi, A.C. Novick, A.W. Partin, & C.A. Peters (Eds.), *Campbell's urology* (9th ed., pp. 2305–2321). Philadelphia: Elsevier Saunders.

[c]Developed by Diane K. Newman.

Key: CHF = congestive heart failure; UTI = urinary tract infection.

Table 4.3   Predisposing conditions causing the development of transient urinary incontinence (UI)

Condition	Approach
Stool impaction—can cause urge UI and may induce fecal incontinence as well.	Disimpaction restores continence in most instances if this was the cause. A bowel regimen must be implemented that would include increased fiber in the diet, with use of stool softeners and laxatives if diet changes are not successful. Adequate mobility and fluid intake should also be considered.
Limited or restricted mobility—can aggravate or precipitate UI because of inability to respond promptly to the urge sensation.	Can frequently be corrected or improved by treating the underlying condition (e.g., arthritis, poor eyesight, stroke). A urinal or bedside commode and scheduled toileting often help resolve the incontinence that results from hospitalization and its environmental barriers (e.g., bed rails, restraints, and poor lighting).
Increased urine production from metabolic conditions such as hyperglycemia, hypercalcemia, Paget's disease, venous insufficiency with edema, and congestive heart failure. Many of these conditions impair sensory awareness and induce a diuresis with polyuria (e.g., hypercalcemia, hyperglycemia, and diabetes insipidus).	Treat underlying condition. Implement bladder training to assist with frequency and urgency.
Atrophic urethritis or vaginitis—can cause atrophic changes of the lower genitourinary tract.	Transvaginal estrogen replacement therapy (cream, tablets, vaginal ring).
Hysterectomy in women—can cause neuromuscular denervation.	Behavioral interventions, including pelvic floor muscle training, bladder training and urge suppression, and neuromuscular electrical stimulation.
Prostate cancer treatment (surgery and radiation) in men—disruption of sphincter mechanisms may or may not be permanent.	
Medications—See Table 4.4.	
Urinary tract infection—can cause dysuria and urgency and, in an older person, impair the ability to reach the toilet in time, causing urge UI.	Treat underlying infection. In patients who have recurrent infections, suggest acidification of urine. Cranberry juice causes urine acidification as a result of increased hippuric acid excretion, which inhibits adherence of gram-negative and gram-positive bacteria (especially *Escherichia coli*) to uroepithelial cells.

restraining long-term care (LTC) residents or homebound people by using various straps and ties, as well as geri-chairs and chemical restraints such as sedating drugs, also increases the potential of an acute episode of incontinence. Mobility problems and decreased function place an older person at risk for acute and chronic UI and are emphasized throughout this chapter. People with conditions such as rheumatoid arthritis should be assessed for toileting capabilities because they often exhibit mobility and dexterity problems that affect their ability to get to the toilet safely and on time.

Table 4.4 Medications that affect bladder function

Medication	Effect
Angiotensin-converting enzyme inhibitors (ACE inhibitors) (captopril, lisinopril, enalapril)	Antihypertensives with a common side effect of cough, which can worsen SUI.
Alpha-adrenergic receptor antagonists (prazosin, terazosin, doxazosin)	Smooth muscle relaxation of the bladder neck and proximal urethral causing SUI (mainly in women).
Alpha-adrenergic receptor agonists (pseudoephedrine and ephedrine, present in many cold and OTC preparations)	Contraction of bladder neck and proximal urethra smooth muscle leading to increased urethral resistance, causing postvoid dribbling, straining, and hesitancy in urine flow.
Anticholinergics	Urinary retention with symptoms of postvoid dribbling, straining, hesitancy in urine flow, overflow incontinence, and fecal impaction.
Antidepressants, tricyclic	Anticholinergic effect and alpha-adrenergic receptor antagonist effect causing postvoid dribbling, straining, and hesitancy in urine flow.
Psychotropics (sedatives, hypnotics)	May decrease afferent input; some may decrease bladder contractility, leading to urinary retention. Can accumulate in the elderly and cause sedation, confusion, and immobility, resulting in functional UI.
Cholinesterase inhibitors	Increase bladder contractility and may cause incontinence. Also, a theoretical interference with antimuscarinic/OAB medications by contributing to DO through increasing acetylcholine levels.
Narcotic analgesics, opioids	Decrease bladder contractility, decrease afferent input.
	Depress the central nervous system, causing sedation, confusion, and immobility, leading to urinary retention and UI. Common side effect is constipation.
Beta-adrenergic receptor antagonists (propranolol, metoprolol, atenolol)	Urinary retention (rare).
Calcium channel blockers (verapamil, diltiazem, nifedipine)	Impair bladder contractility, causing urinary retention.
	Cause constipation, leading to fecal impaction.
Diuretics (loop) (furosemide)	Rapid-acting or loop diuretics overwhelm the bladder with rapidly produced urine, resulting in frequency and urgency for up to 6 hours after ingestion.
	If clinically possible, discontinue or change therapy.
	Dosage reduction or modification can be used (e.g., flexible scheduling of rapid-acting diuretics, such as late afternoon dose, to allow accommodation to sudden increase in urine volume).
Methylxanthines (caffeine, theophylline)	Polyuria, bladder irritation.
Neuroleptics (thioridazine, chlorpromazine)	Anticholinergic effect, sedation.
Nonsteroidal anti-inflammatory drugs (NSAIDs) (gabapentin)	Can cause edema, resulting in nocturnal polyuria and exacerbating nocturia; may impair detrusor contractility.
Other: caffeine, alcohol	Act as diuretics causing rapid diuresis, leading to urgency and frequency; alcohol induces sedation.

Data from Thomas, Woodard, Rovner, and Wein (2003) and Newman (2002).

Key: DO = detrusor overactivity; OAB = overactive bladder; OTC = over the counter; SUI = stress urinary incontinence; UI = urinary incontinence.

Urinary *retention* should be considered in any person who suddenly develops UI, because it can be a cause of overflow UI. Among other causes, urinary retention can be an adverse effect of prescription and over-the-counter drugs that have anticholinergic properties (e.g., diphenhydramine [Benadryl]). Urinary retention can also be caused by bladder outlet obstruction (e.g., caused by an enlarged prostate) or from a urethral obstruction (e.g., from a urethral stricture). In men, one of the most common urological causes of incomplete bladder emptying, urgency, and frequency is obstruction due to an enlarged prostate gland. As men age, the normal prostate gland enlarges (called benign prostatic enlargement). More than 60% of 60-year-old men and more than 90% of 85-year-old men have microscopic evidence of benign prostatic hyperplasia, a slowly progressive condition that is diagnosed by histology (microscopic examination of prostate tissue). Of these men, approximately 50% will have enlargement of the prostate gland and will experience urinary symptoms. The enlarged prostate can cause obstruction at the bladder neck, with narrowing and compression of the urethra. This can lead to incomplete bladder emptying or acute urinary retention. Less serious but bothersome symptoms of frequency and nocturia can also occur. Blockage or an obstruction in the urethra secondary to urethral stricture can lead to retention or temporary overflow incontinence. Treatment depends on the cause of the obstruction and the severity of the medical condition.

A—Atrophic Urethritis or Vaginitis

Atrophic urethritis or vaginitis from a decrease in the hormone estrogen can have detrimental effect on the bladder and pelvic muscles. Vaginal pH increases, thus increasing the likelihood of bacterial growth (Palmer & Newman, 2007). The tissues of the vagina and urethra become thinner, drier, and possibly weaker and more susceptible to irritation. This deficiency weakens pelvic floor and urethral tissue, causing atrophic vaginitis/urethritis—a dry, red, and inflamed condition in a woman's vulval and urethral area. Women may complain of symptoms caused by urogenital atrophy, including atrophic vaginitis (symptoms include vaginal dryness, burning, and vaginal bleeding) and urinary symptoms (such as urinary tract infections [UTIs], frequency, urgency, and incontinence) (U.S. Preventive Services Task Force, 2005). It is also common for women with UI who manage their urine leakage by wearing perineal pads to develop vaginal yeast infections. Atrophic vaginitis/urethritis is frequently missed in frail older women, especially those living in LTC facilities or who are homebound. Usually routine pelvic examinations are neglected in these women.

Despite the relationship between hypoestrogenization and LUTS, research does not support the use of oral hormone replacement therapy to treat UI (Hendrix et al., 2005). The North American Menopause Society's 2004 position statement on the use of estrogen and progestogen in peri- and postmenopausal women recommends local (transvaginal) estrogen therapy for the treatment of vaginal dryness or atrophic vaginitis (North American Menopause Society, 2004), but it makes no recommendations regarding hormone use for urinary symptoms. However, many clinicians continue to successfully prescribe transvaginal estrogen for atrophic urogenital changes (see Chapter 9).

I—Infection

Infection, specifically a UTI, can cause a sudden onset of incontinence. Bacteria irritate the mucous membranes of the bladder wall and urethra, which can trigger urinary urgency, UI, and occasional pain or burning when urinating. UI may be an older person's only symptom of an infection. Other symptoms of UTI in the older adult include fever or increase in temperature; dysuria; change in cognition; alteration in urine color, smell, and consistency; and hematuria. A bladder dysfunction, such as OAB, may be aggravated by a UTI.

Women, particularly those in nursing homes, are at greater risk for symptomatic UTIs than are men because the female urethra is shorter in length and is closer in proximity to the anus, allowing contamination with fecal bacteria. The most common infecting organisms are Enterobacteriaceae: *Esherichia coli* (normal bacteria found in stool) is most common in women and *Proteus mirabilis* in men. UTI is also more common in older women because of changes in the urinary tract that occur with age and less efficient immune systems.

Bacteriuria, the presence of bacteria in the urine, increases with age. It is a common problem in the LTC resident because at least 25%–50% of women and 15%–40% of men in LTC facilities have significant bacteriuria (Warren, 2005). In older women, bacteriuria can be caused by estrogen deficiency. A decrease in estrogen in the pelvis and perineum will lead to atrophic changes, disappearance of colonizing lactobacilli, an increase in vaginal pH, and subsequent colonization with uropathogenic bacteria. Men with prostatitis and benign prostatic hyperplasia have a higher prevalence of UTIs. The presence of bacteria in the urine of an asymptomatic patient is known as *asymptomatic bacteriuria.* Asymptomatic bacteriuria is characterized by the presence of a significant quantity of bacteria in a urine specimen from a person without symptoms or signs of a UTI. Many residents in LTC will have bacteriuria without symptoms of infection. In LTC facilities, the use of an indwelling catheter increases the risk of bacteriuria by 60% (Tambyah, 2004). Residents in LTC with a catheter are more likely to have multidrug-resistant polymicrobic flora (e.g., *Pseudomonas aeruginosa*).

It is believed that cranberry (juice or tablets) has several therapeutic properties, including the prevention of bacterial adherence to mucosa (Gray, 2002). One trial that randomly assigned elderly women ($n = 153$) to consume 300 mL per day of a commercially available standard cranberry beverage or a specially prepared synthetic placebo drink that was indistinguishable in taste, appearance, and vitamin C content but lacked cranberry content demonstrated that cranberry beverage reduces the frequency of bacteriuria with pyuria in older women (Avorn et al., 1994). Other means of preventing UTIs are provided in "Preventing Bladder Infections" on the companion CD under Patient Education Tools.

S—Stool Impaction

Stool impaction secondary to bowel dysfunction may be a cause of an acute on-set of temporary UI. Impacted stool will distend the distal sigmoid and rectum and may inhibit sacral parasympathetic transmission, resulting in inadequate detrusor activity that leads to poor bladder emptying. In addition, constipation and fecal incontinence in women increases the risk of developing UI (Finkelstein, 2002). Constipation or fecal impaction increases pressure on the bladder, changing its position within the pelvic area and causing either UI or urinary retention. Once disimpaction occurs and normal bowel movement is restored, the person is able to void and UI can be resolved. Identification and treatment of constipation (and, under ideal circumstances, prevention through health education) are valuable services that clinicians can provide to patients (see Chapter 5).

E—Excessive Urine Output (Polyuria)

Excessuve urine output (polyuria) is seen in endocrine disorders such as hyperglycemia and in volume-expanded states that cause excessive urinary frequency and nocturia (e.g., congestive heart failure, venous insufficiency) (see Chapter 3). In hyperglycemia, the body attempts to rid itself of excess glucose through diuresis, causing increased fluid volume in the bladder. In congestive heart failure, fluid mobilization may occur at night. As diuresis occurs, the individual may have UI as a result of an excessive volume of urine, inability to wake before enuresis occurs, and inability to reach the toilet. Use of support stockings, leg elevation, and sodium restriction should be considered for patients with congestive heart failure and edema.

D—Dehydration/Delirium

Dehydration is the most common fluid and electrolyte problem among older adults. It is caused by an excessive loss of water, failure to recognize the need to increase water intake, or impaired water ingestion (Bennett, Thomas, & Riegel, 2004). Certain medications such as diuretics, laxatives, and angiotensin-converting enzyme inhibitors can affect fluid balance, contributing to dehydration (Mentes, 2006). Warning signs of dehydration include dark urine, dry mouth, decreased salivation, sunken eyes, frequent falling, weakness and fatigue, decreased urine output, headache, weight loss, muscle cramps, and increased confusion. During an illness, dehydration may mask the urge sensation. The individual's response to bladder sensations may be slow or ignored until the urge sensation becomes uncontrollable. In many cases, a UI incident is the first indication that a bladder problem exists. When hydration occurs, the UI may be resolved.

Dehydration is a significant problem in LTC residents, affecting one third of this population (Mentes, Wakefield, & Culp, 2006). The mean amount of fluid consumed by a resident averages 1,200–1,500 mL per day (Kayser-Jones,

Schell, Porter, Barbaccia, & Shaw, 1999), well below the recommended daily requirement of 30 mL/kg of body weight. Simmons, Alessi, and Schnelle (2001) found that a combination of verbal prompts to drink and offering of beverage preferences can significantly increase daily fluid consumption in LTC residents. Others recommend the use of a beverage cart in LTC (Robinson & Rosher, 2002).

Delirium and confusional states are precipitated by illness or medications and will alter a person's awareness of the urge to urinate. Delirium differs from dementia in that it has an abrupt onset and attention is affected more than memory. Mental confusion occurs frequently in people recovering from a medical illness, surgery, and the like. In older adults, acute confusion may be caused by a UTI. Once the confusion is resolved and the person is able to recognize and respond to the urinary urge sensation, UI typically resolves also.

Chronic Urinary Incontinence

The majority of people with UI have experienced problems for several years. Chronic incontinence occurs because of persistent, long-term abnormalities of the structure or function of the lower urinary tract. When UI develops in functionally independent older people, it is commonly related to a defect or dysfunction of the bladder or the bladder outlet, including

- Bladder overactivity or hypersensitivity (the bladder contracts when it should not or discomfort causes the need to void)

- Bladder underactivity (the bladder fails to contract when or as well as it should); can be related to overflow incontinence

- Urethral obstruction, usually resulting from an enlarged prostate or stricture (narrowing of the urethra); can be related to overflow incontinence

- Urethral incompetence, wherein the resistance is too low, resulting in urine leakage

The most common types of UI are: stress, urgency, or mixed symptomatology of stress and urgency. Chronic UI is classified into five groups: stress incontinence, urgency incontinence, mixed incontinence, overflow incontinence, and functional incontinence (Table 4.5). Common diagnoses associated with persistent UI are outlined in Table 4.6. The symptomatology, underlying pathophysiology, and incidence of the various types of chronic UI are discussed in the following text.

Stress Urinary Incontinence

Does your patient report leakage of small amounts of urine with any type of physical effort or when coughing or sneezing, while playing tennis, or while golfing? Have you ever heard someone say, "I laughed so hard I wet my pants"?

Table 4.5   Summary of classifications of persistent urinary incontinence

Types	Description
Stress (or effort) incontinence	Small amount of urine leakage occurs with coughing, laughing, sneezing, physical activities, exercise, or any action that increases intra-abdominal pressure.
Urgency (or urge) incontinence with overactive bladder	Sudden intense urge to pass urine and the inability to delay voiding after sensation of bladder fullness (urge) is perceived. Moderate to large amounts of urine leakage that usually occurs on the way to the bathroom; urgency and frequent urination.
Mixed incontinence	A combination of stress and urge symptoms.
Overflow incontinence (incontinence with high postvoid residuals)	Sudden overflow of urine when pressure inside the bladder exceeds the pressure of a urethral obstruction. Symptoms include small, frequent voiding; postvoid dribbling; hesitancy; and straining to void.
Functional incontinence	Urine loss due to inability to reach bathroom because of physical disabilities or psychological problems that do not allow self-toileting.

Stress UI (SUI), referred to as effort-related UI or sphincteric UI, is the involuntary leakage of urine with effort or physical exertion, or on sneezing or coughing, as a result of insufficient urethral closure (Abrams et al., 2002). SUI affects approximately 38% of adult women in the United States. Increased intra-abdominal pressure causes an increase in total bladder pressure and results in urine loss when bladder pressure exceeds urethral pressure. Urine escapes because the bladder outlet is inadequate and the urethra does not stay closed tightly during the increases in bladder pressure (Figure 4.1). SUI usually produces only drops or small amounts of urine leakage and may not be a daily occurrence. However, severity of leakage may change, depending on the specific activities that cause the urine loss. Minimal SUI can occur with relatively vigorous activities: coughing, laughing, sneezing, and aerobic exercises. Moderate SUI occurs with activities such as rising from a sitting to standing position, swinging a golf club, or walking across a room. Severe SUI can occur with changing positions (rising from a chair) or just by standing. The patient may also complain that urine loss occurs when getting out of bed in the morning as the abdominal muscles push down on the bladder (Newman, 2003). In rare cases, patients are unable to link urine leakage to any given activity. Usually the patient will start a pattern of frequent urination (usually referred to as "defensive voiding") because an SUI episode is more likely to occur with a full bladder.

Causes of SUI   In SUI, the problem lies with a damaged or weakened urethra, urethral sphincter mechanism, and nerves or connective tissue within

Table 4.6   Common diagnoses and definition of terms for bladder and urethral dysfunctions

Diagnosis	Definition
Underactive bladder (sometimes referred to as hypoactive or hypocontractile bladder)	A bladder that is not able to contract and empty properly, usually because of damage to the nerves that control the bladder or to the bladder smooth muscle. As a result, the bladder fills with urine and remains full, and excess urine that the bladder cannot accommodate leads to urine dribbling through the urethra, causing overflow incontinence.
Neurogenic detrusor overactivity [NDO] (formerly detrusor hyperreflexia)	Overactivity of the bladder muscle causing uncontrolled and involuntary bladder contractions; seen in neurological lesions above the sacral spinal cord.
Detrusor areflexia	Inability of the detrusor muscle to contract (referred to as noncontractile) because of abnormality of neural control, seen in spinal shock or in lesions above the brain stem. Urinary retention generally occurs.
Detrusor–sphincter dyssynergia (DSD)	Bladder outlet dysfunction that causes a lack of coordination between the bladder and the striated sphincter. The sphincter contracts simultaneously with bladder contraction, clamping the urethra closed and interfering with the flow of urine. The bladder attempts to empty against a closed sphincter. Urinary retention can occur. Very high bladder pressures may be generated, which predisposes these individuals to reflux of urine into the ureters and ultimately to kidney damage.
Detrusor hyperactivity with impaired bladder contractility (DHIC)	A condition characterized by frequent but ineffective involuntary detrusor contractions. A person either is unable to empty the bladder completely or can empty the bladder completely only with straining. This abnormality of the bladder was first diagnosed in nursing home residents.
Genuine stress urinary incontinence (SUI)	Incontinence associated with hypermobility of the bladder outlet secondary to poor pelvic support. Mild to moderate SUI occurs with increases in intra-abdominal pressure.
Intrinsic urethral (sphincter) deficiency (ISD) (formerly type III SUI)	Severe SUI in which there is a very poorly functioning bladder neck and proximal urethra at rest. Many times this is referred to as "gravitational" urinary incontinence that worsens when standing. Also referred to as "stovepipe" urethra. Seen in both men and women.

the pelvic floor, or some combination of these. There is reduced outflow resistance because the urethra cannot remain closed under increases in intra-abdominal pressure. It is the urethral support rather than urethral position that is crucial for maintaining continence. In women, the urethra lies in a position where it can be compressed against a supporting hammock consisting

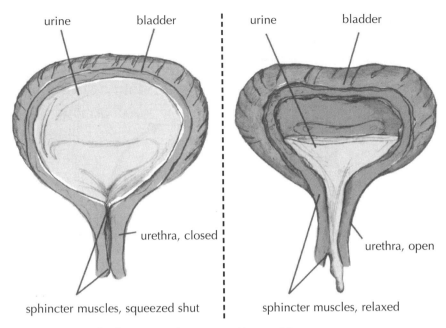

urine   bladder   urine   bladder

urethra, closed   urethra, open

sphincter muscles, squeezed shut   sphincter muscles, relaxed

Figure 4.1.   Weak sphincter muscles as seen with stress UI.

of the connective tissue layer of the anterior vaginal wall and suspension structures connecting to either levator ani muscle. In the continent woman, the bladder base and proximal urethra are supported by endopelvic fascia and the pelvic floor muscles (the levator ani) (see Chapter 3). When faced with a precipitous rise in abdominal pressure, these supportive structures act as a "backboard," preventing the urethra from prolapsing into the vaginal vault while spontaneously complementing urethral closure and continence. Laxity of the pelvic floor muscles or tearing of the endopelvic fascia results in distortion of the proximal urethra and loss of the additional active closure afforded by the backboard.

In a person with a firm supporting layer, the urethra is compressed by abdominal pressure against pelvic fascia in much the same way one can stop the flow of the garden hose by stepping on it against an underlying concrete path (Figure 4.2). The loss of support causes descent of the bladder neck, with loss of bladder neck closure (Figure 4.3). Pelvic descent is thought to create sphincter incompetence by distorting the anatomy of the bladder base and proximal urethra (Abrams, Artibani, Cardozo, Khoury, & Wein, 2005).

Weakness of the muscular elements of the sphincter mechanism may arise from a variety of factors that compromise pelvic floor muscle strength or the integrity of the endopelvic fascia. Potential risk factors include pregnancy, vaginal delivery, extensive abdominopelvic surgery, obesity, genetic factors, and menopausal status. Although these factors may not lead to descent of the bladder base and urethra, they do compromise muscle tone within the sphincter mechanism, predisposing the woman to SUI when abdominal

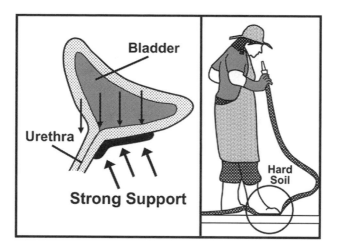

Figure 4.2. Strong urethral support. (Adapted from Abrams, P., Artibani, W., Cardozo, L., Khoury, S., & Wein, A. (2005). *Clinical manual of incontinence in women*. Paris: Health Publications, Ltd.; reprinted by permission.) (Courtesy of Robin Noel.)

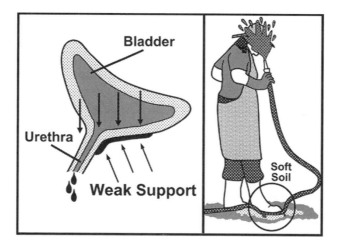

Figure 4.3. Weak urethral support. (Adapted from Abrams, P., Artibani, W., Cardozo, L., Khoury, S., & Wein, A. (2005). *Clinical manual of incontinence in women*. Paris: Health Publications, Ltd.; reprinted by permission.) (Courtesy of Robin Noel.)

pressures rise. Because of the relationship between pelvic descent, weakness of the pelvic floor muscles, and sphincter incompetence, it is possible to mistakenly assume that SUI is exclusively the result of an anatomic problem, and that correction of SUI will be ensured by surgical repair of prolapse. Considering SUI to be a purely anatomic defect ignores issues related to incompetence of the muscular elements of the sphincter mechanism, and to the role of the central nervous system and the importance of neuromodulators in lower urinary tract function (Gray, 2004).

SUI is often associated with multiparity (having delivered a child more than once) or direct anatomic damage to the urethral sphincter, which may lead to severe, continuous leakage. Childbearing stretches and relaxes a woman's pelvic floor musculature and may damage nerves in the pelvic area and tissue in the bladder's neck. As many as 35% of childbearing women experience postpartum SUI for 6–12 months after delivery.

A decline in estrogen levels at menopause and pelvic organ prolapse are associated with SUI in middle-aged women. A woman's estrogen level lowers after menopause and drops dramatically when the ovaries and uterus are removed in a hysterectomy. This further weakens pelvic floor and vaginal area muscles and tissues, increasing the likelihood of SUI. Women with pelvic organ prolapse will complain of a "fallen uterus," one that has shifted within the abdominal cavity. The position of the uterus, bladder, and bladder neck within the abdomen has a direct effect on the control of urine. Pelvic floor muscle exercises can be used to strengthen the pelvic muscles to help prevent or improve pelvic organ prolapse and resulting SUI (see Chapter 8). However, it is estimated that at least 50% of young women are unable to identify the correct muscle for these exercises (Bump, Hurt, Fantl, & Wyman, 1991).

Sphincteric incontinence in men is related to intrinsic sphincter dysfunction. It can be seen after prostatectomy and transurethral resection of the prostate, after pelvic trauma, or in men with certain neurological diseases. Approximately 5%–15% of men experience permanent, bothersome SUI after prostate cancer surgery. The removal of the prostate during prostatectomy eliminates the sphincter action of the bladder neck and exposes the external urethral sphincter to the full task of maintaining continence. In these men, urine leakage occurs mostly after exercise or physical exertion. Fatigue of the striated muscle of the pelvic floor leads to increased loss of urine during the second half of the day. Often UI is temporary, but sometimes it is a prolonged condition that causes anxiety and disruption in a man's life.

Urgency or Urge Urinary Incontinence

Does your patient complain about such a "strong urge" that he or she rushes and leaks on the way to the bathroom? Have you ever heard a patient say, "When I gotta go, I gotta go" or "I lose it every time I reached my front door or go to open my garage door"?

Urge UI, now referred to as urgency UI (UUI), is involuntary urine leakage accompanied by or immediately preceded by urgency—a strong, sudden, and uncontrollable desire to urinate as a result of detrusor muscle overactivity, or an overactive bladder (OAB) (Abrams et al., 2005). OAB is also known as "urgency-frequency" syndrome. Approximately one third of patients with OAB, a symptom complex including urgency generally with daytime and nighttime frequency, experience UUI (Abrams et al., 2002). An additional symptom is nocturia, or voiding more than two times per night. Nocturia is associated

with a profound decrease in quality of life, causes a range of sleep disturbances, and adversely affects daytime functioning. Detrusor overactivity (DO)
refers to demonstrable involuntary detrusor contractions during urodynamics
studies (see Chapter 6). DO can be caused by neurological conditions, termed
neurogenic detrusor overactivity. DO is described as "idiopathic" when there is
no such association. Many "normal" individuals (no symptoms of OAB) will
demonstrate DO on a urodynamic study.

UUI occurs when the detrusor muscle of the bladder involuntarily contracts during bladder filling, forcing urine through the urethra. Ordinarily,
when a person feels the urge to urinate, a detrusor contraction can be inhibited voluntarily through cortical control or contraction of pelvic floor muscles. The patient with UUI senses an urgent need to void, but is unable either
to inhibit detrusor contraction or to prevent loss of urine by adequate closure
of the outlet. Patients will complain that the urine just "gushes" out (Newman
& Giovanni, 2002). The amount of urine lost may be large (greater than 100
mL) because the bladder may empty completely. The volume of urine lost
with urinary "accidents" varies tremendously and does not seem to be dependent on bladder volume.

UUI is the most common pattern of UI in older people and is the most
common type of UI encountered among residents in LTC facilities. In these individuals, UI is often associated with impaired cognitive or physical function
or both. In many elderly patients, it is frequently difficult to determine
whether DO or the functional disability is the predominant cause of the UI
(Resnick & Yalla, 2007).

Causes of UUI and OAB   A common cause of UUI and OAB is a neurological disease or injury (multiple sclerosis [MS], spinal cord injury, cerebrovascular accident, Parkinson's disease) that impairs the normal ability to inhibit
the micturition reflex. Changes in the smooth bladder itself (myogenic) may
also result in OAB through alterations in innervation and excitability resulting in an increase in spontaneous activity and the ability of such activity to
spread from cell to cell, setting up pockets of "micromotion." OAB and UUI
may also be due to increased afferent (sensory) activity or increased sensitivity of the detrusor to acetylcholine. OAB with UUI can also be idiopathic,
which means it has no defined cause (Wein & Rackley, 2006).

Common Triggers   Urinary urgency or leakage can be triggered by certain
events, which is probably due to a conditioned reflex—a reflex that gradually
developed in the body by the frequent repetition of a specific stimulus (e.g.,
a person who burns a finger when touching a hot stove will not touch it
again). A very common trigger is "key-in-the-lock" or "garage door syndrome," terms that characterize the development of a sudden urge to urinate,
with subsequent leakage, when arriving home. If approaching the door to a
house or opening a garage door continues to cause urgency and UI, then the
person will subconsciously begin to associate putting the key in the lock or

opening the garage door with the urge to void, and eventually UUI will happen uncontrollably. Other triggers include urine leakage in response to the sound of running water, washing dishes or clothes, placing hands in warm water, anxiety, pulling down clothes to void, seeing a bathroom sign, or exposure to cold. A person may be aware of the need to urinate and yet cannot seem to get to the toilet before having an incontinence episode. People with OAB and UUI will develop certain behaviors such as "toilet mapping," which involves locating toilets in advance of travel or only visiting places where they know the toilet location. Many may frequent the web site http://www.the bathroomdiaries.com before traveling.

Mixed Incontinence

A large number of people with UI report a combination of both SUI and UUI symptoms, termed *mixed UI* (MUI), consisting of involuntary leakage with both urgency and exertion, effort, sneezing, or coughing. Together, these three types of UI (SUI, UUI, MUI) account for more than 80% of UI in community-dwelling older adults. A common picture is the elderly woman who has been experiencing SUI since her last child was born and is now having UUI episodes as well, secondary to decreased mobility (see Functional Urinary Incontinence later).

Overflow Urinary Incontinence

> *Does your patient complain about urine "dribbling," or a feeling of "bladder fullness," or that the bladder is never completely empty?*

The cause of urine "dribbling" may be overflow UI, which is urine leakage associated with either chronic or acute urinary retention. Although "overflow UI" is often used in clinical practice, overflow is not a symptom or condition, and the International Continence Society (ICS) believes this term may be misleading and has recommended against its use (Abrams et al., 2002). They recommended the use of UUI, SUI, or MUI with "high postvoid residual." Types of overflow UI are usually characterized by the associated pathophysiology causing elevated postvoid residuals. A common complaint is continual urine leakage from a constantly overdistended bladder. When toileting, the individual may have difficulty starting the urine stream and, once started, the stream is weak and postmicturition dribble is common. People with overflow UI often complain that they feel as though their bladder never empties. However, some individuals with overflow UI may not be aware that they are leaking urine because the sensation of bladder fullness is diminished and the stream of urine is weak. This is particularly likely to occur at night when the patient is less likely to inhibit urinary leakage. Overflow incontinence has been termed *paradoxical incontinence* because it often can be cured by relief of bladder outlet obstruction.

Causes of Overflow UI Overflow UI can occur from outflow obstruction secondary to a narrowed or obstructed urethra from a prolapsed pelvic organ, a stricture, an enlarged prostate, chronic constipation, or neurological disease. An enlarged and obstructing prostate can cause overflow UI. The prostate blocks the urethra and the bladder does not empty completely during voiding. The bladder may be underactive or acontractile secondary to drugs, fecal impaction, neurological conditions (i.e., diabetic neuropathy, low spinal cord injury), or radical pelvic surgery. Overflow UI can be precipitated by the use of over-the-counter cold remedies that cause the urethral sphincter to constrict and close. Urethral obstruction with subsequent overflow UI is associated with symptoms of hesitancy, poor or weak urinary stream, and postmicturition dribble. Men report straining while urinating, with small volumes voided, dribbling small amounts of urine all day. They have difficulty starting the urine stream, and once started, the stream is weak. These individuals complain that they feel like their bladders never empty completely. Diabetes and drugs such as narcotics, antidepressants, and smooth muscle relaxants may increase the capacity of the bladder, but they dull the sensation of the need to urinate. Trauma to the spinal cord affects the central nervous system, impairing the ability to control the urinary cycle. Peripheral neuropathy reduces the bladder's ability to contract and release stored urine. All of these problems can cause urinary retention (incomplete bladder emptying) and overflow UI.

Outlet obstruction is rare in women but can occur as a complication of an anti-incontinence operation. Other causes of obstruction in women are severe pelvic prolapse, suprasacral spinal cord injuries, MS, and detrusor–external sphincter dyssynergia, in which the sphincter muscle inappropriately involuntarily contacts rather than relaxes when the detrusor contracts.

Functional Urinary Incontinence

> *Have you had a patient's spouse, daughter, or son complain to you about the loved one's poor toileting habits or inability to get to the toilet?*

Functional UI involves a person's inability or unwillingness to use toilet facilities because of decreased mental awareness, decrease in or loss of mobility, or personal unwillingness to go to the toilet (DuBeau, 2006). The diagnosis of functional UI is problematic because it implies a normal lower urinary tract, which may not be present in older individuals. Functional UI is rarely seen in the absence of bladder or neurological abnormality, and assigning this diagnosis may result in failure to appropriately investigate the patient's condition, leading to misdiagnosis (Fonda et al., 2005). Functional UI can exist with UUI, SUI, or MUI. Patients will have UUI with a functional component, which may be decreased mobility.

Functional UI is a significant problem in frail, elderly patients who are dependent on others for toileting. Functional UI in home care has been related to the use of physical restraints and environmental barriers (Landi et al., 2003).

More than 25% of UI cases found in acute care hospitals and LTC facilities have some component of decrease in function or mobility. Some hospitals have very poor and inconvenient bathroom facilities. Staffing problems, as well as Medicare and insurance company policies regarding length of hospitalization and medical treatment, do not place an activity such as toileting, which is an activity of daily living, as a high priority. LTC facilities may manage UI with absorbent products such as adult briefs. Individual patient needs and assessment of voiding patterns and toileting habits are not usually part of the patient assessment process in LTC facilities. However, it is important to remember that many people who suffer from impaired cognitive function or mobility are not incontinent.

Common factors contributing to functional incontinence include

- Restricted mobility or dexterity—difficulty in getting to the bathroom or in toileting, or inability to do so, because of physical disability

- Environmental barriers—inconvenience of bathroom or toilet equipment, stairs, lack of handrails, and narrow doorways that do not accommodate wheelchairs or walkers

- Mental and psychosocial disability—lack of awareness of the need to urinate, confusion over the location of the bathroom, or individual toileting habits that cause a person to be completely unaware of the need to urinate

- Drugs that affect awareness, mobility, or dexterity

Neurogenic Bladder

Neurogenic bladder, also known as neurogenic bladder dysfunction or neurogenic lower urinary tract dysfunction, is a general term referring to bladder or voiding dysfunction resulting from interrupted innervation caused by a lesion or disease of the central or peripheral nervous system (Figure 4.4). It represents one of the most common problems in individuals with a variety of neurological impairments (Wyndaele et al., 2005). Causes of neurogenic lower urinary tract dysfunctions include, but are not limited to, traumatic and nontraumatic lesions of the spinal cord, demyelinating disease, diabetes mellitus, cerebral palsy, spina bifida, MS, human immunodeficiency virus infection, systemic lupus erythematosus, and Guillain-Barré syndrome. Neurologic disorders may affect the central or peripheral nervous system. Chapter 3 reviews the neurophysiology of the bladder in more detail. The type of bladder dysfunction that occurs from the neurologic disease depends on which area of the central nervous system is affected. Urine leakage can occur without a warning sensation and is often referred to as "unconscious or reflex UI" (Fantl et al., 1996). These patients do not have the urge sensation to urinate when the bladder contracts involuntarily, causing UI.

All neurogenic voiding disorders may be classified in a functional manner as to whether they affect filling/storage, emptying/voiding, or both. Neu-

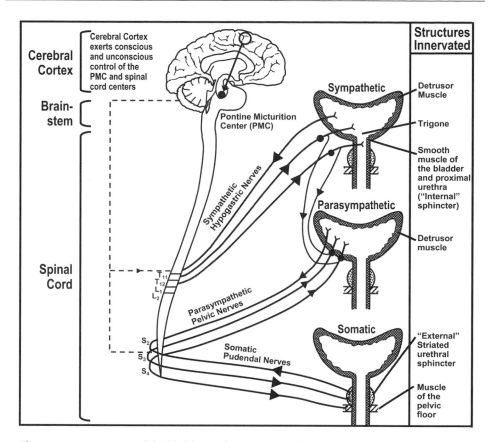

Figure 4.4.   Innervation of the bladder, urethra, and pelvic floor. (Courtesy of Robin Noel.)

rogenic problems generally manifest clinically as either UI (failure to store) or urinary retention (failure to empty) or a combination of both. Table 4.7 reviews the pathophysiology of bladder dysfunction associated with neurologic diseases and site of the injury. If the injury is complete, patients will have both sensory and motor loss; patients with an incomplete injury usually have abnormal motor function but retain sensation.

A flaccid or atonic bladder, which is frequently seen after an acute spinal cord injury, is a result of the phenomenon of spinal shock (a period of decreased excitability of spinal cord segments above and below the lesion). During the stage of spinal shock, which may persist for several weeks to several months after injury, all reflex activity below the level of injury ceases. The bladder becomes acontractile and areflexic. Because the detrusor fails to contract in response to even high levels of filling, the result is acute urinary retention. As spinal shock subsides, reflex detrusor function should return, except when the actual site of the injury involves the S2–S4 segments or cauda equina. When the spinal reflex is permanently disrupted by an injury to this area, the atonic or flaccid bladder persists, resulting in chronic urinary reten-

Table 4.7 Pathophysiology of bladder dysfunction associated with neurologic diseases

Level of lesion/injury	Neurologic disease	Pathophysiology	Dysfunction	Symptoms
Spinal shock	Traumatic SCI	Complete interruption of sensory and motor pathways between sacral spinal cord and brain stem (Wein & Moy, 2007).	No motor or sensory activity below the level of the lesion.	Urinary retention.
Suprapontine lesions (lesions above the brain stem, in the cerebral cortex)	Dementia Parkinson's disease CVA Head injury Brain tumor Cerebral palsy Multiple system atrophy	Often, bladder sensation is retained so that urgency is felt, but the important inhibiting signal is weak or absent, and urgency and UUI can result. This condition is identical to DO, and represents involuntary bladder contractions of neurogenic or idiopathic origin. Delayed sensation may reduce cortical awareness and thus inhibition, and permit incontinence despite a normal lower urinary tract (Mostwin, 2006).	General: NDO without DSD. Specific conditions: Focal brain lesion from tumor and CVA—20%–50% NDO, decreased sensation, impaired voluntary control. Parkinson's disease—35%–70% have NDO, delay in striated sphincter relaxation (bradykinesia—relaxes and contracts slowly). MS—34%–99% have NDO, 30%–65% have coexistent NDO and DSD, and 12%–38% have areflexia or impaired detrusor contractility. Cerebral palsy—NDO, 25% DSD.	Sensation may be deficient or delayed. Urinary frequency, urgency, UUI, and in some cases uninhibited voiding occur, and bladder emptying is generally adequate.

Location	Causes	Description	Effect on bladder	Symptoms
Suprasacral spinal cord lesions (above the S2–S4 segments)	Traumatic spinal cord injury—initially spinal shock; Multiple sclerosis; Compression (e.g. tumors, cervical spondolysis); Myelitis; Spina bifida	In this condition, the voiding reflex is intact but overactive because the normal inhibiting influence of the cerebral centers is blocked at the level of the spinal lesion. Voiding will occur frequently and uncontrollably as a result of bladder contraction and a lack of sensation. The bladder capacity is decreased. The strength of detrusor contractions may be inadequate to promote complete emptying.	Overactive bladder with uncoordinated external sphincter (DSD) and uncoordinated bladder neck if above T_6.	Sensory impairment. Urinary retention.
Sacral spinal cord and peripheral nerve lesions	Sacral agenesis; Pelvic surgery; Childbirth injury; Diabetes mellitus	Diseases of the peripheral nervous system (DM) affect local nerve supply to the bladder, urethra, and pelvic floor muscles (both sensory and motor pathways). Motor damage leads to inefficient bladder emptying, and overflow UI can develop. Childbirth injury and pelvic surgery can disrupt peripheral nerves.	DO or areflexia of the detrusor may be combined. Disc disease—detrusor areflexia is common. Diabetes—5%–59% DO, impaired bladder sensation resulting in detrusor overdistention and decompensation.	Urinary frequency, urgency, UUI. Urinary retention.

Data from Wein and Moy (2007) and Wein (2007).
Key: CVA = cerebrovascular accident; DM = diabetes mellitus; DO = detrusor overactivity; DSD = detrusor–sphincter dyssnergia; NDO = neurogenic detrusor overactivity; SCI = spinal cord injury; UUI = urgency urinary incontinence.

tion. Overflow UI may occur if retention is not periodically relieved through intermittent catheterization. SUI may also be seen when injury to the sacral cord and nerves coming from this area results in a flaccid external sphincter.

People with MS may also experience urinary retention as a result of flaccid bladder. Whether this condition is temporary or chronic depends on the extent to which remyelination occurs. The most common dysfunction seen in MS is involuntary bladder contractions with sensation, and UUI if these cannot be suppressed.

IDENTIFYING INDIVIDUALS AT RISK

Evidence has been growing concerning the risk factors associated with developing UI (Landefeld et al., 2008). A person's UI and OAB may be directly connected to defined internal and external predispositions. These predispositions, or risk factors, affect the anatomy and physiology of the lower urinary tract. Studies have tried to evaluate the risk factors for UI. Daily UI episodes have been associated with increasing age, childbirth and parity, pelvic surgery (e.g., hysterectomy), higher body mass index (BMI), smoking, diabetes, chronic obstructive pulmonary disease (e.g., asthma, emphysema), and poor overall health (Brown, Seeley, Fong, Ensrud, & Grady, 1996; Danforth et al., 2006; Sampselle, Harlow, Skurnick, Brubaker, & Bondarenko, 2002). Risk determinants for OAB without UI include advanced age and obesity but otherwise have not been clearly elucidated. Documented risk factors associated with UI are wide ranging and are described in the following text.

Advancing Age

There is consistent evidence that the frequency of UI, primarily UUI, increases with age, especially in women. Pelvic floor muscle relaxation accelerates rapidly after menopause and may progress with aging in general. This relaxation of the pelvic floor causes prolapse of pelvic organs in women. SUI is believed to be more common in women ages 45–54 years, whereas UUI increases with age between 35 and 64 years. Melville, Fan, and colleagues (2005) conducted a population-based, age-stratified postal survey of 6,000 women between 30 and 90 years of age who were enrolled in a large health maintenance organization in Washington State. The prevalence of UI increased with age (28% for respondents between 30 and 39 years compared with 55% for those between 80 and 90 years). Among all respondents, 9% reported slight UI, 15% reported moderate UI, 18% reported severe UI, and 58% reported no UI. The prevalence of severe UI increased markedly with age because only 8% of women between 30 and 39 years reported severe incontinence compared with 33% of those between 80 and 90 years. The Urologic Diseases in America Project on UI in men (Stothers, Thom, & Calhoun, 2005) found that

17% of men older than 60 years have UI, noting a strong trend toward an increasing prevalence with increasing age. Although aging is associated with increasing incidence and severity of UI, UI is not an inevitable consequence of aging, and elderly patients deserve UI evaluation and treatment.

Sex and Race

Throughout their life spans, women are twice as likely to develop UI as men. It has been suggested that Caucasian women have a shorter urethra, weaker pelvic floor muscles, and a lower bladder neck than African American women, thus making them more likely to have stress incontinence (Duong & Korn, 2001). However, parity and socioeconomic factors may also contribute to the difference. In relationship to race, the prevalence of SUI is thought to be significantly lower in black women than in white, Hispanic, and Asian women (Duong & Korn, 2001). African American women, especially older women, are at significant risk for developing both UUI and MUI. This difference may be related to greater urethral volume and higher urethral closure pressure during a pelvic muscle contraction in black women (Graham & Mallett, 2001; Howard, DeLancey, Tunn, & Ashton-Miller, 2000). There are no data on the relationship between race and UI or OAB in men.

Pregnancy and Childbirth

Over the past three decades, an expanding body of literature has supported the notion that pregnancy and childbirth, even uncomplicated vaginal delivery, has an effect on the pelvic nerves, anal sphincter, and pelvic floor muscles (Thornton & Lubowski, 2006). Rates of SUI reported in the literature range from 20% to 73% during pregnancy and 6% to 31% postpartum (Mason, Glenn, Walton, & Appleton, 1999; Viktrup, 2002; Wilson, Herbison, & Herbison, 1996). Antenatal UI increases the risk of postpartum UI, which increases the risk of long-term chronic UI. The incidence of incontinence at 9 weeks postpartum has been reported as 21% for spontaneous and 36% for forceps delivery (Meyer, Schreyer, DeGrandi, & Hohfield, 1998). The Norwegian Mother and Child Cohort Study (MoBa) is a large population-based study that has reported on women during pregnancy, with several years of follow-up (Wesnes, Rortveit, Bø, & Hunskaar, 2007). The authors noted that UI was reported by 11,294 women (26.2%) before pregnancy. In week 30 UI was reported by 58% of women. SUI was the most common type of incontinence in week 30 of pregnancy, experienced by 31% of nulliparous and 42% of parous women. SUI and MUI were three times more common among parous women as compared with nulliparous women.

Onset of SUI during the first pregnancy or puerperal period carries an increased risk of long-lasting symptoms. Overall, 30% of women will develop SUI within 5 years after their first vaginal delivery, and in many of these women, symptoms persist. Viktrup, Rortveit, and Lose (2006) conducted a longitudinal cohort study of 241 women who answered validated questions about SUI after their first delivery and 12 years later. Twelve years after their first delivery, the prevalence of SUI was 42% (102 of 241 women), and the 12-year incidence was 30% (44 of 146 women). In this study, a cesarean section during the first delivery was significantly associated with a lower risk of incontinence. Other obstetric factors were not significantly associated with the risk of incontinence 12 years later. Patients who were overweight before their first pregnancy were at increased risk. Age at the time of pregnancy and delivery also increases a woman's risk. Rortveit and Hunskaar (2006) reported that the prevalence of any UI was significantly higher among women who had their first delivery after the age of 25. However, in the Study of Women's Health Across the Nation (SWAN) by Waetjen and colleagues (2007), parity was a factor in women in the reproductive years, whereas UI that develops in midlife was more related to other factors (e.g., obesity).

Pregnancy, vaginal delivery, and episiotomy are the most common precipitating events contributing to SUI in women. Bladder dysfunction may become more severe with each additional pregnancy. Vaginal birth, especially with high fetal weight or when the second stage of labor is protracted, imposes a risk of pressure, stretch, and shearing damage to the muscles and denervation of pelvic nerves (Sampselle & Hines, 1999; van Kessel, Reid, Newton, Meier, & Lentz, 2001). Damage sustained from vaginal delivery occurs primarily during the second stage of labor. During the second stage of labor, the infant's head puts the pelvic floor muscles under considerable stretch as the mother times contractions of the abdominal wall and respiratory diaphragm muscles with uterine contraction to drive the fetal head through the levator hiatus (Ashton-Miller & Delancey, 2007). When the baby's head encounters the muscular floor of the pelvis, the mechanical process of extension of the head through the urogenital opening, along with further descent of the baby, causes significant stretching and compression of the nerves to the urethrovesical junction and levator ani muscles (Dietz & Bennett, 2003). Further extension of the baby's head through the urogenital opening causes distention of the pubococcygeus muscle, with similar soft tissue trauma to muscle and nerves, as well as breaks in the adjacent endopelvic fascia that supports the urethra.

Disruption of the sphincter complex is associated with diminished sphincter pressures, and defects occur more frequently in women who have undergone forceps delivery, anal sphincter laceration, and episiotomy (Arya, Jackson, Myers, & Verma, 2001; Dietz & Bennett, 2003; Kearney, Miller, Ashton-Miller, & DeLancey, 2006). Women with clinically recognized anal sphincter tears are more than twice as likely to report postpartum fecal incontinence as women without tears. The injury is caused by descent of the pudendal nerve as it emerges from its fixed site. The pudendal nerve can be stretched by as much as 20% of its length during second-stage labor, which is substantial as only 12% stretch is necessary to damage a nerve. It results in a "pudendal neuropathy" and is also seen in women who have rectal prolapse, chronic straining at stool, and pelvic floor descent. Other pregnancy-related risk factors for UI in women include undergoing the first delivery at an older age, giving birth to a baby weighing over 4 kg (8.8 lb), protracted delivery, and delivering a baby who is in the occiput posterior position (Glazener et al., 2006; Kearney et al., 2006). Vaginal delivery can also cause neuromuscular damage to the pelvic muscles. Traction injury to the pudendal nerve commonly accompanies obstetric sphincter laceration and contributes to UI and fecal incontinence (Abramov et al., 2005).

Most women who have only borne one child and who develop UI in the immediate postpartum period usually regain continence within 3 months. However, it has been suggested that continence function regained in the first postpartum period declines yearly as a result of additional trauma (e.g., additional births), the effects of aging, or the loss of estrogen following menopause.

Controversy currently exists over whether delivery by cesarean section prevents SUI (MacAuthur et al., 2006; Weber, 2007). In the United States, 29.1% of births in 2004 were cesarean, an increase of 40.6% over the 1996 rate of 20.7% (Hamilton, Martin, & Sutton, 2003; Weber, 2007). This increase in cesarean deliveries is a result of many factors: morbid fear of childbirth (tokophobia), breech presentation, more than one previous cesarean section, and physician or patient convenience (Devendra & Arulkumaran, 2003; Land, Parry, Rane, & Wilson, 2001; Quinlivan, Petersen, & Nichols, 1999). The most common reason for choosing elective cesarean delivery, cited by 88% of British obstetricians (Devendra & Arulkumaran, 2003; Land et al., 2001), is protection of the pelvic floor in the hope of preventing future incontinence and related morbidities, such as pelvic organ prolapse. Cesarean delivery may also reduce the risk of subsequent pelvic floor surgery 30 years after delivery (Uma, Libby, & Murphy, 2005).

Systematic review of the literature noted that short-term occurrence of any degree of postpartum SUI is reduced with cesarean section but severe symptoms are equivalent by mode of delivery (Press, Klein, Kaczorowski, Liston, & von Dadelszen, 2007). In a large community-based study of 15,307 Norwegian women, those who had delivered only vaginally had an 8.4% higher prevalence of UI than women who delivered by cesarean section only (Rortveit, Daltveit, Hannestad, & Hunskaar, 2003). A study in twins showed that women delivering vaginally demonstrated a significantly higher likelihood of SUI than their biological counterparts who delivered by cesarean section (Goldberg et al., 2005). This impact of the birth mode was strong enough to nullify the effect of parity. However, among women who had successive elective cesarean deliveries (and no vaginal births), highly significant differences in SUI compared with women who had vaginal births occurred only with the first delivery; protection was only marginally significant with the second, and was lost with three or more deliveries (Wilson et al., 1996).

Clinicians caring for women during pregnancy and postpartum need to address this problem proactively by readily discussing SUI and the treatment options available, and not wait for the woman to raise the issue. Moreover, childbearing women should be taught pelvic floor muscle exercises because there is evidence-based research showing their effectiveness in preventing childbirth-related UI (Newman et al., 2005). Clinicians need to remember that cesarean section is a surgical procedure, and this mode of delivery also carries risks and associated complications.

Menopause

With menopause, the depletion of estrogen hormone receptors found in the lower urinary tract of women contributes to UI (see Chapter 3). Estrogen depletion increases the atrophy rate of the muscosal tissue that lines the urethra and vagina (Ulmsten, 1995). This deterioration and a decline in mucus production within the urethra weaken the urethra's ability to maintain a tight seal, especially when intra-abdominal pressure increases with a Valsalva maneuver. Symptoms of urgency, frequency, and dysuria may also occur, but the exact cause and connection to the estrogen depletion is as yet unknown.

Chronic, Treatable Conditions That Can Cause UI and Other LUTS

Chronic diseases that cause peripheral neuropathy or decreased mobility may place a person at risk for developing OAB with incontinence (Adams, Lorish, Cushing, & Willis, 1994). OAB with incontinence in older men and women is associated with cognitive impairment and impaired mobility (Fantl et al., 1996; Fonda et al., 2005; Hunskaar, Ostbye, & Borrie, 1998).

Dementia (Alzheimer's, multi-infarct, others) is a neurological disorder that causes certain memory, speech, intellectual, and muscular functions, including those of the lower urinary tract, to deteriorate (Skelly & Flint, 1995). As the stages of dementia progress, the ability to perform personal care functions diminishes, and impaired cognition and apraxia interfere with toileting and hygiene. The prevalence of UI in dementia can range from 11% to 90% depending on the methods and definitions used in estimation (Skelly & Flint, 1995). UI occurs in the later stage of Alzheimer's disease because of the changes in the neurological pathways between the brain and bladder.

Cerebrovascular accident (CVA) or stroke initially can cause urinary retention from areflexic bladder, but long-term lower urinary tract dysfunction is experienced as symptomatic DO with urgency, frequency, and UUI. Frontal cortical lesions from a CVA may affect higher cognitive function (Pettersen, Stien, & Wyller, 2007). The patient may have an impaired awareness of the need to void and be unable to suppress a reflex detrusor contraction, resulting in UI (Marinkovic & Badlani, 2001). A stroke may cause impaired mobility, perceptual problems, or communication dysfunction together with specific physiological bladder disturbances, such as DO or urinary retention, any of which may predispose a person to incontinence. Also, many individuals experience a lack of sensory awareness of the need to void or inability to control bladder emptying.

Parkinson's disease and rigidity of muscles contribute to the inability to ambulate to the toilet and self-toilet, especially in the later stages of the disease. Lower urinary tract dysfunction—primarily urgency, frequency, nocturia, and UI—occurs in 35%–70% of patients with Parkinson's disease. Voiding dysfunction secondary to Parkinson's disease is from storage failure secondary to bladder overactivity (Wein, 2007). Associated muscle weakness affects the sphincter muscles, particularly the rectal sphincter, causing urinary and fecal incontinence. In one study, stroke and Parkinson's disease each were associated with an increased risk of subsequent UI in men and women (Thom, Haan, & van den Eeden, 1997). In patients with Parkinson's disease, DO occurs from loss of inhibitory inputs to the pontine micturition center in the brain.

Diabetes mellitus, particularly type 2, has been independently associated with a 30%–70% increased of UI in women, primarily as UUI (Brown et al., 1996; Lifford, Curhan, Hu, Barbieri, & Grodstein, 2005; Sampselle et al., 2002). Diabetic bladder neuropathy causing voiding dysfunction may affect as many as 5% to 59% of people with diabetes mellitus (Wein, 2007). In one study of diabetic women between the ages of 50 and 90, UI was reported by 22% of women, with limitations in any activity of daily living a strong indicator of UI (Lewis, Schrader, Many, Mackay, & Rogers, 2005). Brown et al. (2006) noted that the prevalence of weekly or more UUI was 27% in the diabetic population, of which 25% was seen in those with impaired fasting glucose. Diabetes causes a peripheral autonomic neuropathy that affects afferent pathways. This leads to impaired bladder sensation, causing a gradual increase in the time interval between awareness of urge and voiding because the patient has a decreased sense of urge (Mostwin, 2006). Hyperglycemia or poorly controlled diabetes may cause polyuria, urgency, frequency, and DO. As the diabetes progresses, the individual may develop microvascular complications causing diabetic neuropathic bladder or altering detrusor muscle and sphincter function, leading to urinary retention and a reduced sensation of the need to void. Better control of diabetes can reduce osmotic diuresis and associated polyuria.

Multiple sclerosis (MS) affects multiple layers of the spinal cord, leading to bladder dysfunction. Approximately 10%–15% of patients will have voiding symptoms at the time of diagnosis, and 80% of people with the disease will develop some form of a neurogenic bladder. In early MS, urgency, UUI, and frequency will be the prominent symptoms caused by neurogenic DO; many with DO have detrusor–sphincter dyssynergia. In advanced MS, neurogenic bladder disease probably affects all patients, causing long-term urinary retention (De Ridder et al., 2005). Neurogenic DO and sphincter dyssynergia may yield high intravesical pressures, eventually leading to ureteral reflux and upper urinary tract deterioration. Despite the fact that the risk of upper urinary tract deterioration seems to be lower in MS than in spinal cord injury, special attention needs to be given to people with MS (especially men). The loss of bladder control may be temporary, improving as the symptoms of the disease improve. However, as the MS patient's disease progresses, and the medical condition deteriorates and lower limb and mobility function worsens, symptoms of bladder dysfunction will become more severe and troublesome.

Degenerative joint disease, osteoporosis, and *arthritis* can impair mobility and precipitate UI. People with conditions such as rheumatoid arthritis should be assessed for toileting capabilities because they often exhibit mobility and dexterity problems that affect the ability to get to the toilet safely and on time.

Congestive heart failure and *lower extremity venous insufficiency* can cause nocturnal polyuria, nocturia, and nocturnal enuresis (see Chapter 3). Treatment should include appropriate pharmacological management because changing a rapid-acting loop diuretic from a morning administration to a late afternoon dose may reduce nocturnal polyuria and nocturia. The patient should be instructed on a sodium-restrictive diet, the use of support stockings, and leg elevation in the early afternoon.

Obstructive sleep apnea can increase production of atrial natriuretic peptide, leading to nocturnal polyuria (increased nighttime urine production), nocturia, and nocturnal enuresis. Treatment with continuous positive airway pressure may improve symptoms.

Immobility resulting from confinement to a bed or use of a wheelchair as a result of a disease such as stroke or conditions such as a hip fracture that does not heal properly, or other surgical complications, places individuals at increased risk for developing UI. In addition, there appears to be a relationship between UUI, urinary urgency, and falling (Tinetti, Inouye, Gill, & Doucette, 1995). For example, the presence of a UUI episode at least once a week was independently associated with a 34% increase in fracture risk (Brown, Vittinghoff, et al., 2000). Box 4.1 lists the fall risks and strategies for reducing these risks in a patient with UI.

Prostate Disorders in Men

Symptoms of OAB overlap with those of prostate disorders seen in men. Box 4.2 describes the terminology related to disorders of the prostate. Bladder outlet obstruction, which is a common cause of urinary symptoms in men, may be a result of benign prostatic hyperplasia, although the association is not clearly defined. As the prostate enlarges, it may obstruct the urethra and cause the bladder wall to thicken. LUTS associated with prostatic obstruction include urgency, frequency, hesitancy, nocturia, the feeling of incomplete emptying, decreased or weak urine stream, and postvoid dribbling. The generic phrase "LUTS suggestive of benign prostatic obstruction" is used to describe elderly men with filling/storage or voiding/emptying problems likely to be caused by an obstructive prostate with no evidence of cancer.

Treatment is primarily alpha blockers (e.g., tamsulosin [Flomax], alfuzosin [Uroxatral]) and 5-alpha-reductase inhibitors (e.g., finasteride [Proscar],

Box 4.1   Urinary incontinence and fall risk

Fall Risk Factors

Urinary incontinence can contribute to fall risk in several ways:

- Incontinence episodes may lead to slips on wet floor surfaces.

- Urgency and urge incontinence may increase risk when a patient hurries to the toilet to avoid wetting him- or herself.

- Medications used to treat incontinence, such as anticholinergics or alpha blockers, can cause postural hypotension.

- Nocturia can result in poor sleep, which is associated with increased fall risk.

Factors contributing to increased risk of falling include the following:

- Reduced mobility and balance—impaired ambulation and balance make it difficult to reach the toilet and thereby increase the risk of falling.

- Reduced dexterity (in manipulating undergarments, etc.).

- Impaired vision.

- Need for toileting assistance and impaired cognition (i.e., performing both a primary and a secondary task, such as walking and concentrating on getting to the toilet, may be difficult).

- Need to use a walker—urinary incontinence is a significant risk factor for falling while toileting for those who cannot stand without support.

- Increased episodes of nighttime incontinence.

- Urinary frequency and toileting assistance—the combination of urinary frequency and the need for frequent assistance with toileting is much more of a fall risk factor than incontinence by itself.

Strategies for Reducing Fall Risk

- Identify and treat the cause(s) of incontinence, including medication side effects. Patients may have more than one type of urinary incontinence.

- Identify and address comorbid fall risk factors (gait and balance, transfer ability, reduced dexterity, etc.) that can have an impact on toileting.

- Respond to toileting requests promptly, especially if the patient requires assistance to get to the toilet. Ensure that patients with impaired mobility can reach/use the nurse call bell; if not, consider the use of a **fall alarm** to warn staff of unassisted transfers and the use of a **hip protector** for patients at risk of hip fracture.

- Locate the patient near to the toilet if possible. Consider a bedside commode or urinal if the toilet is not close by.

- Implement a toilet assistance program that best matches the patient's needs and pattern of voiding.

- Ensure that the patient is wearing suitable clothes that can be easily removed or undone by self or staff and that the patient wears footwear to reduce slipping in urine. Consider a nonslip mat on the floor beside the bed for patients who experience incontinence when transferring from bed.

- Keep the pathway to the toilet lighted and obstacle-free.

- Leave a night-light on in the bedroom/bathroom at night.

Box 4.2   Terminology for prostate conditions

- **Benign prostatic hyperplasia (BPH)**—term is used and reserved for the typical histopathological pattern that defines the condition.

- **Benign prostatic enlargement (BPE)**—refers to the size of the prostate, specifically the prostatic enlargement due to a benign cause, generally histological BPH.

- **Benign prostatic obstruction (BPO)**—a form of bladder outlet obstruction (BOO); term may be applied when the cause of the outlet obstruction is known to be BPE due to a benign cause, generally histologic BPH.

Adapted from Wein & Lee (2007).

dutasteride [Avodart]). The latter medications block conversion of testosterone to dihydrotestosterone, the androgen primarily responsible for prostate enlargement; the former relax the smooth muscle in the bladder neck and prostate, thereby reducing LUTS (Roehrborn & Uzzo, 2006). Combination therapy has recently become more popular for those patients suffering from moderate to severe LUTS. This therapy has been thought to rapidly improve symptoms and provide long-term disease management. In patients with persistent symptoms of urgency and frequency, the use of antimuscarinic medications may be considered (Kaplan et al., 2006).

Pelvic Floor Muscle Weakness

Pelvic floor muscle weakness causing pelvic organ prolapse can occur in women with aging. Poor pelvic support of the bladder and urethra by weak muscles can cause prolapse of these organs. When the muscles of the pelvic floor are weak or lax in the absence of a prolapse, the proximal urethra (the portion of the urethra closest to the bladder) does not have the support (backboard) against which the urethra can be compressed with increases in abdominal pressure. Consequently, the urethral pressure does not rise with the rise in the bladder pressure, causing SUI.

Depression

There is a growing body of evidence showing an association between depression and UI (Melville, Delaney, et al., 2005; Melville, Katon, Delaney, & Newton, 2005; Nygaard, Turvey, Burns, Crischilles, & Wallace, 2003). Studies that have used depression diagnostic tools rather than symptom screening measures reveal that many women with UI have serious forms of depression that are often undiagnosed or undertreated (Nygaard et al., 2003). Symptoms of depression are more likely to be reported by adults with UI, and adult women with bladder control problems indicate that they have more emotional distress than continent adults. Adults with UI were more apt to report depression if

UI interfered with their daily lives (Dugan et al., 2000). It is not clear, though, which occurs first, depression or UI, because symptoms and functional impairment associated with a chronic illness such as UI may lead to depression.

Physiologically, the altered neurotransmitter function (specifically serotonin) commonly seen with depression could affect the bladder's complex regulation, leading to the development of involuntary detrusor contractions and UUI (Zorn, Montgomery, Pieper, Gray, & Steers, 1999). Pharmacological agents effective in treating both depression and UI (e.g., serotonin/norepinephrine reuptake inhibitors such as duloxetine [not approved by the FDA for SUI]) have been identified (Viktrup, Pangallo, Detke, & Zinner, 2004). Serotonin at the sacral spinal cord level acts to inhibit bladder contractility and increase sphincter resistance. It is essential that clinicians identify major depression in patients with other medical illnesses because depression causes significant symptomatic distress, and also may adversely impact other disease processes.

Polypharmacy

Numerous medications have been previously discussed as causes of acute UI. Medications can contribute to the development or aggravation/worsening of UI. Furthermore, the pharmacological effects of a drug may be augmented by pharmacokinetic (absorption, distribution, metabolism, clearance) considerations and drug–drug interactions. Drugs can cause functional UI by depressing cognitive function/sensation. They can contribute to urinary retention and precipitate overflow UI by decreasing bladder contractility and increasing outlet resistance. Drugs can worsen or cause UUI by decreasing volume threshold for DO, increasing bladder tone/contractility, and reducing functional bladder capacity for DO. This leads to increased residual urine volume and increasing frequency/intensity of afferent stimulation, leading to increasing rate of bladder filling and adding a bladder irritant. Drugs can cause SUI by decreasing outlet resistance. Older patients who take multiple medications are at increased risk for developing long-term UI as well.

Pelvic Surgery

Pelvic surgery (e.g., hysterectomy in women, prostatectomy in men) probably increases the risk of UI. However, the results of studies showing a relationship between UI, specifically UUI, and hysterectomy in women age 60 years or older are mixed in terms of the role of hysterectomy as a risk factor for UI (Brown, Sawaya, & Thom, 2000; Kjerulff, Langenberg, Greenaway, Uman, & Harvey, 2002; van der Vaart, van der Bom, de Leeuw, Roovers, & Heintz, 2002). In a number of studies, women who had undergone a hysterectomy were at increased risk for all types of UI, whereas in other studies, hysterectomy was not associated with increased risk for SUI (van der Vaart et al., 2002). In a meta-analysis of five previously published studies examining the association between hysterectomy and UI in older women (age > 60 years), Brown, Sawaya, and Thom (2000) estimated that women who had had a prior hysterectomy, as compared with women who had not, were 60% more likely to have UI. The studies reporting that women who had had hysterectomies were at increased risk for developing UI did not differentiate between the type of hysterectomy (abdominal or vaginal) performed.

In men, UI may occur and persist after prostate surgery (e.g., prostatectomy, transurethral resection of the prostate). The historical incidence of UI after radical prostatectomy varies from 2.5% to 87%. These data include patients with both UUI and SUI. However, determining the definition of UI is important when reviewing these data because some authors report UI as being present in patients with very mild SUI, and others only report those patients with severe or total incontinence. The incidence of total UI varies from zero to 12.5%.

Smoking

Smoking increases the risk of developing all forms of UI, and SUI in particular, depending on the number of cigarettes smoked (Hannestad, Rortveit, Daltveit, & Hunskaar, 2003; Fantl et al., 1996). Current smoking, but not previous smoking, has been associated with UI in middle-aged women (Sampselle et al., 2002). It is thought that smoker's cough (more violent and frequent than that of a nonsmoker) promotes the earlier development of SUI (Bump & McClish, 1994). Other investigators have identified chronic coughing, which may be the result of smoking-related diseases such as chronic obstructive pulmonary disease, as a risk factor for SUI (Jackson et al., 2004). In a Norwegian study of women greater than 20 years old (n = 34,755), Hannestad, Lie, Rortveit, and Hunskaar (2004) found that former and current smoking was associated with incontinence, but only for those who smoked more than 20 cigarettes per day. Chronic pulmonary disease is associated with chronic cough that precipitates SUI or worsens existing UI. There may also be an association between nicotine and increased detrusor contractions. Giving the patient information about the contribution of smoking to UI may provide a further deterrent for this unhealthy habit.

Obesity

Obesity has been identified as an independent risk factor for UI in women in cross-sectional and case–control studies (Hunskaar et al., 2005). An analysis of 83,355 participants in the Nurses' Health Study II revealed that middle-aged women with a BMI of 30 kg/m^2 or greater are approximately 3 times more likely to have severe incontinence than their counterparts with a BMI of 22–24 kg/m^2 (95% confidence interval [CI]: 2.91–3.30) (Danforth et al., 2006). Results from the SWAN study (n = 3,302) suggest that each unit of increase in BMI increases the risk of any incontinence by 5% (95% CI: 4%–7%)

(Sampselle et al., 2002). The UI seen in obesity may be secondary to increased intra-abdominal and intravesical pressure on the urethra, leading to greater urethral mobility. Also, obesity may impair blood flow or nerve innervation to the bladder.

Adding support to the importance of weight in the development of UI are findings that weight loss improves or eliminates UI in obese women (Bump, Sugerman, Fantl, & McClish, 1992; Deitel, Stone, Kassam, Wilk, & Sutherland, 1988; Frigg, Peterli, Peters, Ackermann, & Tondelli, 2004; Subak et al., 2002). A significant decrease in symptoms of SUI was seen in morbidly obese women following weight reduction induced by surgery (Deitel et al., 1988; Sugerman, Felton, Salvant, Sismanis, & Kellum, 1995). Subak et al. (2002) reported on 10 moderately obese women (mean baseline BMI, 38.3 kg/m^2) with an average of 13 incontinence episodes per week. Study participants experienced a significant reduction in incontinence episodes (down to an average of 8 episodes per week) with a mean BMI reduction of 5.3 kg/m^2. All six women with a weight loss of 5% or greater had a 50% or greater reduction in incontinence frequency, as compared with only one of four women who had weight loss reduction of less than 5%.

Programs for the prevention and treatment of UI should include education about the association of obesity with UI, and should provide information on diet and weight loss. Maintaining normal weight through adulthood may be an important factor in the prevention of the development of UI. In cases of morbid obesity, surgical intervention may be appropriate.

Physical and Occupational Forces and Activity

Certain physical activities cause increased pressure in the abdomen, thus increasing downward pressure on the bladder. It is thought that at least 50% of women who exercise regularly are at risk for developing SUI (Bo, Stein, Kulseng-Hanssen, & Kristofferson, 1994; Nygaard, DeLancey, Arnsdorf, & Murphy, 1990). College and Olympic athletes participating in high-impact activities are more likely to report the symptoms of SUI during exercise than those participating in low-impact exercise (Eliasson, Nordlander, Larson, Hammarstrom, & Mattsson, 2005; Nygaard, Thompson, Svengalis, & Albright, 1994). Sports associated with causing increased pressure on the bladder include combat sports (karate, judo), team games (basketball, volleyball, and handball), horseback riding, bodybuilding with heavy weights, and track and field (jumping and running). Activities with little risk include swimming, bicycling, walking, rowing, low-impact aerobics, and others in which at least one foot touches the floor at all times. Usually, women wear a tampon or perineal pad, limit fluid intake, change their sport, or stop exercising altogether to cope with the incontinence. Men report SUI when swinging a golf club.

Strenuous exercise on the job does not cause UI but is likely to unmask the symptom of SUI during a provocation (Wilson et al., 2005). Many jobs require heavy lifting, bending, walking, or standing, thus placing women at greater risk for incontinence, urgency, and frequency. Annual work loss due to disability and medically related absenteeism is higher in patients with OAB than it is in the nonaffected population (Wu, Birnbaum, Marynchenko, Williamson, & Mallett, 2005).

Davis and Goodman (1996) described nine female infantry trainees who had never borne children and who developed SUI and pelvic floor defects for the first time during airborne training that included parachute jumping. Sherman, Davis, and Wong (1997) reported that one third of 450 female soldiers reported incontinence during physical exercise, but only 5% reported the incontinence as significantly impacting their work.

Palmer, Fitzgerald, Berry, and Hart (1999) surveyed working women to ascertain the presence of LUTS. Of the 1,113 women surveyed, average age of respondents was 40.3 years, and 21% reported UI at least monthly. Incontinent women were significantly older and had a higher BMI than continent women. The majority thought it was not at all important or just slightly important to get treatment for it, although, overwhelmingly, they wanted more information about the condition.

However, physical activity in general has been shown to reduce the risk of developing UI. In the Nurses' Health Study, women with higher levels of physical activity had a 15% to 20% lower risk of developing UI (Danforth et al., 2007).

Work Environment

Because of the increasing number of women in the workforce, the effect of UI and OAB at work has been the subject of investigation. Nurses, teachers, and women in the military are occupational groups that have demonstrated urinary health problems (e.g., UTIs, urgency) related to toilet access. Approximately 21% of women who worked in a large urban academic setting and 29% of women who worked in a ceramic pottery production facility (average age for both groups was 45 years) reported being incontinent at least monthly. Women in blue-collar jobs (e.g., factory work, sales) may have limited breaks and restricted access to a bathroom (S. Fitzgerald, Palmer, Berry, & Hart, 2000). Very little is known about the occupational impact of UI, but OAB has been associated with voluntary termination or early retirement.

Coping strategies appear to differ depending on the occupation and the availability of work breaks and toilet facilities. Palmer and Fitzgerald (2002) compared the characteristics of women working in a large academic center with those working in a manufacturing facility. Women in the manufacturing setting coped by using self-care practices while at work, including wearing a perineal pad, limiting fluids, and avoiding caffeinated beverages. Women in the academic setting used voiding schedules and pelvic floor muscle exercises to cope. Data are not available about the potential long-term deleterious effects of such self-management strategies as fluid restriction, absorbent pad use, and prolonged periods between voiding. Although scheduling of breaks is an employment practice that research has associated with poor bladder habits and increased UI, no intervention studies have been reported in these at-risk populations.

Increased publicity has focused on the importance of employers providing rest breaks and the right for employees to use these breaks. A 1995 lawsuit by workers at a Nabisco plant in California cited bladder infections and UTIs that stemmed from being unable to urinate when needed due to lack of breaks (Linder, 2003). Women resorted to wearing adult briefs (i.e., diapers) when supervisors ordered them to urinate in their clothes or face suspension (Linder, 2003).

To address the issue of toileting in the workforce, the Occupational Safety and Health Administration (OSHA) has defined "toilet facility," "toilet room," "urinal," and "water closet" for the workforce environment (OSHA, 1998). OSHA interpretation of Regulation 1910.141 states that employers must make toileting facilities available to employees and avoid imposing unreasonable restrictions on employee use of these facilities so that workers will be protected from possible health risks (e.g., UTIs), which can result if the person is unable to use a toilet when needed (OSHA, 1998). Certain states (e.g., California, Kentucky, Nevada, Colorado, Oregon) have regulations mandating rest, relief, and relaxation for employees.

Childhood Incontinence and Familial Risk

A history of childhood nocturnal enuresis has been reported by some women with OAB and other LUTS (Kuh, Cardozo, & Hardy, 1999). M.P. Fitzgerald et al. (2006) found a strong association between reports of frequent daytime voids in childhood and adult urgency and between childhood and adult nocturia. Childhood daytime UI and bed-wetting had a more than twofold increased association with adult UUI. Early identification and intervention, including secondary prevention, may reduce the burden of adult OAB and UI.

UI may also "run in the family." Hannestad et al. (2004) noted that daughters whose mothers were incontinent were 14.6% more likely to have SUI than a daughter whose mother did not have SUI. This study also showed a correlation between sisters.

CONCLUSION

This chapter has outlined the causes of UI, including LUTS, with identification of risk factors. These conditions are seen by clinicians and caregivers in all practice settings and in all patient age groups. Many clinicians accept UI without investigating the underlying reason for the problem. If the clinician can identify those patients at risk for UI through early screening, intervention and treatment can be provided. Also, having a common language for understanding the reason for the UI makes the effort to find solutions that much easier.

REFERENCES

Abramov, Y., Sand, P.K., Botros, S.M., Gandhi, S., Miller, J.J., Nickolov, A., et al. (2005). Risk factors for female anal incontinence: New insight through the Evanston-Northwestern Twin Sisters Study. *Obstetrics and Gynecology, 106,* 726–732.

Abrams, P., Artibani, W., Cardozo, L., Khoury, S., & Wein, A. (2005). *Clinical manual of incontinence in women.* Paris: Health Publications, Ltd.

Abrams, P., Cardozo, L., Fall, M., Griffiths, D., Rosier, P., Ulmsten, U., et al. for the Standardisation Sub-committee of the International Continence Society. (2002). The standardization of terminology of lower urinary tract function: Report from the Standardisation Sub-committee of the International Continence Society. *Neurourology and Urodynamics, 21,* 167–178.

Adams, C., Lorish, C., Cushing, C., & Willis, E. (1994). Anatomical urinary stress incontinence in women with rheumatoid arthritis: Its frequency and coping strategies. *Arthritis Care and Research, 7,* 97–103.

Arya, L.A., Jackson, N.D., Myers, D.L., & Verma, A. (2001). Risk of new-onset urinary incontinence after forceps and vacuum delivery in primiparous women. *American Journal of Obstetrics and Gynecology, 185,* 1318–1323.

Ashton-Miller, J.A., & DeLancey, J.O. (2007). Functional anatomy of the female pelvic floor. *Annals of the New York Academy of Sciences, 1101,* 266–296.

Avorn, J., Monane, M., Gurwitz, J.H., Glynn, R.J., Choodnovsky, I., & Lipsitz, L.A. (1994). Reduction of bacteriuria and pyuria after ingestion of cranberry juice. *JAMA, 271,* 751–754.

Bennett, J.A., Thomas, V., & Riegel, B. (2004). Unrecognized chronic dehydration in older adults: Examining prevalence rates and risk factors. *Journal of Gerontological Nursing, 30*(11), 22–28.

Bo, K., Stein, R., Kulseng-Hanssen, S., & Kristofferson, M. (1994). Clinical and urodynamic assessment of nulliparous young women with and without stress incontinence symptoms: A case-control study. *Obstetrics and Gynecology, 84,* 1028–1032.

Brown, J.S., Sawaya, G., & Thom, D.H. (2000). Hysterectomy and urinary incontinence: A systematic review. *Lancet, 356,* 535–539.

Brown, J.S., Seeley, D., Fong, J., Ensrud, K., & Grady, D. (1996). Urinary incontinence in older women: Who is at risk? *Obstetrics and Gynecology, 87,* 715–721.

Brown, J.S., Vittinghoff, E., Lin, F., Nyberg, L.M., Kusek, J.W., & Kanaya, A.M. (2006). Prevalence and risk factors for urinary incontinence in women with type 2 diabetes and impaired fasting glucose: Findings from the National Health and Nutrition Examination Survey (NHANES) 2001–2002. *Diabetes Care, 29,* 1307–1312.

Brown, J.S., Vittinghoff, E., Wyman, J., Stone, K., Nevitt, M., Ensrud, K., et al. (2000). Urinary incontinence: Does it increase risk for falls and fractures? *Journal of the American Geriatrics Society, 48,* 721–725.

Bump, R.C., Hurt, W.G., Fantl, J.A., & Wyman, J.F. (1991). Assessment of Kegel pelvic exercise performance after brief verbal instruction. *American Journal of Obstetrics and Gynecology, 165,* 322–327.

Bump, R.C., & McClish, D.M. (1994). Cigarette smoking and pure genuine stress incontinence of urine: A comparison of risk factors and determinants between smokers and nonsmokers. *American Journal of Obstetrics and Gynecology, 170,* 579–582.

Bump, R.C., Sugerman, H.J., Fantl, J.A., & McClish, D.K. (1992). Obesity and lower urinary tract function in women: Effect of surgically induced weight loss. *American Journal of Obstetrics and Gynecology, 167,* 392–397.

Coppola, L., Caserta, F., Grassia, A., Mastrolorenzo, L., Altrui, L., Tondi, G., et al. (2002). Urinary incontinence in the elderly: Relation to cognitive and motor function. *Archives of Gerontology and Geriatrics, 35,* 27–34.

Danforth, K.N., Townsend, M.K., Lifford, K., Curhan, G.C., Resnick, N.M., & Grodstein, F. (2006). Risk factors for urinary incontinence among middle-aged women. *American Journal of Obstetrics and Gynecology, 194,* 339–345.

Danforth, K.N., Shah, A.D., Townsend, M.K., Lifford, K.L., Curhan, G.C., Resnick, N.M., et al. (2007). Physical activity and urinary incontinence among healthy, older women. *Obstetrics and Gynecology, 109,* 721–727.

Davis, G.D., & Goodman, M. (1996). Stress urinary incontinence in nulliparous female soldiers in airborne infantry training. *Journal of Pelvic Surgery, 2,* 68–71.

Deitel, M., Stone, E., Kassam, H.A., Wilk, E.J., & Sutherland, D.J.A. (1988). Gynecologic-obstetric changes after loss of massive excess weight following bariatric surgery. *Journal of the American College of Nutrition, 7,* 147–153.

De Ridder, D., Ostl, D., Van der Aal, F., Stagnarol, M., Beneton, C., Gross-Paju, K., et al. (2005). Conservative bladder management in advanced multiple sclerosis. *Multiple Sclerosis, 11,* 694–699.

Devendra, K., & Arulkumaran, S. (2003). Should doctors perform an elective caesarean section on request? *Annals of the Academy of Medicine, Singapore, 32,* 577–581.

Dietz, H.P., & Bennett, M.J. (2003). The effect of childbirth on pelvic organ mobility. *Obstetrics and Gynecology, 102,* 223–228.

DuBeau, C.E. (2006). Functional and overflow incontinence. In C.R. Chapple, P.E. Zimmern, L. Brubaker, A.R.B. Smith, & K. Bo (Eds.), *Multidisciplinary management of female disorders* (pp. 65–74). Philadelphia: Elsevier Saunders.

Dugan, E., Cohen, S.J., Bland, D.R., Preisser, J.S., Davis, C.C., Suggs, P.K., et al. (2000). The association of depressive symptoms and urinary incontinence among older adults. *Journal of the American Geriatrics Society, 48,* 413–416.

Duong, T.H., & Korn, A.P. (2001). A comparison of urinary incontinence among African American, Asian, Hispanic and white women. *American Journal of Obstetrics and Gynecology, 184,* 1083–1086.

Eliasson, K., Nordlander, I., Larson, B., Hammarstrom, M., & Mattsson, E. (2005). Influence of physical activity on urinary leakage in primiparous women. *Scandinavian Journal of Medicine and Science in Sports, 15,* 87–94.

Fantl, J.A., Newman, D.K., Colling, J., DeLancy, J.O., Keeys, C., Loughery, R., et al. for the Urinary Incontinence in Adults Guideline Update Panel. (1996). *Urinary incontinence in adults: Acute and chronic management. Clinical practice guideline No. 2: Update.* (AHCPR Publication No. 96-0682). Rockville, MD: Agency for Health Care Policy and Research.

Finkelstein, M.M. (2002). Medical conditions, medications, and urinary incontinence: Analysis of a population-based survey. *Canadian Family Physician, 48,* 96–101.

Fitzgerald, M.P., Thom, D.H., Wassel-Fur, C., Subak, L., Brubaker, L., van den Eeden, S.K., et al. for the Reproductive Risks for Incontinence Study at Kaiser Research Group. (2006). Childhood urinary symptoms predict adult overactive bladder symptoms. *Journal of Urology, 175,* 989–993.

Fitzgerald, S., Palmer, M.H., Berry, S.J., & Hart, K. (2000). Urinary incontinence: Impact on working women. *AAOHN Journal, 48,* 112–118.

Fonda, D., DuBeau, C.E., Harari, D., Ouslander, J.G., Palmer, M., & Roe, B. (2005) Incontinence in the frail elderly. In P. Abrams, L. Cardozo, S. Khoury, & A. Wein (Eds.), *Incontinence: Proceedings from the Third International Consultation on Incontinence* (pp. 1163–1239). Plymouth, UK: Health Publications, Ltd.

Frigg, A., Peterli, R., Peters, T., Ackermann, C., & Tondelli, P. (2004). Reduction in co-morbidities 4 years after laparoscopic adjustable gastric banding. *Obesity Surgery, 14,* 216–223.

Glazener, C.M., Herbison, G.P., MacArthur, C., Lancashire, R., McGee, M.A., Grant, A.M., et al. (2006). New postnatal urinary incontinence: Obstetric and other risk factors in primiparae. *BJOG, 113,* 208–217.

Goldberg, R.P., Abramov, Y., Botros, S., Miller, J.J., Ghandi, S., Nickolov, A., et al. (2005). Delivery mode is a major environmental determinant of stress urinary incontinence: Results of the Evanston-Northwestern Twin Sisters Study. *American Journal of Obstetrics and Gynecology, 193,* 2149–2153.

Graham, C.A., & Mallett, V.T. (2001). Race as a predictor of urinary incontinence and pelvic organ prolapse. *American Journal of Obstetrics and Gynecology, 185,* 116–120.

Gray, M. (2002). Are cranberry juice or cranberry products effective in the prevention or management of urinary tract infection? *Journal of Wound, Ostomy and Continence Nursing, 29,* 122–126.

Gray, M. (2004, May). Stress urinary incontinence: Myths, misconceptions, and other impediments to the diagnosis and treatment of stress urinary incontinence. *American Journal for Nurse Practitioners, Special Supplement,* pp. 15–22.

Hamilton, B.E., Martin, J.A., & Sutton, P.D., for the U.S. Department of Health and Human Services Centers for Disease Control and Prevention. (2003). Births: Preliminary data for 2002. *National Vital Statistics Reports, 51*(11), 1–20.

Hannestad, Y.S., Lie, R.T., Rortveit, G., & Hunskaar, S. (2004). Familial risk of urinary incontinence in women: Population based cross sectional study. *BMJ, 329,* 889–891.

Hannestad, Y.S., Rortveit, G., Daltveit, A.K., & Hunskaar, S. (2003). Are smoking and other lifestyle factors associated with female urinary incontinence? The Norwegian EPINCONT study. *BJOG, 110,* 247–254.

Hendrix, S., Cochrane, B., Nygaard, I., Handa, V., Barnabei, V., Iglesia, C., et al. (2005). Effects of estrogen with and without progestin on urinary incontinence. *JAMA, 293,* 935–984.

Howard, D., DeLancey, J.O.L., Tunn, R., & Ashton-Miller, JA. (2000). Racial differences in the structure and function of stress urinary incontinence mechanism. *Obstetrics and Gynecology, 95,* 713–717.

Hunskaar, S., Burgio, K., Clark, A., Lapitan, M.C., Nelson, R., Sillen, U., et al. (2005) Epidemiology of urinary (UI) and faecal (FI) incontinence and pelvic organ prolapse. In P. Abrams, L. Cardozo, S. Khoury, & A. Wein (Eds.), *Incontinence: Proceedings from the Third International Consultation on Incontinence* (pp. 255–312). Plymouth, UK: Health Publications Ltd.

Hunskaar, S., Ostbye, T., & Borrie, M. (1998). The prevalence of urinary incontinence in elderly Canadians and its association with dementia, ambulatory function, and institutionalization. *Norwegian Journal of Epidemiology, 8,* 177–182.

Jackson, R.A., Vittinghoff, E., Kanaya, A.M., Miles, T.P., Resnick, H.E., Kritchevsky, S.B., et al. for the Health, Aging, and Body Composition Study. (2004). Urinary incontinence in elderly women: Findings from the Health, Aging, and Body Composition Study. *Obstetrics and Gynecology, 104,* 301–307.

Kane, R.L., Ouslander, J.G., & Abrass, I.B. (1994). *Essentials of clinical geriatrics* (3rd ed.). New York: McGraw-Hill.

Kaplan, S.A. (2006). Update on the American Urological Association guidelines for the treatment of benign prostatic hyperplasia. *Reviews in Urology, 8*(Suppl. 4), S10–S17.

Kaplan, S.A., Roehrborn, C.G., Rovner, E.S., Carlsson, M., Bavendam, T., & Guan, Z. (2006). Tolterodine and tamsulosin for treatment of men with lower urinary tract symptoms and overactive bladder: A randomized controlled trial. *JAMA, 296,* 2319–2328.

Kayser-Jones, J., Schell, E.S., Porter, C., Barbaccia, J.C., & Shaw, H. (1999). Factors contributing to dehydration in nursing homes: Inadequate staffing and lack of professional supervision. *Journal of the American Geriatrics Society, 47,* 1187–1194.

Kearney, R., Miller, J.M., Ashton-Miller, J.A., & DeLancey, J.O. (2006). Obstetric factors associated with levator ani muscle injury after vaginal birth. *Obstetrics and Gynecology, 107,* 144–149.

Kjerulff, K.H., Langenberg, P.W., Greenaway, L., Uman, J., & Harvey, L.A. (2002). Urinary incontinence and hysterectomy in a large prospective cohort study in American women. *Journal of Urology, 167,* 2088–2092.

Kuh, D., Cardozo, L., & Hardy, R. (1999). Urinary incontinence in middle aged women: Childhood enuresis and other lifetime risk factors in a British prospective cohort. *Journal of Epidemiology and Community Health, 53,* 453–458.

Land, R., Parry, E., Rane, A., & Wilson, D. (2001). Personal preferences of obstetricians towards childbirth. *Australian and New Zealand Journal of Obstetrics and Gynaecology, 41,* 249–252.

Landefeld, C.S., Bowers, B.J., Feld, A.D., Hartmann, K.E., Hoffman, E., Ingber, M.J., et al. (2008). National Institutes of Health state-of-the-art science conference statement: Prevention of fecal and urinary incontinence in adults. *Annals of Internal Medicine, 148*(6), 449–458.

Landi, F., Cesari, M., Russo, A., Onder, G., Lattanzio, F., Bernabei, R., et al. for the Silvernet-HC Study Group. (2003). Potentially reversible risk factors and urinary incontinence in frail older people living in community. *Age and Ageing, 32,* 194–199.

Lewis, C.M., Schrader, R., Many, A., Mackay, M., & Rogers, R.G. (2005). Diabetes and urinary incontinence in 50- to 90-year-old women: A cross-sectional population-based study. *American Journal of Obstetrics and Gynecology, 193,* 2154–2158.

Lifford, K.L., Curhan, G.C., Hu, F.B., Barbieri, R.L., & Grodstein, F. (2005). Type 2 diabetes mellitus and risk of developing urinary incontinence. *Journal of the American Geriatrics Society, 53,* 1851–1857.

Linder, M. (2003). *Void where prohibited revisited.* Iowa City, IA: Fanpihua Press.

MacArthur, C., Glazener, C.M., Wilson, P.D., Lancashire, R.J., Herbison, G.P., & Grant, A.M. (2006). Persistent urinary incontinence and delivery mode history: A six-year longitudinal study. *British Journal of Obstetrics & Gynecology, 113*(2), 218–224.

Marinkovic, S.P., & Badlani, G. (2001). Voiding and sexual function after cerebrovascular accidents. *Journal of Urology, 165,* 359–370.

Mason, L., Glenn, S., Walton, I., & Appleton, C. (1999). The prevalence of stress incontinence during pregnancy and following delivery. *Midwifery, 15,* 120–128.

Melville, J.L., Delaney, K., Newton, K., & Katon, W. (2005). Incontinence severity and major depression in incontinent women. *Obstetrics and Gynecology, 106,* 585–592.

Melville, J.L., Fan, M.Y., Newton, K., & Fenner, D. (2005). Fecal incontinence in US women: A population-based study. *American Journal of Obstetrics and Gynecology, 193,* 2071–2076.

Melville, J.L., Katon, W., Delaney, K., & Newton, K. (2005). Urinary incontinence in US women: A population-based study. *Archives of Internal Medicine, 165,* 537–542.

Mentes, J. (2006). Oral hydration in older adults. *American Journal of Nursing, 106*(6), 40–50.

Mentes J., Wakefield, B., & Culp, K. (2006). Use of a urine color chart to monitor hydration status in nursing home residents. *Biological Research for Nursing, 7,* 197–203.

Meyer, S., Schreyer, A., DeGrandi, P., & Hohfield, P. (1998). The effects of birth on urinary continence mechanisms and other pelvic floor characteristics. *Obstetrics and Gynecology, 88,* 470–478.

Mostwin, J.L. (2006) Clinical physiology of micturition. In L. Cardozo & D. Staskin (Eds.), *Textbook of female urology and urogynecology* (2nd ed., pp. 141–156). Abingdon, UK: Informa Healthcare.

Newman, D.K. (2002). *Managing and treating urinary incontinence.* Baltimore, MD: Health Professions Press.

Newman, D.K. (2003). Stress urinary incontinence in women. *American Journal of Nursing, 103*(8), 46–55.

Newman, D.K., Denis, L., Gruenwald, I., Ee, C.H., Millard, R., Roberts, R., et al. (2005). Promotion, education and organization for continence care. In P. Abrams, L. Cardozo,

S. Khoury, & A. Wein (Eds.), *Incontinence: Proceedings from the Third International Consultation on Incontinence* (pp. 35–72). Plymouth, UK: Health Publications, Ltd.

Newman, D.K., & Giovanni, D. (2002). The overactive bladder: A nursing perspective. *American Journal of Nursing, 102*(6), 36–45.

North American Menopause Society. (2004). Recommendations for estrogen and progestogen use in peri-and postmenopausal women: October 2004 position statement of the North American Menopause Society. *Journal of the North American Menopause Society, 11,* 589–600.

Nygaard, I., Turvey, C., Burns, T.L., Crischilles, E., & Wallace, R. (2003). Urinary incontinence and depression in middle-aged United States women. *Obstetrics and Gynecology, 101,* 149–156.

Nygaard, I.E., DeLancey, J.O., Arnsdorf, L., & Murphy, E. (1990). Exercise and incontinence. *Obstetrics and Gynecology, 75,* 848–851.

Nygaard, I.E., Thompson, F.L., Svengalis, S.L., & Albright, J.P. (1994). Urinary incontinence in elite nulliparous athletes. *Obstetrics and Gynecology, 84,* 183–187.

Occupational Safety and Health Administration. (1998, April 6). Interpretation of 29 C.F.R. 1910.141(c)(1)(i): Toilet Facilities. Retrieved from http://www.osha-slc.gov/OshDoc/Interp_data/I19980406.html

Palmer, M.H., & Fitzgerald, S. (2002). Urinary incontinence in working women: A comparison study. *Journal of Women's Health (Larchmont), 11,* 879–888.

Palmer, M.H., Fitzgerald, S., Berry, S.J., & Hart, K. (1999). Urinary incontinence in working women: An exploratory study. *Women and Health, 29*(3), 67–80.

Palmer, M.H., & Newman, D.F. (2007). Bladder matters—urinary incontinence and estrogen. *American Journal of Nursing, 107*(3), 35–36, 37.

Pettersen, R., Stien, R., & Wyller, T.B. (2007). Post-stroke urinary incontinence with impaired awareness of the need to void: Clinical and urodynamic features. *BJU International, 99,* 1073–1077.

Press, J.Z., Klein, M.C., Kaczorowski, J., Liston, R.M., & von Dadelszen, P. (2007). Does cesarean section reduce postpartum urinary incontinence? A systematic review. *Birth, 34,* 228–237.

Quinlivan, J.A., Petersen, R.W., & Nichols, C.N. (1999). Patient preference the leading indication for elective caesarean section in public patients—results of a 2-year prospective audit in a teaching hospital. *Australian and New Zealand Journal of Obstetrics and Gynaecology, 39,* 207–214.

Resnick, N.M., & Yalla, S.V. (2007). Geriatric incontinence and voiding dysfunction. In A.J. Wein, L.R. Kavoussi, A.C. Novick, A.W. Partin, & C.A. Peters (Eds.), *Campbell's urology* (9th ed., pp. 2305–2321). Philadelphia: Elsevier Saunders.

Robinson, S.B., & Rosher, R.B. (2002). Can a beverage cart help improve hydration? *Geriatric Nursing, 23,* 208–211.

Roehrborn, C.G., & Uzzo, R.G. (2006, November). Benign prostatic hyperplasia. *Clinical Advisor, Supplement,* pp. 2–23.

Rortveit, G., Daltveit, A.K., Hannestad, Y.S., & Hunskaar, S. (2003). Urinary incontinence after vaginal delivery or cesarean section. *New England Journal of Medicine, 348,* 900–907.

Rortveit, G., & Hunskaar, S. (2006). Urinary incontinence and age at the first and last delivery: The Norwegian HUNT/EPINCONT study. *American Journal of Obstetrics and Gynecology, 195,* 433–438.

Rosenberg, M.T., Staskin, D.R., Kaplan, S.A., MacDiarmid, S.A., Newman, D.K., & Ohl, D.A. (2007). A practical guide to the evaluation and treatment of male lower urinary tract symptoms in the primary care setting. *International Journal of Clinical Practice, 61,* 1535–1546.

Sampselle, C.M., Harlow, S.D., Skurnick, J., Brubaker, L., & Bondarenko, I. (2002). Urinary incontinence predictors and life impact in ethnically diverse perimenopausal women. *Obstetrics and Gynecology, 100,* 1230–1238.

Sampselle, C.M., & Hines, S. (1999). Spontaneous pushing during birth: Relationship to perineal outcomes. *Journal of Nurse-Midwifery, 44,* 36–39.

Sherman, R.A., Davis, G.D., & Wong, M.F. (1997). Behavioral treatment of exercise-induced urinary incontinence among female soldiers. *Military Medicine, 162,* 690–694.

Simmons, S.F., Alessi, C., & Schnelle, J.F. (2001). An intervention to increase fluid intake in nursing home residents: Prompting and preference compliance. *Journal of the American Geriatrics Society, 49,* 926–933.

Skelly, J., & Flint, A. (1995). Urinary incontinence associated with dementia. *Journal of the American Geriatrics Society, 43,* 286–294.

Standard Number 1910: Sanitation. 29 C.F.R. § 141 (1998).

Stothers, L., Thom, D., & Calhoun, E. (2005). Urologic Diseases in America Project: Urinary incontinence in males—demographics and economic burden. *Journal of Urology, 173,* 1302–1308.

Subak, L.L., Johnson, C., Whitcomb, E., Boban, D., Saxton, J., & Brown, J.S. (2002). Does weight loss improve incontinence in moderately obese women? *International Urogynecology Journal and Pelvic Floor Dysfunction, 13,* 40–43.

Sugerman, H.J., Felton, W.L., III, Salvant, J.B., Jr., Sismanis, A., & Kellum, J.M. (1995). Effects of surgically induced weight loss on idiopathic intracranial hypertension in morbid obesity. *Neurology, 45,* 1655–1659.

Tambyah, P.A. (2004). Catheter-associated urinary tract infections: Diagnosis and prophylaxis. *International Journal of Antimicrobial Agents, 24*(Suppl. 1), S44–S48.

Thom, D.H., Haan, M.N., & van den Eeden, S.K. (1997). Medically recognized urinary incontinence and risks of hospitalization, nursing home admission and mortality. *Age and Ageing, 26,* 367–374.

Thomas, A., Woodard, C., Rovner, E.S., & Wein, A.J. (2003). Urologic complications of nonurologic medication. *Urologic Clinics of North America, 30,* 123–131.

Thornton, M.J., & Lubowski, D.Z. (2006). Obstetric-induced incontinence: A black hole of preventable morbidity. *Australian and New Zealand Journal of Obstetrics and Gynaecology, 46,* 468–473.

Tinetti, M., Inouye, S., Gill, T., & Doucette, J. (1995). Shared risk factors for falls, incontinence, and functional dependency. *Journal of the American Geriatrics Society, 273,* 1348–1353.

Ulmsten, U. (1995). On urogenital ageing. *Maturitas, 21,* 163–169.

Uma, R., Libby, G., & Murphy, D.J. (2005) Obstetric management of a woman's first delivery and the implications for pelvic floor surgery in later life. *BJOG, 112,* 1043–1046.

U.S. Preventive Services Task Force. (2005). *Hormone therapy for the prevention of chronic conditions in postmenopausal women: Recommendation statement.* Retrieved February 10, 2007, from http://www.ahrq.gov/clinic/uspstf05/ht/htpostmenrs.htm

van der Vaart, C.H., van der Bom, J.G., de Leeuw, J.R.J., Roovers, J.P.W.R., & Heintz, A.P.M. (2002). The contribution of hysterectomy to the occurrence of urge and stress urinary incontinence symptoms. *BJOG, 109,* 149–154.

Van Kessel, K., Reed, S., Newton, K., Meier, A., & Lentz, G. (2001). The second stage of labor and stress urinary incontinence. *American Journal of Obstetrics and Gynecology, 184,* 1571–1575.

Viktrup, L. (2002). The risk of lower urinary tract symptoms five years after the first delivery. *Neurourology and Urodynamics, 21,* 2–29.

Viktrup, L., Pangallo, B.A., Detke, M.J., & Zinner, N.R. (2004). Urinary side effects of duloxetine in the treatment of depression and stress urinary incontinence. *Primary Care Companion to the Journal of Clinical Psychiatry, 6,* 65–73.

Viktrup, L., Rortveit, G., & Lose, G. (2006). Risk of stress urinary incontinence twelve years after the first pregnancy and delivery. *Obstetrics and Gynecology, 108,* 248–254.

Waetjen, L.E., Liao, S., Johnson, W.O., Sampselle, C.M., Sternfield, B., Harlow, S.D., et al. (2007). Factors associated with prevalent and incident urinary incontinence in a cohort of midlife women: A longitudinal analysis of data. Study of Women's Health Across the Nation. *American Journal of Epidemiology, 165,* 309–318.

Warren, J.W. (2005). Nosocomial urinary tract infections. In G.L. Mandel, J.E. Bennett, & R. Dolin (Eds.), *Mandell, Douglas, and Bennett's principles and practice of infectious diseases* (pp. 3370–3381). Philadelphia: Elsevier Saunders.

Weber, A.M. (2007). Elective cesarean delivery: The pelvic perspective. *Clinical Obstetrics and Gynecology, 50,* 510–517.

Wein, A.J. (2007). Lower urinary tract dysfunction in neurologic injury and disease. In A.J. Wein, L.R. Kavoussi, A.C. Novick, A.W. Partin, & C.A. Peters (Eds.), *Campbell's urology* (9th ed., pp. 2011–2045). Philadelphia: Elsevier Saunders.

Wein, A.J., & Lee, D.I. (2007). Benign prostatic hyperplasia and related entities. In P.M. Hanno, A.J. Wein, & S.B. Malkowicz (Eds.), *Penn clinical manual of urology* (pp. 479–521). Philadelphia: Elsevier Saunders.

Wein, A.J., & Moy, M.L. (2007). Voiding function, dysfunction and urinary incontinence. In P.M. Hanno, A.J. Wein, & S.B. Malkowicz (Eds.), *Penn clinical manual of urology* (pp. 341–478). Philadelphia: Elsevier Saunders.

Wein, A.J., & Rackley, R.R. (2006). Overactive bladder: A better understanding of pathophysiology, diagnosis and management. *Journal of Urology, 175*(3 Part 2), S5–S10.

Wesnes, S.L., Rortveit, G., Bø, K., & Hunskaar, S. (2007). Urinary incontinence during pregnancy. *Obstetrics and Gynecology, 109,* 922–998.

Wilson, P.D., Berghamns, B., Hagen, S., Hay-Smith, J., Moore, K., Nygaard, I., et al. (2005). Adult conservative management. In P. Abrams, L. Cardozo, S. Khoury, & A. Wein (Eds.), *Incontinence: Proceedings from the Third International Consultation on Incontinence* (pp. 855–964). Plymouth, UK: Health Publications, Ltd.

Wilson, P.D., Herbison, R.M., & Herbison, G.P. (1996). Obstetric practice and the prevalence of urinary incontinence three months after delivery. *British Journal of Obstetrics and Gynaecology, 103,* 154–161.

Wu, E.Q., Birnbaum, H., Marynchenko, M., Williamson, T., & Mallett, D. (2005). Employees with overactive bladder: Work loss burden. *Journal of Occupational and Environmental Medicine, 47,* 439–446.

Wyndaele, J.J., Castro, D., Madersbacher, H., Chartier-Kastler, E., Igawa, Y., Kovindha, A., et al. (2005). Neurologic urinary and faecal incontinence. In P. Abrams, L. Cardozo, S. Khoury, & A. Wein (Eds.), *Incontinence* (pp. 1059–1163). Paris: Health Publications Ltd.

Zorn, B.H., Montgomery, H., Pieper, K., Gray, M., & Steers, W.D. (1999) Urinary incontinence and depression. *Journal of Urology, 162,* 82–84.

5

Bowel Dysfunction
and Its Relationship
to Urinary Incontinence

This chapter reviews the most common bowel disorders that older adults with urinary incontinence (UI) may experience: fecal (anal) incontinence (FI), constipation, fecal impaction, and diarrhea. The chapter is only an overview; for more in-depth information, we recommend *Bowel Continence Nursing* by Christine Norton and Sonya Chelvanayagam (2004). The clinician should have

- Knowledge of the anatomy and physiology of the lower rectum in relation to the normal bowel

- Awareness of common bowel disorders seen in older adults

- Knowledge of stool type by history and physical examination

- Ability to discuss constipation, fecal incontinence (FI), and fecal impaction management options

- A critical synthesis of evidence-based practice and relevant literature

Bowel dysfunction is commonly seen in older adults with UI. Bowel regularity or irregularity has an impact on the bladder and its ability to empty. Therefore, it is important for the clinician to investigate any bowel disorder that is identified in a UI evaluation. The most common types of bowel dysfunction are FI, chronic constipation, fecal impaction, and diarrhea. These conditions can occur alone or together. For example, severe constipation can contribute to FI and fecal impaction. A presenting symptom of fecal impaction may be FI, in which liquid stool can trickle around the impaction and leak out. Chronic and intractable constipation, especially in frail older patients, may lead to fecal impaction. Consequently, fecal impaction and diarrhea can lead to FI, a common sequela in long-term care residents (Akhtar & Padda, 2005).

FI is one of the most common reasons for placing an older person in a nursing facility. Over 50% of nursing home residents are estimated to have some degree of bowel disorder, mainly constipation and FI (Chassagne et al.,

1999; Nelson, Furner, & Jesudason, 1998). Constipation is more prevalent among older adults, women, African Americans, individuals with low income or low levels of education, and individuals with severe pelvic organ prolapse and mental disabilities (Johanson, 1998).

The standard definition of constipation is fewer than three stools per week, which results in a 2%–28% prevalence of constipation in older adults. However, approximately 50% of older adults use over-the-counter laxatives, and more than 3 million prescriptions are written for cathartics yearly (Nelson, Norton, Cautley, & Furner, 1995). Every year, Americans spend $200 million on laxatives, and there are more than 70 commercially produced laxative products (Johanson, 1998).

Taboos regarding bowel function and feces create social and psychological problems for people with FI and other bowel disorders that are even greater than those associated with UI and overactive bladder (Norton, 2004). For many older adults, especially those who are homebound or residing in a nursing facility, constipation and FI represent a humiliating regression in bodily function, severely impairing activity and socialization (Kuehn, 2006). The embarrassment surrounding bowel dysfunction results in significant underreporting (Bano & Barrington, 2007). Therefore, determining the prevalence of these disorders is problematic.

ANATOMY AND PATHOPHYSIOLOGY OF THE BOWEL

Normal anorectal function includes storage and appropriate evacuation of stool. Certain requirements must be met to achieve these functions. The continence component requires normal perception and discrimination of bowel contents, as well as colonic and rectal accommodation of stool.

The large intestine is a hollow, muscular tube about 5 feet in length (Figure 5.1). It is divided into the cecum, colon, rectum, and anus. The colon is subdivided into the ascending, transverse, descending, and sigmoid colon. The large intestine has many functions, all related to the final processing of intestinal contents, or feces. Very little, if any, digestion takes place in the large intestine or proximal half of the colon, whose most important function is the absorption of water and electrolytes. The distal half is for storage. Stool consists of water, indigestible residue from food, and bacteria that aid in breakdown of food. Approximately 600 mL of water is absorbed daily from intestinal contents. The longer the fecal mass stays in the colon, the more water can be absorbed. The faster contents move through the colon, the less opportunity there is for this absorption, leading to loose stool. Transit time through the colon does not change with aging and averages 36–72 hours.

The colon has mass peristalsis, a series of contractions that move stool along the colon in the direction of the rectum. The fecal mass is moved into the sigmoid colon, where it is stored. Peristalsis of intestinal contents in the

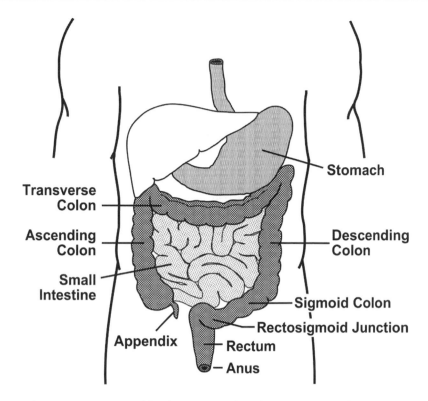

Figure 5.1. Anatomy of the digestive tract, frontal view. (Courtesy of Robin Noel.)

large intestine is slow. A second type of colonic movement is haustrations or "mixing" movements. Stool will distend and stretch the intestinal wall, causing concentric contractions. These slowly dig into and roll over the fecal material, exposing it to the surface of the large intestine, absorbing fluid and dissolved substances. These bowel contractions are more pronounced after eating and drinking (referred to as the gastrocolic reflex), delivering soft, formed stool to the rectum at regular intervals, typically 1 to 3 times per day. The bowel is inactive during sleep, becoming very active in the first few hours after waking, with additional stimulation after mobility and meals (e.g., strongest in the first 15 minutes following breakfast).

The sigmoid colon bends as it joins the rectum (see Figure 5.1). This junction, called the rectosigmoidal junction, plays an essential role in maintaining fecal continence and normal defecation. Not only does this angulation provide a mechanical break for material leaving the colon, but there is also evidence that the sensory response to sigmoidal distention modulates rectal sensation.

The last portion of the large intestine is the rectum (about 6 inches), which extends from the sigmoid colon to the anus. The last inch of the rectum is called the anal canal. It contains the internal and external anal sphincters, which play an important role in regulating defecation (Figure 5.2). Muscle

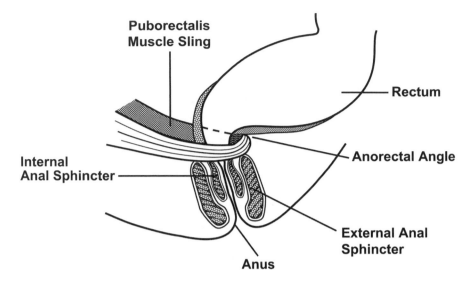

Figure 5.2.   Internal and external anal sphincters with puborectalis muscle. (Courtesy of Robin Noel.)

peristaltic contractions in the colon push stool toward the rectum, causing distention and initiating the defecation reflex. By the time stool reaches the rectum, it is solid because most of the water has been absorbed.

The nerve supply to the large intestine contains both parasympathetic and sympathetic nerves and is not under voluntary control. In general, stimulation of the sympathetic nerve fibers inhibits activity in the gastrointestinal (GI) tract. It also excites the internal anal sphincter. Thus stimulation of the sympathetic fibers can totally block movement of feces through the GI tract both by inhibition of the intestinal wall and by closure of the two anal sphincters. Stimulation of the parasympathetic nerve fibers causes an increase in bowel activity and in the defecation reflexes. Awareness of rectal distention is dependent on both intact nerve pathways and a normal mental status. Normal sensory awareness includes the ability to discriminate among gas, liquid, and solid contents as well as the ability to recognize rectal distention resulting from the presence of stool. Rectal sensation is necessary for bowel continence. Aging causes decreased rectal sensation, reduced sphincter tone, and increased compliance, resulting in bowel disorders such as FI, constipation, and impaction.

The puborectalis muscle component of the pelvic diaphragm (discussed in Chapter 3) is part of the levator ani muscle that stretches from the pubic bone and forms a sling around the rectum (see Figure 5.2). This muscle creates an angle between the lower and the upper parts of the rectum known as the anorectal angle, which is believed to be important in preserving continence. The puborectalis pulls the rectum toward the pubic bone and, when the angle is maintained below 110 degrees, fecal matter from the rectum cannot pass into the anus.

Two distinct anal sphincters are important in maintaining continence. The internal anal sphincter (IAS) is a thin (2- to 3-cm) continuation of the circular smooth muscle of the rectum that begins at the proximal anal canal. It is controlled by the autonomic nervous system. The IAS is normally closed and provides approximately 70% of resting rectal tone, thus preventing the passive seepage of stool. The external anal sphincter (EAS) is composed of voluntary, striated muscle (both slow- and fast-twitch muscle fibers) and, with the puborectalis, functions as one unit to provide voluntary sphincter control. It provides only 30% of resting tone. The EAS surrounds the IAS, and is innervated by the inferior branch of the pudendal nerve. Its main function is to preserve continence during the urge to defecate and during rises in intra-abdominal pressure, such as those that occur during physical activity. The puborectalis muscle is directly innervated by the S_3 and S_4 sacral nerves. As the feces approach the anus, the IAS is inhibited and, if the EAS is relaxed, defecation will occur. Because the EAS is under voluntary control, normal defecatory function is a learned behavior that is amenable to behavior modification.

Process of Defecation

Defecation is a reflex involving the muscles of the anal canal and terminal bowel. Normal defecation occurs only when intra-abdominal pressure increases through a contraction of the chest muscles and simultaneous contraction of the abdominal muscles (Valsalva maneuver or "straining at stool"). At the same time, the puborectalis muscle relaxes, allowing voluntary passage of stool. Entry of the fecal mass into the rectal vault distends the rectal walls and stimulates mass peristaltic movements of the bowel, which move the feces toward the anus. As the stool enters, there is a transient decrease in IAS tone and an increase in EAS tone, known as the "rectoanal inhibitory reflex" (Cundiff & Fenner, 2004). This allows for "sampling," which is when the anal canal determines whether the rectal contents are solid, liquid, or gas. This is followed by accommodation, whereby relaxation of the rectum permits it to accept the increased rectal volume, causing an "urge to defecate."

The defecation reflex may be halted by voluntary contraction of the EAS. When this is done, the defecation reflex ceases, allowing the accommodation of stool to continue, and usually will not return for several hours. If it is not suppressed, defecation of stool is initiated by a Valsalva maneuver. Voluntary inhibition of the EAS and puborectalis enables the rectum to empty. This is assisted by coordinated peristaltic activity of the rectosigmoid colon. Once evacuation is completed, the EAS and puborectalis contract (called the "closing reflex"), and the continence mechanism is initiated again.

A key factor in the defecation process is access to toilet facilities. Repeated inhibition of the defecation reflex is common in people who are immobile and need assistance to toilet. If the urge to defecate occurs and a caregiver is unavailable, the person will inhibit the urge, thus allowing stool to further solidify. Water continues to be absorbed from the fecal mass, causing it to become firmer, so that subsequent defecation is more difficult and constipation may result. If the stool is not passed in a timely manner, the continued absorption of water may cause it to become impacted in the rectum (called fecal impaction), a common problem seen in residents in nursing facilities.

COMMON BOWEL DISORDERS IN OLDER ADULTS

Fecal Incontinence

FI is defined as the involuntary or inappropriate loss of liquid or solid stool, and anal incontinence consists of incontinence of flatus (gas) as well as stool (Hunskaar et al., 2005; Madoff, Parker, Varma, & Lowry, 2004; Norton & Chelvanayagam, 2004). The prevalence of FI in the general population has been estimated to range from 11% to 15% (Hunskaar et al., 2005). In a population-based postal survey of 6,000 women ages 30 to 90 years enrolled in a large health maintenance organization in Washington State, the prevalence of FI was 7.2%, and it increased notably with age (Melville, Fan, Newton, & Fenner, 2005). Associated risk factors for FI in this study were older age, major depression, UI, medical comorbidity, and vaginal delivery (Landefeld et al., 2008). The prevalence of FI is increased among women, the elderly, persons with poor health status or physical limitations, and those residing in nursing homes (Edwards & Jones, 2001). The prevalence of FI in women presenting for routine gynecological care was reported as 28%, and post-childbirth FI has been reported in one of four women (Guise et al., 2007; Nelson, 2004). The prevalence of FI is similar in men and women and depends on the population studied and the definition of FI used. Like UI, it is believed to be underreported because only one third of symptomatic patients discuss their FI with providers. This prevalence increases (20%–24%) in women with pelvic organ prolapse and UI (Altman et al., 2006; Nichols, Ramakrishnan, Gill, & Hurt, 2005). Combined UI and FI is experienced by 3%–6% of older adults in the community (Agency for Healthcare Research and Quality, 2007). FI is a leading cause of nursing home placement, and its prevalence in nursing facilities is reported to be higher than in the community. As many as 43% (Chiang, Ouslander, Schnelle, & Reuben, 2000) to 46% (Nelson, 2004) of nursing home residents experience FI. It is believed that the cost of FI is considerable, but cost estimates are not available (Miner, 2004).

Most cases of FI are acquired; common causes and risk factors are outlined in Table 5.1 (Abramov et al., 2005). In adult women, the most common cause of FI is obstetric or surgical trauma, usually a direct injury to either the anal sphincter (anal sphincter tear) or the pudendal nerves (Jackson, Weber, Hull, Mitchinson, & Walters, 1997). The strongest predictor of FI is chronic diarrhea, and FI is associated with prostate disease in men and hysterectomy in women (Goode et al., 2005). In older adults living in long-term care facilities,

Table 5.1 Common causes and risk factors for fecal incontinence in adults

Causes	Examples
Congenital	Imperforate anus
	Rectal agenesis
	Myelomeningocele
Sphincter or pelvic floor muscle damage	Pregnancy, injury to the sphincter, or nerve damage associated with vaginal delivery
	Chronic straining at stool
	Direct trauma or injury
	Rectal radiation therapy (e.g., for prostate cancer)
	Anal dilation
	History of stress urinary incontinence
Diarrhea states	Inflammatory bowel disease
	Intestinal diarrhea
	Infectious diarrhea
	Laxative abuse
	Irritable bowel syndrome
Iatrogenic/postsurgical	Hemorroidectomy
	Anorectal surgical procedures (e.g., sphincterotomy for anal fissures or anal stretch)
Anorectal pathology	Rectal prolapse
	Anal or rectovaginal fissure
Neurological disease	Stroke
	Spinal cord injury or diseases
	Multiple sclerosis
	Spina bifida
	Parkinson's disease
	Alzheimer's disease/dementia
	Pudendal neuropathy
	Peripheral neuropathies (e.g., diabetes, chronic alcoholism)
Overflow diarrhea	Fecal impaction
	Older adults living in long-term care or with mobility problems
Environmental	Poor toilet facilities
	Inadequate care
	Lack of toileting by caregiver
Idiopathic	Unknown cause

From Wald, A. (2007). Clinical Practice: Fecal incontinence in adults. *New England Journal of Medicine, 356,* 1648–1655; reprinted by permission.

acute diarrhea and fecal impaction are the main causes of FI. In women, FI has also been associated with major depression, UI, and increased medical comorbidity (Melville et al., 2005). People with long-standing constipation can develop FI because the sensation of the movement of feces into the rectum does not occur.

There are three main types of FI: 1) *overflow* FI, which is seen primarily in cognitively impaired, bedridden nursing home residents; 2) *reservoir* FI, which occurs in patients who have diminished colonic or rectal capacity (chronic rectal ischemia, irritable bowel syndrome [IBS]); and 3) *rectosphincteric* FI, which is seen in conditions associated with structural anal sphincter damage (Wald, 2007). Constipation with hard stool decreases the ability to perceive movement of new stool into the sigmoid/rectum and reflexly dilates the IAS, allowing liquid to escape (so-called overflow FI). Fecal or anal incontinence can be described as mild when there is loss of small amounts of gas or liquid stool; or major, when there is intermittent, involuntary loss of large amounts of solid stool. People with mild FI may pass small amounts of stool that is visible on the underclothes, referred to as fecal staining. Mild anal incontinence may occur with a normal anal sphincter and can be caused by anorectal conditions such as hemorrhoids, colitis, or IBS. Poor mental activity caused by dementia or depression can also predispose to incontinence, as can limitations of mobility. Major anal incontinence is usually the result of neuromuscular damage to the anal sphincter mechanism.

Rectal sensation warns of imminent defecation and helps a person discriminate between formed and unformed stool and gas. Impaired rectal sensation may deprive a person of this useful information and result in incontinence. Probably one of the most common causes of FI is damage to one or both anal sphincters. The EAS is responsible for delaying bowel emptying once the rectum fills and the urge to empty the bowel is felt. People with a weak or damaged EAS muscle typically experience urgency and must rush to the toilet as soon as the need to defecate is felt; if the toilet is not reached in time, urge FI can occur. The weakened sphincter muscle is unable to squeeze hard enough to prevent the seepage of stool.

The combination of FI and UI, called *double incontinence,* is seen in 50% (Nelson & Furner, 2005) to 70% (Chiang et al., 2000) of residents in the long-term care setting. Double incontinence is a result of poor mobility and cognitive impairment. It may be also a result of peripheral neural or muscular lesions such as repeated obstetric injuries or severe chronic constipation. FI with UI is an indication of poorer overall health, is associated with increased mortality, and increases the person's risk of urinary tract infections and pressure ulcers (Schnelle & Leung, 2004). The reason both types of incontinence may occur at the same time is that the digestive tract and the lower urinary tract are closely connected, and anything that affects one of them can affect the other. Both systems share common nerves and are supported by the pelvic floor muscles and other structures that play a vital role in maintaining continence. Therefore, anything that causes damage or trauma to the nerves that supply the rectum or pelvic floor can cause UI and FI. Diseases or injuries that affect the spinal cord or the nerves or muscles can affect both systems. Having both types of incontinence is so difficult to manage that people with double incontinence live in a constant state of anxiety and may totally withdraw from society.

To prevent complications from FI, clinicians need to identify those patients at risk and understand causes of FI (see Table 5.1). Among older people, the most common cause of FI is neither loss of mobility nor dementia but simply the natural effects of aging on the body. Muscles and tissues weaken, lose their elasticity, and become lax. Changes in muscle strength, muscle mass, and muscle and nerve reflexes affect the anorectal area. The strength of the EAS and pelvic floor muscles decreases with aging. Thus some older adults cannot retain gas or stool, especially liquid stool, as well as or for as long as they once could. Also, the older adult may not be able to reflexively close the anal sphincter quickly enough to avoid an FI "accident." Compared to continent people, incontinent older adults have less rectal sensation and less sphincter strength.

Chronic Constipation

A decrease in the normal frequency of bowel movements is often associated with increased difficulty in defecation. As mentioned previously, constipation is defined as having fewer than three stools per week. Based on this definition, it has been estimated that at least 17% of the adult population will be constipated at some point in their lives. Usually an individual's definition of constipation is considerably broader, however, and includes straining at stool, painful defecation, dry hard stools, small stools, and incomplete or infrequent stool evacuation. The prevalence of constipation increases with age, and constipation is more common in women than in men, in nonwhites than in whites, in people living in rural areas, and in those with lower family income and lower levels of education (Leoning Baucke, 2007). The steepest increase in reported prevalence rates of constipation occurs in the sixth decade, and ranges from 4% to 30%. Older adults are 5 times more likely than younger adults to report problems with constipation. Up to 45% of frail elderly adults report constipation. Older adults self-medicate for constipation more than any other medical condition (Folden et al., 2002).

The types of constipation (referred to as defecatory disorders) include normal-transit or functional constipation, slow-transit constipation, and rectosigmoidal or obstructed outlet delay. *Normal-transit or functional constipation* is the most common and is seen in patients with normal colon function but who complain of hard stools and poor ability to evacuate. In normal-transit constipation, stools travel through the colon in a normal amount of time, but patients report being constipated because they have difficulty during defecation and must strain because the stools are hard or because they have abdominal bloating or pain (Davis, Rao, Pallentino, & Schiller, 2007). The definition of functional constipation is based on the Rome III criteria, which were developed and updated by an international panel of GI experts (Longstreth et al., 2006) and require that a person have more than two of the following parameters for at least 12 weeks in the preceding 12 months:

1. Fewer than three stools per week

2. Lumpy or hard, pellet-like stools on more than 25% of defecations

3. Straining at defecation more than 25% of the time

4. Sensation of incomplete evacuation in more than 25% of defecations

5. Requires manual maneuvers to facilitate defecations (e.g., digital evacuation, vaginal splinting)

6. Sensation of anorectal obstruction/blockage in more than 25% of defecations

To meet this definition, loose stools should not be present without use of laxatives and IBS should not be present. Causes of functional constipation include inadequate dietary fiber or fluid intake, constipating medications, and defecation inhibition (ignoring the defecation urge or the "call to stool").

Slow-transit constipation (colonic inertia) is characterized by a reduction in frequency of bowel movements to once a week or less and abdominal complaints such as bloating and discomfort. This may be caused by neuropathy. This is usually seen in women, and in two thirds of individuals it is an acquired disorder, with the remaining third developing it in childhood. The colon has marked reduction in peristalsis, or contractions that propel the stool through the colon. This type of constipation causes a decrease in the gastrocolic response following meals and morning awakening. As the stool moves slowly through the colon, it becomes dehydrated, causing difficulty when the patient attempts to defecate.

Rectosigmoidal outlet delay or outlet obstruction constipation (also referred to as anismus, dyssynergic defecation, pelvic floor dyssynergia, or spastic pelvic floor syndrome) occurs when chronically constipated patients are unable to relax the puborectalis muscle and the EAS (Palsson, Heyman, & Whitehead, 2004). Many times these patients will either inhibit defecation or have prolonged defecation—usually more than 10 minutes. The dyssynergia of muscle activity (failure of the levator ani muscle to relax during straining) will cause incomplete or blocked evacuation. The person will report a need to press in or around the anus with a finger to aid in defecation (digital stimulation). Usually, if more than 3 days pass without a bowel movement, feces may harden or may become pellet-like. The person may have difficulty or even pain during elimination and may use excessive straining to pass the stool. This is an acquired behavior disorder that may have been present since childhood. This type of constipation responds well to biofeedback training to learn to relax pelvic floor musculature.

Risk factors for constipation include age, recent abdominal or perianal surgery, general anesthesia, neurological disease (e.g. spinal cord injury, multiple sclerosis, Parkinson's disease), limited physical activity, inadequate diet or fluid intake, history of constipation or laxative abuse, and use of drugs known to cause constipation. Complications of constipation include intestinal impaction, anal fissures, hemorrhoids, volvulus, internal obstruction, fecal seepage, and bowel perforation.

Chronic constipation and straining during defecation can contribute to lower urinary tract symptoms (LUTS) and pelvic organ prolapse (Alling Moller, Lose, & Jorgensen, 2000). Jelovsek, Barber, Paraiso, and Walters (2005) found that 31%–41% of patients presenting with pelvic organ prolapse or incontinence met formal standardized definitions of constipation. Chronic constipation and repeated straining efforts may induce progressive neuropathy in the pelvic floor. The close proximity of the bladder and urethra to the rectum and their similar innervations make it likely that there are reciprocal effects between them. Studies of severely constipated women who have strained during defecation over a prolonged period have demonstrated changes in pelvic floor neurological function (Snooks, Barnes, Setchell, & Henry, 1985). Denervation of the EAS and pelvic floor muscles may occur in association with a history of excessive straining at defecation. Many believe that, if these are lifetime habits, they may have a cumulative effect on pelvic floor and bladder function. Spence-Jones, Kamm, Henry, and Hudson (1994) found that straining excessively at stool was significantly more common in women with stress UI and in women with prolapse. Research has shown that constipation treatment with laxatives (e.g., senna [Senokot], lactulose) can relieve symptoms of urinary urgency and frequency (Charach, Greenstein, Rabinovich, Groskopf, & Weintraub, 2001).

Because there are data to suggest that chronic constipation and straining may be a risk factor for the development of LUTS, self-care practices that promote bowel regularity should be an integral part of any treatment care plan. Combining fluid management, elimination of bladder irritants, and regulation of bowels may yield the maximum benefit.

Constipation may present as a change in bowel habit or as overflow FI. People suffering from constipation may present with acute changes in cognition, urinary retention, UI, and fecal impaction. Fecal impaction is a cause of FI, particularly in older adults and in those in nursing homes. Impaction-associated overflow FI is caused by a combination of decreased anorectal sensation and reduced sphincter pressures. If the person also has UI, once constipation is resolved, improvement in urine leakage usually occurs. Constipation is a symptom, not a disease, but prolonged constipation can lead to urinary retention and incontinence. Also, repeated straining to expel hard stool that occurs over many years can eventually lead to pelvic floor muscle weakness, weakening of the anal sphincter, and rectal prolapse (Newman, 2005).

Many people have misconceptions concerning normal bowel habits. Many times older people become overly concerned with having a daily bowel movement, and constipation may be imaginary. Older individuals are more likely to describe themselves as constipated if they had to strain during defecation or had incomplete evacuation, difficulty or pain with defecation, or hard stools. They believe that a bowel movement is necessary every day. These patients need to be taught that bowel patterns can vary and that having a bowel movement every other day or every third day may be normal. Also, an individual may express concern that, if wastes remain in the bowel, they are absorbed and can shorten the person's life. Therefore, these individuals take large amounts and many different types of laxatives to have daily movements and to get rid of "harmful wastes."

In general, people with constipation commonly use laxatives, enemas, and other invasive procedures such as manual removal of fecal impaction. These interventions are not without risk and may produce undesired side effects such as cramping, bloating, dehydration, diarrhea, rectal bleeding, anal irritation, and FI. Heavy dependence on laxatives can become habit-forming because long-term use of laxatives interferes with the colon, decreasing peristalsis. Mineral oil coats the intestines; blocks absorption of vitamins A, D, E, and K; and also may interact with other medications. Milk of magnesia can increase peristalsis and prevent complete and adequate absorption of vitamins and minerals (Kumar, Yoselovitz, & Gambert, 2007). Habitual use of enemas leads to loss of normal bowel function. Bowel training programs have been shown to be successful in reducing constipation in the chronically constipated person who is at risk for injury from overuse of laxatives and enemas (e.g., soapsuds enemas should not be used as they can cause irritation or hemorrhagic colitis). Ignoring or suppressing the urge to defecate can contribute to constipation (Sanburg, McGuire, & Lee, 1996).

Fecal Impaction

Fecal impaction is defined as the presence of hard stool in the rectum, oozing of liquid stool without the passing of fecal mass, and the absence of a bowel movement for over 3 days (Stern, 2006). Fecal impaction occurs when stool that has not been passed builds up over days and becomes hardened in the rectum. This condition is not very common but may occur in frail, ill, older adults. Fecal impaction usually occurs in the rectum, but approximately 25%–30% of impactions are high impactions (colon and cecum), which may not be easily diagnosed by rectal examination (Figure 5.3). Stool may be seen on abdominal radiographs in the sigmoid colon or higher, even with a negative digital exam or documentation in the clinical record of daily bowel movement. The person with a rectal impaction has a frequent urge to defecate but is unable to do so, and the effort is complicated by rectal pain. It is more common in older adults and in patients with neurogenic bowel.

Fecal impaction may present as diarrhea, FI, or both in the geriatric population. Fecal impaction may be recognized by the paradoxical passage of liquid stool and no normal stools. The portion of stool above the obstructing

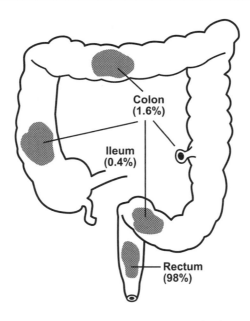

Figure 5.3.   Sites of fecal impaction. (Courtesy of Robin Noel.)

fecal mass becomes liquefied and oozes out around the impacted mass. This condition, sometimes called fecal oozing or fecal staining, commonly presents with semisolid fecal soiling many times daily. Clinical presentation of fecal impaction also may include generalized weakness, mental changes, decreased appetite, abdominal distention and discomfort, severe stomach pain, urinary retention, bloating, and nausea and vomiting. Frail older adults may exhibit changes in cognition and develop a fever. Although impaction may occur in some people regardless of prevention measures taken, it is usually preventable. Impaction is caused by a combination of factors that include poor rectal sensation, immobility, inadequate fluid and food intake, drug side effects, and inability to recognize, delay in recognizing or responding to, or inappropriate responding to the urge to defecate. If fecal impaction is left untreated or unresolved, it can cause intestinal obstruction, ulceration, and urinary problems. Usually, the person is unable to pass this large amount of stool.

If a large impaction is present and enemas have been ineffective in removing the impaction, the feces must be broken up manually. Nurses tend to use enemas initially, followed by laxatives to remove the impaction, using manual removal only as a last resort. The clinician must use caution with manual removal because stimulation of the vagus nerve in the rectal wall can slow the patient's heart rate. For individuals with chronic illness who develop fecal impaction frequently, the nurse may need to teach the caregiver how to remove the impaction. The nurse should slowly insert a lubricated, gloved index finger approximately 5 cm into the rectum. The index finger should be inserted into the rectum using a rotating motion to stimulate relaxation of the IAS and peristaltic contractions in the left colon. If the stool is hard and solid, an attempt should be made to break up the hard stool and remove it. This can be accomplished by pushing a finger into the center, splitting the stool and breaking it up into small sections. Another method that may be successful is mixing 30 mL of water and 30 mL of hydrogen peroxide in a piston syringe, attaching a red-rubber catheter to the tip of the syringe, and injecting this solution directly into the hard fecal mass. This mixture will cause foaming of the stool and will successfully break the mass into small pieces. The person should be encouraged to assist by bearing down using the Valsalva maneuver.

It is recommended that an enema be used to remove stool that remains. The patient education tool "Tips for Keeping Your Bowels Moving" (see the companion CD) discusses the use of a milk-and-molasses enema. A milk-and-molasses enema works as an osmotic enema that helps the patient eliminate stool comfortably. If phosphate-containing Fleet enemas are used, only one enema at a time should be given because the colon may absorb some of the phosphate, which may lead to electrolyte imbalance.

Diarrhea

Diarrhea is defined as the passage of frequent, watery bowel movements and can be seen in people with decreased anal sphincter pressures. The symptoms usually disappear quickly and are more an inconvenience than an illness. In certain cases, however, diarrhea may persist for days, weeks, and even months. If this occurs, the person may have viral or bacterial diarrhea resulting from exposure to the flu, a virus, food poisoning, or, in some cases, a parasite. Diarrhea caused by an infectious process raises particular concern in the institutional setting, such as hospitals or nursing facilities, where an infection may spread among the resident population. Usually the *Clostridium difficile* bacterium, which causes diarrhea, is treated effectively with medications. A stool culture will determine the presence of bacteria or parasites. Diarrhea can also be caused by antibiotic therapy, which can destroy the normal balance of organisms in the intestines, and has the potential to cause a fungal superinfection resulting in liquid stool. Preventive measures include probiotic products (*Lactobacillus* [Lactinex]) or dairy products that contain bacterial cultures (buttermilk, yogurt).

Gastroenteritis is a common cause of diarrhea. Immunocompromised and malnourished people, and older adults, are at risk for bacterial or viral gastroenteritis causing diarrhea. Gastroenteritis should always be considered when a person develops acute diarrhea. Assessment for signs and symptoms of acute illness must be completed. In certain situations, a stool culture may be necessary.

Enteral feedings are commonly associated with diarrhea and FI. Although the diarrhea is usually attributed to the formula, it is more commonly caused by an underlying malnutrition that results in edema of the intestinal wall and malabsorption. Malabsorption and diarrhea associated with enteral feedings may also be caused by atrophy of the intestinal wall and loss of intestinal enzymes, which results in decreased absorptive surface and capacity.

Interventions to prevent or control diarrhea in patients receiving enteral feedings include use of isotonic formula, beginning the feedings at a low rate with gradual increase, possible use of bulk-containing formula, and use of antidiarrheal agents during the adaptation phase. Stopping the feedings in response to diarrhea is not recommended. The underlying cause of the diarrhea (malnutrition, atrophy of intestines, intestinal edema, malabsorption) will be corrected by providing nutritional support and stimulating the GI tract.

Individuals who are lactose intolerant may experience diarrhea after ingestion of milk and dairy products. Another cause of diarrhea, especially in the older adult, is laxative abuse. Regular, frequent use of laxatives dulls the sensation of the need for bowel elimination. Natural emptying mechanisms fail to work as the body becomes dependent on laxatives and enemas. Symptoms such as abdominal cramping, frequent passage of thin watery stool, change in color and odor of stool, nausea and vomiting, and even fever may occur.

Prolonged diarrhea can cause skin irritation and breakdown around the anal, gluteal, and perineal area (see Chapter 10). After each bowel movement, the entire perineum should be cleaned with a "no-rinse" skin cleanser and thoroughly dried. A moisturizing skin care product should be applied following cleansing. Barrier moisture skin products should be considered if any skin irritation or redness occurs. Antidiarrheal medications such as loperamide (Imodium), codeine phosphate, or diphenoxylate and atropine (Lomotil) have been shown to reduce stool frequency. Loperamide, the most commonly used drug, is a synthetic opioid with a low side effect profile. It increases gut transit time, thus increasing the amount of water absorbed from the stool. Diphenoxylate and codeine have central nervous system side effects, so they should be used cautiously in elderly patients. Ingesting medicinal fiber (e.g., Metamucil) mixed with very little fluid allows excess fluid from diarrhea to be reabsorbed, which slows GI motility.

FACTORS THAT CONTRIBUTE TO BOWEL DYSFUNCTION

Several risk factors have been identified as contributing to bowel disorders. Aging and obesity are major risk factors for both UI and FI (Abramov et al., 2005; Richter et al., 2005). This section discusses the most common contributing factors.

Insufficient Dietary Fiber

Dietary fiber is important for the successful long-term management of constipation because extensive studies have shown that it inhibits constipation. The volume of fecal material is related to the amount of ingested fiber. Soluble fiber sources such as oatmeal and peeled fruit can add bulk to liquid stool, absorb excess water in the colon, and increase the ability to form solid stool in people with FI and diarrhea. A diet high in animal fats and refined sugars tends to be low in fiber. Fat delays gastric emptying and slows intestinal motility, which promotes constipation. High-fiber diets result in larger stools, more frequent bowel movements, and less constipation. Oral calcium supplements can also decrease the incidence of diarrhea by improving stool consistency.

Hemorrhoids

Hemorrhoids are dilated anal veins situated within the mucosa and subepithelial tissues of the anal canal. They can be internal (inside the rectum) or external (outside the anal opening). They may develop from chronic straining during defecation. The presence of hemorrhoids causes pain, itching, and discomfort during defecation. Spasms can occur in the anal sphincters, causing the person to delay bowel movements.

Rectal Surgery

Any surgery in the area of the rectum that involves the anal sphincters can contribute to bowel dysfunction, especially if it results in disorders that interfere with defecation. Hemorrhoidectomy may lead to a "keyhole" deformity, which allows the passive seepage of liquid stool. Another common anorectal procedure is a sphincterotomy, in which the lower third of the anal sphincter is divided to relieve an anal fissure. It can inadvertently cause sphincter damage in women.

Poor Fluid Intake

Drinking plenty of fluids, preferably water, helps stimulate intestinal activity. The content of stool is 70%–80% water, and less water content means firmer, smaller stool. Water and other fluids add bulk to stools, making bowel movements softer, more frequent, and easier to pass. For good bowel management, it is very beneficial for patients to consume at least 50% of the volume of their daily intake in the form of water. For the purpose of measuring adequate fluid intake, fluids include liquids and food items that break down into fluid at room temperature (e.g., gelatin dessert, ice cream).

Specific diseases can affect fluid balance. An example is diabetes, which brings on a tendency to constipation if the patient maintains a high glucose level. This is because the unmetabolized sugar cannot be excreted through the kidneys without a solvent, so body water is drawn to the kidneys and this deprives the GI tract of its normal fluid level.

Ignoring the Defecation Urge

As the rectum fills, the defecation sensation (the "call to stool" or "nature's call") is relayed centrally to the cerebral cortex. The sensation lasts 5–20 seconds, with increasing duration as the volume of rectal contents increases. It is possible to defer defecation, and patients with chronic illness, those who have decreased functional mobility, or those with dementia or mental illness may ignore or inhibit the urge to defecate. If defecation is delayed or inhibited, the urge to defecate diminishes within a few minutes and may not return for several hours (Folden et al., 2002). Stool is returned to the rectum, initiating retrograde peristalsis in the rectum and pushing stool back into the sigmoid colon. If the stool stays in the rectum, water reabsorption occurs, causing the stool to harden. If the person repeatedly ignores the call to stool, self-induced constipation occurs. Repeated inhibition or delay of defecation can lead to FI, impaction, or both. Delaying defecation is believed to be one of the main causes of bowel disorders, especially FI and constipation, and especially in older people who are dependent on caregivers or live in long-term care facilities.

Pregnancy

Damage to one or both anal sphincters during delivery is the most common cause of FI in women. This is particularly the case in women with third-degree tears that extend from the vagina through the anal sphincter, but as many as 10% of women complain of new defecatory symptoms after an uncomplicated vaginal birth (Sultan & Kamm, 1997) (see Chapter 4). Women whose first delivery was assisted with forceps are the most likely to develop incontinence. Women who are pregnant often have problems with constipation, possibly as a result of increased pressure from the fetus on the intestines, or hormonal changes.

Medications

Most of the medications commonly prescribed for older adults cause constipation. Drugs that can affect the bowel are those that decrease bowel motility or increase stool consistency. This is especially true with the following types of medications:

* Analgesics and opioids—inhibit GI peristalsis and motility, particularly in the colon, and prolong intestinal transit time. Orally administered opiates are more constipating than parenterally administered agents.

* Anticholinergics, including antihistamines, antiparkinsonian drugs, tricyclic antidepressants, and phenothiazines—inhibit bowel contractility, particularly in the colon and rectum.

* Antacids that contain aluminum and calcium; antibiotics—may cause diarrhea and constipation. This includes over-the-counter medications such as TUMS and iron and calcium supplements.

* Nonsteroidal anti-inflammatory agents.

- Calcium channel blockers—slow intestinal transit time by affecting autonomic nervous system function or smooth muscle contractility.

- Iron supplements; calcium supplements—can slow colonic transit time, leading to constipation.

Diarrhea also can be caused by antibiotics, serotonin reuptake inhibitors, 5-hydroxytryptamine$_4$ agonists, proton pump inhibitors, magnesium-containing antacids, digoxin, and laxatives.

Chronic Diseases

Underlying medical conditions, especially neurological diseases that affect nerves leading to the intestines or rectum and anus, can cause bowel dysfunction. IBS may cause refractory constipation. Parkinson's disease may cause an abnormal response of the rectoanal inhibitory reflex, causing the anal sphincter to contract during defecation. Multiple sclerosis is associated with bowel dysfunction in more than two thirds of people who have this disease. The presence of FI is correlated with the degree of disability, duration of disease, and bladder symptoms. People with multiple sclerosis also develop constipation as a result of slow colonic transit time and the inability to relax the pelvic floor muscles at the time of defecation. Those with diabetes mellitus may suffer chronic diarrhea secondary to IAS neuropathy and impaired sensation, which can also lead to FI. Hypothyroidism may cause hypomotility and slow bowel transit time.

Psychological factors such as depression and cognitive impairment, as seen in people with Alzheimer's disease or other dementias, predispose the older adult to constipation, fecal impaction, and FI. The cause is believed to be neurological impairment that results in

- Inability to recognize or respond to an urge to have a bowel movement

- Inability to control the defecation and use of inappropriate toileting facilities

- Abnormal behaviors such as "parceling" (wrapping or concealing) feces

- Smearing of fecal material

- Denial or avoidance of the urge to defecate

- Loss of social awareness of the need for continence

- Inability to identify toilet facilities appropriately

- In some cases, physical inability to cope with bowel function

Lack of Physical Activity

A decrease in mobility or prolonged bed rest as a result of an accident or illness may contribute to constipation and FI. Decreased physical activity increases both self-reported and objectively measured constipation in older adults. People are more apt to have FI if they cannot get to the bathroom on sensing an urge to defecate. This is even more significant in the individual who has loose stools or diarrhea.

Laxative Abuse

Laxatives are substances that stimulate defecation and aid in the smooth transit of fecal material through the GI tract. However, individuals who habitually take laxatives become dependent on them and may require increasing dosages, until the intestine ultimately becomes refractory (accustomed to the laxatives and does not respond) to them.

Travel

When traveling, individuals often experience diarrhea or constipation, especially during long-distance trips and trips to other countries. This may be due to changes in drinking water, schedule, diet, and lifestyle.

EVALUATION OF BOWEL FUNCTION

The evaluation of a person with bowel dysfunction should include a focused history and physical examination. A bowel profile and a bowel function checklist can be used for this purpose. Patients who report bowel dysfunction may be referring to "blocked bowels," soiling, diarrhea, poor hygiene, or minor anal abnormalities such as hemorrhoids. Some people soil their clothes without knowing that they are about to have a bowel movement.

History of Bowel Function

A detailed history can give important clues to the cause of the bowel dysfunction. This may be difficult because events surrounding defecation involve meaning and social ramifications that may prevent patients from openly discussing problems (Norton, 2004). As with UI, people with bowel disorders are aware of the public stigma surrounding "bathroom issues" (Peden-McAlpine & Bliss, 2002). The clinician must approach the patient with sensitivity for the patient to share his or her bowel habits and rituals. The use of a Bowel Function Evaluation Checklist (Box 5.1) may be helpful (Boreham et al., 2005).

The history should include determining the previous bowel pattern and habits (laxative and enema use) as well as stool consistency, size, and shape (hard, soft, loose, and watery). The use of the Bristol Stool Form Scale

Box 5.1   Bowel Function Evaluation Checklist

History

- Elicit the patient's definition of constipation and of bowel disorder.
- Describe the stool form (see Figure 5.4 for Bristol Stool Form Scale).
- Determine the onset, frequency, and duration of fecal leakage, constipation, or other bowel problem.
- Determine the current bowel management program.
- Determine the patient's ability to distinguish stool and flatus.
- Identify associated symptoms of fecal incontinence:
  - Abdominal pain and cramping
  - Abdominal bloating
  - Gas incontinence
- Identify associated symptoms of constipation:
  - Decreased stool frequency
  - Sense of incomplete evacuation or stool trapping (dyssynergia)
  - Pain and discomfort with defecation
  - Abdominal pain and cramping
  - Rectal pain
  - Postdefecation soiling
  - Straining on defecation
  - Digital help with defecation
  - Frequent laxative use
  - Change in mental status
- Identify associated symptoms of fecal impaction:
  - Anorexia
  - Nausea and vomiting
  - Abdominal pain
  - Acute states of confusion
  - Fecal incontinence
- Determine the effect bowel dysfunction has had on the patient's quality of life.
- Identify all primary and secondary medical problems to determine their impact on the GI tract.
- Specify the type, frequency, and results of laxatives used in the past, as well as stool softeners, mini-enemas, suppositories, and enemas.
- Determine previous problem with fecal impaction and intervention.
- Determine current medication use to identify drugs with side effect profiles that may contribute to bowel disorder.
- Check lifestyle habits:
  - Does the patient smoke (nicotine is a known colonic stimulant)?

Box 5.1 *(continued)*

- Check diet/fluid intake:
  - Is dehydration present?
  - What is the total fluid intake in a 24-hour period?
  - How much caffeinated beverages and food are ingested?
- Check past medical history:
  - Pelvic, urological or GI disorders (e.g., UI, IBS, lactose intolerance)
  - Previous GI or pelvic surgery
  - Neurological diseases (Parkinson's, DM, MS)

Physical Examination

- Abdomen:
  - Listen for the presence of hyperactive or no bowel sounds.
  - Check for the presence of abdominal cramping, bloating or discomfort, masses, or bulges.
  - Percuss to determine the presence of gas.
  - Check for dullness that may indicate a fecal mass.
- Genitalia:
  - Visually inspect the perineal skin for integrity, rashes, and other effects of chronic leakage of stool.
- Pelvic examination (women):
  - Are structural abnormalities present, such as pelvic organ prolapse, particularly rectocele?
  - Can pelvic floor muscle strength be assessed?
- Anorectal examination:
  - Note the color and characteristics of the anal mucosa; note any gaping of the anus, which indicates abnormal external sphincter tone.
  - Note the presence and consistency of stool in the rectal vault—note the presence of fecal impaction.
  - Check for the presence of an anal wink, and note anal sphincter tone, impaired rectal sensation, and the size and condition of the rectum.
  - Note the presence of external or internal hemorrhoids and rectal prolapse.
  - Perform a Hemoccult test to determine the presence of occult blood in the feces.

Functional, Environmental, and Mental Assessment

- Mobility and ability to self-toilet:
  - Are restraints (physical or chemical) used?
  - Is manual dexterity sufficient for self-toileting?
- Environment:
  - Are toilet facilities accessible?
  - Are chairs designed for ease in rising?
  - Are grab bars available and within the resident's reach when toileting?

(continued)

Box 5.1 *(continued)*

- Mental
  - Is a Mini-Mental State Examination needed?
  - Assess mood, affect, and comprehension.

Bowel Record

- Has the defecation pattern been assessed through collection of a 3-day record or some other method?

Other Testing

- Anorectal manometry to provide baseline information on sphincter function and measurement of the rectal inhibitory reflex
- Flexible sigmoidoscopy, especially in those patients with Hemoccult-positive stools or in those who recently became constipated without obvious cause, and in all patients with fecal incontinence
- Plain abdominal radiographs in patients with constipation
- Barium enema if colonic obstruction is suspected
- Colonic transit time and motility testing in those patients with severe constipation that is not amenable to lifestyle modification treatments such as fluids, diet, and exercise
- Defecography to determine aspects of anorectal and pelvic floor function

Key: GI = gastrointestinal; MS = multiple sclerosis; UI = urinary incontinence.

(Figure 5.4) is recommended. Information should be gathered about onset and type of bowel dysfunction, including any pattern to bowel incontinence or constipation. Passive soiling, staining, seepage, or incontinence of gas is likely to be caused by an IAS problem, but it is impossible to be certain of the cause without further tests. The history should note all symptoms (e.g., constipation, diarrhea, bowel impaction, bowel incontinence or prolonged straining before defecation or both, fecal urgency). Rectal urgency is believed to be an important symptom and is defined as the need to "rush to the toilet" often (> 25% of the time) or usually (> 75% of the time) because of an urgent need to empty the bowels (Bharucha et al., 2006). The history should include the degree of rectal sensation and whether the patient identifies fullness in the rectum, has the sensation of passage of stool or gas, and identifies warning symptoms of abdominal cramps and urgency. Associated symptoms (abdominal bloating, nausea, cramping pain, rectal bleeding, and urinary symptoms) are important, as well as exacerbating or relieving factors (mechanical strategies, such as digital disimpaction or vaginal splinting).

The clinician should review the patient's daily diet, including fiber-rich foods and fluid intake, to determine the presence of dehydration. A list of current medications must be obtained, noting use of herbal agents, laxatives, stool softeners, suppositories, and enemas and medications that can cause side effects of constipation and diarrhea. Many commonly used medications, including calcium- and aluminum-containing antacids, beta blockers, calcium channel

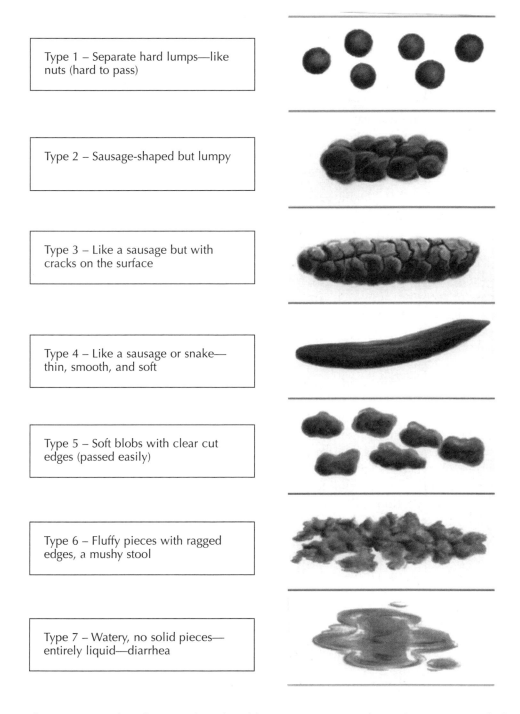

Figure 5.4. Bristol Stool Form Scale. (Adapted from Heaton, K.W., Ravdan, J., Cripps, H., Mountford, R.A., Braddon, F.E.M., & Hughes, A.O. [1992]. Defecation frequency and timing, and stool form in the general population: A prospective study. *Gut, 33,* 818–824.)

blockers, anticholinergic agents, antidepressants, and opiates, also cause constipation. Systemic diseases such as thyroid disease, diabetes mellitus, and neuromuscular and neurological diseases (spinal cord injury, multiple sclerosis, stroke) are yet other potential etiologies. Defecatory dysfunction is often a result of functional obstruction occurring because of pelvic floor muscle weakness with subsequent prolapse, including rectocele and enterocele (Jensen, 1997). Bowel function can also be affected by psychiatric disorders, including depression, dementia, and anorexia. A history of previous back, anorectal, bowel, or pelvic surgery or radiation can also be helpful. In women, bowel dysfunction in association with pregnancy and childbirth should be ascertained.

Physical Examination

The physical examination should include a thorough abdominal, anorectal, and pelvic examination. Distention, pain, or discomfort on abdominal exam may suggest the presence of gas, fluid, or obstruction, which could be due to a mass or feces in the bowel. Abdominal palpation may reveal the presence of stool-filled bowel loops, which can indicate constipation or a high impaction. A pelvic examination may reveal posterior vaginal wall relaxation and presence of a rectocele. Visual inspection of the perineal skin and anus should be performed. Perianal skin should be inspected for erythema, presence of soiling, hemorrhoids, and skin tags (may prevent adequate perianal hygiene). The anus is normally closed circumferentially. Gaping of the anus suggests rectal prolapse, which can usually be demonstrated with a Valsalva maneuver (Madoff, 2004). The examiner should stroke the perianal skin with a finger in the 9 and 3 o'clock positions. This normally elicits the "anal wink," a visible contraction of the anal sphincter—the anus will pucker. The anorectal exam should include an inspection for soiling and an assessment of rectal contents.

After inspection, a digital rectal examination should be performed to determine the presence of a rectal tumor or mass, presence of fecal material, and strength of the anal sphincter. Even in the absence of stool in the rectal vault, a higher impaction may be present. In order to determine overall anal sphincter tone, the strength and symmetry of the sphincter contraction, defects in the sphincter mechanism, and the dynamic changes of the pelvic floor during a Valsalva maneuver, the person is asked to squeeze or strain during digital examination. The puborectalis muscle should pull the examiner's finger toward the pubic symphysis. However, the positive predictive value of digital examination is 67% for detecting decreased anal tone as compared to anal manometry. Bearing down during the digital exam may reveal a rectal prolapse or enterocele. An inability to contract the anal sphincter may indicate neurological deficits.

Daily Bowel Record

Another important part of the evaluation is asking the patient to complete a Bowel Disorders Profile (see the companion CD under Assessment Forms). The person should be asked to discuss the bowel problem in his or her own words (Jensen, 2000). Using a pictorial scale such as the Bristol Stool Form Scale (see Figure 5.4) may aid the clinician in understanding the patient's description of stool consistency (Bliss, Dhamani, Savik, & Kirk, 2003). Stool consistency can vary from hard lumps to very loose or pasty stool; the consistency often depends on how long the stools have been in the colon and how much water has been absorbed. Ideally stool should be formed into a smooth sausage shape, soft and comfortable to pass.

Diagnostic Tests

A simple procedure to detect defecatory disorders is the balloon expulsion test. A latex balloon is inserted in the rectum and 50 mL of water or air is instilled into the balloon. The patient is asked to expel the balloon; most should be able to expel it in 1 minute. If the patient is unable to expel the balloon within 3 minutes, dyssynergic defecatory muscle activity should be suspected.

Additional studies such as anoscopy, proctoscopy, and barium enema radiography may be necessary. A plain abdominal radiograph (kidney, ureters, and bladder) can identify a high impaction, which would be seen as an obstructive pattern. A flexible sigmoidoscopy or colonoscopy can identify colitis, cancer, IBS, colonic or rectal ischemia, laxative abuse, and other structural abnormalities. Anorectal manometry measures liquids or gases and can assess function of anal sphincter tone and strength (both the IAS and EAS), the rectoanal inhibitory reflex, and perception of rectal sensation (Norton, 2004). Imaging examines rectal emptying and can determine structural damage (e.g., rectal prolapse) that may be amenable to surgery. Anal ultrasound (endoanal ultrasonography) or magnetic resonance imaging can identify defects in the IAS and EAS and may be a helpful but expensive diagnostic test in patients with FI. Defecography, or evacuation proctography, can determine defecation and evacuation abnormalities.

TREATMENT

Management of bowel disorders is influenced by many factors, including tradition, culture, and people's expectations of what is "normal" (Coolen, Florisson, Bissett, & Parry, 2006). Because patients are too embarrassed to report their problem to a professional, they tend to "self-treat" using a variety of over-the-counter laxatives or a self-determined bowel regimen (Matthiesen & De Wolff, 2006). Many bowel disorders, especially constipation and FI, that are seen in older people who are dependent on caregivers or live in nursing facilities could be prevented by proper attention to mobility, fluids, diet, medication, and establishment of good bowel habits (Potter & Wagg, 2005). In long-term care facilities, staff attitudes are crucial: Staff should not simply accept the situation as inevitable but rather approach it in an individualized manner (Benton, O'Harra, Chen, Harper, & Johnston, 1997). Box 5.2 describes the elements of a successful bowel program that can be used by staff in long-term care facilities. Although a Cochrane Review of practical management found very few evidenced-based studies, several strategies are often recommended to individuals with bowel disorders (Coggrave, Wiesel, & Norton, 2006). Management of bowel disorders should be tailored to the specific cause when possible, but typically a variety of treatment strategies are used. These include modification of stool consistency and delivery of stool to the anorectum through diet and medications; behavioral interventions, including biofeedback-directed pelvic floor muscle training; and surgery to correct abnormal continence mechanisms.

Maintaining Adequate Fluid Intake

Daily fluid intake should not be less than approximately 30 mL/kg per day of fluids, and a 1,500-mL per day minimum, based on clinical condition, is recommended. Drinking a glass of prune or apricot juice daily or eating prunes may help with bowel regulation. Prune juice has almost no fiber but does have a laxative effect, probably because of its content of magnesium salts. Apricot juice has high fiber content.

There are creative ways to increase fluid intake. Setting the table or tray with two types of liquid at each meal helps increase total intake. If a person is averse to drinking additional amounts of juice and water, the intake of foods that have high water content, such as fruits (e.g., watermelon), soups, ice cream, and flavored ices, can be encouraged. In long-term care, a fluid cart containing water and juices that makes rounds twice during a day shift and once during the early evening (before 7:00 P.M.) shift could be implemented.

Promoting Physical Activity

Physical activity in any form enhances colon peristalsis and motility. Walking for 20–30 minutes once or twice a day has been recommended as an aid to bowel motility, but even a small increase in physical activity has been shown to stimulate the bowel. Exercise together with abdominal massage can result in reduced FI and a significant increase in the number of bowel movements. Chair or bed exercises, such as pelvic tilt, also help.

Increased Fiber Intake

Fiber-Rich Foods

Increasing intake of dietary fiber is widely advocated as first-line treatment for patients complaining of constipation and can be useful in FI (Bliss et al., 2001). Ingesting a soluble fiber supplement, containing either psyllium or

Box 5.2   Elements of a successful bowel program in long-term care

A well-planned bowel management program centers on adequate fluid intake, exercise, inclusion of fiber to stimulate bowel function, and scheduled time for defecation.

1. Increase Fluid Intake

- There are creative ways to increase fluids. Set the table or tray with two types of fluid at each meal to help increase total intake. It may also be helpful to offer popsicles or ice.

- Residents should drink six to eight 8-ounce glasses of fluid daily, or 30 mL/kg. If a resident is averse to drinking additional amounts of juice and water, encourage the intake of foods that have a high water content, such as fruits (e.g., watermelon), soups, ice cream, and flavored ices.

- Encourage residents to drink a large glass of prune and/or apricot juice daily. Prune juice produces catharsis and apricot juice has a high-fiber content.

2. Increase Dietary Fiber

- Residents and staff should be instructed about the need for increased fiber and about foods that have a high fiber content. Fiber will help to form stool that has more bulk and allow it to pass more easily. Consult with dietary staff to develop a high-fiber diet for specific residents.

- High-fiber foods include whole-grain breads and cereals, raw vegetables (especially green leafy ones), and fresh fruits with their skins intact.

- Bran is the most concentrated form of fiber. It mixes with food residue in the colon and dilutes the gut contents, facilitating evacuation and speeding up colon transit time. Bran also favorably influences the microbial flora in the colon. Ingesting unprocessed wheat bran is recommended to increase dietary fiber and restore bowel function. This type of bran is not the same as the commercial bran cereals that are widely advertised. Since wheat bran is a natural substance, it cannot harm the resident. It will not cause diarrhea, but if it causes too frequent stools, the amount should be decreased.

- Team with the facility's dietary department to determine a "creative culinary solution" to get residents to eat bran. One solution is using a bran mixture consisting of

  - 1 cup applesauce

  - 1 cup whole, unprocessed coarse wheat bran

  - ½ to ¾ cup prune juice

- Start by giving 2 tablespoons of the mixture daily in the morning with a glass of water or juice. Increase the bran mixture by 1 tablespoon at a time until the resident's bowel movements become regular. When the necessary amount exceeds 4 tablespoons, give the mixture in divided doses in the morning and evening.

- Some nursing homes find it helpful to place the amount and administration time of the bran directly on the resident's medication card to ensure administration. Instructing the dietary department to prepare the mixture and provide it for the nurses is also helpful.

- Other dietary options include adding bran to cereal in the morning, mashed with bananas, or mixed into applesauce to enhance taste. It may also be added to Jell-O, cottage cheese, ice cream, and puddings.

3. Implement a Defecation Schedule and Procedure

- Sit the resident on the toilet or bedside commode within 15 minutes after eating breakfast. Breakfast is the best meal for triggering the gastrocolic reflex because the reflex

(continued)

Box 5.2 *(continued)*

---

is strongest on an empty stomach. The peristalsis created by this reflex propels feces to the descending colon and rectum.

- Give the resident a warm drink because the warmth of the liquid will stimulate the colon to move.

- The abdomen may be massaged to induce the gastrocolic reflex. Allow 20–30 minutes for evacuation, and maintain privacy.

- Place the resident's body in correct alignment by elevating the feet on a footstool and leaning the body slightly forward. If the resident is unable to sit, position him or her on the left side.

- A glycerin or bisacodyl (Dulcolax) suppository may be used to help establish a normal, regular bowel pattern and facilitate evacuation. The suppository should be inserted within 1 hour after breakfast, the triggering meal.

4. Encourage Exercise

- Resident ambulation is an important component of restorative nursing in long-term care facilities. Walking the resident to the bathroom meets two restorative nursing goals, ambulation and toileting. Exercise in any form stimulates colon peristalsis, assisting in bowel evacuation.

Adapted from Newman, D.K. (2005). *Bladder and bowel rehabilitation program.* Philadelphia: SCA Personal Products; and Newman, D.K. (1999). *The urinary incontinence sourcebook* (2nd ed.). New York: McGraw-Hill.

---

gum Arabic, can decrease incontinent stools. Fiber acts in several ways: It increases water content in the stool, increases fecal bulk, promotes softer consistency of stool, replenishes bacteria in the colon, and can be used to increase or decrease colonic transit, all leading to bulkier stools (Hinrichs, Huseboe, Tang, & Titler, 2001). Inadequate fiber intake is a common reason for constipation in Western society. Recommended daily fiber intake is 20–35 g, and the average American eats only 14–15 g (Lembo & Camilleri, 2003). It may take several weeks of increased dietary fiber to see positive effects.

Dietary fiber includes insoluble and soluble fiber. Insoluble (referred to as bulk-forming) fiber is found in wheat bran, vegetables, apple skin, and whole grains. It binds water and electrolytes, forming a colloid suspension that increases stool volume. This type of fiber, especially wheat bran, is most helpful in preventing constipation. Soluble (also referred to as water-soluble) fiber is found in oat bran, barley, some beans, and certain fruits and pectin. It alters cholesterol and lipoprotein synthesis, producing short-chain fatty acids that decrease colonic transit time. Soluble fiber has minimal benefit in preventing or treating constipation. The most beneficial means to prevent constipation is to take in a combination of insoluble and soluble fiber by increasing dietary intake of bran, fruits, and vegetables.

Fiber acts as a bulk-forming agent and is metabolized by colonic bacteria to nonabsorbable, volatile fatty acids, which act as an osmotic cathartic. As fiber passes through the colon, it acts as a sponge by absorbing water. Fiber may bind with fecal bile salts and thus increase transit of stool through the intestine. While adding bulk, fiber also promotes retention of water in the stool, thus decreasing the amount and frequency of watery liquid stool. It is recommended that fiber be added to the diet gradually (increase by 5 g/day) to prevent the GI tract from overreacting, causing excessive gas, bloating, cramping, and diarrhea. High-fiber foods include

- Whole-grain breads and cereals (e.g., All-Bran [insoluble], oatmeal [soluble]). Whole-grain bread contains 8%–10% dietary fiber, but some fiber-rich breakfast cereals contain 25%.

- Fiber-rich herbal tea (Smooth Move), which has been shown to increase bowel movements in nursing home residents (Bub, Brinckmann, Cicconetti, & Valentine, 2006).

- Brown rice.

- Raw vegetables, especially green leafy ones. Vegetables contain cellulose, hemicellulose, and lignin. Lignin is not digested in the human intestine and, therefore, adds to stool weight.

- Fresh fruits with peels (e.g., apples), and raisins.

For patients on tube feedings, products containing dietary fiber based on 10–15 g per 1,000 calories should be used. Many contain soy fiber, which can be helpful in decreasing severe constipation in elderly patients. Examples of those tube-feeding products with larger amounts of insoluble fiber are Ensure with fiber (9.4 g/L insoluble soy fiber), Jevity (13.5 g/L insoluble soy fiber), Sustacal with fiber (7.4 g/L insoluble and 3.2 g/L soluble fiber), and Glucerna (13.5 g/L insoluble soy fiber).

Addition of Raw Wheat Bran

One solution to bowel dysfunction is the administration of high-fiber mixtures (Khaja, Thakur, Bharathan, Baccash, & Goldenberg, 2005; Wisten & Messner, 2005). If the person is not allergic to wheat products, the use of whole, unprocessed wheat bran, often called miller's bran, can be successful. Raw (unprocessed) bran has 40% fiber content and is the most concentrated form of fiber available. Wheat bran is a natural substance that is harmless to the body. Bran mixes with food residue in the colon, diluting the gut contents, facilitating evacuation, and speeding up colon transit time. Bran can also add bulk to stools that are too liquid. The goal in using bran is to produce one bowel movement daily of soft, well-formed stool. Clinical trials on the efficacy of bran, specifically using a "special bran recipe," have been performed on people with chronic constipation (Badiali et al., 1995; Smith & Newman, 1989). These studies used the combination of bran with applesauce and prune juice to regulate bowel function in nursing facility residents. Howard, West, and Ossip Klein (2000) reported an 80% reduction in total bowel medication use (laxative, suppository, or enema) in men living in nursing facilities who were placed on 4–5 tablespoons per day of a bran mixture.

Unprocessed wheat bran is not the same as the commercial bran cereals that are widely advertised. Unprocessed wheat bran can be purchased very inexpensively at health food stores and local grocery stores. Bran may be added to cereal in the morning, mashed with bananas, or added to applesauce. Bran may also be added to soups, cottage cheese, ice cream, and puddings. Bran will not cause diarrhea, but, if bowel movements become too frequent, the individual should be instructed to decrease the amount (Newman, 2005).

The patient education tool "Tips for Keeping Your Bowels Moving" (see the companion CD) can be used to explain to individuals and caregivers how bran helps to promote bowel regularity. People should be instructed to begin using bran in small amounts, such as 1 tablespoon, and to gradually increase the amount over time. Use of bran can have side effects—flatulence, abdominal bloating, and cramps. However, by starting with small amounts and only gradually increasing the intake, the person can usually avoid any side effects. In any case, if side effects do occur, the adverse effects disappear in a few weeks. In long-term care facilities, it is a good idea for staff to team with the facility's dietary department to determine a "creative culinary solution" to getting residents to eat bran. Some long-term care facilities find it helpful to place the amount and administration time of the bran directly on the resident's medication record to ensure administration.

Establishing a Routine Defecation (Toileting) Schedule

Although there is very little evidence-based research on bowel training or toileting programs (Bliss, Norton, Miller, & Krissovich, 2004), clinicians promote bowel programs that involve a regular timetable for bowel evacuation. It has been shown that patients with a regular bowel pattern empty their bowels at approximately the same time each day (Hsieh, 2005), so patients should always promptly respond to the call to stool, or the urge to defecate. The schedule should be determined by the individual's bowel elimination pattern and previous timing of defecation. The person should be taught never to ignore the feeling that the bowel needs to be emptied. Also, the person must have adequate time to toilet. Ouslander, Simmons, Schnelle, Uman, and Fingold (1996) demonstrated that prompted voiding, commonly used for nursing home residents with UI, increased bowel movement frequency and bowel continence. Staff should always provide privacy because public facilities or toilets in close proximity to other residents may cause the person to suppress the urge to defecate because of embarrassment.

Because the bowel is relatively quiet at night, the optimal times to schedule defecation are in the morning and after a meal, preferably breakfast. The gastrocolic reflex, or the mass propulsion of material through the large intestine, is highest upon awakening and when combined with food (morning breakfast). The peristalsis created by this reflex propels feces to the descending colon and rectum. Normal defecation requires relaxation of the pelvic floor muscles, particularly the anal sphincter; adequate rectal tone; and sensation of rectal filling (Doughty, 1996). Normal sensation of rectal filling is key to providing motivation (a learned response), and underlines the cognitive component of normal defecatory function. This cognitive or behavioral component suggests that, in some cases, constipation may be a learned or conditioned response.

Heeding the urge to have a bowel movement and allowing sufficient time for undisturbed visits to the bathroom are especially important for residents in a long-term care facility who need assistance to toilet. If a regular toileting time is not set aside for residents to empty their bowels, they will have FI accidents. Attention should be paid to body alignment, because a sitting or squatting position is best to allow for an abdominal contraction with pelvic floor relaxation. For bedridden patients, manually pushing the legs toward the abdomen may be helpful, especially when expelling feces is difficult (Folden et al., 2002). Placing the feet on a footstool and leaning the body slightly forward will promote complete evacuation and decrease straining. Massaging the abdomen can induce an increase in peristalsis and stimulate the gastrocolic reflex (Wilson, 2005).

A bedridden person, whether living at home or in a nursing facility, may need to use a bedpan. If the resident is unable to sit, he or she should be positioned on the left side. However, attempting to defecate in a bedpan is very difficult for most people because this position causes undue strain. It forces the extension of the legs, pushes the stomach (abdomen) out, and does not allow the pelvic floor muscles to aid in defecation. The caregiver should try to avoid using a bedpan if at all possible.

Use of Medications

The four main categories of medications used to treat bowel disorders are emollients or softeners, stimulants, hyperosmotic saline, and bulk formers. In many cases, medications are prescribed to complement other strategies such as increased fluid and physical activity, addition of bran, and behavioral strategies. Bulk-forming laxatives have few side effects and minimal systemic effects. Bulk-forming agents have properties similar to those of dietary fiber. Table 5.2 lists common medications used to treat constipation. A typical bowel program for a neurogenic bowel with constipation may consist of the use of a stool softener three times a day with two senna tablets and a bisacodyl enema daily or every other day (useful in spinal cord injury patients) (Stern, 2006).

In patients with diarrhea, reducing the intake of dietary fiber has benefit when combined with the administration of antidiarrheal drugs, which slow colonic transit and decrease intestinal fluid secretion (Wald, 2007). Of the antidiarrheal agents, loperamide (Imodium) is preferred because it has no effects on the central nervous system (Sun, Read, & Verlinden, 1997). In patients with diarrhea associated with IBS, tricyclic antidepressants may also help to alleviate diarrhea by means of their anticholinergic properties. Conti-

Table 5.2 Common medications used for chronic constipation

Classification	Agent	Action & uses	Side effects & considerations
Fiber or Bulk-Forming Agents Soluble	*Dietary fiber—bran* (see special bran recipe in "Tips for Keeping Your Bowels Moving" on the companion CD under Patient Education Tools) *Guar gum* *Medicinal fiber—psyllium (Metamucil, Konsyl, Fiberall)* Powder: 3.4 g per rounded teaspoonful of powder; mix with 8 oz liquid, take 1–4 times per day Wafers: 1–2 in 8-oz glass of water	Are hydrophilic because they absorb water from the intestinal lumen to increase fecal bulk and soften stool consistency. These will decrease transit time. May be most effective in patients with normal transit time. Safest laxatives but can interfere with absorption of some drugs. Tablets should be taken with glass of water or juice. Granules/powder mixed with water or juice should be ingested immediately.	Abdominal cramps, gas, bloating, or diarrhea. Bowel obstruction or fecal impaction can occur, especially in elderly patients, if not taken with enough water. Medicinal fiber may cause less gas than dietary fiber. It can also be titrated more easily than dietary fiber. Psyllium and polycarbophil can decrease the effect of drugs such as warfarin, digitalis, salicylates, tetracyclines, ciprofloxacin, and nitrofurantoin.
Insoluble	*Polycarbophil (Perdiem Fiber Therapy, FiberCon)*: 625-mg tablets; take 2 tablets 1–4 times per day *Methylcellulose (Citrucel)* Powder: 2 g per rounded teaspoonful of powder; mix with 8 oz liquid, take 1–3 times per day. 500-mg tablets: take 2 tablets with 8 oz liquid, up to 6 times per day	Take 12 hours to 3 days to achieve effect. Are not the laxative of choice for immediate relief.	Tablets should be avoided in patients with dysphagia because they can expand and become lodged in the esophagus, causing obstruction.
Stool Softeners or Emollients	*Docusate sodium (Colace)* Capsules: 50, 100 mg; daily dose of 500 mg in 1–4 divided doses Liquid: 150 mg/15 mL Syrup: 60 mg/15 mL Daily dose for liquid or syrup is up to 300 mg. *Docusate calcium (Surfak)*: take two 40-mg capsules daily	Surfactants that cause absorption of water and fat. Provide moisture to the stool and prevent excessive loss of water. Well tolerated and used primarily to prevent constipation. Not as effective for constipation as bulk agents. Stool softeners have few side effects but take 1–3 days to produce a firm, semisolid stool. Recommended for situations in which straining should be avoided.	Abdominal cramping, nausea, diarrhea. Use with caution in patients with decreased rectal tone or bowel motility problems because soft stool may accumulate and be difficult to evacuate. May be more useful for patients with anal fissures or hemorrhoids that cause painful defecation. Capsules should be taken with full glass of water, fruit juice, or milk. Liquid should be given with milk or fruit juice to mask bitter taste.

Osmotic or Saline Agents	*Magnesium hydroxide (Milk of Magnesia)*: liquid (400 mg/5 mL). Adult: 30–60 mL daily as needed. Child: 1–3 mL/kg/day divided twice daily as needed.	Milk of Magnesia and Phospho-Soda are hyperosmolar agents that cause increased intestinal retention of fluid by osmotic activity (draw fluid into the intestines). They are considered safe because they work within the colonic lumen and are not absorbed systemically.	Chronic use of magnesium-containing laxatives may contribute to electrolyte imbalances (hypermagnesemia, hypocalcemia, and hypophosphatemia), especially with prolonged use.
	Sodium biphosphate (Phospho-Soda): liquid (45 mL, 90 mL); mix 2 tablespoons in 4 oz water, then follow with 8 oz water; take 20–45 mL per day.		Magnesium compounds are known to decrease effect of tetracyclines and digoxin, and lactulose may decrease the effect of oral neomycin.
	Lactulose (Kristalose, Chronulac): liquid (10 g/15 mL). Adult: take 15–60 mL/day. Child: 1–3 mL/kg/ day daily or divided twice daily.	Sorbitol and lactulose are undigestible agents that are metabolized by colonic bacteria into hydrogen and organic acids. They produce increased osmotic load within the lumen of the colon, resulting in distention and increased peristalsis. Poor absorption may lead to gas and abdominal distention.	Phosphates should not be administered with ACE inhibitors.
	Sorbitol 70%: Adult: 15–60 mL daily. Child: 1–3 mL/kg/day divided twice daily.		May cause abdominal cramping, gas, nausea diarrhea, and dehydration, particularly in people with chronic renal failure.
	Polyethylene Glycol-electrolyte (PEG) solution (PEG 3350, MiraLax)—similar to bowel prep solution (GoLytely, Colyte): powder (17 g [one capful]); dissolve in 240 mL (8 oz) water or juice.	PEG 3350 may cause less gas and is often used for bowel cleansing prior to GI exam.	Monitor these agents closely in patients with renal failure and CHF as they can lead to fluid and salt overload because of their osmotic effect.
	Adult: 17 g (1 capful) daily. Child: Start at 0.8–1 g/kg/day (15 mL/kg/day) divided twice daily. Adjust dose for two soft painless stools per day. Taper dose over time.		
	Magnesium citrate (Citroma): Adult: 8 ounces daily as needed. Child: 4 mL/kg up to 200 ml daily as needed.	Take 24–48 hours to achieve effect, except magnesium citrate, which produces watery stool in 1–3 hours.	May be unpalatably sweet for certain individuals. Chilled solution may be more palpable.

Docusate sodium is a safe agent in elderly patients but doses less than 200 mg may be ineffective.

(continued)

Table 5.2 (continued)

Classification	Agent	Action & uses	Side effects & considerations
Osmotic or Saline Agents (continued)			
Lubricants	*Mineral oil*: take 15–45 mL twice daily. Maximum dose of 45 mL.	Prevents reabsorption of water and lubricates or softens the stool, allowing it to slip through the intestine more easily. Effects usually noted within 6–8 hours. These are becoming obsolete because of severe abdominal cramping and concern of aspiration.	Mineral oil should be used with caution because it can decrease reabsorption of fat-soluble vitamins (A, D, E, and K) and medications such as warfarin. Used for temporary relief of acute fecal impaction and occasional constipation. May inhibit absorption of drugs such as warfarin, oral contraceptives, and sulfonamides.
Stimulants or Irritants (Cathartics)	*Bisacodyl (Dulcolax, Correctol, Carter's Pills)*: 5-mg tablets; take 5–15 mg daily *Anthraquinones such as senna (Senokot, ExLax)*: Senekot: 8.6-mg tablets; take 2 or 4 tablets once or twice daily *Ex-Lax*: 1–2 tablets daily or twice daily *Cascara sagrada*: Liquid: 1 teaspoon of liquid extract 3 times a day or 1 or 2 teaspoons at bedtime. 325-mg tablets: take 1 daily (early evening to stimulate a bowel movement in the morning).	Stimulate sensory nerve endings upon contact, increasing rhythmic muscular contractions (motility) in the intestines, and increase fluid secretions. Should not be used daily or long term because they can damage bowel and cause electrolyte imbalance with continual use. Effects are usually noted within 6–12 hours.	May cause abdominal cramping because of increased peristalsis. Dermatitis, electrolyte imbalance, diarrhea, dehydration. Prolonged use can lead to colonic inertia as a result of nerve damage. Are known to decrease effect of warfarin and should not be taken with dairy products and antacids (decreases the laxative effect).
Prokinetic Agents	*Misoprostol (Cytotec)*: 200 mcg four times daily with food	Accelerates colonic transit time and increases stool frequency in patients with constipation.	Has not been approved by the FDA for constipation. Should be taken with food with last dose at bedtime. Several drug interactions have been noted, so the use of other

Locally Acting Agent	Lubiprostone (Amitiza): 24 mcg (1 cap) twice daily	Acts in the small intestine by increasing luminal fluid secretion, promoting intestinal motility and peristalsis, and allowing for easy passage of stool. Effective for chronic idiopathic constipation. Effects within a few hours.	medications in combination with prokinetic agents should be avoided. Nausea, diarrhea, abdominal bloating, and headache. Should be taken with food. Can be added to tube feedings.
Suppositories	Oil, glycerin, bisacodyl (Dulcolax): 10 mg	Stimulate the defecation reflex and assist the rectum to empty any stool contents. Glycerin is a hyperosmotic laxative that acts by drawing fluid into the rectum and exerting a mild irritant effect on the rectal mucosa. Bisacodyl stimulates peristalsis by activating parasympathetic pathways. Usually an effect is seen within 30 minutes.	Dehydration, electrolyte imbalance. Prolonged excessive use may lead to electrolyte imbalance and hypokalemia, and may precipitate the onset of rebound constipation.
Enemas	Tap water: 500–1,000 mL up to twice weekly Saline Sodium phosphate (Fleet enema): 120 mL, 1–2 times per week Milk and molasses Mini-enemas (Therevac, Enemeez): 283 mg of the active ingredients (docusate sodium, medicinal soft soap, polyethylene glycol and glycerin)	Rectal stimulants. Fluid is instilled into the rectum to soften stool and to aid in removal. Must be retained for 10 minutes to work.	Sodium phosphate enemas can cause dehydration, hypocalcemia, and hypophosphatemia in people with chronic renal failure.

Data from Newman (2002); Kumar, Yoselovitz, and Gambert (2007); and Hsieh (2005).

Key: ACE = angiotensin-converting enzyme; CHF = congestive heart failure; FDA = Food and Drug Administration.

nence is more easily established for solid than for liquid stools and gas, especially when there is adequate puborectalis muscle function. Alosetron (Lotronex) is approved for women with IBS and diarrhea. Because this drug reduces urgency and the frequency of liquid stool, it may improve FI caused by other conditions.

Avoidance of Bowel Irritants

Caffeine consumption causes an increase of fluid secretion in the intestine, thus increasing the amount of liquid stool, and may contribute to FI. Caffeine is presumed to stimulate the parasympathetic nervous system, thus increasing bowel motility. Avoiding foods that contain caffeine (i.e., tea, coffee, chocolate) is recommended. Some foods contain starches that escape digestion in the small bowel and may cause flatulence (gas) in the colon and lead to "gas" incontinence. Some of the foods commonly thought to cause flatulence include apricots, bananas, beans, Brussels sprouts, cabbage, carrots, celery, dried beans, eggs, lentils, milk and milk products, onions, peas, pretzels, prunes, raisins, salad ingredients (especially cucumber), and wheat germ. Hot, spicy foods can increase the speed with which food travels along the bowel and increase gas production. People with incontinence of flatus can experiment to see if certain foods are affecting them and whether avoiding the offending food helps their condition.

Probiotics

Probiotics are live microorganisms, including *Lactobacillus* species (lactobacilli are normally found in the intestine and vagina), *Bifidobacterium* species, and yeasts. The use of probiotics may be beneficial in improving the balance of the intestinal microflora and is becoming more popular. The probiotics that are marketed as nutritional supplements and added to foods such as yogurts are principally the *Bifidobacterium* and *Lactobacillus* species. The most common adverse reactions with use of probiotics are GI side effects, including flatulence and constipation.

External Stimulation

If the individual is unable to defecate, some form of external stimulation should be considered because some people may need stimulation to initiate defecation. There are two types of external stimulation: use of a suppository and digital stimulation. Suppositories can be used to stimulate defecation until a pattern of regular defecation of soft, formed stools is established (Venn, Taft, Carpentier, & Applebaugh, 1992). The two most commonly used are glycerin and bisacodyl. To be successful, the suppository must be placed against the rectal wall and not into the actual stool.

Digital stimulation is commonly used in rehabilitation centers. Digital stimulation involves inserting a gloved, lubricated finger just inside the anus. Movement of the finger in a circular motion for 1–2 minutes will stimulate the rectum to contract. When the IAS relaxes, the stimulation is stopped. Digital stimulation of the rectum can be performed as long as it does not cause the person pain and discomfort, or is not contraindicated by his or her condition. However, digital stimulation may not be acceptable to the caregiver and/or the individual.

Pelvic Floor Muscle Rehabilitation Using Biofeedback Therapy

Biofeedback therapy that involves tightening the pelvic floor muscles is also very useful for strengthening the anal sphincter and is the treatment of choice for anorectal dysfunction. This treatment modality is an established means of treating people with UI and other types of pelvic floor dysfunction. Biofeedback has been used to improve the perception of rectal sensation and the responsiveness of the sphincter muscle to balloon distention with the use of instruments that monitor sphincter contractions (see Chapter 8) (Wald, 2003). Biofeedback has been shown to have an overall efficacy of 92% for FI and, in individuals with constipation, an efficacy of 80% (Ko et al., 1997; Norton, Chelvanayagam, Wilson-Barnett, Redfern, & Kamm, 2003; Norton, Whitehead, Bliss, Metsola, & Tries, 2005). The goals of biofeedback therapy are to improve the strength of the anal sphincter, improve the coordination between the rectum and the anal sphincter, and improve the sensory awareness for stool perception. In patients with constipation, biofeedback is used to teach correct evacuation techniques (Harari, Norton, Lockwood, & Swift, 2004).

A biofeedback-directed pelvic floor muscle training program consists of instruction to the person regarding training of the pelvic floor muscles. In those individuals with constipation, "constipation exercises" (i.e., learning the "bearing-down" maneuver) are taught. Usually a program consists of a biofeedback session involving the use of anorectal electromyographic monitoring of activity of the pelvic floor muscles or a manometry catheter. Patients receive training on visual or auditory feedback or both by simulation of an evacuation with a balloon or a silicone-filled artificial stool. These programs also include education on proper bowel diet, elimination regimen, and pelvic floor physiological function, and instruction in techniques to retrain these functions.

There is very little research to show efficacy for rectal electrical stimulation using a home unit. Norton, Gibbs, and Kamm (2006) conducted a randomized, controlled trial of 8 weeks of anal stimulation in 90 patients (9 men, 81 women) with FI. Subjects reported modest improvement in bowel control, but there was no difference between the control (sham stimulation) and active treatment groups. The improvement seen may have been caused by sensitization of patients to their anal sphincter function.

Devices for Stool Collection

For FI, use of devices such as a rectal plug, rectal tube, rectal trumpet (Grogan & Kramer, 2002), or fecal collection pouch (Ross, 1993) should be considered to collect feces or to divert feces from coming in contact with skin. An anal plug, which is available in the United Kingdom, is one of the only devices that can prevent involuntary leakage of stool. Even so, its effectiveness in eliminating leakage completely has been reported to be only approximately 50% (Norton & Kamm, 2001). It has been tested for safety, but one of its major disadvantages is discomfort. Only 5 of 20 patients who tested the plug tolerated wearing it, and an additional 8 patients refused to conduct the evaluation after trying one (Norton & Kamm, 2001). Questions remain about the safe duration of insertion of rectal tubes and risk of damage to the rectal mucosa from tubes with or without balloons in critically ill patients, in whom they are often used.

There are fecal containment devices that can be used with individuals with high-volume liquid diarrhea and FI (Echols et al., 2007). The Zassi Bowel Management System (Hollister, Libertyville, IL) has a low-pressure retention cuff that assists in holding a tube in place in the rectal vault (Figure 5.5). The FlexiSeal Fecal Collection Device (Convatec, Princeton, NJ) consists of a silicone catheter, a retention balloon that is inserted into the rectum, and a connector for attaching the collection bag (Figure 5.6). Both of these are temporary containment devices, indicated for bedridden or immobilized, incontinent patients with diarrhea and/or FI (Padmanabhan et al., 2007). Stool must be of liquid consistency for it to drain through the tubing. These devices are designed to divert fecal matter, protect patients' wounds from fecal contamination, and reduce both the risk of skin breakdown and spread of infection. These should be considered as a management option for people with FI resulting from prolonged immobility or other chronic neurological causes. When properly applied, these devices can reduce the risk of skin breakdown secondary to *Escherichia coli* from liquid stool.

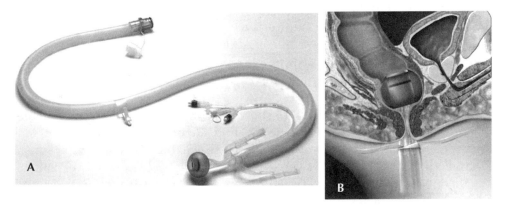

Figure 5.5.   (A) Zassi Bowel Management System (Hollister, Libertyville, IL). (B) Zassi system in the rectum with retention cuff.

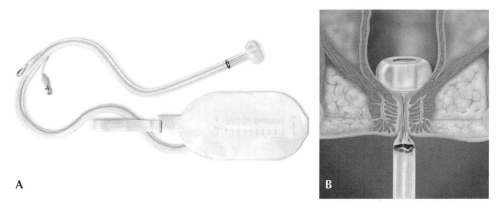

A   B

Figure 5.6.   (A) FlexiSeal Fecal Collection Device (Convatec, Princeton, NJ). (B) FlexiSeal in the rectum with retention balloon.

The use of skin care products is integral to the use of fecal containment devices (e.g., ConvaTec's FlexiSeal, Hollister's Zassi, rectal tubes, rectal trumpets) in people who have incontinence secondary to liquid stool. Based on the current research-based evidence, an external anal device can be an effective diversion and containment system while reducing the risk of skin breakdown and spreading of infection (Newman, Fader, & Bliss, 2004).

The least invasive product is the external perianal pouch (Fecal Collector; Hollister) (Figure 5.7). This is a drainable pouch that is attached to the skin using a synthetic, adhesive skin barrier. Application of the perianal pouch is similar to application of an ostomy pouch. Stool of any consistency can be collected by this pouch. The skin should be clean and dry before application. To prevent skin breakdown, a pectin-based powder (Stomahesive) is applied, followed by a plasticizing agent (skin prep). Once the opening to the pouch is sized relative to the anal opening, the pouch is pressed into place. The pouch spout can be clamped or connected to a drainage bag. The pouch will usually need to be changed every 2 days.

Bowel Irrigation

Irrigation of the rectum is used by certain patients with FI (Norton & Chelvanayagam, 2004). It is similar to a high-colonic enema in that several milliliters of fluid are instilled into the rectum to allow for complete evacuation. Companies are developing products and specific equipment for irrigation.

Surgery

Surgery is reserved for persistent and intractable constipation in patients who have been evaluated and proven to have slow-transit constipation. Surgical procedures are usually reserved for people with FI and include anal sphincter

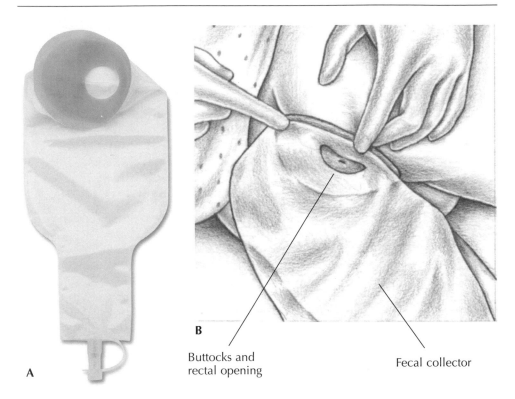

B

A

Buttocks and
rectal opening

Fecal collector

Figure 5.7.   (A) Fecal Collector (Hollister, Libertyville, IL). (B) Application of Fecal Collector.

repair or replacement and fecal diversion (Jensen, 2000). However, in older people, surgical intervention may worsen existing symptoms. In general, surgery for constipation is not very successful. Surgery for structural anal sphincter damage aims to restore anatomic continuity. One such procedure is an anal sphincter repair (anal sphincteroplasty), which repairs a disrupted anal sphincter and is best performed with the use of a technique that overlaps the two ends of the sphincter muscles. Other surgery includes implantation of an artificial anal sphincter (Acticon Neosphincter; AMS). Several small studies report fecal continence rates of 24%–78% following surgery (Madoff, Pemberton, Mimura, & Laurberg, 2005).

CONCLUSION

Bowel dysfunction, especially FI, is an embarrassing, usually debilitating disorder and often coexists with UI and LUTS. Constipation usually worsens symptoms of UI and overactive bladder, and treatment can improve these symptoms. As seen with UI, bowel disorders are mostly underreported, and patients are not aware of treatments options. Once the specific dysfunction is identified, conservative interventions can successfully treat these conditions.

REFERENCES

Abramov, Y., Sand, P.K., Botros, S.M., Gandhi, S., Miller, J.J., Nickolov, A., et al. (2005). Risk factors for female anal incontinence: New insight through the Evanston-Northwestern Twin Sisters Study. *Obstetrics and Gynecology, 106,* 726–732.

Agency for Healthcare Research and Quality. (2007, December). *Prevention of urinary and fecal incontinence in adults* (Evidence Report/Technology Assessment No. 161, Contract No. 290-02-0009). Rockville, MD: Author. Retrieved from http://www.ahrq.gov/downloads/pub/evidence/pdf/fuiad/fuiad.pdf

Akhtar, A.J., & Padda, M. (2005). Fecal incontinence in older patients. *Journal of the American Medical Directors Association, 6,* 54–60.

Alling Moller, L., Lose, G., & Jorgensen, T. (2000). Risk factors for lower urinary tract symptoms in women 40 to 60 years of age. *Obstetrics and Gynecology, 96,* 446–451.

Altman, D., Zetterstrom, J., Schultz, I., Nordenstam, J., Hjern, F., Lopez, A., et al. (2006). Pelvic organ prolapse and urinary incontinence in women with surgically managed rectal prolapse: A population-based case-control study. *Diseases of the Colon and Rectum, 49,* 28–35.

Badiali, D., Corazziari, E., Habib, F.I., Tomei, E., Bausano, G., Magrini, P., et al. (1995). Effect of wheat bran in treatment of chronic nonorganic constipation—a double-blinded controlled trial. *Digestive Diseases and Sciences, 40,* 349–356.

Bano, F., & Barrington, J.W. (2007). Prevalence of anorectal dysfunction in women attending health care services. *International Urogynecology Journal and Pelvic Floor Dysfunction, 18,* 57–60.

Benton, J.M., O'Harra, P.A., Chen, H., Harper, D.W., & Johnston, S.F. (1997). Changing bowel hygiene practice successfully: A program to reduce laxative use in a chronic care hospital. *Geriatric Nursing, 18,* 12–17.

Bharucha, A.E., Zinsmeister, A.R., Locke, G.R., Seide, B.M., McKeon, K., Schleck, C.D., et al. (2006). Risk factors for fecal incontinence: A population-based study in women. *American Journal of Gastroenterology, 101,* 1305–1312.

Bliss, D.Z., Dhamani, K.A., Savik, K., & Kirk, K. (2003). Tool to classify stool consistency: Content validity and use by persons of diverse cultures. *Nursing and Health Sciences, 5,* 115–121.

Bliss, D.Z., Jung, H., Savik, K., Lowry, A., LeMoine, M., Jensen, L., et al. (2001). Supplementation with dietary fiber improves fecal incontinence. *Nursing Research, 50,* 203–213.

Bliss, D.Z., Norton, C.A., Miller, J., & Krissovich, M. (2004). Directions for future nursing research on fecal incontinence. *Nursing Research, 53*(6 Suppl.), S15–S21.

Boreham, M.K., Richter, H.E., Kenton, K.S., Nager, C.W., Gregory, W.T., Aronson, M.P., et al. (2005). Anal incontinence in women presenting for gynecologic care: Prevalence, risk factors, and impact upon quality of life. *American Journal of Obstetrics and Gynecology, 192,* 1637–1642.

Bub, S., Brinckmann, J., Cicconetti, G., & Valentine, B. (2006). Efficacy of an herbal dietary supplement (Smooth Move) in the management of constipation in nursing home residents: A randomized, double-blind, placebo-controlled study. *Journal of the American Medical Directors Association, 7,* 556–561.

Charach, G., Greenstein, A., Rabinovich, P., Groskopf, I., & Weintraub, M. (2001). Alleviating constipation in the elderly improves lower urinary tract symptoms. *Gerontology, 47,* 72–76.

Chassagne, P., Landrin, I., Neveu, C., Czernichow, P., Bouaniche, M., Doucet, J., et al. (1999). Fecal incontinence in the institutionalized elderly: Incidence, risk factors, and prognosis. *American Journal of Medicine, 106,* 185–190.

Chiang, L., Ouslander, J., Schnelle, J., & Reuben, D. (2000). Dually incontinent nursing home residents: Clinical characteristics and treatment differences. *Journal of the American Geriatrics Society, 48,* 673–676.

Coggrave, M., Wiesel, P.H., & Norton, C. (2006). Management of faecal incontinence and constipation in adults with central neurological diseases [Review]. *Cochrane Database of Systematic Reviews,* (2), CD002115.

Coolen, J.C.G., Florisson, M.G., Bissett, I.P., & Parry, B.R. (2006). Evaluation of knowledge and anxiety level of patients visiting the colorectal pelvic floor clinic. *Colorectal Disease, 8,* 208–211.

Cundiff, G.W., & Fenner, D. (2004). Evaluation and treatment of women with rectocele: Focus on associated defecatory and sexual dysfunction. *Obstetrics and Gynecology, 104,* 1403–1421.

Davis, R.H., Rao, S.S., Pallentino, J., & Schiller, L.R. (2007, September). Managing the chronically constipated adult: Emerging approaches to diagnosis and treatment. *Clinical Advisor,* pp. S1–S16.

Doughty, D. (1996). Physiologic approach to bowel training. *Journal of Wound, Ostomy, and Continence Nursing, 23,* 46–56.

Echols J, Friedman BC, Mullins RF, Hassan Z, Shaver JR, Brandigi C, et al. (2007). Clinical utility and economic impact of introducing a bowel management system. *Journal of Wound, Ostomy, and Continence Nursing, 34,* 664–670.

Edwards, N.I., & Jones, D. (2001). The prevalence of faecal incontinence in older people living at home. *Age and Ageing, 30,* 503–507.

Folden, S.L., Backer, J.H, Maynard, F., Stevens, K., Gilbride, J.A., Pires, M., et al. (2002). *Practice guidelines for the management of constipation in adults.* Retrieved December 31, 2007 from http://www.rehabnurse.org/profresources/BowelGuideforWEB.pdf

Goode, P.S., Burgio, K.L., Halli, A.D., Jones, R.W., Richter, H.E., Redden, D.T., et al. (2005). Prevalence and correlates of fecal incontinence in community-dwelling older adults. *Journal of the American Geriatrics Society, 53,* 629–635.

Grogan, T.A., & Kramer, D.J. (2002). The rectal trumpet: Use of a nasopharyngeal airway to contain fecal incontinence in critically-ill patients. *Journal of Wound, Ostomy, and Continence Nursing, 29,* 193–201.

Guise, J.M., Morris, C., Osterweil, P., Li, H., Rosenberg, D., & Greenlick, M. (2007). Incidence of fecal incontinence after childbirth. *Obstetrics & Gynecology, 109,* 281–288.

Harari, D., Norton, C., Lockwood, L., & Swift, C. (2004). Treatment of constipation and fecal incontinence in stroke patients: Randomized controlled trial. *Stroke, 35,* 2549–2555.

Hinrichs, M., Huseboe, J., Tang, J.H., & Titler, M.G. (2001). Research-based protocol: Management of constipation. *Journal of Gerontological Nursing, 27*(2), 17–28.

Howard, L.V., West, D., & Ossip Klein, D.J. (2000). Chronic constipation management for institutionalized older adults. *Geriatric Nursing, 21,* 78–82.

Hsieh, C. (2005). Treatment of constipation in older adults. *American Family Physician, 72,* 2277–2284.

Hunskaar, S., Burgio, K., Clark, A. Lapitan, MC., Nelson, R., Sillen, U., et al. (2005). Epidemiology of urinary incontinence (UI) and faecal incontinence (FI) and pelvic organ prolaspe (POP). In P. Abrams, L. Cardozo, S. Khoury, & A.J. Wein (Eds.), *Incontinence: Proceedings from the Third International Consultation on Incontinence* (pp. 255–312). Plymouth, UK: Health Publications, Ltd.

Jackson, S., Weber, A., Hull, A.T., Mitchinson, A., & Walters, M. (1997). Fecal incontinence in women with urinary incontinence and pelvic organ prolapse. *Obstetrics and Gynecology, 89,* 423–427.

Jelovsek, J.E., Barber, M.D., Paraiso, M.F.R., & Walters, M.D. (2005). Functional bowel and anorectal disorders in patients with pelvic organ prolapse and incontinence. *American Journal of Obstetrics and Gynecology, 193,* 2105–2111.

Jensen, L. (1997). Fecal incontinence: Evaluation and treatment. *Journal of Wound, Ostomy, and Continence Nursing, 24,* 277–282.

Jensen, L.L. (2000). Assessing and treating patients with complex fecal incontinence. *Ostomy/Wound Management, 46*(12), 56–60.

Johanson, J.F. (1998). Geographic distribution of constipation in the United States. *American Journal of Gastroenterology, 93,* 188–191.

Khaja, M., Thakur, C.S., Bharathan, T., Baccash, E., & Goldenberg, G. (2005). 'Fiber 7' supplement as an alternative to laxatives in a nursing home. *Gerontology, 22,* 106–108.

Ko, C.Y., Tong, J., Lehman, R.E., Shelton, A.A., Schrock, T.R., & Welton, M.L. (1997). Biofeedback is effective therapy for fecal incontinence and constipation. *Archives of Surgery, 132,* 829–834.

Kuehn, B.M. (2006). Silence masks prevalence of fecal incontinence. *JAMA, 295,* 1362–1363.

Kumar, V., Yoselevitz, S., & Gambert, S.R. (2007). Laxative use and abuse in the older adult: Part II. *Clinical Geriatrics, 15*(4), 37–42.

Landefeld, C.S., Bowers, B.J., Feld, A.D., Hartmann, K.E., Hoffman, E., Ingber, M.J., et al. (2008). National Institutes of Health state-of-the-art science conference statement: Prevention of fecal and urinary incontinence in adults. *Annals of Internal Medicine, 148*(6), 449–458.

Lembo, A., & Camilleri, M. (2003). Chronic constipation. *New England Journal of Medicine, 349,* 1360–1368.

Leoning Baucke, V. (2007). Prevalence rates for constipation and faecal and urinary incontinence. *Archives of Disease in Childhood, 92,* 486–489.

Longstreth, G.F., Thompson, W.C., Chey, W.D., Houghton, L.A., Mearin, F., & Spiller, R.C. (2006). Functional bowel disorders. *Gastroenterology, 130,* 1480–1491.

Madoff, R.D. (2004). Treatment options for fecal incontinence. *Gastroenterology, 126*(1 Suppl. 1), S48–S54.

Madoff, R.D., Parker, S.C., Varma, M.G., & Lowry, A.C. (2004). Faecal incontinence in adults. *Lancet, 364,* 621–632.

Madoff, R.D., Pemberton, J.H., Mimura, T., & Laurberg, S. (2005). Surgery for faecal incontinence. In P. Abrams, L. Cardozo, S. Khoury, & A. Wein (Eds.), *Incontinence: Proceedings from the Third International Consultation on Incontinence* (pp. 1565–1588). Plymouth, UK: Health Publications, Ltd.

Matthiesen, V., & De Wolff, D. (2006). Constipation and fecal incontinence. *ADVANCE for Nurse Practitioners, 14*(10), 41–44, 90.

Melville, J.L., Fan, M.Y., Newton, K., & Fenner, D. (2005). Fecal incontinence in US women: A population-based study. *American Journal of Obstetrics and Gynecology, 193,* 2071–2076.

Miner, P.B. (2004). Economic and personal impact of fecal and urinary incontinence. *Gastroenterology, 126*(1 Suppl. 1), S8–S13.

Nelson, R., Furner, S., & Jesudason, V. (1998). Fecal incontinence in Wisconsin nursing homes: Prevalence and associations. *Diseases of the Colon and Rectum, 41,* 1226–1229.

Nelson, R., Norton, N., Cautley, E., & Furner, S. (1995). Community-based prevalence of anal incontinence. *JAMA, 274,* 559–561.

Nelson, R.L. (2004). Epidemiology of fecal incontinence. *Gastroenterology, 126*(Suppl. 1), S3–S7.

Nelson, R.L., & Furner, S.E. (2005). Risk factors for the development of fecal and urinary incontinence in Wisconsin nursing home residents. *Maturitas, 52,* 26–31.

Newman, D.K. (2002). *Managing and treating urinary incontinence.* Baltimore: Health Professions Press.

Newman, D.K. (2005). Behavioral treatments. In S.P. Vasavada, R. Appell, P. Sand, & S. Raz (Eds.), *Female urology, urogynecology, and voiding dysfunction* (pp. 233–266). New York: Marcel Dekker.

Newman, D.K., Fader, M., & Bliss, D.Z. (2004). Managing incontinence using technology, devices and products. *Nursing Research, 53*(6 Suppl.): S42–S48.

Nichols, C.M., Ramakrishnan, V., Gill, E.J., & Hurt, W.G. (2005). Anal incontinence in women with and those without pelvic floor disorders. *Obstetrics and Gynecology, 106,* 1266–1271.

Norton, C. (2004). Nurses, bowel continence, stigma and taboos. *Journal of Wound, Ostomy, and Continence Nursing, 31,* 85–94.

Norton, C., & Chelvanayagam, S. (Eds.). (2004). *Bowel continence nursing.* Beaconsfield, UK: Beaconsfield Publishers Ltd.

Norton, C., Chelvanayagam, S., Wilson-Barnett, J., Redfern, S., & Kamm, M.A. (2003). Randomized, controlled trial of biofeedback for fecal incontinence. *Gastroenterology, 125,* 1320–1329.

Norton, C., Gibbs, A., & Kamm, M. (2006). Randomized, controlled trial of anal electrical stimulation for fecal incontinence. *Diseases of the Colon and Rectum, 49,* 190–196.

Norton, C., & Kamm, M.A. (2001). Anal plug for faecal incontinence. *Colorectal Disease, 3,* 323–327.

Norton, C., Whitehead, W.E., Bliss, D.Z., Metsola, P., & Tries, J. (2005). Conservative and pharmacological management of faecal incontinence in adults. In P. Abrams, L. Cardozo, S. Khoury, & A. Wein (Eds.), *Incontinence: Proceedings from the Third International Consultation on Incontinence* (pp. 1521–1564). Plymouth, UK: Health Publications, Ltd.

Ouslander, J.G., Simmons, S., Schnelle, J., Uman, G., & Fingold, S. (1996). Effects of prompted voiding on fecal continence among nursing home residents. *Journal of the American Geriatrics Society, 44,* 424–429.

Padmanabhan, A., Stern, M., Wishin, J., Mangino, M., Richey, K., & DeSane, M., for the Flexi-Seal Clinical Trial Investigators Group.(2007). Clinical evaluation of a flexible fecal incontinence management system. *American Journal of Critical Care, 16,* 384–393.

Palsson, O.S., Heymen, S., & Whitehead, W.E. (2004). Biofeedback treatment for functional anorectal disorders: A comprehensive efficacy review. *Applied Psychophysiology and Biofeedback, 29,* 153–174.

Peden-McAlpine, C., & Bliss, D.Z. (2002). The experience of women managing FI. *The Gerontologist, 42,* 143.

Potter, J., & Wagg, A. (2005). Management of bowel problems in older people: An update. *Clinical Medicine, 5,* 289–295.

Richter, H.E., Burgio, K.L., Clements, R.H., Goode, P.S., Redden, D.T., & Varner, R.E. (2005). Urinary and anal incontinence in morbidly obese women considering weight loss surgery. *Obstetrics and Gynecology, 106,* 1272–1277.

Ross, V. (1993). The fecal containment device: One answer to a dreaded procedure. *Ostomy/Wound Management, 39*(7), 42–45.

Sanburg, A.L., McGuire, T.M., & Lee, T. (1996). Stepping out of constipation: An educational campaign. *Australian Journal of Hospital Pharmacy, 26,* 350–355.

Schnelle, J.F., & Leung, F.W. (2004). Urinary and fecal incontinence in nursing homes. *Gastroenterology, 126*(1 Suppl. 1), S41–S47.

Smith, D.A., & Newman, D.K. (1989). The bran solution. *Contemporary Long-Term Care, 12,* 66.

Snooks, S.J., Barnes, P.R.H., Setchell, M., & Henry, M.M. (1985). Damage to the innervation of pelvic floor musculature in chronic constipation. *Gastroenterology, 89,* 977–981.

Spence-Jones, C., Kamm, M.A., Henry, M.M., & Hudson, C.N. (1994). Bowel dysfunction: A pathogenic factor in ureterovaginal prolapse and urinary stress incontinence. *British Journal of Obstetrics and Gynaecology, 101,* 147–152.

Stern, M. (2006). Neurogenic bowel and bladder in the older adult. *Clinics in Geriatric Medicine, 22,* 311–330.

Sultan, A.H., & Kamm, M.A. (1997). Faecal incontinence after childbirth. *British Journal of Obstetrics and Gynaecology, 80,* 393–394.

Sun, W.M., Read, N.W., & Verlinden, M. (1997). Effects of loperamide oxide on gastrointestinal transit time and anorectal function in patients with chronic diarrhea and fecal incontinence. *Scandinavian Journal of Gastroenterology, 32,* 34–38.

Venn, M.R., Taft, L., Carpentier, B., & Applebaugh, G. (1992). The influence of timing and suppository use on efficiency and effectiveness of bowel training after stroke. *Rehabilitation Nursing, 17,* 116–120.

Wald, A. (2003). Biofeedback for fecal incontinence. *Gastroenterology, 125,* 1533–1535.

Wald, A. (2007). Clinical Practice: Fecal incontinence in adults. *New England Journal of Medicine, 356,* 1648–1655.

Wilson, L.A. (2005). Understanding bowel problems in older people: Part 2. *Nursing Older People, 17,* 24–29.

Wisten, A., & Messner, T. (2005). Fruit and fibre (Pajala porridge) in the prevention of constipation. *Scandinavian Journal of Caring Sciences, 19*(1), 71–76.

6

Clinical Assessment and Evaluation

A systematic evaluation and identification of urinary incontinence (UI) is essential to identify possible transient and reversible causes and potential risk factors, to determine the effect of UI on the person's quality of life, to address current and potential complications, and to identify appropriate interventions. Despite current age, age at onset of UI, length of time incontinent, medical condition, and care setting, all patients should be offered a UI assessment. Treatment decisions should be based on a diagnosis made after a reasonably thorough evaluation of genitourinary anatomy and the physiology of bladder storage and emptying. Physical and mental status, patient expectations for treatment outcomes, motivation, and environmental and functional barriers are important determinants of interventions, so an assessment of these parameters is important. Figure 6.1 is a diagnostic algorithm for the evaluation of UI that may be helpful for primary care clinicians.

The basic evaluation of UI should incorporate recommendations outlined in the 1996 Agency for Healthcare Research and Quality (AHRQ) Clinical Practice Guidelines on "Urinary Incontinence in Adults" (Fantl et al., 1996) and the Third International Consultation on Incontinence (Abrams, Cardozo, Khoury, & Wein, 2005). The baseline evaluation of UI in long-term care (LTC), and particularly nursing home, residents is detailed in the Centers for Medicare & Medicaid Services (CMS) Tag F315 surveyor guidance on "Urinary Incontinence and Catheters" (CMS, 2005) and the Resident Assessment Program (RAP), and is supported by recommendations from the AHRQ and the American Medical Directors Association (AMDA, 2005) guidelines.

Nursing facilities have a federal mandate to conduct a comprehensive assessment and screening of residents on admission, and whenever there is a change in the resident's cognitive or medical condition, physical ability, or bladder function. For newly admitted residents, it is important to determine what the person's bladder function was prior to admission, which may involve gathering information from family members, a previous caregiver, or both. Tag F315 and the RAP recommend evaluation for reversible/transient factors that may cause UI, such as a urinary tract infection (UTI), environmental factors, certain medical conditions, and medications (see Chapter 4). Nursing facility staff must uncover the types of chronic UI and bladder dysfunction experi-

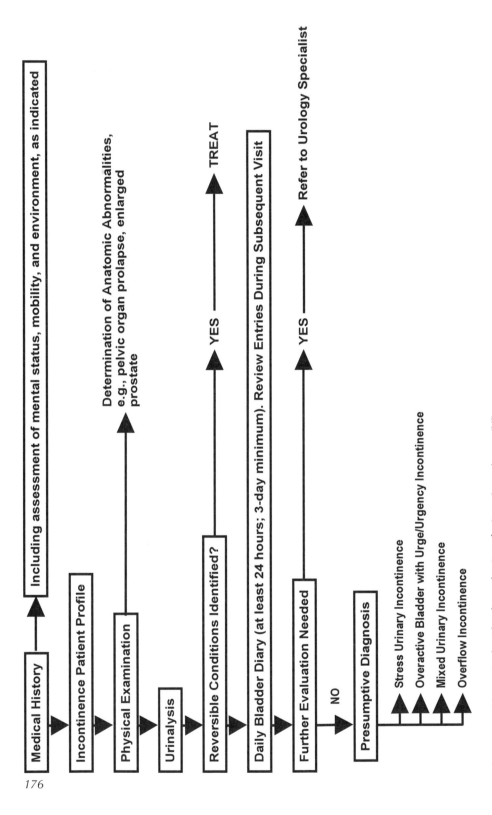

Figure 6.1. Diagnostic algorithm for evaluation of urinary incontinence (UI).

176

enced by the resident to diagnose the type of UI. A physician (e.g., primary care practitioner, internist, geriatrician, gynecologist) and nurse (nurse practitioner, physician assistant, clinical nurse specialist, or registered nurse) can perform an evaluation for UI as part of an interdisciplinary team (Klay & Marfyak, 2005; Maloney & Cafiero, 1999; Newman, 2006). In this setting, as well as home care settings, the evaluation can be performed at the bedside. The facility may document assessment information in any of several places throughout the medical record. Specific areas for documentation include the admission assessment, hospital records, history and physical, physician's orders, social service or psychological history, Minimum Data Set, RAP, laboratory results, and any nursing flow sheets, care plans, or forms the facility uses.

CLINICAL ASSESSMENT

Incontinence can be the result of many dysfunctions in the lower urinary tract or the nervous system, or lack of coordination between the systems; cognitive and functional impairments; lack of motivation; or barriers in the environment. The assessment for identifying the problem, or identifying the person at risk for incontinence problems, should include a detailed history with a review of symptoms (a subjective indicator of disease or change in condition as perceived by the patient, family member, and/or caregiver) related to both storage and emptying functions of the lower urinary tract. In addition to symptoms, signs will be determined by physical examination, by mental, functional, and environmental assessment, and by testing as needed (Newman, 2005a). The symptom of UI is generally thought of as the patient's complaint of involuntary urine loss. The sign is the objective demonstration of urine loss (Wein & Moy, 2007). Box 6.1 presents a comprehensive checklist that can be used when assessing the individual in a community-based, ambulatory practice. Screening, as part of an overall assessment of the patient's general health, requires minimal time from a provider because a self-administered screener or premailed questionnaire can be used in most clinical settings.

The following paradigm or classification system has been developed by the International Consultation on Incontinence (Fonda et al., 2005) to understand how to effectively manage UI, especially when dealing with frail older adults:

Independent continence—the person is able to maintain continence without treatment. He or she may have successfully undergone an intervention (e.g., anti-incontinence surgery).

Dependent continence—the person has physical or mental impairment and is kept dry through the efforts of others. A recurrence of incontinence would occur if management was withdrawn (Abrams et al., 2006). Caring for the person with dependent continence is a high labor cost for the LTC and home settings because staff or caregivers are needed to provide assistance with

---

Box 6.1   Evaluation checklist

History

- Obtain a history of the person's usual bladder or voiding habits.

- Ascertain incontinence/voiding symptoms, time of day symptom occurs, and relationship to activities, events, triggers, or antecedents.

- List symptoms, to include storage versus emptying (e.g., urgency, frequency, nocturia, nocturnal enuresis, straining, hesitancy, dysuria, episodes of leakage).

- Determine onset of the incontinence/voiding symptoms, length of time with current symptoms.

- Awareness of need to urinate:

  – Is the person aware or does he or she have a feeling (urge to void sensation) of the need to urinate?

  – What is the degree of urge or is urgency present (e.g., awareness but easily tolerated; interferes with tasks; extreme, causing person to stop all activity in order to hurry to urinate)?

  – From the first sensation of urge, how long is the person able to defer voiding (warning time) or leaking?

- Urine leakage:

  – When does the leakage occur? With standing (changing position), coughing, sneezing, laughing, lifting objects; with urgency; with seemingly no provocation?

  – How frequently does it occur? Every time, sometimes, daily, once or twice a week?

  – How severe is leakage or quantity of urine loss? Is there use of products to contain the urine (e.g., Kleenex tissues, pads, and briefs)? How often are they changed per day? Percentage of urine saturation?

- Characteristics of the urinary stream (note the following):

  – Character of the stream:

    - When and how does the stream start once the voiding is initiated?

    - Does the stream go continuously or start and stop?

    - How strong is the stream?

  – Is the patient straining or "bearing down" to get the urine out?

  – Is there pain or discomfort (e.g., grimacing, wincing, and moaning) with urination? If present, is it relieved with voiding?

  – Is postvoid dribbling present?

- Initiation of urination:

  – Once at the toilet, can the patient initiate the stream within a minute?

  – Does it take coaxing (e.g., running water or other triggers)?

  – What is the number of times that the patient actually urinates when at the toilet?

- Emptying of the bladder:

  – Does the bladder feel completely empty once voiding is completed?

  – Does the patient "push down" on the lower abdomen to ensure bladder emptying?

- Characteristics of the urine:

  – Color

  – Odor

  – Presence of blood, sediment, or mucus

Box 6.1   *(continued)*

- Assess all acute/transient causes of UI that can be reversed.

- Identify all primary and secondary medical problems to determine impact on lower urinary tract.

- Mental status:

  - Is the patient motivated to self-toilet or regain continence?

  - Is cognition intact—alert enough to recognize bladder fullness (urge sensation)?

  - Can the patient identify the location of, and is he or she able to ambulate to, a toileting facility (bathroom)?

- Bowel history:

  - Symptoms of constipation, diarrhea, fecal incontinence, abdominal bloating

  - Type of laxatives used in the past (e.g., stool softeners, suppositories, enemas)

  - Previous problem with fecal impaction, incontinence, or both, and intervention

- Observe toileting (if possible or appropriate):

  - Is the patient able to suppress or delay urge long enough to ambulate to the bathroom?

  - What is the distance from the bed/chair to the bathroom/toilet?

  - Is the patient able to self-toilet or toilet with minimal assistance?

  - Does the patient use a toileting device such as a bedside commode, urinal, or other container?

  - Does the patient use an absorbent product or other containment product (e.g., external catheter)?

  - Is the patient able to remove the incontinence product to self-toilet?

- Diet/fluid intake:

  - Are signs of dehydration present during physical exam (e.g., dry skin, poor skin turgor, dry mouth)?

  - What is the total fluid intake in a 24-hour period?

  - Amount of caffeinated beverages and food ingested.

- Relationship of incontinence to medical diagnoses:

  - Is patient diabetic? (Glycosuria may cause incontinence.)

  - Neurological diseases (e.g., Parkinson's disease, multiple sclerosis)

  - Prostate problems (cancer or benign prostatic hyperplasia)

  - History of chronic urinary tract infection

  - Psychiatric disorder

- Medications prescribed that may affect bladder function:

  - Psychotropic drugs can accumulate in the elderly and cause sedation, confusion, and immobility, resulting in functional incontinence.

  - Anticholinergics can cause urinary retention, urinary frequency, and overflow incontinence.

(continued)

Box 6.1   (continued)

- – Calcium channel blockers can reduce smooth muscle contractility, causing urinary retention and overflow incontinence.

- – Narcotics can depress the central nervous system, causing sedation, confusion, and immobility, leading to urinary retention and incontinence.

- – Rapidly acting diuretics, such as furosemide, can overwhelm the bladder with rapidly produced urine, resulting in frequency and urgency.

- – Alpha antagonists can relax the smooth muscle of the bladder neck and proximal urethra, causing or worsening stress incontinence.

- – Alpha agonists (common ingredients in cold preparations) can contract the smooth muscle of the bladder neck, the prostate, and the proximal urethra, causing difficulty emptying and even urinary retention.

Bladder and Bowel Diary—Objective Information

- Maintain a diary for at least 3 days (form provided on companion CD under Assessment Forms).

Functional and Environmental Assessment

- Mobility:
  - – How is toileting accomplished?
  - – Would toileting assistive devices such as a bedside commode or urinal be helpful?
  - – If the patient uses a wheelchair, is he or she able to propel the chair to the toilet in a timely fashion?
  - – Are restraints (physical or chemical) being used that are causing urinary incontinence?
  - – Is equipment that can enhance mobility, such as a cane, walker, or wheelchair, available?

- Environment:
  - – Can improved access to toilets improve urinary symptoms?
  - – Are toilets at least 19 inches high, with arms or bars to assist in lowering or rising?
  - – Are chairs designed for ease in rising?
  - – Are grab bars available and within reach when toileting?

Physical Examination

- Abdominal examination:
  - – Presence of bowel sounds, organomegaly, masses
  - – Complaints of abdominal or suprapubic tenderness, discomfort, or fullness

- Genitalia examination:
  - – Dryness, redness, and thinning of the perineal and gluteal skin (e.g., presence of atrophy or perineal dermatitis)
  - – In men, condition of foreskin, glans, penile shaft
  - – Abnormalities of scrotal sac (size) and testes (masses)

- Pelvic examination (women):
  - – Dryness, redness, and thinning of the vaginal mucosa (indicates atrophic vaginitis)
  - – Presence of structural abnormalities, such as pelvic organ prolapse
  - – Assessment of pelvic floor muscle strength (if possible)

Box 6.1   (continued)

- Rectal examination:
  - Presence of fecal impaction
  - Assessment of rectal sphincter tone
  - In men, size of prostate, presense of nodularity, induration, or tenderness

Urological Testing

- Urinalysis results:
  - Are leukocytes, nitrites, red blood cells, bacteriuria, pyuria, and/or glucose present?
  - Is there a need for urine culture?
- Postvoid residual (PVR) urine:
  - Determine residual urine volume within 15–20 minutes after voiding.
    - Risk factors: suprapubic distention or tenderness, history of prostate disorders, diabetes, drugs that interfere with bladder emptying, neurological disease; history of surgery for stress UI or prolapse or other pelvic surgery
  - Method—ultrasound preferred.
    - "Normal" < 50 mL
    - "Abnormal" > 100 mL
    - If volume is between 150 and 200 mL, monitor PVR volumes on several occasions to determine clinical situation and if elevated measure after a double void.
  - Is a referral to a specialist needed?

Adapted from Newman, D.K. (2005b). *Bladder and bowel rehabilitation program.* Philadelphia: SCA Personal Products; and Newman, D.K. (2007). *Program of excellence in extended care.* Bothell, WA: Verathon Medical Corporation.

toileting. People with dependent continence also include those dependent on UI medications.

Contained incontinence (previously referred to as "social" continence)—the person depends on absorbent products and other devices to contain urine leakage. This person is unable to maintain continence independently or through assistance with regular toileting by caregivers. This is probably the fastest growing group of people with UI—older, frailer, and more functionally and cognitively dependent. Currently, the use of incontinence absorbent products is the first choice for management of UI in this population.

Palmer (1996) added another category to this classification system that is often seen in residents in LTC:

Partial continence—the person has the potential for improving or maintaining dryness levels but is unable to attain total continence. These individuals may use a combination of a scheduled toileting program and containment of urine leakage with devices or products.

Continence requires cognition (mental awareness and attention sufficient to recognize the urge sensation, ability to find the toilet, and motivation to stay continent), physical functional ability (mobility to reach a toilet, manual dexterity to remove clothing), and environmental access (accessible toilets) (DuBeau, 2006).

Cognitive Assessment

Mental status or cognition is an important assessment in elderly people because dementia frequently affects areas of the frontal cortex important for continence. Assessment of mood, affect, orientation, and comprehension, as well as a determination as to whether cognition is sufficient to recognize the urge to urinate, is part of this assessment (Newman 2005b; Voytas, 2002). Cognitive impairment can interfere with the ability to recognize the need to go to the toilet, ability to delay voiding until it is appropriate, ability to find and recognize the toilet, and ability to disrobe and use the toilet appropriately (Yap & Tan, 2006). Mental status examination should include assessment of mood, affect, orientation, speech pattern, memory, and comprehension. Table 8.2 reviews possible contributing factors and solutions to UI in patients with dementia or cognitive impairment. Cognitive status will determine if the person is a candidate for an educational bladder training program.

Cognition is assessed by response to questions or through the use of a mental status exam. The Folstein Mini-Mental State Examination is often used (Folstein, Folstein, & McHugh, 1975). The Clock Drawing Test is a useful tool to use in combination with the Mini-Mental State Examination to determine mild stages of cognitive decline (Harvan & Cotter, 2006). The Clock Drawing Test involves a patient drawing a clock, putting in all the numbers, and setting a specific time given by the clinician administering the test. The scoring is based on the Alzheimer's disease cooperative scoring system, which is based on a score of five points: 1 point for the clock circle, 1 point for all the numbers being in the correct order, 1 point for the numbers being in the proper special order, 1 point for the two hands of the clock, and 1 point for the correct time. A normal clock drawing score (4–5 points) almost always predicts that a person's cognitive abilities are within normal limits. Assessment for depression is important to determine the presence of this mental disorder and its effect on motivation. The Beck Geriatric Depression Scale Short Form can be found online at http://www.stanford.edu/~yesavage/GDS.html.

Functional Assessment

An assessment of the person's functional abilities should focus on self-care tasks or activities of daily living (ADLs)—for example, the ability to ambulate, transfer to the toilet, disrobe, and use any necessary assistive devices. Mobility problems and the inability to transfer to a commode are stronger predictors for developing UI than cognitive impairment. The upper extremities should be assessed for strength. A timed "Up and Go" test can be helpful in determining lower extremity impairment (Podsiadlo & Richardson, 1991). The clinician should time (in seconds) the person as he or she rises from a chair, walks 3 meters, turns around, and sits back down again. A time of 20 seconds or less indicates no impairment, 21–29 seconds moderate impairment, and greater than 30 seconds definite impairment. The individual should be assessed for the ability to perform more instrumental ADLs (e.g., cooking, shopping, driving, attending senior center activities). The person also should be rated on his or her level of dependence, according to the following classifications:

1. Able to do the task without human assistance

2. Able to perform the task with some assistance (noting one- or two-person assist)

3. Unable to perform the task even with assistance

The use of chemical or physical restraints causes decreased mobility and contributes to UI. Physical restraints include various straps and ties, as well as geri-chairs. In addition, sedating drugs can act as chemical restraints.

In nursing facilities, UI is partially iatrogenic in nature and is related to the atrophy of motor skills such as walking; therefore, nursing interventions need to enhance mobility skills. Difficulty ambulating increases the time required to reach the toilet, contributing to the severity of UI (Engberg et al., 1997). Slow ambulation has the potential to affect interventions such as prompted voiding and bladder training. Direct observation of toileting will yield critical information that can direct interventions. Observing toileting skills can be accomplished using POTTI (Performance On Timed Toileting Instrument), developed by Ouslander et al. (1987) for use with residents in LTC. The instrument consists of five tasks that simulate toileting: the ability to walk or move 15 feet, transfer to a toilet, unfasten hooks or snaps, unzip a zipper, and pull down garment/pants.

Environmental Barriers

The following factors should be considered when performing an assessment of the individual's environment:

- *Change in living situation:* A change in continence status may occur if a person has a new environment (moved from home to an extended care setting such as assisted living, senior apartments, or a nursing home), changed rooms, or has a new roommate.

- *Nighttime hours:* Nighttime UI can occur if the bed is too high and the person is unable to get out of the bed, the bathroom is inaccessible, or the individual is fearful of falling. Because aging causes a decrease in muscle mass and strength, falling while attempting to meet elimination needs is a serious problem in the older adult. Aging also causes a decrease in pupil size and visual acuity, decreasing the person's ability to adjust to changes in lighting. People who have mobility or balance problems may be unable to suppress a strong urge to urinate until a caregiver arrives to help them with toileting. If they are independent, they may be unable to walk or propel themselves to the toilet in time when using a wheelchair or walker.

- *Clothing:* Clothing that is difficult to remove can contribute to the development of UI. Aging causes overall decrease in bone mass and degenerative joint disease. This can affect hand dexterity, causing an inability to manipulate belts, suspenders, zippers, and buttons on clothing. Often sweatpants without underwear or pants with elastic bands and the use of fabric that is fastened by Velcro rather than buttons and zippers can be very helpful in these cases.

- *Visual cues:* Inability to recognize the toilet (visual agnosia) is a frustrating situation for an individual. Visual cues such as a picture of a toilet on the bathroom door or of a man standing and voiding into a toilet might aid people with visual agnosia in identifying the proper location and use of the toilet. Also, painting the bathroom door a bright, eye-catching color that is different from the color of other doors may be helpful for some people with dementia.

- *Furniture:* Chairs with good back support, with a seat height of at least 19 inches, allow people to get to their feet more independently, quickly, and easily. The use of a chair lift should be considered for those people who are having difficulty with rising from a chair.

In addition, bathrooms themselves must be assessed for potential barriers to toileting. Adequacy and availability of bathroom facilities and presence of toileting aids such as bedside commodes or urinals are important in promoting continence. (Toileting aids are discussed in Chapter 10.) The bathroom should also be assessed for ease of toileting. The bathroom is considered the most hazardous room with respect to the chance of an older person falling. Size and layout of bathrooms are of paramount importance. The bathroom should have good lighting. The bathroom mirror can be covered if individuals with cognitive impairment become confused and agitated when looking in the mirror.

Distance required to get to the bathroom may also be important. Many older people who reside in metropolitan areas live in narrow multistory, older homes (e.g., row houses) in which the bathroom is on a second floor. People who live in these houses may experience urine leakage while ascending stairs to get to the bathroom, or the bathroom may be inaccessible to the person who spends the majority of the day on the first floor. Construction of a bathroom on the main living floor will promote continence. Agencies that provide elder services will often pay for construction of a bathroom or "water closet" (sink and toilet) in the corner of a downstairs room to aid the person in self-toileting.

In the LTC setting, bathrooms may be adequate but residents may spend a large part of the day in public areas such as the dining room or in activities where access to and assistance in the bathroom are limited.

EVALUATION

The standard of care for evaluation of UI based on practice guidelines recommends a history, physical examination, urinalysis, and, in certain cases, determination of postvoid residual as part of the baseline evaluation to be performed before treatment can be instituted (Abrams et al., 2005; AMDA, 2005; CMS, 2005; Fantl et al., 1996; Viktrup, 2005; Viktrup, Summers, & Dennett, 2004). The companion CD includes samples of medical record forms the authors use when completing a history and physical examination for people in specific care settings. Box 6.2 is a comprehensive checklist that can be used when evaluating residents in nursing homes (Newman, 2005b, 2007). These forms employ cue words because such a format results in higher levels of documentation than open-format forms (Palmer, McCormick, Langford, Langlois, & Alvaran, 1992).

Obtaining a History

The history should determine the characteristics of UI, noting the onset, duration, frequency, severity, and progression of incontinence, and should assist in the differentiation of the cause and type of UI. The severity of urine leakage may vary depending on the type of incontinence because severe UI is generally less common in women who report stress UI (SUI) as opposed to urgency UI (UUI) and mixed UI (Hunskaar et al., 2003). It is important to include family members and caregivers when taking a history because they can add depth to the description of the impact UI is having on the person's daily routine.

Many people will report situational antecedents or "triggers" that may be visual, auditory, or tactile (e.g., hearing running water, seeing a bathroom sign, washing dishes or clothes, placing hands in warm water, anxiety or stressful situations) (Newman & Wein, 2004). In addition to symptoms of urgency, frequency, and incontinence, additional lower urinary tract symptoms (LUTS) relating to filling or storage symptoms (e.g., urgency, frequency, nocturia, dysuria, suprapubic or perineal pain) or obstructive or voiding symptoms (e.g., hesitancy, poor or interrupted stream, straining during voiding) are also an integral part of the history. LUTS are defined in Chapter 4. The distinction among symptoms is important because this will guide treatment options.

Determining the symptom(s) most bothersome to the individual is especially important in guiding intervention and determining response. An example is women with overactive bladder (OAB), UUI, and SUI who report urinary urgency. This is the hallmark symptom of OAB, and these women will

---

Box 6.2   Evaluation checklist in long-term care residents

History

Urinary History

- Determine usual bladder and/or voiding habits.

- List signs and symptoms (e.g., urgency, frequency, nocturia, nocturnal enuresis, and episodes of urine leakage).

- Determine onset, severity, and pattern of urine leakage. The Centers for Medicare & Medicaid Services definition of UI is "any wetness on the skin."
  The Minimum Data Set criteria are as follows:

  - **0.** Continent: Complete bladder control (including control achieved by care that involves prompted voiding, habit training, reminders, etc.)

  - **1.** Usually continent = 1 bladder incontinence episode per week

  - **2.** Occasionally incontinent = 2 (but not daily) bladder incontinence episodes per week

  - **3.** Frequently incontinent: Daily bladder incontinence episodes, but some control is present (e.g., on day shift)

  - **4.** Incontinent: Multiple daily episodes of bladder incontinence

- Determine resident's perception of UI as a problem.

- If UI was present before admission, investigate previous treatments (e.g., medications, surgery) and management of urine leakage (e.g., absorbent products, toileting devices).

- Observe the resident toileting to determine:

  - Usual routine for toileting

  - Resident's self-performance of toileting:

    Level 1—supervision

    Level 2—limited assistance

    Level 3—extensive assistance

    Level 4—total dependence

  - Awareness of the urge sensation and need to void

  - Holding time: when the bladder feels full, how long can the resident hold urine and delay voiding before leakage becomes impossible to prevent? Able to delay voiding or urine leakage long enough for the staff to arrive and offer toileting assistance?

  - When does the leakage occur? With standing (changing position), coughing, sneezing, laughing, lifting objects; with urgency; with seemingly no provocation?

  - How frequently does it occur? Every time, sometimes, daily, once or twice a week?

  - Assessment of urine stream for associated LUTS such as weak stream, hesitancy, postvoid dribbling, feeling of incomplete bladder emptying, and intermittency

- Assess all acute/transient causes of UI.

Other Pertinent History

- Check for diagnoses of primary and secondary medical problems.

Box 6.2 *(continued)*

- Determine daily diet/fluid intake:
  - Total fluid intake, including types (e.g., caffeinated beverages)
  - Whether resident is voluntarily restricting fluid intake to avoid urine leakage
- Obtain bowel history (history of persistent constipation, fecal impaction, diarrhea, fecal incontinence).
  - Defecation frequency and pattern, straining at stool, painful defecation
  - Strategies used to maintain bowel regularity
  - Use of laxative or enemas
- Check for previous pelvic surgery (hysterectomy, prostate surgery).
- In men, determine history of benign prostatic hyperplasia or other prostate conditions.
- Assess for relationships of incontinence to other chronic neurological conditions: stroke, Alzheimer's disease, multi-infarct dementia, other dementias, Parkinson's disease, multiple sclerosis, cervical or lumbar stenosis or disk herniation and spinal cord injury, diabetic neuropathy, nerve injury.

Cognitive, Functional, and Environmental Assessment

Cognitive and physical impairments are primary risk factors for UI, but not good predictors of a resident's responsiveness to toileting programs. Mobility problems, impaired cognitive functioning, or both can interfere with independent toileting and bladder training, so the following are important components to a UI assessment.

- Cognitive Ability Assessment:
  - Ability of the resident to understand instructions; motivation and affect
  - Ability to recognize bladder fullness (urge sensation)
  - Knows location of toileting facility/bathroom
  - Motivated to self-toilet, or to regain continence and normal bladder function
- Functional Ability Assessment:
  - Ability to accomplish toileting (e.g., manual dexterity, ability to disrobe). Consider use of POTTI assessment (see p. 183).
  - Risk for falls (see Box 4.1)
  - Need for or benefit of toileting devices such as bedside commode or urinal
  - Ability of resident who uses a wheelchair or a walker to propel the equipment to the toilet in a timely fashion
  - Whether restraints (physical or chemical) are preventing normal bladder function. (Physical restraints include various straps and ties, as well as geri-chairs. In addition, sedating drugs can act as chemical restraints.)
- Environmental Barrier Assessment:
  - Distance from bed to bathroom
  - Access (e.g., less distance, is visible) to toilet/bathroom is unimpeded
  - Toileting facilities promote privacy
  - Toilets at least 17 inches high, with arms to aid in lowering or rising

(continued)

Box 6.2   *(continued)*

– Call lights available and accessible

– Chairs designed for ease in rising

Other disciplines besides nursing (e.g., dietary, social services, and especially the physical/occupational therapy department) can assist in gathering these data.

Physical Observation and Examination

- General:

  – Assess for presence of dehydration (dry mouth, frequent falls, weakness and fatigue, decreased urine output, headache, weight loss, and increased confusion).

  – Assess for pedal and peripheral edema.

- Abdominal Observation and Examination:

  – Determine presence of bowel sounds.

    ■ Normal sounds consist of clicks or gurgles every 5–15 seconds.

    ■ More frequent bowel sounds are hyperactive, which indicates increased bowel motility. Prolonged gurgling sounds may result from increased motility seen with diarrhea.

    ■ Sluggish bowel sounds, three or fewer per minute, indicate decreased motility.

    ■ No bowel sounds heard for 5 minutes in any quadrant are described as absent.

  – Palpate for presence of masses or organomegaly. If a mass is felt, note its size, shape, consistency, texture, and location. Note if resident complains of tenderness, discomfort, or fullness during palpation.

  – Determine presence of suprapubic distention indicating urinary retention. A distended bladder may rise above the symphysis pubis (pelvic bone), and it may be possible to palpate or percuss the bladder above the level of the symphysis pubis if it contains 150 mL or more of urine. In general, palpation is not accurate in determining postvoid residual (PVR).

- Genitalia Observation and Examination:

  – An internal pelvic examination may not be appropriate or well tolerated if the female resident is severely confused, but external observation of the perineum in both male and female residents is always appropriate.

  – External perineal skin observation—women

    ■ Assess for rash, skin lesions, odor, and discharge.

    ■ Separate the labia and visualize the urinary meatus.

    ■ Note any redness, inflammation, erythema, ulceration, urethral or vaginal discharge, swelling, or nodules.

    ■ Observe the vulva for signs of hypoestrogenism (urogenital atrophy).

  – External perineal skin observation—men

    ■ Note penile discharge, redness, or rash along the penile shaft.

    ■ In the uncircumcised man, the foreskin should be retracted and the glans and meatus should be assessed.

    ■ Inspect the scrotum for abnormalities such as masses or swelling.

Box 6.2   (continued)

- Pelvic Observation and Examination—women:

  - Assess for the presence of structural abnormalities such as pelvic organ prolapse (POP). Women with POP will complain of urinary urgency and frequency and describe a bulging feeling in their vagina or perineum. Assessment of POP should be performed by having the woman strain or bear down like she is having a bowel movement. The following are the descriptions of the organs prolapsing:

    - Bladder—**cystocele:** when the anterior wall of the vagina, together with the bladder above it, bulges into the vagina and sometimes out the introitus

    - Uterus—**uterine prolapse:** weakness of the supporting structures of the pelvic floor causes descent of the uterus and cervix into the vagina

    - Vagina—**vaginal vault prolapse:** the walls of the vagina fall in on themselves and out of the vagina

    - Rectum—**rectocele:** protrusion of the posterior vaginal wall and the rectum behind it

  - Grading scale is used for documentation and is found in Chapter 12.

  - If the resident is a candidate for pelvic floor muscle (PFM) exercises, a PFM assessment should be part of the pelvic examination. Digital measurement of the PFM strength can be performed by inserting the index finger into the vagina to the level of the first knuckle. The resident is asked to tighten or pull in and upward with her vaginal or rectal muscles, or both. If able to contract the PFMs, proceed to having her repeat contracting the muscles, holding the contraction for a count of 5, then relaxing the muscle for a count of 5. Repeat this several times until resident learns this exercise.

- Rectal Observation and Examination:

  - Inspect outside of the anus, noting any fecal smearing or liquid stool seepage. Inspect the perianal areas for lumps, ulcers, inflammation, rashes, or excoriation.

  - Assess rectal sphincter tone. As the sphincter relaxes, gently insert index finger into the anal canal in a direction pointing toward the umbilicus. Note if the resting sphincter tone is weak, moderate, or strong. To assess the strength of the sphincter muscle, ask the resident to tighten the rectum around the examiner's finger. The examiner should feel a gripping sensation around the entire circumference of the finger. This is another method for determining if the resident can perform a PFM contraction.

  - Note the presence and consistency of stool in the rectal vault, which may indicate bowel impaction.

  - An enlarged or abnormal consistency of the prostate gland in men should be noted, and abnormal findings should be discussed with the physician to determine if the resident should be referred to a urologist.

Bladder and Bowel Record

- To determine voiding pattern and incontinence frequency rate, nursing staff observe the resident every hour, noting the following on a Bladder and Bowel Record:

  - Time and frequency of each void

  - If resident is "wet" or "dry," and, if wet, an estimate of the quantity of urine loss

  - Whether absorbent incontinence pad was saturated or dry

  - Frequency of bowel movements

(continued)

Box 6.2   *(continued)*

- The resident is monitored usually for 72 hours (3 consecutive days).

- When reviewing the record, staff should attempt to determine patterns: during the day, during the night, frequency of urination and incontinent episodes.

Diagnostic Testing

All residents with UI should have a urinalysis if possible. Because many residents (approximately 30%–50%), especially female residents, have chronic asymptomatic bacteriuria, the research-based literature suggests treating only symptomatic urinary tract infections (UTIs). Therefore, continued bacteriuria without clinical and diagnostic symptoms does not warrant repeat or continued antibiotic therapy.

- Urinalysis:

  - Obtain a "clean-catch" urine specimen. Only use a catheterized specimen if unable to obtain clean catch. Note urine characteristics: color, odor, presence of sediment.

  - Perform a dipstick urinalysis. If the dipstick urinalysis is positive for nitrites (indicating bacteriuria), white blood cells (WBCs), and leukocyte esterase (an enzyme present in WBCs indicating pyuria) and the resident shows signs and symptoms of a UTI, send a urine specimen for urine culture. A negative leukocyte esterase or the absence of pyuria (increased leukocytes in the urine) strongly suggests that a UTI is not present. A positive leukocyte esterase test alone does not prove that the individual has a UTI.

- Urine culture and sensitivity:

  - A positive urine culture will show bacteriuria, but that alone is not enough to diagnose a symptomatic UTI. However, several test results (urinalysis with a urine culture), in combination with clinical findings, can help to identify UTIs.

  - A urine culture result of a single predominant pathogen is sufficient for the microbiological diagnosis of UTI based on the following result:

    - 1,000 (or 10^3) colony-forming units/mL—clean-catch, midstream specimen

  - The most common infecting organisms are Enterobacteriaceae, *Escherichia coli* (most common in female residents), and *Proteus mirabilis* (most common in male residents).

  - In addition to a positive urine culture, the resident *without* an indwelling (urethral or suprapubic) catheter has to have at least *three* of the following signs and symptoms to treat for a UTI:

    - Fever (2.4°F above the baseline temperature) or chills

    - New or increased burning pain on urination, frequency or urgency

    - New flank or suprapubic pain or tenderness

    - Change in character of urine (e.g., new bloody urine, foul smell, or amount of sediment) or as reported by the laboratory (new pyuria or microscopic hematuria)

    - Worsening of mental or functional status (i.e., confusion, decreased appetite, unexplained falls, incontinence of recent onset, lethargy, decreased activity)

  - In addition to a positive urine culture, the resident *with* an indwelling (urethral or suprapubic) catheter has to have at least *two* of the following signs and symptoms to treat for a UTI. Symptoms are:

    - Fever (2.4°F above the baseline temperature) or chills

    - New flank pain or suprapubic pain or tenderness

Box 6.2   *(continued)*

- ■ Change in character of urine (e.g., new bloody urine, foul smell, or amount of sediment) or as reported by the laboratory (new pyuria or microscopic hematuria)

- ■ Worsening of mental or functional status (i.e., confusion, decreased appetite, unexplained falls, incontinence of recent onset, lethargy, decreased activity)

- ■ Local findings such as catheter obstruction, leakage, or mucosal trauma (may also be present)

- • Postvoid residual urine:

  - – The PVR should be determined in residents with risk factors for urinary retention (history of prostate disorders, neurological diseases [e.g., diabetes, spinal cord injury, Parkinson's, etc.], or pelvic surgery or POP; or on drugs that interfere with bladder emptying).

  - – PVR volume must be measured no more than 20 minutes after the resident voids.

  - – PVR can be obtained by sterile in-and-out catheterization. The use of a portable ultrasonographic device (e.g., BladderScan™, Verathon Medical) permits noninvasive identification of clinically significant residual urine with an accuracy rate of more than 90%.

  - – Normal PVR is between 50 and 100 mL, and findings of between 100 and 200 mL bear repeat measurement. Abnormal PVR in elderly residents is ≥ 200 mL, and those residents should be referred to the urologist.

- • Bladder function tests:

  - – Determine bladder capacity by having resident drink water and then scanning bladder by ultrasound at initial urge sensation.

  - – Is resident a candidate for additional bladder function tests? (Should be considered for residents with recurring UTI that cannot be cleared and for continued urinary retention.)

Adapted from Newman, D.K. (2005b). *Bladder and bowel rehabilitation program.* Philadelphia: SCA Personal Products; and Newman, D.K. (2007). *Program of excellence in extended care.* Bothell, WA: Verathon Medical Corporation.

---

report the fear of or "being worried" about urine leakage if they do not void soon after urgency. The most helpful component of the assessment for determining the presence of urgency UI in women is a history of urine loss associated with urinary urgency (Holroyd-Leduc, Tannenbaum, Thorpe, & Straus, 2008). However, men with benign prostatic enlargement and OAB without UUI do not seem to experience the same fear with the urgency symptom. Also, the first complaint may not be the "chief" complaint or the most bothersome symptom to the individual. The clinician needs to be a sleuth to determine the most distressing symptom. Timing of symptoms is important because women with nighttime incontinence are more likely to experience a greater quality-of-life impact (Huang et al., 2006). Because of the reduced time interval between urgency and the occurrence of UI, a common complaint reported is "no bladder control."

Lower abdominal pain associated with an intense need to urinate may be a clue to urinary retention resulting from obstruction, which may be the presenting sign of a serious underlying disorder. Often people with obstruction, such as that caused by an enlarged prostate in men, describe difficulty initiating urination, voiding small volumes, or a sensation of incomplete bladder emptying or postmicturition (postvoid) dribbling.

Precipitants of incontinence (e.g., previous pelvic surgery, previous pelvic radiation therapy, trauma, new onset of diseases, new medications) should also be explored. Initially, the clinician should determine if the UI is of recent onset and could therefore be caused by acute medical problems. Neurological conditions such as diabetes or multiple sclerosis are risk factors that cause mixed symptomatology and are discussed in Chapter 4. If one of these problems is identified, treatment to correct or lessen the problem should be instituted. A current drug review will identify drug-related causes of UI. Medications that can affect the lower urinary tract include diuretics, sedatives, hypnotics, analgesics, and antidepressants, and a list of these is found in Chapter 4. If the person requires a particular class of drugs, substituting another drug in the same class with a different side effect profile should be considered. Over-the-counter drugs such as cold remedies can also cause or contribute to UI.

An important area to explore is the woman's obstetric history because more than 50% of women experience some degree of urine leakage during pregnancy and postpartum. Information on the mode of delivery, weight of the child at birth, and specifics of the delivery is important. Persistent postpartum SUI may be the result of vacuum extraction or the use of an instrument, such as forceps, or the need for and extent of an episiotomy.

Other components of the medical history that may help in the identification of UI are bowel function, fluid intake (includes liquids and food items that break down into fluids at room temperature), and consumption of known bladder irritants. Chronic constipation, especially straining during defecation, can contribute to UI (see Chapter 5). There is also a strong correlation between pelvic organ prolapse (POP) and constipation (Jelovsek, Barber, Paraiso, & Walters, 2005). Instituting a bowel regimen and ensuring adequate fluid intake can improve urinary symptoms. Questions about bowel function should include frequency and consistency of bowel movements. Patients should be asked about the use of laxatives, enemas, and other bowel medications. Women with constipation who strain during defecation may report "splinting" (pressing on the vagina or the perineum with a finger to aid in stool evacuation). This may also be a sign of the presence of a rectocele. Determination of adequate fluid intake is an important component of the review of diet. Recommendations for changing diet, modifying fluid intake, and regulating bowels are detailed in Chapter 7. It is also important to ask the person questions regarding sexual practices (e.g., urine leakage during intercourse, erectile function in men).

Finally, the clinician should determine how the person is handling the reported urinary symptoms and what has been used to solve his or her problems (e.g., incontinence pads, toilet mapping, medications, etc.).

Screening Tools and Voiding Logs

Screening Tools

The use of a screening tool or gender-specific questionnaire or both may be helpful (Brown et al., 2006; Naughton & Wyman, 1997; Robinson & Shea, 2002; Uebersax, Wyman, Shumaker, McClish, & Fantl, 1995). One of the authors (DKN) conducted a mail survey and was surprised by the findings (Newman, 2004). Regarding the availability of self-administered screening questionnaires to providers: only 18% of respondents said they filled out a form that contained questions about bladder control when they were seen by a provider for a routine medical visit. Although the best way for providers to broach the subject of bladder control appears to vary by the individual situation and type of doctor with whom the person is consulting, 69% of the respondents said they thought it would be very helpful in prompting discussion if their doctor provided a form for them to check off symptoms of UI, 24% thought it would be somewhat helpful, and only 6% did not feel it would be helpful at all.

Box 6.3 lists examples of simple questions about bladder control, designating specific questions for UI and OAB and for SUI. One of the authors (DKN) has used an "Incontinence Patient Profile" (on the companion CD under Assessment Forms) for many years in all patients presenting with bladder control symptoms. Patients are asked to complete this profile along with a 3-day voiding diary (Newman, 2005a) prior to the initial visit. The OAB-q, shown in Table 6.1, is an OAB-specific screening tool that can also be used by

---

Box 6.3   Simple UI-related questions

Symptoms of UI and OAB

- Do you get a sudden feeling that you need go to the bathroom immediately and you cannot ignore it?

- Do you experience such a strong and sudden urge to void that you leak before reaching the toilet?

- How often do you go to the bathroom? Is it more than eight times in a 24-hour period?

- Do you get up at night to go to the bathroom? If so, how often? Does the urge to urinate wake you up?

- Do you avoid places you think won't have a nearby restroom?

- When you're in an unfamiliar place, do you make sure you know where the restroom is?

- How many pads do you change because of wetness during the day? During the night?

Symptoms of SUI

- Do you experience a loss of urine when you are doing physical activities, such as lifting heavy objects or exercising?

- Do you sometimes lose or leak urine when you sneeze, cough, or laugh?

- Do you use pantiliners or pads in your underwear to keep from wetting your clothes?

Table 6.1   OAB-q (Courtesy of Pfizer)

Please circle the number that best describes how much you have been bothered by each symptom.

During the past 4 weeks, how bothered were you by. . .	Not at all	A little bit	Somewhat	Quite a bit	A great deal	A very great deal
1. Frequent urination during the daytime hours	1	2	3	4	5	6
2. An uncomfortable urge to urinate	1	2	3	4	5	6
3. A sudden urge to urinate with little or no warning	1	2	3	4	5	6
4. Accidental loss of small amounts of urine	1	2	3	4	5	6
5. Nighttime urination	1	2	3	4	5	6
6. Waking up at night because you need to urinate	1	2	3	4	5	6
7. An uncomfortable urge to urinate	1	2	3	4	5	6
8. Urine loss associated with a strong desire to urinate	1	2	3	4	5	6
Are you a male?	If male, ☐ add **2** points to your score					

Please add up your responses to the questions above: _____

A score greater than 8 may indicate overactive bladder.

Box 6.4   Patient Perception of Bladder Condition (PPBC)

Which of the following statements describes your bladder condition best at this time? Please check one box only.

☐ 1. My bladder condition does not cause me any problems at all.

☐ 2. My bladder condition causes me some very minor problems.

☐ 3. My bladder condition causes me some minor problems.

☐ 4. My bladder condition causes me some moderate problems.

☐ 5. My bladder condition causes me severe problems.

☐ 6. My bladder condition causes me many severe problems.

---

providers in detecting symptoms of OAB (Coyne et al., 2002). An additional OAB measure is the Patient Perception of Bladder Condition (PPBC), a single-item global subjective measure found in Box 6.4 (Coyne, Matza, Kopp, & Abrams, 2006) that asks the patient to rate the severity of their bladder condition. This measure is also useful over time to judge the efficacy of a therapeutic intervention.

Additional questionnaires include the Urogenital Distress Inventory 6 (UDI-6), a short form developed for women with mixed symptoms of OAB with UUI and SUI to determine which symptoms were bothersome (Uebersax et al., 1995); the Incontinence Impact Questionnaire-7 (IIQ-7) to determine impact on quality of life (Gray & Wyman, 2004); and the International Consultation on Incontinence Questionnaire (ICIQ) (Avery et al., 2004). The ICIQ was also created to assess UI and its impact on quality of life. It is simple, so completion rates would be high and useful across a general patient population. The ICIQ consists of four questions and numeric scales:

1. How often do you leak urine? (check one box)

   ❑ 0 Never   ❑ 3 About once a day
   ❑ 1 About once a week or less often   ❑ 4 Several times a day
   ❑ 2 Two or three times a week   ❑ 5 All the time

2. We would like to know how much urine <u>you</u> <u>think</u> leaks. How much urine do you <u>usually</u> leak? (whether you wear protection or not) (check one box)

   ❑ 0 None   ❑ 4 A moderate amount
   ❑ 2 A small amount   ❑ 6 A large amount

3. Overall, how much does leaking urine interfere with your everyday life? (circle a number between 0 and 10)

       0   1   2   3   4   5   6   7   8   9   10
     Not at all   A great deal

The ICIQ score is the sum of questions 1–3.

4. When does urine leak? (Please check all that apply)

   ❑ Never – Urine does not leak
   ❑ Leaks before you can get to the toilet
   ❑ Leaks when you cough or sneeze
   ❑ Leaks when you are asleep
   ❑ Leaks when you are physically active/exercising
   ❑ Leaks when you have finished urinating and are dressed
   ❑ Leaks for no obvious reason
   ❑ Leaks all the time

Because these are simple assessments that require little time for completion, clinicians have many opportunities to distribute screening tools or questionnaires to men and women during annual medical office visits, especially those involving a gynecological examination; outpatient procedure; home visit to patients with chronic illnesses; and routine assessment of elderly patients residing in LTC settings (Newman, 2005a). These assessments can be self-administered, completed prior to scheduled medical visits, or administered in-office while the patient is in a waiting room or while awaiting a provider in an examination room. Clinical staff (office nurses, medical technicians, and certified nurse assistants) can be trained to participate, as suitable to their credentials and positions, in distribution and completion of these questionnaires. If the patient answers in the affirmative to any of the screening questions, the provider should ask the patient about his or her answers and determine the need to move forward with a more detailed history and examination.

Fultz and Herzog (2000) noted that self-reporting of incontinence can be influenced by the survey tool or questionnaire used. For example, if women are given a brief description of UI and respond "no," but then are subsequently asked probing questions, the reported prevalence is higher than in surveys that omit the follow-up questions. Open-ended questions may yield more information. Clinicians should avoid questions that use the phrase "incontinence" because many women who leak urine and are bothered by their symptoms do not consider themselves to be "incontinent."

Voiding Log or Bladder Record

Asking the person or caregiver to complete a voiding log or a bladder record (bladder diary) is an essential component of the evaluation of UI. Self-monitoring on a daily basis using a bladder diary is a simple and practical method of obtaining information on voiding behavior (Sampselle, 2003). Many experts believe that the act of keeping a daily bladder diary is therapeutic and a type of "behavioral intervention" because, once patients identify correlations between type of fluid intake and urinary symptoms, for example, they may reduce then eliminate fluid intake or the dietary cause. It is not uncommon for clinicians to hear comments from patients such as "I did not know I was drinking so much coffee" or "Look at my record, I am always in the bathroom in the morning." Samples of voiding logs are available on the companion CD under Assessment Forms. Figure 6.2 is a sample of a completed bladder diary of a man with SUI.

A daily diary can provide an objective picture of the time of each void; subjective information regarding sensation of urgency and urine leakage episodes; and a record of the events, triggers, or antecedents surrounding these episodes (e.g., on the way to the bathroom, during the night, cold temperature trigger) (Dmochowski, 2005). Having the patient record the degree of urgency, a very bothersome OAB symptom, may be very helpful in subjectively determining improvement following treatment. The Urgency Perception Scale (Cardozo, et al., 2005) can be incorporated into a diary and asks the patient to choose one of the following that best describes the urgency:

- ❏ I am usually not able to hold urine
- ❏ I am usually able to hold urine until I reach the toilet if I go immediately
- ❏ I am usually able to finish what I am doing before going to the toilet.

Because fluid intake and type of liquid consumed can be contributing factors to incontinence, most bladder records request that the person list daily intake, noting type and amount. A well-kept voiding log can help the clinician assess overall voiding patterns, possible triggers, or if the person might be practicing what is sometimes called "defensive voiding," in which the individual uses the toilet to prevent an actual urgency episode.

1st column, time of day

2nd column, place a checkmark (✓) next to the correct time you urinate in the toilet.

3rd column, mark each time you have urine leakage and indicate whether the amount was **L** (large), **M** (moderate), or **S** (small).

4th column, record the reason for the urine leakage (e.g., sneezing, lifting, coughing, laughing, couldn't make it to the bathroom, etc.).

5th column, place a checkmark (✓) each time a wet pad was changed. Mark "how wet," **D** if the pad is slightly wet or damp, **W** if wet, and **S** if the pad is saturated or very wet.

6th column, in the correct time interval, describe your liquid intake (e.g., coffee, water, orange juice, etc.) and estimate the amount (e.g., one cup/8 oz).

1	2	3			4	5			6
Time Interval	**Urinated in Toilet**	**Amount of Urine Leakage**			**Reason for Urine Leakage**	**Changed Wet Pad**			**Type/Amount of Liquid Intake**
		L	**M**	**S**		**D**	**W**	**S**	
6 am		L	M	S		D	W	S	5 oz water
7 am	✓	L	M	✓ S	coughing	✓ D	W	S	8 oz coffee, 6 oz juice
8 am		L	M	S		D	W	S	
9 am	✓	L	M	S		D	W	S	
10 am		L	M	S		D	W	S	
11 am		L	M	S		D ✓ W		S	
Noon	✓	L	✓ M	S	changing position	D	W	S	8 oz soda, 5 oz soup
1 pm		L	M	S		D	W	S	
2 pm		L	M	S		D	W	S	6 oz water
3 pm	✓	L	✓ M	S	golfing	D ✓ W		S	
4 pm		L	M	S		D	W	S	
5 pm		L	M	S		D	W	S	
6 pm		L	M	S		D	W	S	
7 pm		L	M	S		D	W	S	5 oz rum with 6 oz coke
8 pm	✓	L	M	✓ S	bending over	✓ D	W	S	
9 pm	✓	L	M	S		D	W	S	6 oz water
10 pm to Midnight	✓	L	M	S		D	W	S	
Midnight to 2 am		L	M	S		D	W	S	
2–4 am		L	M	S		D	W	S	
4–6 am		L	M	S		D	W	S	

Analysis: 62 yo male, 6 months postprostatectomy, whose diary indicates stress UI symptoms that occur with physical effort. Most of the urine leakage (4x/day) is in small amounts. Urinary frequency is within normal limits, evening alcohol triggered frequency. Fluid intake inadequate at 49 oz—may be limiting intake to minimize urine leakage.

Figure 6.2. Sample bladder diary.

Data are usually collected in 24-hour intervals, with these periods further segmented into smaller time blocks to determine the frequency of diurnal and nocturnal voiding. In one study that evaluated the need for voiding diaries as a diagnostic tool for men, the results demonstrated that this tool was essential in keeping track of the actual number of nightly episodes (Jaffe, Ginsberg, Silverberg, & Harkaway, 2002). The need for a voiding diary appeared to be more important as the number of nighttime voiding episodes increased. Evidence has indicated that 3-day diaries are representative of a person's voiding pattern (Dmochowski, Sanders, Appell, Nitti, & Davila, 2005). If the person is able to fill out a diary, that is preferred; however, the caregiver or LTC staff may need to assist in filling out or completing the record.

Eliciting examples of incontinence episodes helps to objectively diagnose the type of incontinence and frequency and severity of voiding symptoms. An estimate of the volume of leakage during UI episodes is helpful. The following description of urine leakage can be used:

- Small volume (< 30 mL)—enough to make underwear wet if no protective pad is worn

- Moderate volume (31–100 mL)—enough to wet or soak underwear and leak down the legs if no protective pad is worn

- Large volume (101 mL)—soaks through clothing and onto floor or furniture and usually is the entire bladder volume

The clinician should discuss the bladder diary with the patient to determine its accuracy but also to note abnormalities and associations. A person may recognize the cause of the UI by the pattern of urinary accidents and their correlation with events. If more than eight episodes of voiding per day are noted, teaching the individual bladder training will improve this situation. A bladder diary can also identify the most bothersome symptom and generally guide appropriate treatment.

Some records include measurement of voided volume in a 24-hour period using a frequency–volume chart to determine an approximation of bladder capacity. Figure 6.3 shows a 1-day frequency–volume chart of a woman with mixed UI and OAB. The volume of voided urine is an important measure to determine functional and maximal bladder capacity, and daily and nocturnal urine volumes. In the elderly woman, nocturnal urine volumes can be increased by at least 35% because of nocturnal polyuria (see Chapter 3) (Pfisterer, Griffiths, Schaefer, & Resnick, 2006). An OAB contracts at variable degrees of distention before full capacity, resulting in low voided volumes. Frequent voiding of small volumes during both day and night suggests an overactive or low-compliance bladder.

However, despite the value of this simple monitoring tool, patient compliance can be very low. These records can be invaluable sources of information if completed, but one of the authors (DKN) has found compliance in her practice to be less than optimal. Young working women have very busy lives

Time	Amount Voided	Activity	Urine Leakage (Yes/No)	Urgency Present (Yes/No)	Fluid Intake Type/Amount
2:30 am	6 oz	awakening to go to bathroom	no	slight	
5:00 am	7 oz	rushing to bathroom	yes	strong	12 oz coffee 6 oz orange juice
7:45 am	6 oz	brushing teeth	yes	yes	
8:20 am	4 oz	waited too long	yes	strong	8 oz coffee
9:15 am	5 oz			no	10 oz water 12 oz diet soda
12:25 pm	6 oz	washing clothes	yes	yes	12 oz soda
2:45 pm	8 oz			yes	4 oz water
4:15 pm	8 oz	coughing	yes	no	8 oz water
5:30 pm	5 oz			no	
6:30 pm	8 oz	washing dishes	yes	no	12 oz diet soda
7:45 pm	8 oz			no	4 oz wine, 8 oz water
8:20 pm	6 oz			no	4 oz water
10:50 pm	5 oz			no	

Type of Pad: _Serenity large pads & underwear_   # Pads Used _5-6_

Comments: _usually wear the underwear product for added protection when I go out_

Analysis: 70 yo female whose record indicates both urge and stress UI symptoms (mixed UI) with OAB symptoms of urgency that are present 5 times in the morning and frequency that occurs 12 times, 10 during waking hours with nocturia × 2. Large intake averaging 80 ozs with a large caffeinated beverage intake. Client voids frequently and in small amounts (82 ozs).

Figure 6.3.   Sample frequency–volume chart.

and are less likely to comply, whereas older retired men and women may have more severe LUTS symptoms and have more time to monitor their problem.

Bladder Records in LTC

The determination of a resident's voiding pattern and frequency of incontinence can assist staff in identifying interventions (e.g., identifying a voiding pattern for implementing prompted voiding). CMS guidance to surveyors in Tag F315 recommends the use of a bladder and bowel diary (see companion CD under Assessment Forms) kept over 3 days or 72 consecutive hours. To complete this record accurately, staff must check the resident hourly to determine wet or dry status. This method is cumbersome, has many inaccuracies, and usually lacks staff compliance. Again, however, these records are invaluable in determining voiding and incontinence patterns and can be instrumental in planning a successful toileting program.

> *Recently, one of the authors (DKN) discussed the use of bladder records with a director of nursing (DON) from Missouri, when attending a meeting on LTC. When the DON learned that this author had been one of the experts on the 2005 CMS Tag F315 guidance to surveyors on "Urinary Incontinence and Catheters," she felt she could voice her frustration over further "unrealistic federal mandates" such as the requirement of a 3-day bladder record on residents with bladder dysfunction. Nevertheless, she made an effort to comply by asking staff to complete these records on five male residents with dementia who tended to socialize together. Once the records were completed, she was able to observe a pattern to the voiding and incontinence of these residents and designed a prompted voiding program based on the observed pattern. Outcomes of the program were surprising to her and the staff because these residents had less UI, which was determined by less incontinence pad usage.*

New technology that includes moisture detection devices and bladder volume instruments (BladderScan™, Verathon Medical) may prove to be more accurate in reporting, documenting, and tracking incontinence and voiding status automatically (Colling, Ouslander, Hadley, Eisch, & Campbell, 1992; Colling, Owen, McCreedy, & Newman, 2003; Newman, Gaines, & Snare, 2005; Woolridge, 2000). However, because of cost, this technology has not been readily accepted by LTC staff.

Physical Examination

A modified physical examination for men and women with UI and related pelvic floor disorders includes a general assessment, an examination of the abdomen and genitalia, a pelvic examination in women, an evaluation of the pelvic floor muscles (PFM), a pelvic pain assessment, and anorectal and neurological examinations. Prior to the physical examination, the authors use visual guides (anatomy pictures) to show the patient the areas of the examination, noting possible abnormalities.

General Examination

A general examination should be performed to detect conditions such as lower extremity edema, which may contribute to increased renal perfusion in recumbent individuals as the fluid is absorbed back into the circulation, causing nocturia and nocturnal enuresis. The finding of +2 or greater lower extremity edema in a frail, less mobile elderly person should raise a concern about possible nocturnal polyuria. A general assessment can detect neurological abnormalities that may suggest multiple sclerosis, stroke, spinal cord compression, or other neurological conditions. It also can determine mobility, cognition, and manual dexterity related to toileting skills among frail older adults and those with functional impairments.

Abdominal Examination

The abdominal examination is best carried out with the patient in the supine position. The exam is performed to detect the presence of bowel sounds, ascites (accumulation of fluid in the abdominal cavity), organomegaly (abnormal enlargement of organs), surgical incisions, lower abdominal masses, and suprapubic bladder fullness or tenderness, which can influence intraabdominal pressure and urinary tract function. Accurate palpation and percussion for determining incomplete bladder emptying is possible only if the bladder is above the level of the symphysis pubis. If the bladder volume is 500 mL, the bladder will generally rise midway between the symphysis pubis and umbilicus; if 1,000 mL or greater, it will rise above the umbilicus. The finding of a palpable bladder may indicate incomplete bladder emptying or urinary retention. Significant obesity interferes with the ability to palpate the distended bladder and an abnormal mass.

Examination of the Genitalia—Women

Before examining the genitalia, the clinician should explain the procedure to prevent embarrassment. The woman should empty her bladder. Several positions are used, with the lithotomy position considered ideal. This position requires that the patient be supine, with hips and knees bent and abducted; most clinicians choose this position because PFM assessment is usually part of a bimanual, speculum pelvic examination. Ideally, the legs should be supported and the woman should be made as comfortable as possible. If appropriate and acceptable, the examiner should consider the use of a mirror to demonstrate the findings to the woman.

Excuses for not performing the examination include discomfort associated with pelvic pain and atrophic vaginitis, patient and examiner embarrassment with the examination, time constraints of the clinician, and procedural difficulty because of the need for assistance with confused or elderly patients. A speculum exam is optimal, but in older frail women, especially those residing in a nursing home, a digital exam may be more feasible.

External Genitalia   Assessment of the external genitalia includes inspection of the urinary meatus, vulva, labia majora and minora, introitus, and perineum, including the buttocks and anus (Figure 6.4). An inspection of the genitalia is performed to evaluate perineal skin condition, color, and structural abnormalities, to determine the presence of atrophic tissue changes, and to check for the presence of POP. The normal length of the perineum is 3 cm

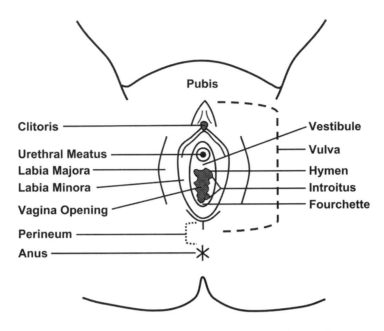

Figure 6.4. External female genitalia. (Courtesy of Robin Noel.)

between the inferior part of the introitus and the superior part of the anus. Congenital shortening of the area between the fourchette (fold of skin that forms the posterior margin of the vulva) and urethra is accompanied by a firm perineum, a thick hymen, and a small introitus (Bourcier, Juras, & Villet, 2004). The examiner should note the size of the genital hiatus, which is the distance from the urinary meatus to the posterior hymen (fold of mucous membrane that surrounds or partially covers vaginal opening) in the midline. A hiatus that is larger than 4 cm may indicate a weak pelvic floor or POP. Special attention should be given to any scars noted in the anterior or posterior lower quadrants or perineum.

Each portion of the vulva from outermost to innermost aspects should be examined. The labia minora contain sebaceous glands that trap oil, causing small inclusion cysts that abate over time (Kellogg-Spadt & Albaugh, 2003). The inner labia, called "interlabial sulci," will contain a thin yellow-white exudate called *smegma*, which is also seen in men between the foreskin and the glans penis. Inspection will determine the presence of dermatological lesions and evidence of irritative or inflammatory conditions (e.g., perineal dermatitis, erythema, excoriation). The combination of UI and fecal incontinence results in increased skin wetness (caused by urine) and permeability (caused by bowel enzymes), thus promoting perineal skin breakdown (Newman, Preston, & Salazar, 2007). Excoriation and maceration of the vulva may occur with constant wetness and may cause secondary infections. The presence of excoriation may give an indication of the severity of incontinence. Redness and soreness extending from the perineum to the upper thighs may indicate a perineal dermatitis from an almost continuous state of wetness. The clinician

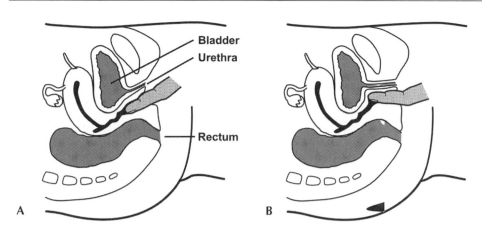

Figure 6.5. Urethral assessment. (A) Palpation of the urethra. (B) Assessing elevation of the urethra during a pelvic floor muscle contraction. (Courtesy of Robin Noel.)

should note other signs of urine leakage, such as wet clothing or the odor of urine on the patient or when examining the perineum.

Internal Genitalia   The internal genitalia, including the urinary meatus, vaginal introitus, and distal vagina, should be examined for evidence of estrogen deficiency, urine or abnormal vaginal secretions, POP, and abnormal pelvic masses. The urethral (urinary) meatus should be examined for size, location, discharge, inflammation, and fixation. An erythematous, tender cherry-red lesion arising from the dorsal (toward the back) aspect of the meatus usually represents a benign urethral caruncle but may represent a possible urethral carcinoma. If the patient reports a discharge or had recent onset of urgency and frequency, it may be useful to obtain swabs to culture for infections of *Chlamydia* or gonococcus.

Palpation of the urethra to the level of the bladder neck and trigone may be accomplished during examination of the anterior vaginal wall (Figure 6.5). Bimanual palpation is useful to define the internal genitalia and to define further the size and consistency of the bladder. Pain or discomfort may be reported in women with suspected interstitial cystitis/painful bladder syndrome and in men with chronic prostatitis or chronic pelvic pain syndrome (see Chapter 2). Palpation of a urethral diverticulum in a woman will often cause pain as well. Both men and women should be asked to assign a number to their pain using a scale of 1 to 10 with 1 being "no pain" and 10 "the worst pain" (see Figures 6.6 and 6.10).

Measurement of urethral mobility, called a "Q-Tip test," is believed by some to be a useful, though optional test in the evaluation of UI in women only, especially when the history suggests SUI. Box 6.5 outlines the procedure for performing a Q-Tip test. Urethral hypermobility is said to be present when the straining angle is greater than 30 degrees, and indicates a deficiency in the support of the urethra. A negative cotton-tipped swab test (straining angle < 30 degrees) in the presence of severe SUI may suggest that the patient has intrinsic urethral sphincter dysfunction (ISD) (discussed in Chapter 4), also

---

Box 6.5   Q-Tip procedure

1. Cleanse the external urethral meatus with an antiseptic solution, such as povidone-iodine (Betadine).

2. Apply an anesthetic jelly (e.g., lidocaine) to the end of a sterile cotton-tipped swab.

3. Gently place the swab through the urethra and into the bladder. Pull the swab back until resistance is met, which indicates entry into the urethra. At this point, ask the patient to strain maximally. Record the angle between the stem of the cotton swab and the floor.

4. Ask the patient to "bear down." The change in the angle between the stem of the cotton swab and the floor (the straining [bearing down] angle) is measured by eyeball estimate or with a goniometer (an instrument that measures angles) and recorded. A change of angle greater then 30 degrees indicates urethral hypermobility.

---

known as a "lead pipe," "stovepipe," or "drainpipe" urethra. PFM exercises are rarely effective in a patient with ISD, and surgical treatment with periurethral injection or suburethral sling may be needed (see Chapter 12). The presence of urethral hypermobility supports the diagnosis of SUI, although it is certainly not diagnostic, because urethral hypermobility may occur in patients with OAB as well as in asymptomatic continent women.

If the woman has vulvar pain, a careful vulvar examination, including the use of a "pain map" (Figure 6.6), will be helpful. In women with vulvodynia, the vulva may be erythematous, but the presence of a rash or altered mucosa or skin is not consistent with vulvodynia and may indicate perineal dermatitis. The posterior introitus and the posterior hymenal remnants are the most common sites of increased sensitivity. The clinician should use a cotton-tipped swab to apply mild pressure (approximately 3- to 5-mm indentation) to various parts of the vulvar vestibule (at 2, 4, 6, 8, and 10 o'clock), asking the women to quantify the pain as mild, moderate, or severe (Bachmann et al., 2006). This pressure should not elicit discomfort unless pelvic pain or vulvodynia is suspected.

The presence of POP, urethrocele, cystocele, uterine prolapse, and rectocele can be initially observed in the lithotomy position. The examination for POP is reviewed in Chapter 11. To clarify this, the woman is asked to bear down or perform a Valsalva maneuver or cough. The presence of rectal prolapse and hemorrhoids is noted. In women with advanced pelvic relaxation, the perineum bulges downward; the vaginal introitus opens, exposing redundant mucosa; and the anus often appears everted. Vulvar episiotomy scars are commonly associated with dyspareunia.

Pelvic Examination   All women who present with UI or related conditions should have a pelvic examination (with or without a speculum). Vaginal dysfunction as a result of obstetric trauma or gynecological causes should be assessed during a careful inspection of the vagina. Because it is the weakest portion of the pelvic floor, the vagina is subjected to all forces of gravity, and may be damaged by vaginal childbirth, estrogen deficiency, or pelvic surgery. The

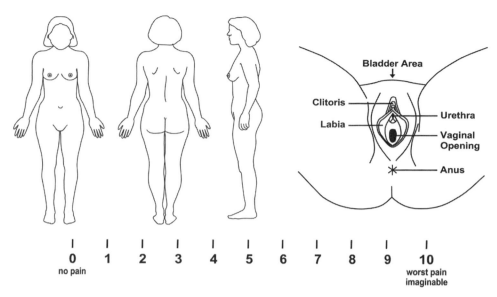

Figure 6.6.   Female body map and a pain scale for patient to mark pelvic pain. (Courtesy of Robin Noel.)

appearance of vaginal secretions may suggest a vaginal infection; urine within the vagina suggests a genitourinary fistula or an ectopic ureter.

Assessment of Estrogen State or Hypoestrogenization   Inspection can determine if the vaginal tissues are atrophic and estrogen deficient. Atrophic vaginitis affects up to 40% of postmenopausal women. Examination of the introitus and distal vagina will identify the presence of atrophic vaginitis or urogenital atrophy, indicating estrogen deficiency. Vaginal mucosa has a high density of estrogen receptors that respond to estrogen stimulation. The vaginal introitus (entrance to the vagina) will become less pliable and narrower (called vaginal stenosis) with estrogen deficiency. Some think that, because the urethra and trigone are also estrogen-dependent tissues, estrogen deficiency can contribute to some of the symptoms of OAB (Batra & Iosif, 1983). The well-estrogenized vagina has a thickened epithelium, with transverse rugae in its lower two thirds. The poorly estrogenized vagina has a thinned epithelium, with loss of transverse rugae. Assessment of the vagina may reveal a pale, thin, shiny, and poorly vascularized mucosa indicating atrophy (atrophic vaginitis and urogenital atrophy). Symptoms of urogenital atrophy can include both vaginal symptoms (burning/soreness, malodorous discharge, dryness, dyspareunia, itching) and urinary symptoms (frequency, urgency, dysuria, UI, nocturia, recurrent UTIs).

Testing of the vaginal pH also serves as an accurate indicator of the vaginal mucosa state. Using a pH paper, the clinician can touch the paper to vaginal discharge. Vaginal pH is usually 5 or lower in women with no infection and other definitive signs of good estrogen effect (Maloney, 2002). A vaginal pH of 5.5 to 7 is consistent with atrophic vaginitis. The healthy, premenopausal vagina is colonized with lactobacilli that produce bactericins, hydrogen peroxide, and lactic acid, all substances that lower the pH. The low pH creates a hostile environment for bacteria other than lactobacilli (Mashburn, 2006). If lactobacilli decrease, the vaginal pH increases, causing overgrowth of bacteria. An alkaline environment correlates with atrophic symptoms. Vaginal pH can be tested using an indicator tape (Baxter diagnostic tape), which is placed inside the vagina past the introitus. In postmenopausal women with recurrent UTIs, the vaginal pH is considerably higher and warrants the use of a topical estrogen preparation. For women who cannot use topical transvaginal estrogen, many believe that over-the-counter products (e.g., Replens, other intravaginal gels) may gradually reduce the symptoms of urogenital atrophy and atrophic vaginitis, although there is no evidence to support this use.

Assessment for Pelvic Organ Prolapse   The next part of the genital examination in women is an assessment of the presence and extent of POP. This condition is discussed in Chapter 11, and information on assessment can be found there.

Examination of the Genitalia — Men

Inspection of the penis will reveal obvious lesions of the skin and will define whether the man has been circumcised. The normal meatus should be located at the tip of the glans penis. In the uncircumcised man, the foreskin or prepuce should be retracted, and the glans and meatus should be assessed. Retracting the foreskin is a very important component of personal hygiene in the uncircumcised man (Ceo, 2006). The size and position of the meatus should be noted. A cheesy, whitish material called smegma may accumulate normally under the foreskin. In uncircumcised men, a condition called *phimosis* can occur if the orifice of the foreskin is constricted, preventing retraction of the foreskin over the glans or tip of the penis. Once the foreskin is cleaned and dried, it should be replaced back over the glans to prevent paraphimosis, an inability to advance the uncircumsized foreskin over the glans penis (Figure 6.7).

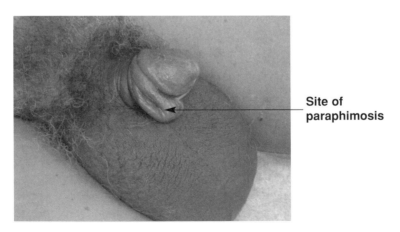

Site of paraphimosis

Figure 6.7.   Paraphimosis.

The scrotum is a loose, wrinkled pouch that holds two testicles. The left sac may be lower than the right. Each testis has a soft, comma-shaped epididymis applied to its posterolateral surface. The contents of each scrotal sac should be palpated in an orderly fashion; first the testes should be examined, then the epididymides. When palpated, the contents of each sac should slide easily. The presence of an abnormal mass within the testes is best defined by careful palpation. Each testis and epididymis should be palpated between the examiner's thumb and first two fingers. Size, shape, consistency, and tenderness are noted. Next, the cord structures should be examined, and finally the area of the external inguinal ring should be checked for the presence of an inguinal hernia during a cough or strain in the standing position.

Pelvic Floor Muscle Evaluation

A very important part of the physical examination in both men and women is assessment of the PFM to determine strength through volitional contraction, tone, and sensitivity to pressure (Fletcher, 2005; Newman & Laycock, 2008). The PFM consist of the levator ani group and include the pubococcygeus, puborectalis, and iliococcygeus muscles (see Chapter 3). The external urethral and anal sphincters are in continuity with these muscles, and both receive pudendal nerve innervation. The PFM provide support to all pelvic organs, and loss of pelvic muscle tone and strength can lead to both UI and OAB. The PFM are innervated by motor efferents from the sacral nerve roots, which originate in S2–S4, and by branches of the pudendal nerve, which has sensory fibers that can contribute to perineal and pelvic pain. A comprehensive review of PFM anatomy and physiology is found in Chapter 3.

Evaluation of the PFM is done through manual intravaginal (or transrectal) examination and may include the use of measuring devices (electromyography or pressure) for complementary assessment. Functional testing of PFM strength by digital examination is a reliable assessment (Brink, Wells, Sampselle, Tallie, & Mayer, 1994; Kerschan-Schindl et al., 2002). A PFM contraction may be assessed by visual inspection or by palpation, electromyography, or perineometry. Factors to be assessed include strength, duration, and repeatability (Abrams et al., 2002). PFM function can be qualitatively defined by the tone at rest and the strength of a voluntary or reflex contraction as strong, weak, or absent, or by a grading system.

Women   The woman should be placed in the semisupine position with the hips flexed at about 45 degrees and the knees flexed at about 120 degrees. Ideally the legs should be abducted with the soles of the feet in contact with each other. This will prevent adductor muscle contraction. If the woman is unable to be placed in this position, then ask her to allow her knees to separate and fall to the side (see Box 6.6). Evaluation begins with a single-finger digital examination with light pressure against the inferior lateral wall of the vagina. It is extremely helpful for the examiner to place a hand on the

Box 6.6   Examiner instructions on how to perform a pelvic floor muscle (PFM) contraction during digital pelvic examination of female patients

1. Explain the purpose of the PFMs and use an illustration when doing this review (see Chapters 3 and 8).

2. Explain that the examination will help her identify the correct muscles and learn how to exercise them properly. This will be a digital examination, inserting a finger in the vagina or anal opening. Determine if the woman has any concerns about this examination (e.g., older women who may be uncomfortable with a pelvic exam).

3. Ask patient to empty bladder prior to examination.

4. Position the patient supine with hips and knees flexed and draped. Avoid use of stirrups, which are usually uncomfortable and may cause the woman to tense her legs.

5. Position a lamp on the perineum (if available).

6. A small amount of lubricant should be applied to the gloved finger.

7. Position yourself to view the perineum from the side of the patient. Rest the leg closest to you against your chest and the other leg abducted and externally rotated on a pillow. This will relax the hip adductors during the exam. Alternatively, the lithotomy position can be used.

8. Separate labia and identify perineal structures, urinary meatus, clitoris, vaginal introitus, and anus. If you feel it would be helpful and accepted by the patient, position a mirror and point out these structures to the patient.

9. The index finger is placed over the middle finger and inserted into the vagina. Then rest your other hand lightly on the patient's abdomen in order to determine whether she contracts the correct muscles during a PFM contraction.

10. First ask the patient to relax. Then instruct her to contract: "Squeeze around my finger(s), lifting in and up."

11. As soon as you feel a perivaginal muscle contraction, tell the patient that this is the correct muscle. Have her relax and then contract again. Repeat several times to establish that she can contract reliably.

12. If you cannot feel any compression of the muscle on your finger, then press slightly on the posterior wall of the vagina and try again. If this is not successful, press simultaneously against the anterior and posterior walls to detect contraction. Try alternate instructions to help her find the muscle.

    •   "Imagine that you are in an elevator with your friends and you are trying to keep from passing gas."

    •   "Imagine that you are trying to hold in a bowel movement."

    •   "Imagine that you are trying to hold in a tampon."

13. Make sure she relaxes completely between contractions.

14. Observe any accessory muscle contraction (buttocks, thighs, abdominals). If she does contract these muscles, teach her that these muscles will not help with bladder control and to try to keep them relaxed.

15. Observe whether the patient is holding her breath during muscle contraction. If she is, remind her to take slow, regular breaths. Have the patient talk to you as she contracts her muscle, because she cannot hold her breath and talk at the same time.

Box 6.6   *(continued)*

16. Give her feedback with each attempted PFM contraction.

17. Next, assess the external anal sphincter.

    • Position the patient in the left lateral or lithotomy position. A pillow can be placed between the legs if needed for comfort if the left lateral position is used.

    • Use lubricant liberally.

    • Place your index finger, palm side back, on the lower edge of the external sphincter. Press slightly (this will help relax the muscle). Proceed by slowing inserting your finger to the first knuckle.

18. Take every opportunity to reinforce PFM contraction, even if weak.

19. Reinforce any observed progress or improvement.

20. If you detect muscle fatigue, give the patient a rest and just converse while waiting for the muscle to recover (at least 1 minute).

21. Provide feedback at the end of the examination.

    • Praise the patient for her ability to correctly perform a PFM contraction (if true).

    • Remind the patient about the use of PFM contractions to control urgency. Be positive that use of PFM contraction can improve her incontinence and/or urgency.

woman's lower abdomen so that abdominal straining can be detected, and feedback may be given to her in an effort to prevent this counterproductive contraction of the abdominal muscles. This simple type of examination not only provides essential biofeedback to the woman (which we have found to be significantly more effective than verbal or written instructions) but also reassures the clinician that the woman is contracting the correct muscle.

Digital measurement of PFM strength in women can be done transvaginally. The clinician should use either one or two digits. The PFM of a parous woman are usually assessed using two fingers, but this technique may be unsuitable for nulliparous women because of their narrower vaginas, or for elderly women with atrophic vaginitis and vaginal stenosis (Newman & Laycock, 2008). Box 6.6 provides instructions on how to perform a digital PFM examination and how to teach a woman to contract the muscle (Figure 6.8). The pubococcygeus muscles are palpated just inside the introitus at 5 and 7 o'clock. Normally, the pubococcygeus muscle is felt as a distinct 1- to 2-cm band that can be palpated on the lateral vaginal wall when the examiner's finger is introduced to a depth of 3–5 cm beyond the vaginal introitus and rotated 360 degrees while palpating the perivaginal muscles. The examiner should then proceed to full-finger depth and palpate the left and right levator ani muscles at 3 and 9 o'clock along the vaginal wall. The strong levator ani muscles of a young woman will be felt as a thick, firm band of muscle, compared with the weak levator ani muscles of an elderly woman. A weak or attenuated pubo-

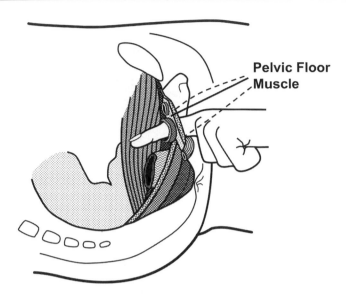

Figure 6.8. Digital (one finger) assessment of pelvic floor muscles (PFM). (Courtesy of Robin Noel.)

coccygeus muscle may be indistinguishable from the surrounding tissues. The woman is then asked to perform a contraction, squeezing the muscle around the examiner's finger to "lift up" the floor of the vagina. The woman is asked to contract the PFM around the examiner's finger with as much force and for as long as she is able; this is repeated several times.

The obturator muscles are deep within the vagina and can be palpated along the lateral aspect of the pelvic sidewalls (Newman & Laycock, 2008). To palpate the obturators, the examiner's hand should be on the outside of the patient's knee and the patient should be instructed to externally rotate the hip. By palpating deeply and laterally within the vagina, the right and left side of this muscle can be palpated.

It is important to realize that, when asked to contract the PFM, over 30% of women believe they are performing the contraction correctly but will use the wrong muscle, strain down, perform a Valsalva maneuver, or fail to activate all layers of the PFM (Bø & Sherburn, 2005; Bump, Hurt, Fantl, & Wyman, 1991). Most women are largely unaware that these muscles exist, and simple instruction in technique may not be adequate preparation. Women who are unable to contract the PFM will often contract other muscles in addition to the PFM. They will adduct the thighs and elevate the buttocks off the exam table (the examiner will hear the exam table paper move) in an attempt to aid PFM contraction through the use of accessory muscle contraction. During a strong contraction, the main observation is a puckering and cephalad in-drawing of the vaginal introitus, anus, and perineum. A weak contraction may only demonstrate a slight puckering, and some patients are unable to produce any movement of the perineum. Observation of a downward movement suggests that the patient is straining and not producing a correct PFM contraction (Newman & Laycock, 2008).

Abdominal, gluteal, and adductor muscle recruitment should be observed as a general assessment of muscle isolation (Newman, 2003). Muscles rarely work in isolation, and the PFM are no exception. Research has shown that the abdominal muscles, in particular the transversus abdominis muscles, are always recruited during a PFM maximum voluntary contraction (Neumann & Gill, 2002). The PFM and transversus abdominis muscles work in conjunction with the lumbar multifidi (a group of deep spinal muscles that stabilize the spine and prevent excessive rotation of the vertebrae) and the respiratory diaphragm to stabilize the lumbar spine. Voluntary relaxation of the PFM should occur after each contraction as the muscle returns to its resting state. A voluntary relaxation can be absent, partial, or complete (Messelink et al., 2005).

The clinician should also have the woman perform certain maneuvers to determine PFM strength. The impact of a cough on a healthy, strong pelvic floor produces little or no movement, either at the vaginal introitus or in the perineum as a whole. In some cases, an anticipatory pre-cough PFM contraction is noted. Conversely, a woman with a very weak pelvic floor may demonstrate perineal descent, possibly below the level of the ischial spines, and the vaginal introitus may bulge and gape. There may also be caudal movement of any prolapse and, in addition, this may generate a positive stress test (small squirt or stream of urine at the time of the cough). The clinician should instruct the woman to perform a quick, hard, and fast PFM contraction to measure PFM coordination and to determine fast-twitch fiber capability. This is important because it is thought that the reflex response of the fast-twitch fibers to coughing is the mechanism that maintains continence, by lifting the proximal urethra and increasing the urethral occlusive pressure (Miller, Ashton-Miller, & DeLancey, 1996).

When the woman is contracting the PFM, three criteria of muscle strength should be noted: pressure, duration of contraction, and whether the contraction causes the examiner's finger to change position; in addition, the examiner should note whether the woman used accessory muscles (Brink et al., 1994). The amount of pressure or strength of the muscle contraction can range from imperceptible to a firm squeeze. Duration involves the number of seconds that the examiner feels the muscle contraction. The woman should be asked to prolong the duration of the contraction to better assess the slow-twitch fibers because the external urethral sphincter is solely, and the levator ani muscle mainly, composed of these fibers. In women with a well-supported PFM group, the muscle contraction can lift the base of the examiner's fingers. The use of an assessment tool for documentation is advised; Figure 6.9 presents a scale for grading digital evaluation of PFM strength that one of the authors (DKN) developed. Using this scale, the authors have found that, if a woman is unable to perform a one-out-of-three muscle contraction, then she is a poor candidate for PFM training. When using the scale, the examiner should

CIRCLE ONE   ☐ Vaginal Exam   ☐ Rectal Exam

Scale	Grade	Description
None	0	No duration of muscle contraction, pressure, displacement
		Recruitment of large muscle group (e.g., gluteals, adductors, abdominals)
Trace	1/5	Slight but instant contraction: < 1 second
		Recruitment of large muscle group (e.g., gluteals, adductors, abdominals)
Weak	2/5	Weak contraction: with or without posterior elevation of fingers, held for > 1 second but ≤ 3 seconds
Moderate	3/5	Moderate contraction: with or without posterior elevation of fingers, held for at least 4–6 seconds, repeated 3 times
Good	4/5	Strong contraction: with posterior elevation of fingers, held for at least 7–9 seconds, repeated 4–5 times
Strong	5/5	Unmistakably strong contraction with posterior elevation of fingers, held for at least 10 seconds, repeated > 5 times

USAGE OF ACCESSORY MUSCLE GROUPS

Abdominal	☐ **YES**	☐ **NO**
Gluteal	☐ **YES**	☐ **NO**
Thigh/abductor	☐ **YES**	☐ **NO**

EVALUATION—MUSCLE HYPERTONUS/SPASM

CIRCLE ONE:	0	No pressure, tenderness, or pain associated with exam
	1	Comfortable pressure associated with exam, slight tenderness but bearable
	2	Uncomfortable pressure associated with exam, slight pain
	3	Moderate pain associated with exam that intensifies with muscle contraction
	4	Severe pain associated with exam, patient unable to perform contraction because of pain

EMG Muscle Evaluation   ☐ No   ☐ Yes

Results _____

Diagnosis:	Muscle disuse atrophy/muscle wasting	☐ 728.2
	Muscle spasm	☐ 728.85
	Anal spasm	☐ 564.6

COMMENTS: _____

SIGNATURE: _____ DATE: _____

Figure 6.9. Pelvic floor muscle strength assessment. © 2007 Diane K. Newman

note the type of exam performed (vaginal, rectal, both). If the woman has pelvic muscle spasms, the examiner should note the degree of spasm.

There is a relative paucity of data regarding digital scoring systems in the evaluation of high-tone pelvic floor dysfunction, which refers to the clinical condition of hypertonic, spastic pelvic floor musculature (Newman & Laycock, 2008). Most scales seem to address a woman's ability to contract her pelvic floor musculature without an assessment of tenderness or impaired relaxation (Fletcher, 2005). The levator ani can be palpated in the 4 and 8 o'clock positions, just superior to the hymeneal ring. Pain or discomfort during palpation may indicate high-tone pelvic muscles. The same examination is performed for both the right and left PFM. The woman is then asked to relax her muscles, and tenderness (hypertonus) is graded on a 0–4 scale (see Figure 6.9).

Men   PFM examination is performed transrectally in men. The man should tighten or squeeze the muscles around the anus and try to lift the anus toward his head, as he would if he were trying to prevent the passing of flatus (gas). The clinician should be able to see and feel the anus contracting and lifting. The man should then attempt to lift the scrotum and draw up both testicles; this can also be felt and seen. The examiner should feel and observe the area around the base of the penis because it will move toward the abdomen. Verbal feedback noting the presence of a voluntary contraction can also encourage and assist in enhancing the man's effort.

Pelvic Pain Assessment

Women   After assessing the PFM, the clinician should palpate anteriorly and posteriorly the iliococcygeus, pubovaginalis, puborectalis, and coccygeus muscles by simply pressing into the middle of each muscle with moderate pressure while observing the woman for signs of tenderness, pain, and trigger points. If there is no resistance, the clinician's finger should be able to push easily into the muscle, which will feel like an overripe, soft tomato. Muscle resistance (feels like pushing into a hard, not-yet-ripe tomato) is felt in a woman with a short PFM that is the source of the pain. Trigger points will manifest as areas of hyperirritability or hypersensitivity in a muscle that generates pain. If the woman complains of pelvic pain (e.g., seen in painful bladder syndrome), assessment of the obturator internus muscle is recommended. This is performed by palpating the pubovaginalis muscle at the 9 o'clock position (right muscle) and 3 o'clock position (left muscle). To ensure palpation of the correct muscle, the examiner should have the woman bend her knee and abduct her right knee against resistance (examiner's outstretched right arm) while keeping her foot on the exam table or in the stirrup. If pain is present, the woman should be asked to rate the pain on a scale from 1 to 10, with 10 being the most severe pain (see Figures 6.6 and 6.10). It should also be characterized by type, frequency, duration, precipitating and relieving factors (e.g., relieved by voiding), and location (bladder, urethral, vulva, vaginal, perineal).

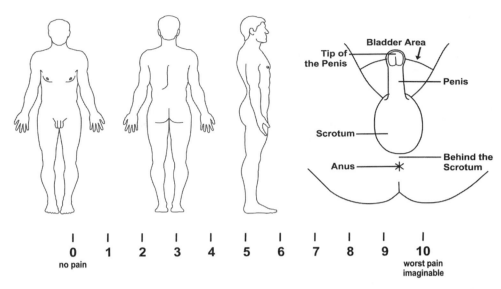

Figure 6.10. Male body map and a pain scale for patient to mark pelvic pain. (Courtesy of Robin Noel.)

Men   Pelvic pain in men is usually centered behind the scrotum toward the anus, but physical examination may not be helpful. Clinicians can ask the man to point to the location of the pain on a body map (Figure 6.10).

Anorectal Examination

A digital rectal examination is performed in both men and women to assess for fecal impaction, and to evaluate anal sphincter tone. A rectal exam should also be performed to determine the presence of a fecal mass, fecal impaction, or rectal mass. Despite its importance in a frail, elderly population, this exam is often neglected in nursing home residents; in one study, only 15% of residents had a digital rectal examination (Watson, Brink, Zimmer, & Mayer, 2003). Assessment of the rectal sphincter can be performed by evaluating the anal sphincter contraction and resting tone of the anal canal, derived primarily from the internal anal sphincter (70%) with contributions from the external anal sphincter (30%) (Wald, 2007).

   In the rectum, the distal external sphincter is felt just inside the anal canal. The puborectalis portion of the levator ani muscle can be palpated about 2.5–4 cm from the anal verge. The examiner should feel a symmetrical circumferential resistance (a gripping and pulling in around the entire circumference of his or her finger) when inserting a finger in the anus if the sphincter tone is normal. As the sphincter relaxes, the examiner should gently insert a gloved, lubricated index finger into the anal canal in a direction pointing toward the umbilicus and note the resting sphincter tone of the anus (e.g., weak, moderate, or firm). Normally, the muscles of the anal sphincter close snugly around the entire circumference of the examiner's finger. Tension should be felt. The individual should be asked to perform a voluntary sphincter contraction by first relaxing and then contracting the anal sphincter by pulling in the anus as if holding back gas and to try to maintain that contraction. The patient is also asked to relax and "bear down" as if having a bowel movement or to push out the examiner's finger. This will allow the clinician to assess the overall sphincter tone and the strength and symmetry of the sphincter and to identify defects in the sphincter mechanism. When the patient is asked to squeeze, the strength and duration of the contraction of the external anal sphincter may be assessed.

To assess the puborectalis muscle, the examining finger is advanced and oriented posteriorly. When the patient is asked to squeeze, the contraction of the puborectalis muscle is felt as an anterior and upward tug as the muscle shortens. Simultaneously, the external anal sphincter contracts to increase the pressure in the anal canal. The clinician should note any weakness in the pelvic floor, such as the presence of a rectocele or enterocele in women.

In men, the size, consistency, and contour of the prostate gland are determined. The prostate can be palpated by inserting a gloved, lubricated finger 2.5–4 cm into the rectum. The normal prostate gland is walnut sized, with a flattened, heart-shaped configuration. The normal prostate has a consistency referred to as "rubbery." Abnormalities include the presence of nodules or areas of induration, or areas of "bogginess." The normal consistency is similar to the fleshy part below the thumb of a clenched fist. A knuckle defines "nodularity." Induration is diffuse firmness of an area without a discrete nodule. A man with an abnormal or enlarged prostate should be referred to a urologist. If bladder outlet obstruction is suspected, an appropriate prostate exam should be performed, along with a prostate-specific antigen determination, urinalysis, and postvoid residual (PVR) measurement.

Prostatic massage may be performed with gentle digital (index finger) pressure, moving from the lateral margin of the superior portion of a selected lobe of the prostate toward the apex, for approximately 1 minute (longer massage may inhibit the fluid outflow). Several drops of expressed prostatic secretion should emerge from the urethral meatus within 2–3 minutes after the massage is completed. The expressed prostatic secretion and the first 10 mL of urine voided after prostatic massage can be cultured as a prostate specimen.

Neurological Examination

A focused neurological examination is divided into four parts: 1) mental status, 2) sensory function, 3) motor function, and 4) reflex integrity.

A sensory function neurological examination includes testing specific dermatomes (areas of the skin that are supplied by certain spinal nerves) for response to position, vibration, pinprick, light touch, and temperature. Relevant dermatomes include

- Lumbosacral nerve roots

    - L1 (innervates base of penis, upper scrotum, labia majora)

    - L1–L2 (innervate midscrotum, labia minora)

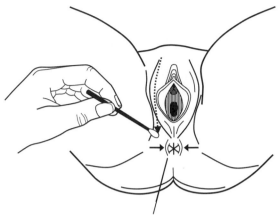

Figure 6.11. Contraction of anal sphincter (anal "wink"). (Courtesy of Robin Noel.)

- Sacral nerve roots
  - S3–S5 (innervate perineum and perianal skin)
  - S2–S4 (innervate the striated muscles of the bladder and pelvic floor [external urethral and anal sphincters])

Tests used to evaluate the sacral nerve root reflexes include deep tendon reflexes, lower extremity strength, sharp/dull sensation, and stimulation of the anal "wink" reflex (S2–S5) and the bulbocavernosus reflex (BCR). Evaluation of deep tendon reflexes provides an indication of segmental spinal cord function:

- Hyperactivity is associated with an "upper motor neuron lesion"—brain and anterior horn cells
- Hypoactivity is associated with a "lower motor neuron lesion"—anterior horn cells to periphery

The tip of a cotton-tipped swab can be used to test for sharp versus dull sensation over the S2–S4 dermatomes. The test for the anal wink reflex involves lightly stroking the anus with a gloved finger or cotton-tipped swab while the clinician observes for anal contraction—the anus puckers or "winks" (Figure 6.11). An intact reflex indicates normal function of S2–S4. The anal wink may be absent in older women, and this is not considered pathological in that population. The BCR refers specifically to the contraction of the bulbocavernosus muscle, but is also used to test the innervation (S2–S4) of all perineal striated muscles. To test the BCR, the examiner gently squeezes the clitoris in women or the glans penis in men while checking for anal contraction. The BCR may be absent in up to 20% of neurologically normal women.

Urological Testing

Several practice guidelines on UI recommend basic tests that should be completed to identify bladder dysfunction (AMDA, 2005; CMS, 2005; Fantl et al.,

1996; Viktrup et al., 2004). They include a urinalysis and determination of bladder emptying.

Urinalysis Testing the urine for bacteriuria, pyuria, and hematuria is an essential component of the UI evaluation. A clean-catch, midstream urine specimen should be obtained, and a dipstick urinalysis (UA) is performed. The clinician should remember that false-positive and false-negative results are not unusual in dipstick UA (Simerville, Maxted, & Pahira, 2005).

Midstream urine is collected by cleansing the vulva (women) and meatus (men and women) and having the individual start to urinate into the toilet and subsequently insert a sterile container into the urinary stream to collect a urine sample. Prior cleansing of the glans in men and external genitalia in women is recommended, but it may not be necessary in women (Lifshitz & Kramer, 2000). However, a clean-catch urine specimen in women is frequently contaminated by vaginal flora. Urine should be refrigerated if it cannot be examined immediately (Simerville et al., 2005).

The color of urine is generally clear yellow, and changes in color may be due to foods and medications (e.g., pyridium can cause urine to turn orange). Urine color can indicate hydration status because urine darkens with dehydration (Mentes, Wakefield, & Culp, 2006). Low specific gravity may indicate diabetes insipidus. The normal pH of urine ranges from 4.5 to 8.0; an acidic pH is between 4.5 and 5.5 and an alkaline pH is between 6.5 and 8.0 (VanArsdalen, 2007). A pathogen that produces urease (e.g., *Proteus mirabilis* and *Pseudomonas*) can result in a pH greater than 7.0–7.5 (alkaline). A strong urine odor does not necessarily imply infection (Gray, 2003).

A positive nitrite test indicates that bacteria may be present in significant numbers (Wallace & Sadovsky, 2005). The test is specific but not very sensitive, so it is helpful when it is positive. Bacteria without reductases, such as enterococci and streptococci, cannot be detected by nitrate testing. Leukocyte esterase is produced by neutrophils and may signal pyuria associated with UTI. It has a better positive predictive value for bacteriuria when considered with nitrite testing. A negative leukocyte esterase probably means that infection is unlikely. If tests for leukocyte esterase or nitrites are positive and the patient is symptomatic, a separate specimen should be sent for culture and sensitivity testing. A UA positive for leukocytes does not always require antibiotic treatment in older women because it is not useful diagnosing UTI in an asymptomatic patient.

Hematuria without leukocytes or nitrites may be a sign of urinary tract pathology, including nephrolithiasis, glomerulonephritis, or tumor. However, exercise-induced hematuria may occur and may be associated with long-distance running. A more extensive workup, including urine cytology, computed tomographic urography, intravenous urography or renal ultrasound, and referral for cystoscopy (test that utilizes a fiberoptic scope with a light source to examine the internal surfaces of the bladder and urethra), should be considered, however, if microscopic hematuria is discovered. The presence of glycosuria should raise the possibility of diabetes, which, if unrecognized, may be responsible for polydipsia, polyuria, or both, thereby mimicking some of the symptoms of OAB. The clinician should realize that a patient will not spill glucose into the urine until the blood sugar is greater than 180 mg/dL. Consequently, a dipstick UA may fail to pick up on intermittently high sugars or mild diabetes.

Gross, microscopic, and culture examinations of the urine may help distinguish between a noninfectious condition and the presence of an infectious agent. Bacterial counts between 10^2 and 10^5 colony-forming units/mL of catheterized urine and 10^5 in a clean catch, midstream urine specimen are indicative of a UTI in symptomatic patients.

Frequency, urgency, dysuria, lower abdominal or pelvic pain, nocturia, pyuria, UI, and low back pain are common symptoms suggestive of bacterial involvement of the lower urinary tract. In the nursing facility resident, symptoms of UI are often nonspecific and may include low-grade fever or change in temperature, increased confusion or delirium, worsening of incontinence, anorexia, and functional decline (CMS, 2005; Ouslander, Shapira, Schnelle, & Fingold, 1996). Bacteriuria is common in nursing facility residents; the prevalence is 30%–50% among female residents. However, in older patients and in residents in nursing facilities, there is no benefit from screening or antimicrobial treatment of asymptomatic bacteriuria. The accuracy of a rapid, enzyme-based screening test for nitrite and leukocyte esterase using a dipstick has been demonstrated in nursing facility residents with UI (Ouslander, Schapira, & Schnelle, 1995). Box 6.2 lists the criteria for determining UTI in nursing home residents as detailed in the CMS Tag F315. This testing can be performed easily by nursing facility staff using a clean-catch urine specimen. Therefore, most clinicians believe that nursing facility residents do not need to be catheterized to obtain a urine specimen for culture.

Postvoid Residual Urine Volume   A PVR determination should be performed on at-risk individuals to eliminate the possibility of urinary retention. At-risk individuals include those with suprapubic distention or tenderness, a feeling of incomplete bladder emptying, men with prostate enlargement or a history of prostate disease, women with a history of pelvic surgery, diabetics, those taking anticholinergic drugs that may interfere with bladder emptying, and those with neurological disease (CMS, 2005; Newman, 2005b, 2006, 2007). It remains a point of contention whether all individuals presenting with symptoms of UI and OAB require a PVR measurement prior to the initiation of treatment. It is desirable to measure the PVR in some individuals, particularly older people with voiding symptoms, recurrent or persistent UTIs, or both; those with neurological disease and voiding dysfunction; and those with symptoms that suggest poor bladder emptying.

Specific PVR measurement can be accomplished either by catheterization or preferably by ultrasound within 10–20 minutes of voiding. Portable ultrasound scanners are quick, easy to use, reasonably sensitive, very specific for determining elevated PVRs (Newman et al., 2005). The authors use the BladderScan™ to determine PVR in at-risk patients. Goode, Locher, Bryant,

> **Box 6.7   Applications of a portable ultrasound machine (the BladderScan™) in long-term care**
>
> 1. **During assessment:** The instrument can be used to properly assess the resident's bladder function to determine incomplete bladder emptying through the measurement of the bladder volume and postvoid residual urine volume (required by the Resident Assessment Protocol and Tag F315 guidance).
>
> 2. **During management:** Residents with urinary retention will be assessed to determine actual bladder volume versus "blind" scheduled catheterization times in residents who require intermittent catheterization.
>
> 3. **During treatment:** Scanning can be used to prevent the onset of urinary retention following indwelling catheter removal, after hospitalization, and in those residents with risk factors for developing urinary retention (e.g., diabetes; neurological conditions such as Parkinson's disease, multiple sclerosis, spinal cord injury, or stroke; suprapubic tenderness or distention; prescribed anticholinergic or other medications that interfere with bladder emptying; history or possibility of prostate disorder in men; history of pelvic surgery in women).
>
> 4. **During toileting assistance programs:** Toileting assistance can be provided based on critical bladder volume versus "blind" toileting. A toileting schedule can be planned according to volume, rather than time.
>
> 5. **During residents' bladder training programs:** The instrument can be used to demonstrate bladder volume in specific residents in whom the goal is to stop obsessive or unnecessary toileting requests.
>
> Adapted from Newman, D.K. (2007). *Program of Excellence in Extended Care.* Bothell, WA: Verathon Medical Corporation; and Newman, D.K., Gaines, T., & Snare, E. (2005). Innovation in bladder assessment: Use of technology in extended care. *Journal of Gerontological Nursing, 31*(12), 33–41.

Roth, and Burgio (2000) compared portable ultrasound to catheterization in ambulatory women. They found the portable ultrasound to have a sensitivity of 66.7% and a specificity of 96.5% in detecting PVR of 150 mL or greater. In acute care and rehabilitation hospitals, the use of a portable ultrasound machine (a common one used is the BladderScan™ [Verathon Medical, Bothell, WA]) is the preferred method of obtaining a PVR and has become the standard of care for "best practices" of bladder management (Colling, 1996; Newman et al., 2005; Ouslander et al., 1994; Wagner & Schmid, 1997; Woolridge, 2000). In acute care, the use of a noninvasive bladder volume instrument has been shown to decrease unnecessary catheterizations (Lee, Tsay, Lou, & Dai, 2006; Stevens, 2006) and decrease UTIs (Phillips, 2000). Box 6.7 lists the many applications in LTC of a portable ultrasound machine. Despite these applications, this instrument has not been as readily embraced in LTC and home care, settings that have significant numbers of "at-risk" individuals.

There is also controversy regarding the amount of PVR that should be considered abnormal. Complete or near-complete emptying of the bladder generally occurs during voiding. A PVR of greater than 100 mL obtained on at least two separate occasions should arouse concern. Individuals who have abnormal volumes should be referred for further studies.

An 85-year-old male LTC resident with a history of urinary frequency, frequent episodes of small amounts of UI, and UTIs was falling frequently on the way to the bathroom. This resident could perform self-toileting. Bladder scans performed over 2 weeks revealed incomplete bladder emptying with PVRs ranging from a low of 93 mL to a high of 446 mL. Average scan volume was 330 mL. The resident was referred to a local urologist, who diagnosed bladder outlet obstruction and severe prostatitis. An enlarged prostate was causing urethral obstruction, leading to incomplete bladder emptying with overflow UI. The urologist prescribed an alpha-adrenergic blocking agent; bladder emptying improved, UI decreased, and the resident's comfort increased. Quality of life increased with the addition of a 6-week course of antibiotic treatment for the prostatitis.

Cough Test   An optional test is the "cough" or provocative stress test. With a known quantity of fluid in the bladder (e.g., > 150 mL), the patient is asked to cough forcefully several times while the clinician observes for urine loss from the urethra. The patient should be in a supine or standing position. This testing should not be performed if the urge to void is present. If an instantaneous leakage occurs with cough, then SUI is a likely diagnosis. If the leakage is not instantaneous, then other types of UI may be present. If a woman has a significant POP (grade 3 or 4), the prolapse should be reduced before performing the stress test. A delayed or prolonged urine leak following the cough may actually indicate the presence of "cough-induced detrusor overactivity." A cough test is very difficult to perform in people with cognitive and functional disabilities, and its usefulness in this population is questionable.

Pad Test   Pad testing is a simple and objective method for quantifying urine leakage. It can be done in two ways. In the "home" pad test, the patient is asked to save incontinence pads or products used over a 24- to 48-hour period. The pads are placed in a plastic bag and are brought into the clinician's office to be weighed to measure urine loss. The patient education tool "Doing a Pad Test" on the companion CD contains information for individuals performing a home pad test. The second method is performed in the clinician's office and is called a "1-hour" test. A patient with a full bladder and wearing an absorbent pad is asked to perform various provocative maneuvers such as coughing and jumping over a 1-hour period. The pad is then removed and weighed to determine the amount of urine lost. It is believed that the home pad test is more accurate in detecting urine loss.

Urodynamic Studies   Individuals requiring further evaluation include those who meet the following criteria (Fantl et al., 1996; Newman, 2002; Newman, Burgio, & Sand, 2004; Ouslander, 2004):

1. Uncertain diagnosis and inability to develop a reasonable treatment plan based on unclear correlation between symptoms and clinical findings

2. Failure to respond to an adequate therapeutic trial (e.g., bladder training, PFM exercises, and drug therapy); may be based on patient's satisfaction with treatment

3. Consideration of surgical intervention

4. Presence of comorbid conditions such as

   a. Recurrent symptomatic UTIs

   b. Persistent symptoms of difficult bladder emptying

   c. Severe (beyond the introitus) POP

   d. Abnormal PVR

   e. Neurological condition (e.g., multiple sclerosis, spinal cord lesions) in which a component of neurogenic bladder is suspected

When diagnosis is uncertain or one of the previous criteria is met, urodynamic studies (UDS) may be indicated. UDS are one or more of a series of tests that allow direct assessment of lower urinary tract function by the measurement of relevant parameters (Carcio, 2005). These tests include filling cystometry or cystometrography (storage function of the bladder), uroflow and pressure flow studies (voiding function), urethral pressure profilometry and determination of leak point pressures (function of the urethra), and electromyography (function of the PFM) (Dmochowski, 2005). Box 6.8 reviews UDS terminology, and Table 6.2 provides a description of the specific tests. Proper interpretation of urodynamic testing results requires that, ideally, UDS should reproduce the patient's symptoms for the test to be diagnostic, so false-

---

Box 6.8   Urodynamics terminology

- P_{abd}—the abdominal pressure (pressure outside of and around the bladder), measured by a rectal (or occasionally a vaginal) catheter.

- P_{ves}—the total bladder (intravesical) pressure.

- P_{det}—the pressure generated by the bladder wall, usually as detrusor contractions; measured as the difference between the total intravesical and the abdominal pressure (subtracting $P_{ves} - P_{abd}$).

- P_{ura}—the intraurethral pressure, or the pressure within the urethra.

- $P_{ura} - P_{ves}$—the difference between the bladder (intravesical) pressure and the urethral pressure. Pressure in the bladder is automatically subtracted from the intraurethral pressure; the urethral closure pressure is the difference between P_{ura} and P_{ves} at that time.

- UPP—the urethral pressure profile, which measures intraluminal pressure along the length of the urethra.

- MUCP—the maximum urethral closure pressure, which is the maximum difference between the peak urethral pressure and the intravesical pressure at that time.

- ALPP—the abdominal leak point pressure, or the resistance of the urethra during abdominal stress (cough) or Valsalva maneuver producing leakage (may refer to this as VLPP) in the absence of detrusor contraction.

- DLPP—the detrusor leak point pressure, or the measure of P_{det} required to induce leakage across the urethra when the bladder is the main expulsive force; this is an important measurement when a neurogenic bladder is suspected.

- $Q_{average}$—average flow rate, measured as voided volume divided by flow time.

- Q_{max}—maximum flow rate, or the maximum measured value of the flow rate after correction for artifacts.

Table 6.2 Description of specific urodynamic studies

Test	Description	Indications	Procedure
Cystometrogram (CMG) Simple (only bladder pressure during filling is measured) Complex (pressure–flow study in which bladder and abdominal pressures are measured)	Measures bladder pressure during controlled filling and subsequent voiding, with measurement of the synchronous flow rate (called a pressure–flow study or voiding pressure study). It can be used to measure: • Activity during bladder filling (normal: no bladder contractions, normal compliance, normal sensation; abnormal: involuntary contractions, decreased compliance, hypersensitivity, pain). • Sensations during filling. • Bladder capacity. • Bladder compliance: describes the pressure–volume relationship, or the bladder's response to being filled, by looking at the change in bladder volume and change in detrusor pressure (in mL/cm H_2O). Compliance is reduced if the bladder is unable to stretch during filling, leading to a steady increase in detrusor pressure. Simple cystometrography can detect abnormal detrusor compliance and measure volume and intravesical pressure, whereas the complex multichannel, or subtracted, cystometrogram simultaneously measures intra-abdominal (P_{abd}) and total bladder (intravesical) (P_{ves}) pressures. Electronic subtraction of the former from the latter ($P_{ves} - P_{abd}$)	Cystometrography is indicated under certain circumstances, including diagnosing detrusor overactivity and mixed UI, in patients with neurological disorders, after pelvic surgery or radiation treatments, in the event of failed medical or surgical therapy, as part of planning for invasive surgery, to rule out emptying disorder, or to clarify a diagnosis. Cystometrography can also be combined with urinary sphincter electromyography, which can then determine normal or abnormal detrusor–sphincter physiology during bladder filling and emptying.	It involves the passage of two small catheters into the bladder, one to fill it with fluid. The bladder is slowly filled with sterile saline or water through one of the catheters placed in the urethra. Bladder pressure is measured with a transducer system that varies with different types of catheters and is recorded on a graph during filling. In order to account for increases in abdominal pressure (such as coughing or bearing down), which may be misinterpreted as bladder contractions, the abdominal pressure is recorded separately using a pressure transducer placed in the patient's vagina or rectum. It is this pressure graph that is used in looking for abnormal bladder contractions and compliance problems. The patient is asked to state the bladder sensation during filling in the following manner: • **First sensation**—feeling when the patient first becomes aware of the filling. • **First desire to void**—feeling that the patient would pass urine if conveniently possible but that voiding could still be delayed. • **Strong desire to void**—a persistent desire to void without fear of leakage.

(continued)

- **Maximum cystometric capacity—** reached when the patient had a very strong urge to void and can no longer delay micturition.

enables the detrusor pressure (P_{det}) to be determined and provides a clearer picture of true bladder activity.

Test	Definition	Clinical significance	Methodology
Urethral pressure profile (UPP)	Defined as the fluid pressure needed to open a closed (collapsed) urethra. UPP is represented as a graph indicating the pressure along the length of the urethra. Measurements are carried out along the whole length of the urethra. The functional urethral length is the length of the urethra along which urethral pressure exceeds intravesical pressure. The intravesical pressure (P_{ves}) and the intraurethral pressure (P_{ura}) are recorded, which enables the calculation of the urethral closure pressure ($P_{ura} - P_{ves}$). The maximum urethral closure pressure (MUCP), or the maximum difference between P_{ura} and P_{ves}, is also measured. The pressures can be measured at rest and during stress (e.g., coughing or straining).	Urethral function is an important factor in the determination of stress incontinence. Some experts believe that a MUCP < 20 cm H_2O is indicative of intrinsic urethral sphincter deficiency (ISD). If the difference between P_{ura} and P_{ves} is minimal or low (< 20 cm H_2O), then the patient may leak urine with minimal exertion, such as standing up from the sitting position or bearing down slightly. These patients are said to have ISD (see Chapter 4, Table 4.6). A low UPP may indicate outlet resistance. False "positives" (low readings) can be produced by having an indwelling urinary catheter (especially of large size) in place for a period of time.	A pressure transducer with a special catheter system is inserted into the bladder through the urethra and then pulled out, at a constant rate, in order to measure pressures along the length of the urethra. It can be measured during bladder filling, during a cough or Valsalva maneuver, or during voiding. The measurements are prone to artifacts caused by the catheters (stiffness, direction of the tip) and by the patient (movement, etc.). An alternate methodology for UPP is to infuse fluid through a small catheter with radially drilled sideholes at the end as it is slowly withdrawn from the bladder through the urethra at a fixed rate. The infusion pressure is measured, thus the name "infusion urethral profilometry."
Abdominal leak point pressure (ALPP)	Assesses the competence of the urethral sphincter. Measures the ALPP caused by abdominal stress producing leakage. The abdominal stress may be induced by a cough but is	An ALPP > 90 cm H_2O is considered to represent a normal urethral sphincter, whereas ALPP values lower than 60 cm H_2O are considered indicative of ISD.	The bladder is filled with a standard volume of fluid, and the patient is asked to slowly bear down in an incremental manner until leakage is noted from the external urethral meatus. The lowest

Table 6.2 *(continued)*

Test	Description	Indications	Procedure
Abdominal leak point pressure (ALPP) *(continued)*	more commonly measured during a Valsalva maneuver.	There are disagreements about what constitutes a pressure that indicates ISD. This is an important distinction because a patient with ISD often does not respond well to conservative treatment.	pressure at which leakage occurs is recorded as the ALPP.
Uroflowmetry (flowmeter)	Indicates a quantity of fluid passed per unit time (expressed in mL/sec). It measures: • Voided volume • Flow pattern (should be a smooth, bell-shaped curve)	Poor detrusor function with outlet obstruction will cause a reduction in flow rate.	The patient should have a comfortably full bladder. The patient voids into a flow-meter, which gives a graphical representation of the urine flow over time. Voided volumes of < 100–125 mL can lead to erroneous results.
Electromyography (EMG)	Study of electrical activity in the striated muscles of the sphincter to assess PFM activity during bladder filling and emptying.	To determine detrusor–sphincter dyssynergia (the PFM will contract simultaneously with detrusor contraction) or the presence of a learned dysfunctional voiding pattern in neurologically normal patients.	Surface patch electrodes are placed around the anus at 10 and 2 o'clock. Needle electrodes can be inserted into the muscle. This latter technique is typically reserved for those patients with neurological abnormalities (e.g., spinal cord injury).
Video-urodynamics	Multichannel testing with fluoroscopic visualization of the bladder and urethra, utilizing contrast material instilled in the bladder.	Increases the ability to easily document opacified urine leakage, to identify provocative maneuvers such as straining, and to observe urine leakage and bladder descent with Valsalva maneuver. Also enables determination of the site of obstruction if present.	A fluoroscopic (x-ray) and pressure measurement study that simultaneously evaluates the appearance and function of the urinary bladder and urethra. All the previously listed urodynamic tests will be performed.

Adapted from material developed by Tamara Dickinson, RN, CURN, CCCN, BCIA-PMDB, Senior Research Nurse, Continence and Voiding Dysfunction, Department of Urology, University of Texas Southwestern Medical Center, Dallas, Texas.

negative or false-positive tests may occur. Furthermore, UDS testing must be interpreted in the context of patient history, physical exam, and preliminary testing, including ultrasound. Pressure–flow UDS and video-UDS are useful in men to determine bladder outlet obstruction and in women with POP. Video-UDS combine the techniques of urodynamics and fluoroscopy. The International Continence Society has published standardized definitions and measurements (Abrams et al., 2002; Schäfer et al., 2002).

In the LTC and home care settings, UDS are rarely justified or needed for diagnosis unless the results may change management (Fonda et al., 2005). A simple or "eyeball" cystometrogram may be performed at the bedside in selected individuals to determine bladder compliance and detrusor activity. Box 6.9 describes the procedure for performing this test. One must be careful,

---

Box 6.9   Procedure for bedside or "eyeball" cystometrogram

1. Insert a 14-French red-rubber catheter into the bladder, note the PVR, and obtain a specimen for possible UA.

2. Using a 60-mL catheter-tipped syringe with the plunger (piston syringe) placed on the end of the catheter, slowly pour room-temperature sterile water or saline in 50-mL aliquots into the syringe. (A 1000-mL bag of sterile water connected to IV tubing can be substituted if a 60-mL syringe is not available.)

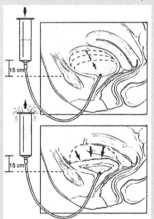

3. The patient is asked to report various sensations experienced during filling, and the volumes at which these sensations occur are recorded. Note:

    a. First desire to void (normally experienced at between 100 and 250 mL)

    b. Normal desire to void (usually felt at 300–400 mL)

    c. A strong or "must" urge or desire to void (usually occurs at 400–600 mL)

4. During the test, the water level (meniscus) within the syringe should be carefully inspected because an increase in the level may indicate an involuntary bladder contraction, which is diagnostic of detrusor overactivity. A sudden reverse in the flow of fluid or water expelled around the catheter or actual expulsion of the catheter suggests a spontaneous bladder contraction. It should be kept in mind, however, that abdominal straining will produce a false-positive rise in the meniscus; therefore, the patient should be asked not to strain during the procedure, and an examiner's hand may be placed gently on the lower abdomen during filling in order to detect such a response. Uncontrollable bladder contractions or incontinence during the procedure is not normal.

5. When the patient's bladder reaches capacity, the catheter is removed and the patient is asked to perform a cough stress test. If the results of this test are negative, the patient is asked to stand and repeat the same maneuver, because there is a greater likelihood of SUI occurring in the standing position.

6. The PVR may be repeated.

Key: IV = intravenous; PVR = postvoid residual; SUI = stress urinary incontinence; UA = urinalysis.

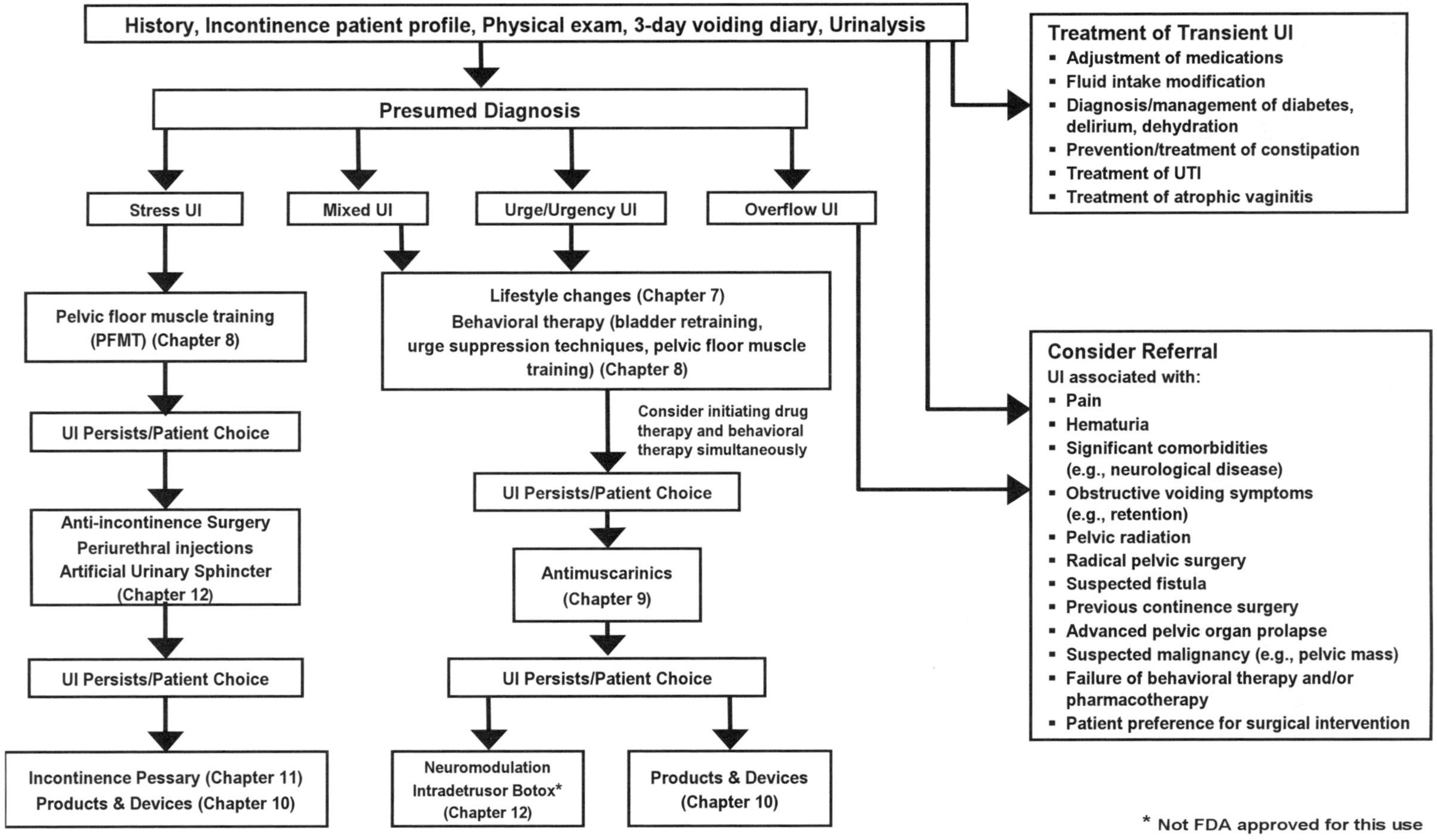
History, Incontinence patient profile, Physical exam, 3-day voiding diary, Urinalysis
Presumed Diagnosis
Stress UI
Mixed UI
Urge/Urgency UI
Overflow UI
Pelvic floor muscle training (PFMT) (Chapter 8)
UI Persists/Patient Choice
Anti-incontinence Surgery
Periurethral injections
Artificial Urinary Sphincter (Chapter 12)
UI Persists/Patient Choice
Incontinence Pessary (Chapter 11)
Products & Devices (Chapter 10)
Lifestyle changes (Chapter 7)
Behavioral therapy (bladder retraining, urge suppression techniques, pelvic floor muscle training) (Chapter 8)
Consider initiating drug therapy and behavioral therapy simultaneously
UI Persists/Patient Choice
Antimuscarinics (Chapter 9)
UI Persists/Patient Choice
Neuromodulation
Intradetrusor Botox*
(Chapter 12)
Products & Devices (Chapter 10)
Treatment of Transient UI
Adjustment of medications
Fluid intake modification
Diagnosis/management of diabetes, delirium, dehydration
Prevention/treatment of constipation
Treatment of UTI
Treatment of atrophic vaginitis
Consider Referral
UI associated with:
Pain
Hematuria
Significant comorbidities (e.g., neurological disease)
Obstructive voiding symptoms (e.g., retention)
Pelvic radiation
Radical pelvic surgery
Suspected fistula
Previous continence surgery
Advanced pelvic organ prolapse
Suspected malignancy (e.g., pelvic mass)
Failure of behavioral therapy and/or pharmacotherapy
Patient preference for surgical intervention
* Not FDA approved for this use

Figure 6.12. UI care pathway.

however, to rule out abnormal straining as a cause for an increase in bladder pressure.

CONCLUSION

A detailed history and physical examination including symptom review is necessary to determine the etiology and to obtain an effective diagnosis of OAB and/or UI. Symptom-specific questionnaires and voiding diaries are helpful in understanding the extent of the problem. Other tests are necessary depending on the presenting symptoms and severity of the problem. The evaluation of UI will lead to a presumed diagnosis, allowing the clinician to make treatment recommendations. Figure 6.12 is a simple care pathway for bothersome UI that can be used for informing patients of treatment options that are detailed in the following chapters.

REFERENCES

Abrams, P., Artibani, W., Cardozo, L., Dmochowski, R., van Kerrobroeck, P., & Sand, P. (2006). Reviewing the ICS 2002 terminology report: The ongoing debate. *Neurourological Urodynamics, 25,* 293.

Abrams, P., Cardozo, L., Fall, M., Griffiths, D., Rosier, P., Ulmsten, U., et al. for the Standardisation Sub-committee of the International Continence Society. (2002). The standardization of terminology in lower urinary tract function: Report from the Standardisation Sub-committee of the International Continence Society. *Neurourology and Urodynamics, 21,* 167–178.

Abrams, P., Cardozo, L., Khoury, S., & Wein, A. (Eds.). (2005). *Incontinence: Proceedings from the Third International Consultation on Incontinence.* Plymouth, UK: Health Publications Ltd.

American Medical Directors Association. (2005). *Urinary incontinence clinical practice guideline.* Columbia, MD: Author.

Avery, K., Donovan, J., Peters, T., Shaw, C., Gotoh, M., & Abrams, P. (2004). ICIQ: A brief and robust measure for evaluating the symptoms and impact of urinary incontinence. *Neurourology and Urodynamics, 23,* 322.

Bachmann, G.A., Rosen, R., Pinn, V.W., Utian, W.H., Ayers, C., Basson, R., et al. (2006). Vulvodynia: A state-of-the-art consensus on definitions, diagnosis and management. *Journal of Reproductive Medicine, 51,* 447–456.

Batra, S.C., & Iosif, C.S. (1983). Female urethra: A target for estrogen action. *Journal of Urology, 129,* 418–420.

Bø, K., & Sherburn, M. (2005). Evaluation of female pelvic-floor muscle function and strength. *Physical Therapy, 85,* 269–282.

Bourcier, A.P., Juras, J.C., & Villet, R.M. (2004). Office evaluation and physical examination. In A.P. Bourcier, E.J. McGuire, & P. Abrams (Eds.), *Pelvic floor disorders* (pp. 133–148). Philadelphia: Elsevier Saunders.

Brink, C., Wells, T.J., Sampselle, C.M., Tallie, E.R., & Mayer, R. (1994). A digital test for pelvic muscle strength in women with urinary incontinence. *Nursing Research, 43,* 352–356.

Brown, J.S., Bradley, C.S., Subak, L.L., Richter, H.S., Kraus, S.R., Brubaker, L., et al. for the Diagnostic Aspects of Incontinence Study (DAIsy) Research Group. (2006). The sensitivity and specificity of a simple test to distinguish between urge and stress urinary incontinence. *Annals of Internal Medicine, 144,* 715–723.

Bump, R.C., Hurt, W.G., Fantl, A., & Wyman, J.F. (1991). Assessment of Kegel pelvic muscle exercise performance after brief verbal instruction. *American Journal of Obstetrics and Gynecology, 165,* 322–329.

Carcio, H. (2005). Urodynamic testing. *ADVANCE for Nurse Practitioners, 13*(10), 45–48, 50–52, 54.

Cardoza, L., Coyne, K.S., & Versi, E. (2005). Validation of the urgency perception scale. *BJU International, 95*(4), 591–596.

Centers for Medicare and Medicaid Services. (2005). *State Operations Manual, Appendix PP—Guidance to Surveyors for Long-Term Care Facilities, Tag F315, §483.25(d) Urinary Incontinence* (Rev. 8, Issued: 06-28-05, Effective: 06-28-05, Implementation: 06-28-05) Retrieved November 11, 2007, from http://www.cms.hhs.gov/transmittals/downloads/R8SOM.pdf

Ceo, P.D. (2006). Assessment of the male reproductive system. *Urologic Nursing, 26,* 290–297.

Colling, J. (1996). Noninvasive techniques to manage urinary incontinence among care-dependent persons. *Journal of Wound, Ostomy, and Continence Nursing, 23,* 302–308.

Colling, J., Ouslander, J., Hadley, B.J., Eisch, J., & Campbell, E. (1992). The effects of patterned urge response toileting (PURT) on urinary incontinence among nursing home residents. *Journal of the American Geriatrics Society, 40,* 135–141.

Colling, J.C., Owen, T.R., McCreedy, M., & Newman, D.K. (2003). The effects of a continence program on frail community-dwelling elderly persons. *Urologic Nursing, 23,* 117–122, 127–131.

Coyne, K., Matza, L.S., Kopp, Z., & Abrams, P. (2006). The validation of the Patient Perception of Bladder Condition (PPBC): A single-item global measure for patients with overactive bladder. *European Urology, 49,* 1079–1086.

Coyne, K., Revick, D., Hunt, T., Corey, R., Stewart, W., Bentkover, J., et al. (2002). Psychometric validation of an overactive bladder symptoms and health related quality of life questionnaire: The OAB-q. *Quality of Life Research, 11,* 563–574.

Dmochowski, R.R. (2005). Urinary incontinence: Proper assessment and available treatment options. *Journal of Women's Health, 14,* 906–916.

Dmochowski, R.R., Sanders, S.S., Appell, R.A., Nitti, V.M., & Davila, G.W. (2005). Bladder-health diaries: An assessment of 3-day vs 7-day entries. *BJU International, 96,* 1049–1054.

DuBeau, C.E. (2006). Functional and overflow incontinence. In C.R. Chapple, P.E. Zimmern, L. Brubaker, A.R.B. Smith, & K. Bo (Eds.), *Multidisciplinary management of female disorders* (pp. 65–74). Philadelphia: Elsevier Saunders.

Engberg, S.J., McDowell, B.J., Weber, E., Brodak, I., Donovan, N., & Engberg, R. (1997). Assessment and management of urinary incontinence among homebound older adults: A clinical trial protocol. *Advanced Practice Nursing Quarterly, 3*(2), 48–56.

Fantl, J., Newman, D., Colling, J., DeLancey, J.O.L., Keeys, C., Loughery, R., et al. for the Urinary Incontinence in Adults Guideline Update Panel. (1996). *Urinary incontinence in adults: Acute and chronic management. Clinical practice guideline No. 2: Update* (AHCPR Publication No. 96-0692). Rockville, MD: Agency for Health Care and Policy Research.

Fletcher, E. (2005). Differential diagnosis of high-tone and low-tone pelvic floor muscle dysfunction. *Journal of Wound, Ostomy, and Continence Nursing, 32*(3 Suppl. 2), S10–S11.

Folstein, M.F., Folstein, S.E., & McHugh, P.R. (1975). "Mini-mental state": A practical method for grading the cognitive state of patients for the clinician. *Journal of Psychiatric Research, 12,* 189–198.

Fonda, D., DuBeau, C.E., Harari, D., Ouslander, J.G., Palmer, M., & Roe, B. (2005). Incontinence in the frail elderly. In P. Abrams, L. Cardozo, S. Khoury, & A. Wein (Eds.), *Incontinence: Proceedings from the Third International Consultation on Incontinence* (pp. 1163–1239). Plymouth, UK: Health Publications, Ltd.

Fultz, N.H., & Herzog, A.R. (2000). Prevalence of urinary incontinence in middle-aged and older women: A survey-based methodological experiment. *Journal of Aging and Health, 12,* 459–469.

Goode, P.S., Locher, J.L., Bryant, R.L., Roth, D.L., & Burgio, K.L. (2000). Measurement of postvoid urine with portable transabdominal bladder ultrasound scanner and urethral catheterization. *International Urogynecology Journal and Pelvic Floor Dysfunction, 11,* 296–300.

Gray, M. (2003). The importance of screening, assessing, and managing urinary incontinence in primary care. *Journal of the American Academy of Nurse Practitioners, 15,* 102–107.

Gray, M., & Wyman, J. (2004). Is the Incontinence Impact Quesionnaire short form (IIQ-7) a clinically useful tool for WOC nursing practice? *Journal of Wound, Ostomy, and Continence Nursing, 31,* 317–324.

Harvan, J.R., & Cotter, V. (2006). An evaluation of dementia screening in the primary care setting. *Journal of the American Academy of Nurse Practitioners, 18,* 351–360.

Holroyd-Leduc, J.M., Tannenbaum, C., Thorpe, K.E., & Straus, S.E. (2008). What type of urinary incontinence does this woman have? *Journal of the American Medical Association, 299*(12), 1446–1456.

Hornick, L., & Slocumb, J.C. (2008). Treating chronic pelvic pain. *ADVANCE for Nurse Practitioners, 16*(2), 44–54.

Huang, A.J., Brown, J.S., Kanaya, A.M., Creasman, J.M., Ragins, A.I., van den Eeden, S.K., et al. (2006). Quality-of-life impact and treatment of urinary incontinence in ethnically diverse older women. *Archives of Internal Medicine, 166,* 2000–2006.

Hunskaar, S., Burgio, K., Diokno, A.C., Herzog, A.R., Hjalmas, K., & Lapitan, M.C. (2003). Epidemiology and natural history of urinary incontinence in women. *Urology, 62*(Suppl. 4A), 16–23.

Jaffe, J.S., Ginsberg, P.C., Silverberg, D.M., & Harkaway, R.C. (2002). The need for voiding diaries in the evaluation of men with nocturia. *Journal of the American Osteopathic Association, 102,* 261–265.

Jelovsek, J.E., Barber, M.D., Paraiso, M.F.R., & Walters, M.D. (2005). Functional bowel and anorectal disorders in patients with pelvic organ prolapse and incontinence. *American Journal of Obstetrics and Gynecology, 193,* 2105–2111.

Kellogg-Spadt, S., & Albaugh, J.A. (2003). External genital and dermatologic examination Part I: The female patient. *Urologic Nursing, 23,* 305–306.

Kerschan-Schindl, K., Uher, E., Wiesinger, G., Kaider, A., Ebenbichler, G., Nicolakis, P., et al. (2002). Reliability of pelvic floor muscle strength measurements in elderly incontinent women. *Neurourology and Urodynamics, 21,* 42–47.

Klay, M., & Marfyak, K. (2005). Use of a continence nurse specialist in an extended care facility. *Urologic Nursing, 20,* 1–4.

Lee, Y.Y., Tsay, W.L., Lou, M.F., & Dai, Y.T. (2006). The effectiveness of implementing a bladder ultrasound programme in neurosurgical units. *Journal of Advanced Nursing, 57,* 192–200.

Lifshitz, E., & Kramer, L. (2000). Outpatient urine culture: Does collection technique matter? *Archives of Internal Medicine, 160,* 2537–2540.

Maloney C. (2002). Estrogen & recurrent UTI in postmenopausal women. *American Journal of Nursing, 102*(8), 44–52.

Maloney, C., & Cafiero, M. (1999). Implementing an incontinence program in long-term care settings. *Journal of Gerontological Nursing, 25*(6), 47–52.

Mashburn, J. (2006). Etiology, diagnosis and management of vaginitis. *Journal of Midwifery and Women's Health, 51,* 423–430.

Mentes, J., Wakefield, B., & Culp, K. (2006). Use of a urine color chart to monitor hydration status in nursing home residents. *Biological Research for Nursing, 7,* 197–203.

Messelink, B., Benson, T., Berghmans, B., Bo, K., Corcos, J., Fowler, C., et al. (2005). Standardisation of terminology of pelvic floor muscle function and dysfunction. Report from the Pelvic Floor Clinical Assessment Group of the International Continence Society. *Neurourology and Urodynamics, 24,* 374–380.

Miller, J., Ashton-Miller, J.A., & DeLancey, J.O.L. (1996). The Knack: Use of precisely timed pelvic muscle exercise contraction can reduce leakage in SUI. *Neurourology and Urodynamics, 15,* 302–393.

Naughton, M.J., & Wyman, J.F. (1997). Quality of life in geriatric patients with lower urinary tract dysfunction. *American Journal of the Medical Sciences, 314,* 219–227.

Neumann, P., & Gill, V. (2002). Pelvic floor and abdominal muscle interaction: EMG activity and intra-abdominal pressure. *International Urogynecology Journal and Pelvic Floor Dysfunction, 13,* 125–132.

Newman, D.K. (2002). *Managing and treating urinary incontinence.* Baltimore: Health Professions Press.

Newman, D.K. (2003). *Clinical manual—pelvic muscle rehabilitation* (pp. 89–98). Dover, NH: The Prometheus Group.

Newman, D.K. (2004). Report of a mail survey of women with bladder control disorders. *Urologic Nursing, 24,* 499–507.

Newman, D.K. (2005a). Assessment of the patient with an overactive bladder. *Journal of Wound, Ostomy, and Continence Nursing, 32*(3 Suppl. 2), S5–S9.

Newman, D.K. (2005b). *Bladder and bowel rehabilitation program.* Philadelphia: SCA Personal Products.

Newman, D.K. (2006). Urinary incontinence, catheters and urinary tract infections: An overview of CMS Tag F 315. *Ostomy/Wound Management, 52*(12), 34–36, 38, 40–44.

Newman, D.K. (2007). *Program of excellence in extended care.* Bothell, WA: Verathon Corporation.

Newman, D.K., Burgio, K.L., & Sand, P.K. (2004). Key challenges in the diagnosis and management of overactive bladder. *Journal of the American Academy of Nurse Practitioners, 16*(10 Suppl), 1–12.

Newman, D.K., Gaines, T., & Snare, E. (2005). Innovation in bladder assessment: Use of technology in extended care. *Journal of Gerontological Nursing, 31*(12), 33–41.

Newman, D.K., & Laycock, J. (2008). Evaluation of the pelvic floor. In B. Schussler, F. Baessler, K. Moore, P. Norton, K. Burgio, & S. Stanton (Eds.), *Pelvic floor reeducation—principles and practice* (2nd ed.). London: Springer-Verlag.

Newman, D.K., Preston, A.K., & Salazar, S. (2007). Moisture control, urinary and fecal incontinence and perineal skin management. In D.L. Krasner, G. Rodeheaver, & R.G. Sibbald (Eds.), *Chronic wound care: A clinical source book for healthcare professionals* (4th ed., pp. 609–627). Wayne, PA: HMP Communications.

Newman, D.K., & Wein, A.J. (2004). *Overcoming overactive bladder.* Los Angeles: New Harbinger.

Ouslander, J.G. (2004). Management of overactive bladder. *New England Journal of Medicine, 350,* 786–799.

Ouslander, J.G., Morshita, L., Blaustein, J., Orzeck, S., Dunn, S., & Sayre, J. (1987). Clinical, functional, and psychological characteristics of an incontinent nursing home population. *Journal of Gerontology, 42,* 631–637.

Ouslander, J.G., Schapira, M., & Schnelle, J.F. (1995). Urine specimen collection from incontinent female nursing home residents. *Journal of the American Geriatrics Society, 43,* 279–281.

Ouslander, J.G., Schapira, M., Schnelle, J., & Fingold, S. (1996). Pyuria among chronically incontinent but otherwise asymptomatic nursing home residents. *Journal of the American Geriatrics Society, 44,* 420–423

Ouslander, J.G., Simmons, S., Tuico, E., Nigam, J.G., Fingold, S., Bates-Jensen, B., et al. (1994). Use of portable ultrasound device to measure post-void residual volume among incontinent nursing home residents. *Journal of the American Geriatrics Society, 42,* 1189–1192.

Palmer, M.H. (1996). A new framework for urinary continence outcomes in long-term care. *Urologic Nursing, 16,* 146–151.

Palmer, M.H., McCormick, K.A., Langford, A., Langlois, J., & Alvaran, M. (1992). Continence outcomes: Documentation on medical records in the nursing home environment. *Journal of Nursing Care Quality, 6*(3), 36–43.

Pfisterer, M.H., Griffiths, D.J., Schaefer, W., & Resnick, N.M. (2006). The effect of age on lower urinary tract function: A study in women. *Journal of the American Geriatrics Society, 54,* 405–412.

Phillips, J.K. (2000, March). Integrating bladder ultrasound into a urinary tract infection-reduction project. *American Journal of Nursing,* (Suppl.), 3–15.

Podsiadlo, D., & Richardson, S. (1991). The timed "Up & Go": A test of basic functional mobility for frail elderly persons. *Journal of the American Geriatrics Society, 39,* 142–148.

Robinson, J.P., & Shea, J.A. (2002). Development and testing of a measure of health-related quality of life for men with urinary incontinence. *Journal of the American Geriatrics Society, 50,* 935–945.

Sampselle, C.M. (2003). Teaching women to use a voiding diary. *American Journal of Nursing, 103*(11), 62–64.

Schäfer, W., Abrams, P., Liao, L., Mattiasson, A., Pesce, F., Spangberg, A., et al. for the International Continence Society. (2002). Good urodynamic practice: Uroflowmetry, filling, cystometry, pressure-flow studies. *Neurourology and Urodynamics, 21,* 261–274.

Simerville, J.A., Maxted, W.C., & Pahira, J.J. (2005). Urinalysis: A comprehensive review. *American Family Physician, 71,* 1153–1162.

Stevens, E. (2006). Bladder ultrasound: Avoiding unnecessary ultrasounds. *MEDSURG Nursing, 14,* 249–453.

Uebersax, J.S., Wyman, J.F., Shumaker, S.A., McClish, D.K., & Fantl, J.A., for the Continence Program for Women Research Group. (1995). Short forms to assess life quality and symptom distress for urinary incontinence in women: The Incontinence Impact Questionnaire and the Urogenital Distress Inventory. *Neurourology and Urodynamics, 14,* 131–139.

VanArsdalen, K.N. (2007). Signs and symptoms: The initial examination. In P.M. Hanno, S.B. Malkowicz, & A.J. Wein (eds.), *Penn clinical manual of urology* (pp. 37–74). Philadelphia: Elsevier Saunders.

Viktrup, L. (2005). Addressing the need for a simpler algorithm for the management of women with urinary incontinence. *MedGenMed, 7*(3), 62.

Viktrup, L., Summers, K.H., & Dennett, S.L. (2004). Clinical practice guidelines on the initial assessment and treatment of urinary incontinence in women: A US focused review. *International Journal of Gynaecology and Obstetrics, 86*(Suppl. 1), S25–S37.

Voytas, J. (2002). The role of geriatricians and family practitioners in the treatment of overactive bladder and incontinence. *Reviews in Urology, 4*(Suppl. 4), S44–S49.

Wagner, M., & Schmid, M. (1997). Exploring the research base and outcome measures for portable bladder ultrasound technology. *MEDSURG Nursing, 6,* 304–314.

Wald, A. (2007). Clinical Practice: Fecal incontinence in adults. *New England Journal of Medicine, 356,* 1648–1655.

Wallace, M., & Sadovsky, R. (2005, April). What clinicians should know about urinalysis. *Clinical Advisor,* pp. 39–47.

Watson, N.M., Brink, C.A., Zimmer, J.G., & Mayer, R.D. (2003). Use of the Agency for Health Care Policy and Research Urinary Incontinence Guideline in nursing homes. *Journal of the American Geriatrics Society, 51,* 1779–1786.

Wein, A.J., & Moy, M.L. (2007). Voiding function and dysfunction: Urinary incontinence. In P.M. Hanno, S.B. Malkowicz, & A.J. Wein (eds.), *Penn clinical manual of urology* (pp. 314–478). Philadelphia: Elsevier Saunders.

Woolridge, L. (2000, June). Ultrasound technology and bladder dysfunction. *American Journal of Nursing,* (Suppl.), 3–14.

Yap, P., & Tan, D. (2006). Urinary incontinence in dementia—a practical approach. *Australian Family Physician, 35,* 237–241.

7

Self-Care Practices and Lifestyle Changes to Reduce Urinary Symptoms

Self-care, as the term implies, involves techniques that a patient with urinary incontinence (UI) may use to lessen symptom severity. Self-care practices such as regulation of fluid intake, elimination of bladder irritants, bowel regulation, smoking cessation, and weight reduction—referred to as lifestyle changes or behavior modification—are thought to be ways to prevent or reduce UI and associated lower urinary tract symptoms (LUTS) (Box 7.1). These interventions improve symptoms through the identification of lifestyle habits and aspects of a patient's behavior, environment, or activity that are contributing factors or triggers (Nygaard, Bryant, Dowell, & Wilson, 2002). These treatments are frequently recommended by health care providers and are supported by a growing body of research (Fantl et al., 1996; Wilson et al., 2005). People can take control of UI and overactive bladder (OAB) symptoms of urgency and frequency by identifying daily lifestyle practices that have a detrimental effect on the urinary system. If these individuals learn to alter certain lifestyle habits through self-care practices, further treatments may not be necessary. Lifestyle modifications are most successful in cognitively intact, motivated patients with stress, urgency, and/or mixed UI and should be offered as first-line therapy because these interventions may decrease symptoms without significant side effects. In addition, some have been proven as effective as drug therapy for urgency and urgency-predominant mixed UI and surgical interventions for stress UI. Finally, lifestyle modifications may be preferred by patients over other interventions. This chapter targets those behaviors that, if altered, can have a positive impact on bladder function. Providers in all settings can easily teach the methods described in this chapter (also refer to the companion CD).

Box 7.1   Key components of lifestyle changes

- Adjust daily fluid intake to approximately 2,500 mL or 30 mL/kg per day. Modifying excessively low or high fluid intake may be helpful for some individuals.

- Modify the diet to reduce potential bladder irritants such as carbonated beverages, artificial sweeteners (particularly aspartame), spicy foods, citrus juices and fruits, and highly spiced foods. Alcohol intake is related to worsening of overactive bladder symptoms.

- Reduce caffeine intake to less than 400 mg per day. Caffeine reduction should be tapered slowly to avoid severe headache by reducing by 4–6 oz per day or 3–5 cups per week.

- Regulate bowel function to prevent constipation and straining during bowel movements through use of dietary fiber, fluid intake, and exercise.

- Limit fluid intake 2–3 hours prior to bedtime if nocturia is a problem.

- Quit smoking.

- Lose weight if moderately or morbidly obese.

DIETARY RESTRICTIONS AND MODIFICATIONS

Dietary changes have become a fundamental and first-line approach of self-care for many people with UI. Unknown urinary metabolites of certain foods are postulated to traverse the bladder mucosa, thereby further stimulating hypersensitive nerves, eliciting an inflammatory response, or both. This may precipitate or worsen urinary symptoms of urgency, frequency, and incontinence. People can decrease these symptoms through modification of certain diet habits (Bryant, Dowell, & Fairbrother, 2000). (See the patient education tool "What You Eat and Drink Can Affect Your Bladder" on the companion CD.)

Fluid Intake

Individuals with UI or OAB may exhibit either restrictive or excessive fluid intake behavior. At both extremes, these practices can cause or exacerbate urinary symptoms. This is of concern because adequate fluid intake is needed to eliminate irritants from the bladder. In studies of the urinary habits of typical adults (M. P. Fitzgerald, Stablein, & Brubaker, 2002), urinary frequency is significantly correlated with fluid intake. There is evidence from animal studies to suggest that distribution of fluid intake over time is clinically reasonable. During normal bladder filling at a rate of approximately 1 mL/kg per hour, there is no rise in bladder pressure (Klevmark, 2002), and stimulation of bladder wall A-delta stretch receptors during filling is thought to be the normal trigger for micturition, rather than a change in vesical (bladder) pressure (Ruggieri, Whitmore, & Levine, 1990).

Many people who have bladder control problems reduce the amount of liquids they drink because they fear urinary frequency, urgency, and incontinence. It is known that certain professionals (e.g., teachers) will limit fluid intake while working to decrease voiding frequency, placing them at increased risk of urinary tract infection (UTI) (Nygaard & Linder, 1997). Fluid restriction is also a commonly recommended treatment for symptoms of OAB (Brown, van der Meulen, Mundy, & Emberton, 2003). Fluid restriction and the avoidance of caffeinated beverages were strategies reported by women who worked for a large academic center to avoid urinary symptoms (S. Fitzgerald, Palmer, Berry, & Hart, 2000). Although drinking less liquid does result in less urine in the bladder, the smaller amount of urine may be more highly concentrated and irritate the bladder lining, perhaps causing urgency and frequency. Underhydration may play a role in the development of UTIs and decreases the functional capacity of the bladder (Dowd, Campbell, & Jones, 1996). Other individuals drink large quantities of fluids to "flush" the kidneys or to avoid UTIs. Many women who are dieting may drink excessive amounts of fluids that may total or exceed 4 L per day.

Surveys of community-residing elders report self-care practices to include the self-imposed restrictions of fluids because they fear UI, urinary urgency, and frequency (Engberg, McDowell, Burgio, Watson, & Belle, 1995; Johnson, Kincade, Bernard, Busby-Whitehead, & DeFriese, 2000). Adequate fluid intake is very important for older adults who already have a decrease in their total body weight and are at increased risk for dehydration. Long-term care residents are chronically dehydrated because most require assistance from staff to eat and drink (Colling, McCreedy, & Owen 1994; Gaspar, 1999). Also, as long-term care (LTC) facilities attempt to limit the number of times medication is dispensed, there are fewer times that residents are offered liquids. Lack of staffing is also a factor in dispensing fluids to nursing home residents (Kayser-Jones, Schell, Porter, Barbaccia, & Shaw, 1999). In these settings, the majority of fluids tend to be given between 6:00 A.M. and 6:00 P.M.

Approaches that have been successful in increasing hydration in LTC residents include offering more between-meal snacks, supervision of residents at mealtimes to ensure adequate ingestion of liquids, designating a certified nurse assistant who is responsible for offering fluids every 2 hours from a "beverage cart," and switching to a five-meal plan that provides a more even distribution of fluids over a longer period of time.

However, the research showing the relationship of quantity of fluid intake to urinary symptoms is inconclusive. The reference fluid intake for adults has recently been revised, and there are recommendations for water, tea and coffee, milk, and sweetened and unsweetened beverages (Panel on Dietary Reference Intakes for Electrolytes and Water, 2004; Popkin et al., 2006). Generally, it is recommended that women have a total fluid intake (from foods and all types of beverages) of approximately 2.7 L per day (30 mL/kg per day, or 2,500 mL for a 180-lb woman) and men a total of 3.7 L per day (Panel on Dietary Reference Intakes, 2004; Popkin et al., 2006). Of this fluid, water should average at least 20–50 fl oz per day. Drinking water is the preferred method to fulfill daily water needs. Typically, much of that total is obtained from food, and most adults can adequately meet their daily hydration needs by letting thirst be their guide.

Bladder Irritants

Certain dietary factors that are considered common bladder irritants, such as caffeine, artificial sweeteners, spicy foods, and citrus fruits, may influence continence status (Wyman, 2000). Caffeine, a central nervous system stimulant that is found in many beverages, foods, medications, and dietary supplements, reaches peak blood concentrations within 30–60 minutes after ingestion. Research in animals has shown that caffeine increases calcium release, causing smooth muscle contraction that can have an excitatory effect on detrusor muscle contraction (J. G. Lee, Wein, & Levin, 1993), and this could lead to urinary urgency and frequency, and exacerbate urgency UI. Caffeine is also believed to have a diuretic effect (Riesenhuber, Boehm, Posch, & Aufricht, 2006). It can also stimulate the central nervous system, and can stimulate bowel motility.

Caffeine occurs naturally in coffee beans, tea leaves, and cocoa beans. More than 80% of the U.S. adult population consumes caffeine (at least 200 mg/day) on a daily basis in the form of coffee, tea, or soft drinks (R. A. Lee & Balick, 2006). A 12-ounce cup of brewed coffee contains 200 mg of caffeine. Tea has approximately 30–50 mg of caffeine for each 8-ounce serving but holds second place to coffee in global consumption. Caffeine is found in liquids such as sodas (e.g., Mountain Dew, Pepsi, Coca-Cola) and foods and candy that contain milk chocolate. Energy drinks boosted with caffeine are the newest caffeine beverage to enter the marketplace, and they have significantly raised the level of caffeine ingested (80 mg/8 oz). A common favorite energy drink, Red Bull, contains caffeine, vitamins, and amino acids. In addition, many over-the-counter (OTC) drugs (e.g., Excedrin, Anacin) and prescription medications (e.g., Darvon compounds, Fiorinal) contain caffeine (Newman, 2002). Nutritional supplements, puddings, and cakes that contain cocoa are favorite foods and daily staples in LTC facilities. However, cocoa is also a source of caffeine. Intake of cocoa among nursing facility residents is estimated to average approximately 200 mg daily, which is equivalent to two 7.5-oz cups of brewed coffee (Lamarine, 1994). Additionally, the U.S. Food and Drug Administration has listed more than 300 drugs that are purchased off the shelf (OTC) in pharmacies and retail drug stores that contain caffeine. (This is usually listed on the labels of the products.)

The patient education tool "Caffeine Count" (see the companion CD) lists the caffeine content of many drinks, foods, and medications. Patients should be advised about the possible adverse effects caffeine may have on the detrusor muscle and the possible benefits of reduction of caffeine intake (Gray, 2001). It is recommended that people with incontinence and OAB avoid excessive caffeine intake (e.g., no more than 200 mg per day or no more than 2 cups of caffeinated drinks per day). Research has shown that urine leakage decreased (63%) when caffeine consumption was reduced from 23 to 14 g per day (Tomlinson et al., 1999). Even though current research is not conclusive, providers should assess all patients with LUTS for amount of daily caffeine intake (Arya, Myers, & Jackson, 2000; Holroyd-Leduc & Straus, 2004).

The individual should be taught to restrict caffeine through behavior modification. Patients should be instructed to switch to caffeine-free beverages and foods or eliminate beverages and foods with caffeine and see if symptoms decrease or resolve. For people who ingest large quantities of caffeine, total elimination may be unrealistic. Because caffeine works primarily on the central nervous system by crossing the blood–brain barrier and causing vasoconstriction of blood vessels in the brain, a sudden withdrawal from caffeine can cause headaches, nervousness, nausea, and muscular tension. Symptoms of withdrawal have been recorded when caffeine consumption per day is reduced to as little as 100 mg. A simple strategy to deal with this problem is the "elimination diet." Patients are encouraged to eliminate foods one by one to see if symptoms change. If a patient is sensitive to a particular food or beverage, symptoms will worsen within 30 minutes to 6 hours when he or she puts that food or beverage back into the diet.

People also need to read product labels. Herbal teas, which are believed to be more "natural," may contain caffeine unless the label indicates otherwise. Many people seem to think that iced tea (referred to as "sweet tea" in the southern United States) has less caffeine than hot tea. Sweet tea is usually brewed, which increases the caffeine content. Caffeine content in certain beverages such as coffee and tea can be decreased by adding extra water when preparing them. Switching to decaffeinated or "decaf" liquids is an option; however, patients need to understand that these have less caffeine but are not "caffeine-free."

Alcohol also has a diuretic effect that can lead to increased frequency. Alcohol inhibits the release of antidiuretic hormone from the posterior pituitary (Creighton & Stanton, 1990). Alcohol with dinner may be a contributing factor for nocturia. Anecdotal evidence suggests that eliminating dietary factors such as artificial sweeteners (those that contain aspartame) and certain foods (e.g., highly spiced foods, citrus juices, and tomato-based products) also may play a role in OAB symptomatology (Newman, 2002).

Bowel Irregularity/Chronic Constipation

Dietary changes should also be recommended to people who have constipation because chronic constipation can contribute to incontinence. The use of bran and other approaches to improve bowel regularity are outlined in Chapter 5.

MANAGEMENT OF NOCTURIA

Nighttime voiding and incontinence are major problems for many older adults. Nocturia, or nighttime voiding, is variously defined as awakening to void more than one or two times per night. The loss of urine during sleep is called nocturnal enuresis (nighttime incontinence). Aging causes an increase in nocturia, defined as the number of voids recorded from the time the individual goes to bed with the intention of going to sleep, to the time the individual wakes with the intention of rising. Nocturia can be due to nocturnal polyuria, a condition in which the largest amount of urine production occurs at rest while the patient is supine. Chapter 3 provides a review of aging changes in the lower urinary tract. During the night, there is a lower level of physical activity and body fluid moves more quickly from one part of the body to another, causing an increase in the amount of urine in the bladder. Chronic medical conditions such as congestive heart failure, venous stasis with peripheral edema, hypoglycemia and excess urine output, obstructive sleep apnea, and diuretics, as well as evening/nighttime fluid consumption, are causes of nocturnal polyuria. Because greater quantities of potassium, sodium, and solute are excreted into the urine at night, nighttime incontinence may also lead to skin irritation in older people with nighttime UI. In a geriatric population, there appears to be a strong relationship between evening fluid intake, nocturia, and nocturnal voided volume (Griffiths, McCracken, Harrison, & Gormley, 1993).

The timing of fluid ingestion may be important in people who have problems with nocturia. The largest amount of urine production occurs at rest, usually between the hours of midnight and 8:00 A.M. (Colling et al., 1994). To decrease nocturia precipitated by drinking fluids primarily in the evening or with dinner, the patient should be instructed to reduce fluid intake after 6 P.M. and shift intake toward the morning and afternoon. The issues surrounding continence care during the night for long-term care residents are complex and will require coordination of the efforts of all nursing staff. Staff who are responsible for the purchase of care products must be aware of improved absorbent products and the correct use of skin cleansers, moisturizers, and moisture barrier products (see Chapter 10).

The following preventive measures can be employed to decrease nighttime UI (Newman & Wein, 2004):

- People with peripheral edema should be advised to elevate the lower extremities for several hours during the afternoon. This will help to stimulate a natural diuresis by promoting the movement of extravascular fluid back into the blood vessels and limit the amount of edema present at bedtime. These individuals may also want to consider wearing support stockings or using fluid compression devices.

- The use of diuretics has been associated with nighttime urine volumes. Altering the timing of the administration of short-acting or "loop" diuretics (e.g., giving diuretics at 2:00 P.M. rather than 6:00 or 7:00 P.M.) may decrease nocturia (Ouslander, Schnelle, Simmons, Bates-Jensen, & Zeitlin, 1993). Individuals taking diuretics should maintain adequate fluid intake by drinking the bulk of their liquids before dinner and restricting fluids in the evening.

- Elimination of caffeine-containing beverages and foods in the evening hours, especially with dinner, will decrease the frequency of nighttime UI.

- Residents in nursing facilities who are put to bed after dinner, usually around 6:00 or 7:00 P.M., will need to toilet before midnight. This may be a task for the night shift nursing staff. (See the patient education tool "Ways to Prevent Bladder Problems During the Night" on the companion CD.)

TECHNIQUES TO FACILITATE VOIDING AND BLADDER EMPTYING

Many elderly men and women will complain of feelings of incomplete bladder emptying and alterations in micturition with obstructive symptoms of hesitancy and decreased urinary stream. Men will report postmicturition voiding (referred to as "postvoid dribbling"). Manual techniques are available that can assist the bladder and urethra to completely empty. These techniques can also be helpful for the individual with urinary retention and overflow incontinence. The following maneuvers can be used to teach the patient how to completely empty the bladder manually:

- Postvoid dribbling, or postvoid micturition in men, is caused by a pooling of urine in the bulbar urethra or by residual urine in the bladder, or both. This may be the result of sphincteric weakness and is seen primarily in men who have bladder outlet obstruction (e.g., benign prostatic hyperplasia). Men will report that a small amount of urine leaks from the urethra immediately following voiding. In some cases, the man may not be aware that the urine is leaking. Urine can be expressed from the urethra by either "milking" the urethra or tightening the pelvic floor muscle to increase urethral resistance to continued seepage of urine from the postvoid residual volume in the bladder. (See the patient education tool "How to Prevent Postvoid Dribble" on the companion CD.) Double voiding (see below) may also be helpful.

- A program of double voiding may be effective in cases of mild to moderate urinary retention. The individual is taught to void twice during each trip to the bathroom to reduce residual urine volumes. The patient is instructed to void, to remain at or on the toilet, and to void again after a rest period of 2–10 minutes. Another method of double voiding is to have the patient void, then stand up and sit back down (or move away from and then back to the toilet), and attempt to void again.

- Patients with a spinal cord injury may be able to identify a "trigger" point to initiate a bladder contraction. One common method is called "suprapubic tapping," which involves drumming the abdomen overlying the bladder with the fingers. Other trigger mechanisms include pulling on pubic hairs, stroking the abdomen or inner thigh, digital anal stimulation, running water in the sink, placing the hands in a basin of warm water, drinking warm fluids, and pouring warm water on the perineal area. The patient should try all methods to discover which technique works best and is easiest. (See the patient education tool "Helping Your Bladder to Empty" on the companion CD.)

- The Credé maneuver or bladder expression is a means of direct manual compression to empty the bladder and is often recommended. However, this does not promote bladder emptying unless there is decreased outlet resistance. It may not be safe because it can cause reflux into the upper urinary tracts.

Suprapubic or bladder tapping and Credé or Valsalva maneuvers to enhance voiding are relatively contraindicated in the presence of detrusor–sphincter dyssynergia because these maneuvers can cause increased bladder pressure, leading to reflux and upper urinary tract damage.

SMOKING CESSATION

Chronic coughing secondary to smoking and pulmonary diseases such as asthma and emphysema increases intra-abdominal pressure and may promote the development of UI and urinary urgency, particularly in women. (Nuotio, Jylha, Koivisto, & Tammela, 2001). Smoking increases the risk of developing all forms of UI, and stress UI in particular, depending on the number of cigarettes smoked. There may be several causes of the increased risk of stress UI in smokers. Smokers have stronger, more frequent and violent coughing, which may lead to earlier development of anatomic and pressure damage to the urethral sphincteric mechanism and to vaginal supports (Bump & McClish, 1994). Violent and frequent, prolonged coughing can increase downward pressure on the pelvic floor, causing repeated stretch injury to the pudendal and pelvic nerves. Nicotine has been shown to contribute to large phasic bladder contractions in animal studies through the activation of purinergic receptors, and has been postulated to similarly affect the human bladder (Koley, Koley, & Saha, 1984; Ruggieri et al., 1990). This could lead to urinary urgency in both women and men.

Smoking is also the most important etiological factor in other LUTS and in the development of bladder cancer. An increased risk of LUTS, specifically incomplete bladder emptying and hesitancy, daily frequency, nocturia, urgency, and urgency UI, was reported in men who smoked (Koskimaki, Hakama,

Huhtala, & Tammela, 1998) and hypothesized to be mediated through the development of benign prostatic hyperplasia.

No data have been reported examining whether smoking cessation in women resolves incontinence. However, in clinical practice, women who smoke are educated on the relationship between smoking and UI, and strategies designed to discourage women from smoking are often suggested, although no evidence supports their effectiveness.

WEIGHT REDUCTION

Obesity (defined as a body mass index [BMI] $\geq$ 30) has been identified as a risk factor for the presence or severity of stress UI and mixed UI in women (Hunskaar et al., 2005). It is thought that the excess abdominal weight, as in pregnancy, may increase pressure on pelvic tissues, leading to weakening of the muscles, nerves, and other pelvic structures. The stress UI seen in obesity may be secondary to increases in intra-abdominal pressure on the bladder and greater urethral mobility. Also, obesity may impair blood flow or nerve innervation to the bladder. Richter et al. (2005) found a particularly high prevalence of urinary and anal incontinence in a group of 178 morbidly obese (BMI 40 kg/m^2 or more) women undergoing consultation for bariatric surgery. The prevalence of UI was 66.9% and that of anal incontinence 32% (17.4% when considering liquid and solid stool and not flatus).

Weight loss is an acceptable treatment option for morbidly obese women. Research has shown that stress UI symptoms decreased in morbidly obese women who experienced extreme weight loss after gastric bypass surgery (Bump, Sugerman, Fantl, & McClish, 1992) and that the prevalence of both UI and fecal incontinence can decrease after laparoscopic gastric bypass surgery (Burgio, Richter, Clements, Redden, & Goode, 2007). Research has shown that weight loss of 5%–10% of baseline weight can cause a 50%–60% reduction in frequency of weekly UI episodes (Subak et al., 2005). The effect of weight loss on urinary symptoms is comparable to what has been reported in patients undergoing surgery for stress UI. Providers should suggest self-care weight loss programs such as Weight Watchers or, depending on the BMI, refer patients to supervised weight loss programs.

REFERENCES

Arya, L.A., Myers, D.L., & Jackson, N.D. (2000). Dietary caffeine intake and the risk for detrusor instability: A case-control study. *Obstetrics and Gynecology, 96,* 85–89.

Brown, C.T., van der Meulen, J., Mundy, A.R., & Emberton, M. (2003). Lifestyle and behavioural interventions for men on watchful waiting with uncomplicated lower urinary tract symptoms: A national multidisciplinary survey. *BJU International, 92,* 53–57.

Bryant, C.M., Dowell, C.J., & Fairbrother, G. (2000). A randomized trial of the effects of caffeine upon frequency, urgency and urge incontinence. *Neurourology and Urodynamics, 19,* 501–502.

Bump, R.C., & McClish, D.M. (1994). Cigarette smoking and pure genuine stress incontinence of urine: A comparison of risk factors and determinants between smokers and nonsmokers. *American Journal of Obstetrics and Gynecology, 170,* 579–582.

Bump, R.C., Sugerman, H., Fantl, J.A, & McClish, D.M. (1992). Obesity and lower urinary tract function in women: Effect of surgically induced weight loss. *American Journal of Obstetrics and Gynecology, 166,* 392–399.

Burgio, K.L., Richter, H.E., Clements, R.H., Redden, D.T., & Goode, P.S. (2007). Changes in urinary and fecal incontinence symptoms with weight loss surgery in morbidly obese women. *Obstetrics and Gynecology, 110,* 1034–1040.

Colling, J., McCreedy, M., & Owen, T. (1994). Urinary tract infection rates among incontinent nursing home and community dwelling elderly. *Urologic Nursing, 14,* 117–119.

Creighton, S.M., & Stanton, S.L. (1990). Caffeine: Does it affect your bladder? *British Journal of Urology, 66,* 613–614.

Dowd, T.T., Campbell, J.M., & Jones, J.A. (1996). Fluid intake and urinary incontinence in older community-dwelling women. *Journal of Community Health Nursing, 13,* 179–186.

Engberg, S.J., McDowell, B.J., Burgio, K.L., Watson, J.E., & Belle, S. (1995). Self-care behaviors of older women with urinary incontinence. *Journal of Gerontological Nursing, 21,* (8), 7–14.

Fantl, J., Newman, D., Colling, J., DeLancey, J.O.L., Keeys, C., Loughery, R., et al. for the Urinary Incontinence in Adults Guideline Update Panel. (1996). *Urinary incontinence in adults: Acute and chronic management. Clinical practice guideline No. 2: Update* (AHCPR Publication No. 96-0692). Rockville, MD: Agency for Health Care and Policy Research.

Fitzgerald, M.P., Stablein, U., & Brubaker, L. (2002). Urinary habits among asymptomatic women. *American Journal of Obstetrics and Gynecology, 187,* 1384–1388.

Fitzgerald, S., Palmer, M.H., Berry, S.J., & Hart, K. (2000). Urinary incontinence: Impact on working women. *AAOHN Journal, 48,* 112–118.

Gaspar, P.M. (1999). Water intake of nursing home residents. *Journal of Gerontological Nursing, 25,* (4), 22–29.

Gray, M. (2001). Caffeine and urinary continence. *Journal of Wound, Ostomy, and Continence Nursing, 28,* 66–69.

Griffiths, D.J., McCracken, P.N., Harrison G.M., & Gormley, E.A. (1993). Relationship of fluid intake to voluntary micturition and urinary incontinence in geriatric clients. *Neurourology and Urodynamics, 12,* 1–7.

Holroyd-Leduc, J., & Straus, S. (2004). Management of urinary incontinence in women: Scientific review. *JAMA, 291,* 986–995.

Hunskaar, S., Burgio, K., Clark, A., Lapitan, M.C., Nelson, R., Sillen, U., et al. (2005). Epidemiology of urinary (UI) and faecal incontinence (FI) and pelvic organ prolapse (POP). In P. Abrams, L. Cardozo, S. Khoury, & A. Wein (Eds.), *Incontinence: Proceedings from the Third International Consultation on Incontinence* (pp. 257–312). Plymouth, UK: Health Publications, Ltd.

Johnson, T.M., Kincade, J.E., Bernard, S.L., Busby-Whitehead, J., & DeFriese, G.H. (2000). Self-care practices used by older men and women to manage urinary incontinence: Results from the National Follow-up Survey on Self-Care and Aging. *Journal of the American Geriatrics Society, 48,* 894–902.

Kayser-Jones, J., Schell, E.S., Porter, C., Barbaccia, J.C., & Shaw, H. (1999). Factors contributing to dehydration in nursing homes: Inadequate staffing and lack of professional supervision. *Journal of the American Geriatrics Society, 47,* 1187–1194.

Klevmark, B. (2002). Volume threshold for micturition: Influence of filling rate on sensory and motor bladder function. *Scandinavian Journal of Urology and Nephrology: Supplementum, 210,* 6–10.

Koley, B., Koley, J., & Saha, J.K. (1984). The effects of nicotine on spontaneous contractions of cat urinary bladder in situ. *British Journal of Pharmacology, 83,* 347–355.

Koskimaki, J., Hakama, M., Huhtala, H., & Tammela, T.L.J. (1998). Association of smoking with lower urinary tract symptoms. *Journal of Urology, 159,* 1580–1582.

Lamarine, R.J. (1994). Selected health and behavioral effects related to the use of caffeine. *Journal of Community Health, 19,* 449–466.

Lee, J.G., Wein, A.J., & Levin, R.M. (1993). The effect of caffeine on the contractile response of the rabbit urinary bladder to field stimulation. *General Pharmacology, 24,* 1007–1011.

Lee, R.A., & Balick, M.J. (2006). Rx: Caffeine. *Explore, 2,* 55–59.

Newman, D.K. (2002). *Managing and treating urinary incontinence.* Baltimore: Health Professions Press.

Newman, D.K., & Wein, A.J. (2004). *Overcoming overactive bladder.* Los Angeles: New Harbinger.

Nuotio, M., Jylha, M., Koivisto, A.M., & Tammela, T.L.J. (2001). Association of smoking with urgency in older people. *European Urology, 40,* 206–212.

Nygaard, I., Bryant, C., Dowell, C., & Wilson, P.D. (2002). Lifestyle interventions for the treatment of urinary incontinence in adults. Cochrane Incontinence Group. *Cochrane Database of Systematic Reviews,* (2), CD003505.

Nygaard, I.E., & Linder, M. (1997). Thirst at work—an occupational hazard? *International Urogynecology Journal, 8,* 340–343.

Ouslander, J., Schnelle, J., Simmons, S., Bates-Jenson, B., & Zeitlin, M. (1993). The dark side of incontinence in nursing home residents. *Journal of the American Geriatrics Society, 41,* 371–376.

Panel on Dietary Reference Intakes for Electrolytes and Water, Standing Committee on the Scientific Evaluation of Dietary Reference Intakes. (2004). *Dietary reference intakes for water, potassium, sodium, chloride, and sulfate* (pp. 146–147). Washington, DC: National Academy Press.

Popkin, B.M., Armstrong, L.E., Bray, G.M., Caballero, B., Frei, B., & Willett, W.C. (2006). A new proposed guidance system for beverage consumption in the United States. *American Journal of Clinical Nutrition, 83,* 529–542.

Richter, H.E., Burgio, K.L., Clements, R.H., Goode, P.S., Redden, D.T., & Varner, R.E. (2005). Urinary and anal incontinence in morbidly obese women considering weight loss surgery. *Obstetrics and Gynecology, 106,* 1272–1277.

Riesenhuber, A., Boehm, M., Posch, M., & Aufricht, C. (2006). Diuretic potential of energy drinks. *Amino Acids, 31,* 81–83.

Ruggieri, M.R., Whitmore, K.E., & Levine, R.M. (1990). Bladder purinergic receptors. *Journal of Urology, 144,* 176–181.

Subak, L.L., Whitcomb, E., Shen, H., Saxton, J., Vittinghoff, E., & Brown, J.S. (2005). Weight loss: A novel and effective treatment for urinary incontinence. *Journal of Urology, 174,* 190–195.

Tomlinson, B.U., Dougherty, M.C., Pendergast, J.F., Boyington, A.R., Coffman, M.A., & Pickens, S.M. (1999). Dietary caffeine, fluid intake and urinary incontinence in older rural women. *International Urogynecology Journal and Pelvic Floor Dysfunction, 10,* 22–28.

Wilson, P.D., Berghamns, B., Hagen, S., Hay-Smith, J., Moore, K., Nygaard, I., et al. (2005). Adult conservative management. In P. Abrams, L. Cardozo, S. Khoury, & A. Wein (Eds.), *Incontinence: Proceedings from the Third International Consultation on Incontinence* (pp. 855–964). Plymouth, UK: Health Publications, Ltd.

Wyman, J.F. (2000). Management of urinary incontinence in adult ambulatory care populations. *Annual Review of Nursing Research, 18,* 171–195.

Behavioral Treatments

Implementing Toileting, Bladder Training, and Pelvic Floor Muscle Rehabilitation Programs

Conservative treatments such as behavioral treatments or behavioral interventions (sometimes referred to as behavior modification) are now recommended as the first-line treatment for urinary incontinence (UI) and overactive bladder (OAB) (Fantl et al., 1996; Shamliyan et al., 2008; Wilson et al., 2005). These interventions involve education, toileting programs such as prompted voiding (PV) and bladder training (BT), and pelvic floor muscle training or rehabilitation (PFMT). Most behavior modification protocols for lower urinary tract dysfunction combine timed voiding practices with other components such as urge suppression techniques and PFMT designed to help individuals control the physiological responses of the bladder and pelvic floor muscles (PFM) that mediate continence. Toileting and BT programs are part of behavioral methods that target restoration or maintenance of bladder function with the goal of returning an individual to continence. These interventions usually include lifestyle changes or self-care practices, including adjusting the intake of fluids and eliminating bladder irritants—all discussed in Chapter 7 (Newman, 2004).

The Third International Consultation on Incontinence (ICI) has labeled these interventions as "packages" because most of them are usually recommended in different combinations (Wilson et al., 2005). They attempt to decrease UI and OAB symptoms through increasing awareness of the function and coordination of the bladder detrusor and PFM to decrease bladder overactivity and gain muscle identification, control, and strength. They involve learning new skills through intensive one-on-one individual instruction on strategies for preventing urine loss, urgency, and other symptomatology (Newman, 2004, 2005a).

BEHAVIOR MODIFICATION

The best way to learn new behavior or to relearn old behavior is by identifying the desired or optimal behavior and outlining the steps to be taken to gradually achieve it. Experience shows that the most successful behavioral treatments are multicomponent programs that combine several elements into a program tailored to the individual (Figure 8.1). One of the original researchers in this area has been Dr. Kathy Burgio, a behavioral psychologist. However, there are two major overlapping approaches to behavior management of incontinence and OAB that incorporate one or more of the following techniques: BT, which focuses on voiding habits; urge control; and behavioral training with physical therapy, which focuses on PFM exercises and managing detrusor or bladder overactivity (Figure 8.2). This shaping of desired behavior is achieved through goal setting and positive reinforcement or reward. For example, toilet training of toddlers involves providing rewards as a motivating factor for the child to void appropriately—in the toilet. An additional component of any behavioral treatment program for UI is monitoring voiding patterns and specified behavior, accomplished through the use of a Bladder Diary (discussed in Chapter 6). A critical part of any behavior program is the feedback from the clinician or from a caregiver in settings such as long-term or in-home care. Feedback should be provided about compliance, progress with the program, and positive reinforcement for success.

Behavioral interventions can be categorized as "patient-dependent" or "patient-independent" and "caregiver-dependent" therapies. Patient-dependent interventions necessitate adequate function, learning capability, and motivation

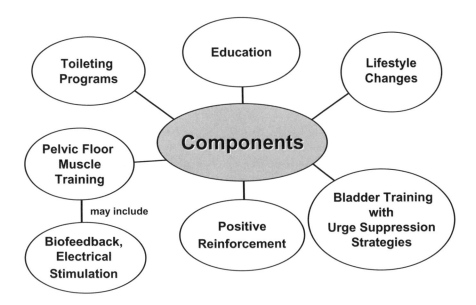

Figure 8.1.   Behavioral treatments for urinary incontinence.

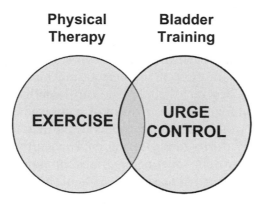

Figure 8.2. Overlapping approaches to behavior management of incontinence.

of the individual. Scheduled voiding regimens, which are patient- or caregiver-dependent therapies, have been the mainstay of treatment for decades for managing UI and symptoms of OAB. Caregiver-dependent interventions (regular toileting, PV) are useful in people with functional disabilities. The success of these interventions is largely dependent on caregiver knowledge and motivation, rather than on the person's physical function and mental status. In the frail elderly population, the clinician may find it helpful to consider the "Paradigm for Continence" classification of management options developed by Fonda et al. (2005) (Figure 8.3). Most ambulatory, cognitively intact adults can learn or can relearn to regulate bladder or bowel performance sufficiently to achieve and maintain clinically significant, improved function through BT and PFMT, both patient-independent therapies.

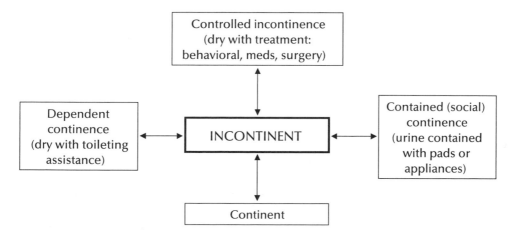

Figure 8.3. A paradigm for continence in frail older adults. (From Fonda, D., DuBeau, C.E., Harari, D., Ouslander, J.G., Palmer, M., & Roe, B. [2005]. Incontinence in the frail elderly. In P. Abrams, L. Cardozo, S. Khoury, & A. Wein (Eds.), *Incontinence: Proceedings from the Third International Consultation on Incontinence* [pp. 1163–1239]. Plymouth, UK: Health Publications, Ltd; reprinted by permission.)

TOILETING PROGRAMS

The initial treatment approach to someone with incontinence and OAB depends on the overall condition of the person and his or her ability to participate in a toileting program. People who can benefit from such programs may have mobility or cognitive impairment or may need assistance (e.g., one- to two-person assist) but are able to cooperate with toileting. A caregiver-dependent program that provides toileting on a scheduled time basis may be the simplest initial approach. Toileting programs can impact caregiver burden, especially in the community. At least 47%–68% of these individuals' informal caregivers provide assistance with toileting, and 29%–53% provide incontinence-related care (National Alliance for Caregiving and AARP, 2004). In studies examining the impact of toileting intervention programs for UI, there is some evidence that the interventions may decrease incontinence-related caregiver burden (Colling, Owen, McCreedy, & Newman, 2003) and decrease or at least not increase caregiver workload (Engberg, Sereika, McDowell, Weber, & Brodak, 2002).

If residents in long-term care (LTC) facilities or people living at home have an available and willing caregiver, a timed toileting program should be established. At least one third of care-dependent individuals with incontinence can benefit from a toileting assistance program. The premise of these programs is that, if the person is taught to void frequently, incontinence will not occur. The programs most commonly used are routine or scheduled toileting, habit training, and PV. Table 8.1 provides an overview of the different types of bladder programs that are described in more detail in this chapter.

Prior to determining which program is the most appropriate in the LTC resident, assessment, determination of the underlying pathophysiology, and identification of the expected outcomes must be done. Also, the assessment should determine which individuals would not benefit from either a scheduled toileting or BT program and should be just "checked and changed" (see Figure 8.1). With the recent implementation of the Centers for Medicare & Medicaid Services (CMS) Tag F315 interpretive guidance (CMS, 2005), assessment becomes all the more critical. Staff will need to develop a "management pathway" for UI in LTC; Figure 8.4 is an example. Tag F315 identifies four specific toileting programs—scheduled toileting, habit training, PV, and BT—that staff can implement. Therefore, nursing facility staff, especially the direct caregivers, such as certified nurse assistants (CNAs), must be aware of the key components of these programs and be able to identify which residents are appropriate candidates for each program so that optimal bladder function is achieved. Most experts recommend combining toileting programs with other interventions such as antimuscarinic drug therapy (van Houten, Achterberg, & Ribbe, 2007).

Some form of a toileting program is part of timed scheduled toileting, habit training, PV, and BT. Systematic reviews have been performed on timed or scheduled voiding (Ostaszkiewicz, Johnston, & Roe, 2004b); on habit training

Table 8.1 Description of types of bladder programs

Program	Other terms	Definitions	Changes in intervoid intervals (times between voiding)	Patient profile	Approach
Scheduled or timed voiding	Timed toileting	A fixed voiding schedule that remains unchanged	Unchanged	Neurogenic* bladder. Cognitively impaired. Available and compliant caregiver.	Fixed voiding regimen (e.g., every 3 or 4 hours). Techniques to facilitate or "trigger" voiding may be helpful (e.g., double voiding, running water at the sink, placing hands in a basin of warm water, drinking warm fluids, and pouring warm water on the perineum). Usually not followed during sleep hours.
Habit	Habit training (including patterned urge response toileting [PURT]) Bladder drill	A toileting schedule that is matched to the patient's voiding pattern	Increased or decreased	Neurogenic bladder*. Cognitively impaired. Available and compliant caregiver.	Assigned toileting schedule (every 3–4 hours). Schedule should be determined by voiding pattern determined from a voiding diary. Person is encouraged to defer toileting until the set times unless urge is unbearable. Usually not followed during sleep hours.
Prompted voiding	Bladder training	Promotion of continence through the use of timed verbal toileting reminders and positive social feedback for successful toileting	Prompting schedule	Ability to state name, transfer from bed or chair independently or with at the most a 1-person assist, has fewer than 4 UI episodes over a day (12 hours). Available and compliant caregiver.	Prior to implementing a PV program, a trial should be done for 3 consecutive days using the following approaches: • Focus attention on continence by asking if individual (resident) is wet or dry. • Check for wetness and give feedback. • Ask if individual (resident) would like to use toilet and, if refused, prompt 3 times. • Provide toileting assistance and encourage voiding.

(continued)

Table 8.1 (continued)

Program	Other terms	Definitions	Changes in intervoid intervals (times between voiding)	Patient profile	Approach
					• Provide positive feedback for dryness and appropriated toileting. • Remind individual (resident) of next toileting time. Predictors of a good response include those who • Respond to prompts when toileting • Have appropriate number of voids (voiding at least 50% of the time into a toileting receptacle) • Have < 4 episodes of UI in 12 hours (baseline incontinence rate) • Have normal PVR urine volume (< 100–150 mL) Usually not followed during sleep hours.
Bladder training	Bladder training Bladder reeducation Behavioral training Urge suppression or inhibition	An education program that aims to restore normal bladder function through a process of education along with a mandatory or self-adjustable voiding regimen with gradually increasing time intervals between voidings	Increased	Cognitively and neurologically intact individual who is motivated to change symptoms.	Individual is instructed to resist the urge to void during a specific interval (e.g., 30 minutes or 1 hour). If urge occurs during the interval, distraction or relaxation techniques or self-affirming statements are used to decrease urgency. Over time, the voiding interval is increased in comfortable units of time until a maximum interval of 3–4 hours is reached. Self-adjustable schedules are allowed so that individuals can void off schedule if experiencing severe urgency and fearful of an incontinence episode occurring. Education on urge suppression strategies such as distraction and relaxation techniques, use of pelvic floor muscle contraction to control urgency episodes, or both are used.

Key: PV = prompted voiding; PVR = postvoid residual; UI = urinary incontinence.
*Assuming normal PVR, if elevated, may also need intermittent catheterization (see Chapter 10).

250

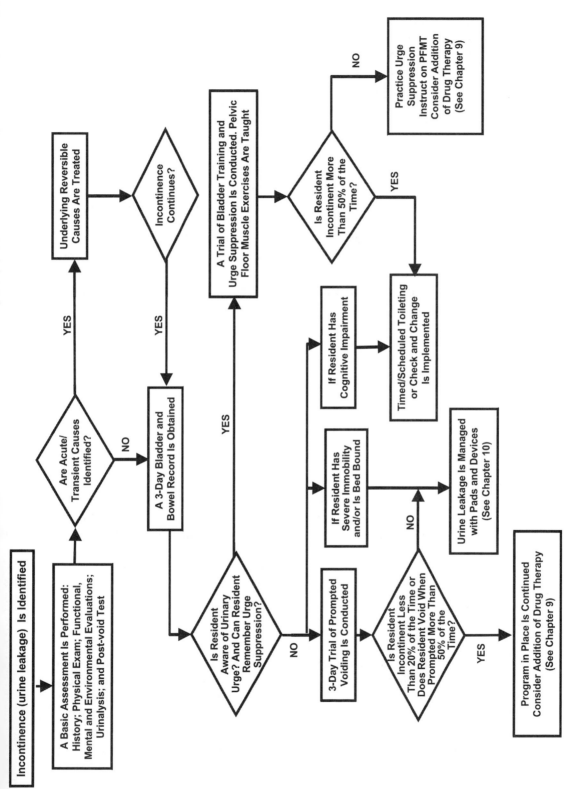

Figure 8.4. Management pathway for urinary incontinence in a long-term care setting. (Developed by Newman, D.K.)

(Ostaszkiewicz, Johnston, & Roe, 2004a); on PV (Eustice, Roe, & Paterson, 2002); and on BT (Roe, Milne, Ostaszkiewicz, & Wallace, 2007; Roe, Ostaszkiewicz, Milne, & Wallace, 2007; Roe, Williams, & Palmer, 2003; Wallace, Roe, Williams, & Palmer, 2004). This section discusses the care-dependent toileting programs: timed or scheduled toileting/habit training and PV.

Timed or Scheduled Toileting

Scheduled voiding/habit training is toileting a person on a rigid, fixed schedule (every 3–4 hours) (Ostaszkiewicz, Roe, & Johnston, 2005). Toileting takes place whether or not a sensation to void is present, but the schedule is usually only followed during waking hours. It is a passive toileting program with no element of patient education (as used in BT programs) or alterations of the person's behavior (Fonda et al., 2005). The goal is to keep the person dry, and no effort is made to alter an individual's voiding pattern or to motivate the person to resist the urge to urinate and delay urination. The premise of these programs is that, if the person is toileted on a preplanned schedule, the bladder will be emptied before incontinence occurs. Regular voiding prevents chronic bladder distention and its sequelae (e.g., compromised detrusor contractility resulting from overstretching of the muscle fibers), urinary tract infection (caused by urine stasis and a poorly perfused bladder wall), and urine leakage with detrusor overactivity (the threshold for detrusor overactivity is reached less frequently) (Newman, 2007b). These individuals may have mobility or cognitive impairments, and may need assistance (e.g., one-person assist), but are able to cooperate with toileting.

Pre-fixed times such as every 2 hours have been adopted for toileting programs in some institutions, particularly in LTC facilities. However, a more realistic schedule may be related to certain daily routines such as on awakening, before or after meals, and at bedtime. A schedule is usually determined by administrative staff for those residents who cannot toilet themselves. If the person self-toilets independently, then scheduled times are readjusted.

Ideally, the schedule for toileting is based on the Bladder Diary or on data collected using a bladder volume recording instrument or from an electronic device used to monitor and record incontinence episodes, providing a more accurate record. The following are components of a habit training toileting program in LTC facilities:

- Identify specific times the resident is likely to void by recording the voiding pattern for 3 days using a Bladder and Bowel Diary (on the companion CD under Assessment Forms) per CMS regulations (CMS, 2005). Based on the pattern/times observed, efforts are made to schedule toileting opportunities around these times. Assess residents with cognitive impairment and dementia as to whether they have "passive" UI (wet on chair/bed with no attempt to urinate in toilet or assistive device) or "active" UI (attempt to toilet but are unsuccessful or use inappropriate facility or receptacle) (Yap & Tan, 2006). If the person is taking a diuretic, the toileting schedule may need to be altered because the urine volume will be increased at the diuretic's peak action time. A common toileting interval used is every 3–4 hours. An example is to toilet:

> After breakfast
>
> After lunch
>
> After dinner
>
> Before bedtime—in settings such as nursing facilities, the person should toilet on the last incontinence rounds or on awakening

- Negotiate the voiding interval and toileting times with people who are cognitively intact to increase compliance.

- Observe possible contributors to UI in patients with cognitive impairment. Table 8.2 provides factors contributing to and possible solutions for UI in patients with dementia.

- Observe body language for cues about need to use the toilet. Look for fidgeting, nervousness, and pacing or increased anxiety.

- Ensure complete bladder emptying by having the person toilet upright at a bathroom commode or a bedside commode rather than on a bedpan.

- Facilitate voiding by using a raised toilet seat or bedside commode to avoid having the person sitting too low (see Chapter 10). Have the person slowly back up to the toilet until he or she can feel the back of the knees touching it. After placing both hands on the commode armrests or the grab bar and edge of the seat, the person lowers him- or herself slowly by bending at the knee and hip. Reverse the procedure by having the person stand up by grasping the grab bars and seat or commode armrests with one hand and perhaps a walker with the other. Instruct the person to keep the knees bent and the feet firmly on the floor when attempting to stand.

This type of toileting program is helpful for residents in nursing facilities who are not incontinent more often than every 2 hours and in homebound people living with a caregiver, usually a family member, who can assist with toileting. Research has shown that, with nursing facility residents, a timed, scheduled toileting program can be successful in decreasing the number of incontinence episodes. This is probably also true in people being cared for in their homes. This pattern may or may not be followed during sleep hours.

In the LTC setting, behavioral interventions such as timed voiding and scheduled toileting use a caregiver-dependent delivery system to achieve the goal of continence. In the home care setting, the need for a caregiver to provide teaching, assistance, and feedback is a problem unless a family member is available throughout the day or a hired paraprofessional is in place. However,

Table 8.2 Possible contributions and solutions to UI in patients with dementia

Contributing factors	Solutions
Cognitive effects • Geographic disorientation (does not know location of toilet even in own home; if bathroom door is shut, bathroom "doesn't exist" behind it) • Agnosia (inability to recognize objects, persons, sounds, shapes, or smells; cannot read words; usual pictorial signs of man or woman that depict a toilet may be meaningless) • Aphasia (inability to produce and/or comprehend language) • Visuospatial deficit (inability to visually perceive spatial relationships among objects; e.g., men stand too far away from toilet bowl and have an inaccurate aim)	• Remind or take to toilet at least every 3 hours. • Leave door of bathroom open so toilet can be seen. • Place picture of toilet on the door. • Show a picture of a man/woman using a toilet. • Make the door of the bathroom a different color. • Write out consistent and clear instructions on voiding and have staff read to resident to prompt voiding. • Gently steer male resident forward, give help to aim penis into toilet bowl. • Consider having male resident sit down.
Behavioral problems • Active—disinhibition, restlessness, anxiety (e.g., distaste, even phobia of using communal toilets) • Passive—apathy, depression, over-dependency, attention seeking (may be caused by embarrassment over urinary and fecal incontinence problems)	• Approach the resident with a calm and reassuring attitude. • Replace white toilet seat with a colored one (these could be colored "disposable" seat covers). • Maintain continuity and familiarity of caregiver staff. • Respect resident's dignity and be aware of personal preferences.
Mobility problems • Impaired mobility, dexterity, and clothing manipulation • Impaired vision (may not be able to see toilet seat) • Apraxia (loss of the ability to execute or carry out learned purposeful movements)	• Simplify clothing: sweatpants, elasticized waistbands. • Replace white toilet seat with a colored one (these could be colored "disposable" seat covers).

Adapted from Yap, P., & Tan, D. (2006). Urinary incontinence in dementia—a practical approach. *Australian Family Physician, 35,* 239.

the following tips can be used by home caregivers (family and professional) to promote safe and independent toileting:

• Try to give the person a private bathroom so someone else is never using it. If a bathroom is inaccessible, use a bedside commode, urinal, or bedpan.

• Ensure that bed height is sufficient so that, when the person sits on the edge of the bed, the feet are flat on the floor and the person can easily accomplish going from sitting to standing.

• Keep a clear, unobstructed, direct walking path to the bathroom and place night-lights along the path.

- Make sure the person can easily use the toilet (e.g., raised toilet seat, grab bars).

- Make sure the person's clothing is easy to remove. Encourage the use of underwear whenever possible. Underwear serves as a reminder to stay dry and as a stimulus to use the toilet and not to wet oneself if it can be avoided.

- Encourage the person to void before going to bed.

- Locate bathroom facilities when traveling, or bring a portable urinal. Choose seats in restaurants, theaters, and other such locations that are near a bathroom.

- Use underpads (reusable or disposable) under bedsheets, on chairs, and in the car. Avoid use of garbage bags, rubber pads, or shower curtain liners because these may be too slippery or may irritate the skin.

- Open windows or use deodorizers to cut down on odors. (A cut-up onion will absorb odors in a room without leaving its own smell. Also, an open box of baking soda will reduce odors.)

A caregiver-dependent program that provides toileting on a scheduled time basis may be the simplest initial approach for many frail older adults. Studies suggest that, although fewer than 20% of frail, incontinent older adults become completely dry, between 30% and 50% improve, with a reduction in the number of incontinence episodes and amount of urine leaked. These programs can be utilized to improve continence especially in frail older adults who are homebound or reside in LTC facilities (Lekan-Rutledge & Colling, 2003). Excluded from these programs are nursing facility residents with mobility impairment necessitating a mechanical or multiple-person transfer, those who are terminally ill or comatose, and residents with severe behavior disturbances. However, currently the frequency of toileting assists by nursing staff in LTC facilities in the United States is inadequate to maintain continence. Therefore, there is a need to combine toileting programs with interventions geared to nursing staff.

Prompted Voiding

PV is a scheduled toileting program that employs behavior modification to reinforce both appropriate toileting behaviors and the individual's desire to stay dry. PV is used with people who are able to recognize urine leakage and are able to respond, voiding when prompted. PV stresses active communication and interaction between a caregiver and the individual, allowing the person to take an active part in his or her incontinence and toileting behavior. A PV program tries to increase the person's awareness of the need to void and to ask for assistance to toilet. Like habit training, this program is used with more frail, ill people who require assistance from family members, professional caregivers, or both.

Research in the area of PV has been conducted mostly in nursing facilities and has shown that from 25% to 40% of incontinent residents respond well to toileting assistance, while approximately 38% cannot successfully toilet even when provided assistance by research assistants (Ouslander et al., 1995). In one study of 191 incontinent residents in seven nursing facilities, 25%–40% responded well to prompted voiding during the day, with incontinence episodes decreasing from three to four during the day to one or none. Responsive residents can be easily identified during a 3-day trial, and principles of continuous quality improvement, such as periodic wet checks of responsive residents, should be applied to determine the program's ongoing effectiveness. Wet checks are examination of pads or adult briefs at regular intervals to identify episodes of incontinence. A decrease in UI rates can be seen within 3 days, but maximal response may not be realized until after several weeks of treatment. Characteristics of "high responders" (Lekan-Rutledge, 2000; Ouslander et al., 1995) include those residents who are able to

- State their name
- Reliably point to one of two objects
- Ambulate independently or with the assistance of one or two people

The CMS's Tag F315 surveyor guidance on urinary incontinence (CMS, 2005) recommends that residents who meet these criteria be given a 3-day therapeutic trial of PV. Other parameters to consider when determining if this type of toileting program will be successful include whether the individual

- Has a bladder capacity of at least 100 mL (can be determined by measuring patient's voided volume or by "scanning" bladder prior to voiding)
- Has a low number of incontinent episodes per day (<4 in 12 hours)
- Has a postvoid residual urine volume of less than 200 mL
- Responds to caregivers if prompted (asked and taken to the toilet) to void
- Can control urination until the toilet is reached

Steps of a Prompted Voiding Program

There are five major steps in a prompted voiding program as used in an LTC facility.

1. *Checking*—Scheduled checking of the resident is done on a regular basis. The caregiver (e.g., CNA) gives the resident a chance to request to toilet. Clothes, linens, and absorbent products are checked by the caregiver. It is important that both the inside and outside of clothes and absorbent products are checked. The caregiver should inform the resident of what is being done and why.

2. *Talking*—The resident is encouraged to discuss the bladder/incontinence problem. The caregiver should ask the resident if he or she knows whether he or she is wet or dry (to determine accuracy and to see if the resident is in denial). The caregiver should verbally verify the accuracy of the resident's response. These efforts will increase the resident's awareness about his or her condition. If the resident is dry, the caregiver should indicate approval or praise the resident. If the resident is wet, the caregiver should provide corrective verbal feedback such as disappointment; for example:

    > "That's right, Mrs. Ellis, you did not have an accident since I was here last time. That is good." (praise)
    > "Oh, dear, Mrs. Ellis, you had a bladder accident. Maybe next time that won't happen." (corrective feedback)

    The caregiver should inquire as to the resident's need to void prior to going anywhere (e.g., before meals, physical therapy). In addition, the caregiver should make sure the resident knows how to communicate with staff the need to void or toilet if he or she is in a new room or area in the facility, and should show the resident the location of and how to access and use the toilet in that area.

3. *Prompting*—Because the goal is to have the resident take an active part in the voiding process, he or she is asked or "prompted" to try to use the toilet and void regardless of continence status. The caregiver should "prompt" the resident three times if he or she refuses. The caregiver should be very persuasive to get the resident to void by offering assistance and providing privacy during toileting. The caregiver should turn on the bathroom faucet because the sound of running water is usually a trigger for voiding. Residents should not be rushed, but rather allowed at least 15 minutes to relax and void. Relaxation is needed to allow the external urinary sphincter to open. However, if the resident does not want to void, the caregiver should not attempt to toilet him or her because more than likely voiding will not occur. Sample prompts include:

    > "Mrs. Ellis, would you like to use the bathroom?"
    > "Mrs. Ellis, maybe you'd better try because I won't be back to help you to the bathroom for 3 hours."

    If the resident is still not sure:

    > "Mrs. Ellis, please give it a try, okay?"

4. *Praising*—The caregiver should praise the resident for 1) being dry (continence) or 2) making an effort to use the toilet. The resident should be informed of the time of the next scheduled prompted voiding; for example:

    > "Very good, Mrs. Ellis. You tried to use the bathroom."
    > "Mrs. Ellis, it has been 3 hours, and you have not had a bladder accident. I will be back in 3 hours. Please try to be dry again."

5. *Correcting*—If the resident has an incontinence episode, the caregiver should indicate to him or her that the expectation is that he or she will stay dry; for example:

> "Mrs. Ellis, you were incontinent this time. Please ask me (push on your call bell) before you have to go to the bathroom the next time."

Outcomes of Prompted Voiding Programs

The outcomes of prompted voiding have been identified through clinical trials and include

- Identification of individual patterns of UI

- Decrease in average urine volume of incontinent episodes

- Increased recognition of urge to void

- Increase in daily average number of dry checks and nonwet (continent) episodes

However, key elements must be in place if these practices are to be transferred effectively to a clinical setting and LTC population. Elements identified include

1. Assessment to determine if the patient is a candidate for a toileting program. Residents in LTC facilities with high baseline incontinence rates (usually incontinent more than every 2 hours), who have small voided urine volumes, and who were unsuccessful at reported toileting regimens using PV techniques are usually not responsive to toileting programs.

2. Ability of the individual to ambulate independently or with the assistance of one person.

3. Ability of the individual to void into a toileting receptacle at least 50% of the time when prompted.

A more successful program called Patterned Urge Response Toileting or "PURT" may involve prompting LTC residents, home care patients, and other care-dependent individuals to void at times when they are most likely to need to void, which is determined by tracking voiding and UI and determining patterns using such techniques as computerized recordings of wetness (Colling, Ouslander, Hadley, Eisch, & Campbell, 1992; Colling et al., 2003). Another use of technology would be to toilet residents based on actual bladder volume (Newman, 2005b, 2007b; Newman, Gaines, & Snare, 2005). Many LTC facilities have instituted the use of a portable ultrasound scanner (BladderScan™; Verathon Medical, Bothell, WA) to determine bladder volume when attempting to toilet a resident (Newman, 2007b; Newman et al., 2005). The following is an example of one facility's approach to prompted voiding using a BladderScan™:

1. Anticipate the needs of the resident related to voiding.

2. Listen to the resident for complaints of pain, discomfort, and need to urinate.

3. When the resident requests toileting, determine bladder volume using the BladderScan™ device. Inform the resident of the scan results, explaining what the volume means.

4. If the amount is greater than 200 mL, toilet the resident using PV techniques.

5. If the amount is 150 mL or less, explain to the resident that the volume is not sufficient to necessitate voiding. If amounts are consistently low (<150 mL) for a given resident and the resident does not appear to be voiding adequate amounts, or voiding at least 4 to 5 times per day, consider increasing fluid intake.

Despite the availability of such new technologies, LTC facilities have not seemed to embrace their use. Unfortunately, with regard to toileting programs, there is a wide gap between what is known and what is actually used. Despite documented research of positive outcomes, PV interventions largely have not been adopted in LTC settings. Improvement in continence on the part of residents can only be maintained if the prompting continues, because the residents do not achieve complete independence from staff. Research has documented the success of a staff training program called the behavioral supervision model, which defines responsibilities of staff members for the PV intervention, gives staff feedback regarding performance, and establishes consequences based on staff performance evaluation.

A novel staffing model that employed a "designated" versus "integrated" role in nursing facilities of the CNA in the delivery of restorative care (walking program, exercise therapy) may have application to delivery of continence care (Schnelle et al., 2002). Specifically, the functional incidental training (FIT) intervention, which combines PV with functionally oriented low-intensity endurance and strength-training exercises, has repeatedly been noted to improve physical function and UI in nursing facility residents (Ouslander et al., 2005).

Combining Toileting with Drug Therapy

Clinicians should consider combining treatments to maximize the effects in residents in LTC. In female residents diagnosed with atrophic vaginitis, topical estrogen cream may improve urogenital atrophy. In residents clinically diagnosed with urgency UI (UUI) and other symptoms of OAB, a combination of an antimuscarinic (see Chapter 9) and a toileting program may maximize the benefit. Ouslander, Maloney, Grasela, Rogers, and Walawander (2001) instituted a quality improvement program at five LTC facilities. Key people in each facility—the director of nursing and a "continence champion"—were trained in assessment and PV protocols and when to consider adding drug therapy in treating incontinence. Of the 377 incontinent residents, 254 had a trial of a toileting program after assessments were done. Of those 254 residents, 151 were believed to be benefiting and were maintained on some type of toileting program for

16 weeks. Of these 151 residents, 48 were believed to be appropriate for a trial of tolterodine (2 mg twice daily) in addition to PV. Of the 151 residents who benefitted, 81 were considered "clinically stable" and had 16%–29% improvement in dryness rates. The conclusion of the program was that, out of the 377 incontinent residents, 81 seemed to have some benefit from a toileting program, with or without drugs. Those on the drugs had no severe side effects.

If PV programs are instituted correctly, nursing facility residents and families should benefit from improvement in incontinence rates, a lowered incidence of complications secondary to UI, less absorbent product (e.g., adult briefs) use, and greater dignity. Nursing facility chains or consortiums should consider using a central data collection process and a program coordinator to produce graphs of outcomes and to provide ongoing feedback to facilities and staff. For a toileting program to be successful, facilities must be motivated, have in place an efficient training process, provide good oversight, continuously monitor the process, and identify "program champions" who will take ownership of the program (Ouslander et al., 2001).

Bladder Training or "Retraining"

Bladder training (BT), also commonly referred to as bladder retraining, bladder discipline, bladder drill, and bladder reeducation, controls urgency through the use of a behavioral strategy called "urge suppression." BT consists of three main components: 1) patient education about the bladder, incontinence, and urgency control (or suppression) strategies; 2) a scheduled voiding regimen that gradually extends the intervoid intervals; and 3) positive reinforcement techniques provided by a health care professional (Fantl et al., 1996). BT goals are adherence to prescribed voiding intervals, improved control over urge, development of greater bladder capacity, reduction of UI episodes, and restoration of the individual's bladder control (Hines et al., 2007). The return to normal bladder function is achieved by gradually increasing the intervals between voiding in an attempt to correct urinary frequency and eventually diminish urgency. It involves learning and independent individual voiding behavior. By practicing urge suppression to diminish urgency, the patient is able to gradually increase the intervals between voiding, correct the habit of frequent voiding, and suppress bladder overactivity.

Mechanisms of action are not well understood, but it is thought that BT improves cortical brain inhibition of bladder contractions, facilitates cortical control over urethral closure during bladder filling, strengthens pelvic floor striated muscles, and alters behaviors that affect continence (e.g., frequent response to urgency) (Wilson et al., 2005). The individual is provided information about normal bladder control and given urge suppression strategies to control the urgency. The main outcomes for a BT program (Newman, 2005a, 2007a) are to

1. Improve bladder overactivity by controlling urgency and decreasing frequency

2. Increase bladder capacity

3. Reduce urgency or mixed incontinence episodes

This type of intervention is most appropriate for individuals with

*   Urgency, frequency, or urgency and/or mixed incontinence

*   Intact cognition

*   Ability to sense the urinary urge sensation

*   Ability to comprehend and follow instructions

*   Willingness to comply with a structured education program

Jeffcoate and Francis (1966) originally introduced BT, which was called "bladder drill," by implementing the program in hospitalized patients with bladder dysfunction secondary to psychological disorders. At that time, it was prescribed for functional disorders of the bladder for which surgical intervention was not expected to be successful. The management regimen included education followed by a strict schedule of voluntary voiding with specific instructions to avoid responding prematurely to urinary urgency. This type of BT was the basis of a randomized, controlled clinical trial of 123 women, who were 55 years of age or older, with detrusor instability, stress UI (SUI), and mixed UI (Fantl et al., 1991). Results of the group taught BT indicated reduction in the number of incontinent episodes by 57% and reduction in the quantity of urine loss of 54%. Although BT was developed originally as a treatment for UUI (e.g., related to detrusor overactivity), in this study, it was effective for SUI (e.g., related to sphincter insufficiency) as well. In addition, BT significantly improved the quality of life, specifically in regard to the ability to carry out activities and relationships, the ability to tolerate and control symptoms, and an improved ability to cope. Subak, Quesenberry, Posner, Cattolica, and Soghikian (2002) conducted a 6-week BT class in community-dwelling women ages 55 and over. After the class, the treatment group had a significant (40%) reduction in mean weekly UI episodes when compared with controls. This improvement persisted for 6 months.

Most BT programs are based on the work of nurse researcher Dr. Jean Wyman, who is currently at the University of Minnesota. Dr. Wyman's Minnesota Continence Associates clinical practice is described in Chapter 13. Prior to beginning a BT program, the individual should be educated about the lower urinary tract, causes of UI, and concepts of bladder urgency using easy-to-understand visual instructions and aids such as "the urgency wave" (Figure 8.5; see also the patient education tool "Bladder Training—Controlling Urgency and Frequency" on the companion CD). Education should include the fact that "continence" is a learned behavior and the importance of the brain's control over lower urinary tract function.

A key component of BT is a scheduled toileting program, which is individualized based on results of a bladder or voiding diary. The voiding diary, completed by the individual before starting treatment, allows the clinician

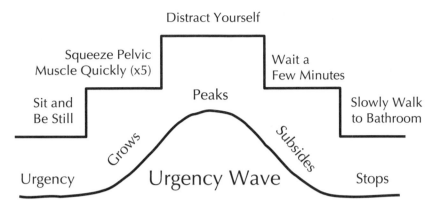

Figure 8.5. Urgency suppression wave.

to assess how often the individual is voiding and to determine the longest interval between voiding that is comfortable. That interval becomes the starting point, which will vary with each patient. Individuals are instructed to empty the bladder on waking and then every hour on the hour, and are asked to increase the duration between voids by 15–30 minutes each week until they feel comfortable with their urinary frequency. If they feel they have to void during the interval, they are instructed to use urge suppression techniques. The initiation of BT with very short voiding intervals is particularly important for people who are experiencing urgency because the shorter intervals will decrease or eliminate these symptoms (Wyman, 2005). The goal is for the patient to void "before" the urge sensation of bladder fullness. Over time, the voiding interval is increased in comfortable units of time until a maximum of every 3–4 hours is reached. It may be unrealistic to expect patients seen in clinical practice to comply with a strict voiding schedule for any length of time.

As mentioned previously, another essential part of BT patient education focuses on the cortical ability to delay voiding and strategies for distraction or relaxation techniques or self-affirming statements to get the individual through to the scheduled voiding time. These should be used to assist the patient in adhering to the assigned voiding times. Concentration on a task that demands close attention is useful in distracting the individual from the sensation of urgency (Wyman, 2005). The patient is taught methods to resist or inhibit the urge sensation so an expanded voiding interval can be adopted. Improving the ability to suppress the urge sensation and eventually diminish urgency will enable the individual to adopt a more normal voiding pattern. Several strategies or techniques are used to control and inhibit the urge sensation (Wyman, 2005):

- Slow, deep breathing to consciously relax the bladder and thereby combat a stressful rush to the toilet.

- Performing five or six rapid, deliberate, and intense PFM contractions, or "quick flicks," which are 2–3 seconds in duration.

- Using self-statements (e.g., "I can wait," "I can take control.")

As mentioned, the scheduled interval between voiding is increased by 30 minutes until the patient can achieve a goal of voiding every 3–4 hours (Wyman & Fantl, 1991). In many cases, people find this schedule difficult. Therefore, the patient should be told to adhere to this schedule at least 75% of the day; it is not realistic to expect people to maintain this voiding schedule during the night. The use of reminders such as a kitchen timer or stopwatch can be beneficial in helping the patient keep on a schedule. Self-monitoring through a Bladder Diary is used to evaluate adherence and to determine the next weekly voiding interval.

Most experts believe that combining behavioral interventions with treatments such as drug therapy will increase symptom reduction. Mattiasson, Blaakaer, Hoye, and Wein (2003) reported on a multicenter, single-blind Scandinavian study of 505 subjects, predominantly women (mean age 63), with symptoms of OAB with and without UUI. The subjects were treated either with tolterodine 2 mg twice a day or with tolterodine 2 mg twice a day and BT. Subjects in the BT group were provided with a written information sheet that outlined the principles of BT and explained simple techniques that could be used to help improve bladder control. Both groups received Bladder Diaries to track outcomes. Seventy-eight percent of subjects completed 24 weeks of treatment. The median percent reduction of voiding frequency for those receiving drug therapy plus BT was 33% compared with 25% reduction in those subjects on drug therapy alone. There was no significant difference between the groups in relation to reduction in incontinence episodes or urgency. The authors termed this a "minimalist" approach because no physician or other professional was involved.

Bladder Training in LTC

BT can be very successful in the LTC setting if the appropriate resident is identified. A BT program in an LTC facility must be flexible enough to be modified to the resident's needs. The following are the components of a BT program for LTC residents:

- When usual voiding times have been established, arrange for the resident to be toileted one-half hour prior to the next expected time. If there is no observable voiding pattern, toilet the resident at 1-hour intervals, beginning at 7:00 or 8:00 A.M. and continuing hourly until bedtime. The resident should be awakened to void at less frequent intervals during the night.

- Timing is crucial to success. Teach the resident to control the urge to void by teaching the following:

  Explain to the resident that urgency is that strong desire to void that occurs suddenly and is difficult to defer. It can lead to sudden urine leakage or UUI. Urgency follows a wave pattern: it starts, grows, peaks, and then subsides until it stops (see Figure 8.5).

The key to controlling urinary urgency is not to respond by rushing to the bathroom. Rushing may precipitate a bladder contraction, which in turn increases urgency, so teach the resident never to rush or run to the bathroom or toilet. Substitute walking slowly. The ultimate goal of BT is to have the resident go to the bathroom every 3–4 hours.

- Staff must give the resident consistent encouragement and positive feedback. If UI continues, focus the resident's attention on successes that are achieved each day.

- When the resident has remained dry most of the time for 1 week, the toileting interval should be increased to 2 hours, and finally to 3 hours. Some residents will never be able to retain urine longer than 2–3 hours, but others will regain more extended control.

- Institute the self-care strategies discussed in Chapter 7.

- Continue to record intake and voiding times on the Bladder and Bowel Diary (on the companion CD under Assessment Forms). Progress can be monitored, and adjustments can be made to the voiding schedule and fluid intake as necessary.

Decreasing Obsessive Toileting

Some individuals request toileting as frequently as every 20–30 minutes. These people fear that, if they do not void, they will be incontinent. It is thought that at least 5% of LTC residents exhibit obsessive toileting behavior. This includes residents who

- Have been diagnosed with "neurogenic" bladder

- Frequently request toileting assistance (every 15, 20, or 30 minutes, or every hour)

- Frequently self-toilet (every 20 minutes, 30 minutes, 1 hour)

The goals for such residents are

- To stop obsessive toileting behavior

- To educate the resident about normal bladder volumes through the use of a portable bladder volume instrument

- To expand and increase intervals between voiding

- To decrease the time the staff spend with frequent toileting of the same resident

The resident is taught to reduce the number of incontinence episodes through combining "dependent" continence and "independent" continence. In "dependent" continence, the staff toilet the resident based on an adequate bladder volume as determined by ultrasound scanning. In "independent" continence, the resident takes a more active role in developing awareness of the need to void based on adequate bladder volume and is able to delay void-ing through urge inhibition techniques.

The portable ultrasound (e.g., BladderScan™) may be a helpful tool with the resident who has an obsession with toileting (Newman, 2007b). Knowledge about bladder volume at any given time helps eliminate unnecessary toileting and allows for accurate assessment of the resident's hydration state. With the resident who repeatedly asks to be toileted before the scheduled time (or before an adequate volume of urine is present in the bladder), the following techniques can be used (Newman, 2007b):

1. Scan the bladder using a portable ultrasound scanner (BladderScan™); if urine volume is under 100–150 mL, show the resident the results. Usually these individuals will have 50- to 75-mL volumes. Include the resident in the scanning process by encouraging the resident to look at the bladder scanner screen and explain what the numbers indicate. Show the resident the printout of the bladder volume.

2. Ask the resident if he or she understands that there is actually very little urine in the bladder and encourage the resident to not go to the bathroom at this time to void, thus extending toileting times. If the resident is cog-nitively intact, teach him or her urge suppression techniques to delay voiding (see previous section on Bladder Training or "Retraining"). Ask the resident to delay voiding for 15–20 minutes.

3. Monitor fluid intake because these residents often intentionally decrease fluid intake for fear of becoming incontinent or having to use the bath-room too often. Education and demonstration with the portable ultra-sound help residents realize that increasing fluid intake actually improves bladder function.

Amelia, an 88-year-old female resident, was noted as a 2 on the Minimum Data Set (occasionally incontinent: > 2 [but not daily] bladder inconti-nence episodes per week) for incontinence of bladder but who was con-tinent of bowel, put on her call light every 15 minutes requesting assis-tance to the toilet. When taken to the bathroom, Amelia was unable to void. The resident reported to the staff that she was not drinking liquids because she feared being incontinent and not being able to make it to the bathroom in time. The staff were able to convince Amelia to let them scan her bladder before toileting to show her the amount of urine that was in her bladder and whether she needed to void. Amelia was reluctant at first and stated, "When I've gotta go, I've gotta go. There ain't no contraption that's gonna tell me when to go to the bathroom." Through much persua-sion and visual education regarding the bladder scanner, the staff were able to get her to agree to allow them to scan her bladder to measure vol-ume. Amelia slowly increased her fluid intake and was able to use the toi-let on a more regular schedule. The staff used the scanner to show Amelia her increasing bladder volumes and when those volumes necessitated voiding. Within a couple of weeks, she was more comfortable, and the staff did not have to answer the resident's call bell every 15 minutes. Amelia's fear of incontinence decreased, incontinence products were eliminated, and the voiding interval improved to every 3–4 hours.

PELVIC FLOOR MUSCLE REHABILITATION

The primary technique of behavioral treatments is pelvic floor muscle training (PFMT) with or without biofeedback. PFMT consists of repetitive episodic contractions of the pelvic floor muscles (PFM) taught by a health care provider (physician nurse or physical therapist) and performed over time (Newman, 2005a, 2007b). This training program is based on "Kegel" exercises. In the late 1940s, Dr. Arnold Kegel, an obstetrician gynecologist, implemented a comprehensive program of progressive contractions of the PFM—specifically the levator ani muscle. During Dr. Kegel's time, most of the medical community believed that UI in women was a physical defect that needed surgery for correction, but Dr. Kegel put forth the idea that it was functional and could be corrected with muscle rehabilitation. Dr. Kegel demonstrated in several clinical trials that repeated, high-intensity contractions of the muscles of the pelvic floor with scheduled exercises increased ability to control urethral activity and decreased SUI in childbearing women (Kegel, 1948). He recommended an exercise program that included isometric contractions of the PFM, conducted under direct supervision by a trained nurse and incorporating biofeedback technology in the form of a perineometer. These Kegel exercises—or, as they have become known, PFM exercises (PFMEs) or more recently PFMT—have been shown to decrease lower urinary tract symptoms of incontinence, urgency, and frequency (Fantl et al., 1996). Evidence-based reviews support the recommendation that PFMT be included in first-line conservative management programs for women with SUI, UUI, or mixed UI (Hay-Smith & Dumoulin, 2006; Wilson et al., 2005).

Dr. Kegel described four phases in the performance of the exercises:

1. Awareness of the function and coordination of the PFM. For older adults and individuals whose muscles are severely relaxed, this may require daily PFMEs of at least 6 weeks to several months in duration (Choi, Palmer & Park, 2007).

2. Gains over muscle identification, control, and strength. Muscle strength is the maximal force that can be generated by the PFM (called a "maximal voluntary contraction [MVC]"). Because the PFM must adapt to different or changing requirements, they must have contractibility and build force quickly when contracting.

3. Firmness, thickening, broadening, and bulking of the muscles to increase muscle endurance. Muscle endurance is a performance characteristic that

indicates the ability of the PFM to execute repeated contractions to an initial level of strength often called a "submaximum" contraction.

4. Improvements of the symptoms, indicating that the muscles are strengthening.

As part of a rehabilitation program, PFMT increases support to the urethral sphincter and detrusor muscle, thereby preventing all types of UI and decreasing urgency. PFMT is most appropriate in people who

- *Do not* have cognitive impairments
- Are motivated to comply with the program
- Have a pelvic floor that is neurologically intact

Mechanism of Action

The rationale for PFMT is that mastering a voluntary contraction of the PFM will help to increase pressure in the urethra, inhibit detrusor contractions, and control leakage of urine. It is a skill that individuals seldom master on their first try, but with repeated training, it can be used successfully and can provide significant improvement in reducing incontinence episodes. The goal of PFMT is to isolate the PFM, specifically the levator ani. The PFMs are a striated, skeletal muscle group under voluntary control whose function is to maintain urinary and fecal continence and to provide support to the pelvic organs (Figure 8.6A and B). The functional demands on the fibers of the PFM (Ashton-Miller, Howard, & DeLancey, 2001) include

- Sustaining force over time, especially during increases in intra-abdominal pressure
- Developing force quickly
- Contracting and relaxing voluntarily

During voiding, the patient must relax the PFM to open the external urethral sphincter to allow voiding. When these muscles do not function properly, women in particular may develop SUI, fecal incontinence, and pelvic organ prolapse. PFMT promotes strength training of these skeletal muscles to improve neuromuscular function and muscle tone.

The PFM consist of two types of muscle fibers: type I, or slow-twitch muscle fibers, and type II, or fast-twitch muscle fibers (see Chapter 3). The majority of the levator ani muscle consists of type I muscle fibers. These fibers maintain a resting tone, produce less force on contraction, and assist in improving muscle endurance by generating a slower, more sustained, but less intense contraction. Over time, the continuous though lower intensity contraction of these muscle fibers maintains a general level of support and urethral closure pressure. Type I muscle fibers are also fatigue resistant. Type II, or fast-twitch, fibers aid in strong and forceful contractions. These fibers come

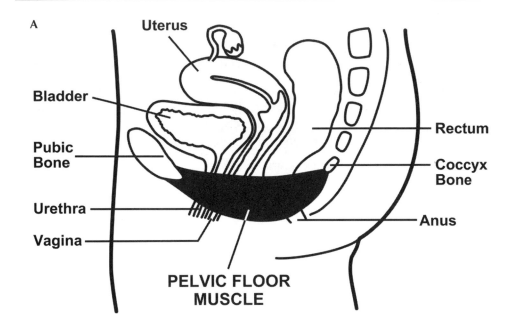

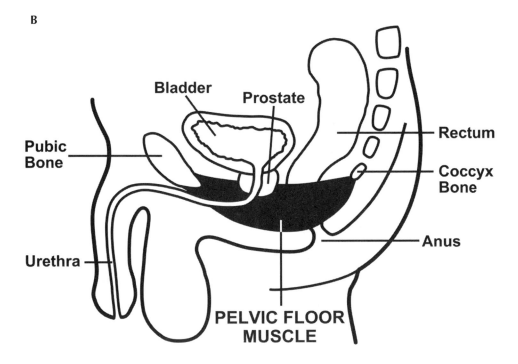

Figure 8.6. *A,* Location of pelvic floor muscles in women. (Courtesy of Robin Noel.) *B,* Location of pelvic floor muscles in men. (Copyright Diane K. Newman.)

into play during sudden increases in intra-abdominal pressure by contributing to urethral closure. These fibers are like the leg muscles used during a sprint; they are powerful and explosive. Exercising these fibers will increase PFM strength. Because these type II fibers fatigue easily, people with UI are taught to perform a small number of "quick" muscle contractions.

The actual effects of PFMT on lower urinary tract function are not completely understood. There appears to be a relationship between changes in various measures of PFM strength, such as anal sphincter strength or increased urethral closure pressure, and resistance, all of which will prevent urine leakage (Bø & Sherburn, 2005). The success of PFMT is based on the presumption that it is possible to both increase the capacity of existing muscle and hypertrophy the muscle. The proposed mechanisms of action for a strong and fast PFM contraction include the following:

1. A strong and fast pelvic muscle contraction closes the urethra and increases urethral pressure to prevent leakage during a sudden increase in intra-abdominal pressure (e.g., during a cough).

2. Contraction of the levator ani prevents peritoneal descent by exerting a counterbalancing upward (cephalic) force through the lifting of the endopelvic fascia on which the urethra rests (Bø, 2004a). The levator ani presses the urethra upward toward the pubic symphysis, creating a mechanical pressure rise.

3. Urethral closure or compression is achieved through increases in urethral pressure, which can be maximized by timing the muscle contraction at the exact moment of intra-abdominal force (called the "Knack") (Miller, 2002; Miller, Ashton-Miller, & DeLancey, 1998; Miller, Perucchini, Carchidi, DeLancey, & Ashton-Miller, 2001).

4. Muscle contraction may reflexively inhibit bladder overactivity (Newman, 2005a). Performing several successive rapid PFM contractions, termed *quick flicks,* at the time of urgency will inhibit or suppress urgency, allowing more time to void.

Identifying the PFM

One of the first steps in teaching PFMEs is instruction on the correct technique of PFM contraction. Many people may have a difficult time identifying and isolating these muscles. Most women do not receive formal instructions on how to identify and train the PFM. Fine et al. (2007) attempted to determine how women learned about performing PFMEs. Women enrolled in a prospective cohort study of the effect of childbirth on fecal and urinary continence were asked if and how they were taught PFMEs. Participants were primiparous women. Methods of PFME instruction included giving women instruction during pregnancy (64%), with 26% of the women given instruction both before and after childbirth. Less than one half (41%) of the women were taught PFMEs by a doctor, nurse, or midwife. Women (59%) reported learning about PFMs from other sources, such as books, videotapes, childbirth classes, friends, or family. Most teaching was by verbal or written instruction, and only 10% of women reported that they learned by demonstration during a pelvic examination. This is disturbing because, without adequate instruction, 30%–50% of women perform the maneuver of PFM contraction incorrectly, with potentially one quarter of women substituting a straining-down maneuver, which threatens to worsen the very condition the contractions are intended to prevent or treat (Sampselle & DeLancey, 1992).

More than one third of women report not feeling confident about their ability to do PFMT correctly (Chiarelli, Murphy, & Cockburn, 2003). Inability to isolate and identify the PFM will usually cause contraction of accessory muscles, primarily the gluteal and abdominal muscles. Contractions of other muscle groups such as the gluteals, hip adductors, and abdominals cause co-contractions of the PFM in healthy volunteers (Bø & Stien, 1994; Peschers, Gingelmaier, Jundt, Leib, & Dimpfl, 2001; Sapsford et al., 2001). However, none of these other muscles can act as a structural support to the pelvic organs, prevent descent of the bladder and the urethra during increases in abdominal pressure, or increase urethral closure pressure by their own isolated contractions, so most PFM specialists prefer patients to isolate the PFM and avoid contraction of these accessory muscles (Bø, 2004b). The gluteal muscles attach to the posterior aspect of the pelvis as well as the femur. Because they are a large muscle group, they can overpower the PFM. For this reason, the gluteal muscles should be relaxed. The abdominal muscles attach to the pubic bone. If contracted, they will increase pressure on the bladder, pelvic, and urogenital muscles, which will make pelvic muscle contraction more difficult. However, the transverse abdominus (TrA) and diaphragm muscles in the abdomen have been shown to co-contract during PFM contraction (Sapsford, 2001). There is controversy concerning the benefit of contracting the TrA when contracting the PFM.

The Pelvic Floor Clinical Assessment Group of the International Continence Society has defined a voluntary contraction of the PFM as when the patient is able to contract the PFM on demand (Messelink et al., 2005). A contraction is felt as a tightening, lifting, and squeezing action under the examining finger. Voluntary relaxation of these muscles means that the patient is able to relax the PFM on demand, after a contraction has been performed. Relaxation is felt as a termination of the contraction. The PFM should return at least to their resting state.

In addition to contracting the PFM, some individuals may benefit by combining contraction of both the PFM and the internal obturator muscle. This can be accomplished by having the patient stand with the feet turned outward and slightly more than hip-width apart. The individual is taught to do a plié by bending the knees 2–3 inches as he or she pulls up and in with the PFM. The patient should hold this position for 10 seconds, then return to an upright position and relax for 10 seconds. This may be a difficult exercise for older, unsteady women. Without sufficient information, the patient may mistakenly bear down or exercise ineffectively. Individuals are encouraged to aim for a high level of concentrated effort with each PFM contraction because greater contraction intensity is associated with improvement in pelvic muscle strength. Also important for control is to learn to sustain the PFM contraction, because the duration of the contraction builds strength. For muscle contractility to improve, the initial muscle strength, power, endurance, repetitions, and fatigue must be considered together with the principles of muscle training. Definitions of these terms are discussed in later in this chapter.

There are several ways to find the PFM, and the clinician should determine which way is most appropriate for any given patient (Newman & Wein, 2004). Among the techniques shown to be successful for this step are biofeedback (which requires instrumentation), verbal feedback during a pelvic examination (using vaginal or anal palpation), or pelvic floor electrical stimulation. A less time-consuming, but also less satisfactory, approach is to distribute a booklet or handout for the patient to read at home (Burgio et al., 2002). Without feedback, people may identify the wrong muscles, or exercise the correct muscles incorrectly. The following techniques for finding the PFM are recommended by the authors and should be considered:

- Everyone, at one time or another, has been in a crowded room and felt as if he or she were going to pass gas or "wind." Ask the patient to imagine that this is happening to him or her. Most will try to squeeze the muscles of the anus to prevent the passing of gas. In most of the individuals seen by one of the authors (DKN), especially in older women with decreased vaginal sensation, this has been found to be the most successful technique. Another example would have the patient imagine they have an egg in their rectum and they are trying to break it. In both cases, the muscles being squeezed are the PFM. If the patient feels a "pulling" sensation at the anus, he or she is using the correct muscles.

- A woman can lie down and insert a finger into the vagina. Tell her to tighten the muscle or "squeeze" around her finger using the vaginal muscles. The woman should be able to feel the sensation in the vagina and pressure on her finger. If she cannot detect any movement, then suggest she insert two fingers and repeat the technique.

- A sexually active woman can contract her PFM around her partner's penis during intercourse. If the correct muscles are contracted, the partner should feel the contraction pressure on his penis.

- A man can stand in front of a mirror and watch his penis, which should move up and down when contracting the PFM.

- Men and women can insert the tip of a finger into the anus and contract around the finger as though they are preventing a bowel movement or the release of gas. The patient should be able to feel the sensation in the anus, as well as the pressure on the finger.

Individuals should be cautioned not to perform regularly these exercises during voiding and not to stop and start urine flow as a form of exercising (see the patient education tool "Exercising Your Pelvic Floor Muscles" on the companion CD). This start/stop exercise has good face validity for effectiveness because many people initially report an inability to stop the urine flow when it begins. However, there is some controversy over this practice because it is nonphysiological, can affect bladder and urethral pressures during voiding, and can be harmful. It mimics detrusor–sphincter dyssynergia and may lead to urine being forced back up the ureters. Also, women should not overexercise the PFM because they can develop levator ani myalgia by performing excessive exercises (DeLancey, Sampselle, & Punch, 1993).

Implementing a PFMT Program

To be effective, PFMT (in the form of either repetitive exercise or an intentional contraction—the Knack) must include repeated correct contractions of the PFM, strengthening them in a regular, intensive, and long-lasting training program. For PFMT to be performed correctly, careful and specific training must occur. Two components are essential to success with PFMT:

1. Following a structured exercise program on a daily basis

2. Gradual increases of the amount and intensity of the exercises

It is important to select relevant starting positions, tailored to the individual, and training and functional activities must be incorporated into the training program as soon as possible. A process of advancement from awareness of isolated contractions to fully automatic controlled function of the pelvic floor during multiple complex tasks and activities is required. An individually tailored home exercise program focused on incorporation of activities of daily living is essential. In general, intensive training shows better results than a low-intensity program.

Individuals are given verbal and written instructions for a daily exercise home program that is based on the baseline assessment of the individual's PFM strength, contraction, and endurance during the initial assessment session. Most clinicians in this field have relied on the use of verbal and written instructions for people to use for home practice of PFMEs, not the use of a home biofeedback device (Figure 8.7). However, research on the benefits of the use of a biofeedback device to aid in performing these exercises at home is not conclusive (Mørkved, Bø, & Fjørtoft, 2002). Visual aids are helpful and should always be used when educating individuals (see Figure 8.6A and B).

Many protocols of training exist and can be selectively chosen for use. Although protocols differ in intensity, in group versus individual exercise sessions, and in degree of biofeedback assistance, all of the existing protocols have proved to be successful in fostering muscle strength and skill development (Borello-France, Zyczynski, Downey, Rause, & Wister, 2006; Chiarelli et al., 2003; Mørkved, Bø, Schei, & Salvesen, 2003; Newman, 2005b, 2007a).

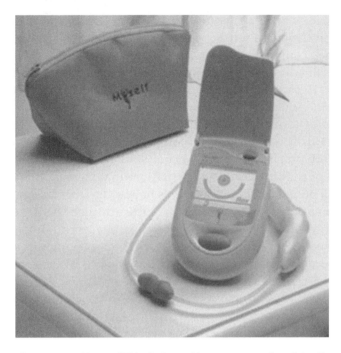

Figure 8.7. Home PFM device with pressure probe. (Myself-Dechutes Medical, Courtesy of *http://www.seeekwellness.com/.*)

Siu, Chang, Yip, and Chang (2003) demonstrated that a program of 30 contractions performed 3 times daily resulted in a reduction in mean monthly incontinence episodes from 79.7 to 19.9. Ultimately, protocol choice depends on individualized needs such as access to exercise groups and biofeedback, ability to allot time, and individual muscle capacity. Perhaps more important is the education of women about this hidden muscular structure—demystifying its function and building awareness both during and after pregnancy of potential disuse atrophy and childbirth-related injury.

Once the patient is able to identify the correct muscles, he or she is instructed to perform a series of quick flicks, or 2- to 3-second contractions, followed by sustained contractions of 5 seconds or longer (endurance contractions) as part of a daily exercise regimen. At least 10 seconds of relaxation is recommended between each sustained contraction. Extrapolation of exercise prescription guidelines suggests that PFMT should include both short- and long-duration exercises because both type I and type II muscle fibers need to be exercised with overload strategies. The frequency and the number of repetitions of exercises should be selected following assessment of the PFM. Daily regimens of increasing repetitions to the point of fatigue are most often recommended. The individual is encouraged to aim for a high level of concentrated effort with each PFM contraction because greater contraction intensity is associated with improvement in PFM strength. Muscle demands may be influenced by body position, because most people with UI will report urine leakage when performing the exercises while standing.

We prescribe a very structured and intense PFMT program. Patients are taught PFMT in the office setting where they can see their muscle contraction on a biofeedback computer screen (called biofeedback-assisted PFMT) (see Figure 8.9B). Initially, individuals are instructed to perform 30 quick (2-second) and sustained (10-second) exercises twice daily, divided over three positions: lying, sitting, and standing (see "Pelvic Floor Muscle Exercise Prescription" on the companion CD under Assessment Forms). Learning to control the PFM in different positions is essential because urgency can occur in any position, and people should be prepared to use their pelvic floor muscles whether sitting at a table or desk or walking around a shop. A gradual increase in number of contractions over a period of PFME practice is believed to increase muscle strength significantly and decrease urine loss. One of the authors (DKN) gives patients either an audiocassette tape or a CD that walks them through an additional 15 sustained (10-second) exercises (Figure 8.8). Self-monitoring through the use of a calendar record and audio- and videotaped material that cues the patient to perform the exercises can improve protocol compliance. Providing the individual with other "cues" to remember to perform these exercises can be helpful. The clinician can suggest that the patient practice the exercises at the same time of the day to establish a routine, or perform some exercises when waiting at a red light or watching television. Once the patient has mastered performing the exercises and is seeing an improvement in symptoms, one of the authors (DKN) recommends use of "the Knack."

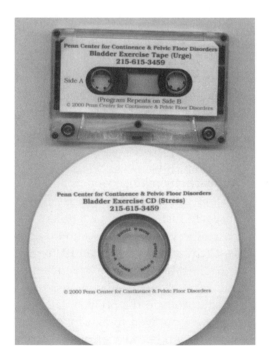

Figure 8.8.   Pelvic floor muscle exercise (PFME) audiocassette tape and CD.

Use of "the Knack"

Recognizing the correct use of a voluntary PFM contraction to prevent leakage prior to and during the activity or "stressor" triggering the incontinence is an acquired motor skill. Miller and colleagues called this contraction "the Knack" because the word *knack* means a clever way of doing a task that requires dexterity (Miller et al., 1998, 2001). Some women refer to this as "holding back." Miller et al. (1998) demonstrated that, during a deep or hard cough, the Knack reduced UI by 73.3%. A more recent study demonstrated that approximately 76.6% of women were able to reduce leakage during coughing by using the Knack maneuver and 18.8% of these women eliminated leakage (Miller et al., 2008). The Knack is the skill of consciously timing an intentional contraction of the PFM just before and throughout the activity that causes an increase in intra-abdominal pressure (Miller, Ashton-Miller, & Delancey, 1996). A strong, fast, well-timed voluntary PFM contraction will compress the urethra, preventing urethral descent and leakage during an increase in intra-abdominal pressure. This technique requires the patient to anticipate the urine leakage. Contracting the PFM before sneezing, coughing, lifting, standing up, or swinging a golf club can prevent SUI from occurring (see the patient education tool "Getting the 'Knack' for Stopping Urine Leaks" on the companion CD). This learned maneuver emphasizing skill and timing in functional performance (rather than strength development) is designed to complement an exercise program.

Some clinicians will instruct individuals on the Knack at the beginning of PFMT; the authors institute this technique once the patient has been exercising for a period of time and has seen symptoms improve. Usually at this point, patients may believe that their incontinence and OAB are so improved that regular exercising is no longer needed; however, they need to incorporate exercises into routine daily activities. Instructing them to perform the Knack is one way to incorporate these exercises because the goal would be that the muscles act automatically during increases in abdominal pressure, similar to a reflex action.

Use of the PFM to Decrease Urgency

The PFM also can be contracted when the individual feels a strong urge to void (called "urge suppression"). The patient is taught to relax the body, perform 5 quick PFM contractions (quick flicks), and focus concentration on the pelvic floor to suppress the sensation of urgency. When the detrusor contraction (and urgency) subsides, the patient is taught to walk at a normal pace to the bathroom. The patient can also combine PFM contractions with the distraction methods discussed in the section on bladder training. The goal is to interrupt the cycle of urgency and rushing, which, in addition to contributing to physical accidents (e.g., falling), also adds pressure on the bladder, increasing urgency and detrusor contractions and the probability of an incontinence accident.

Use of Biofeedback for PFMT

Biofeedback uses instrumentation to provide information regarding physiological processes. It is used with conservative treatments to show PFM contraction and relaxation and bladder contraction or relaxation to control urinary urgency, and when performing pelvic floor electrical stimulation. Biofeedback-assisted PFMT with urge suppression techniques has been shown to improve the psychological burden of UUI in older, community-dwelling women with a history of depression (Tadic et al., 2007). Biofeedback-assisted PFMT teaches the patient how to control the external sphincter by measuring the action of the PFM and "feeding back" to the patient information about how well the muscles are performing. This information is displayed in a form understandable to the patient to permit self-regulation of these events, and relayed back to the patient in the form of sound, lights, or images (Figure 8.9). There are several manufacturers of biofeedback systems (e.g., Prometheus, Dover, NH; Hollister, Libertyville, IL; Laborie, Burlington, VT) (Figures 8.9A and 8.10), and some systems have been specifically developed for pediatric use (Figure 8.11).

Biofeedback can be multichannel, which allows the simultaneous display of the contractions of the PFM and the inhibition of accessory muscles (e.g., abdominal muscle contractions). These measurements are immediately accessible and can be interpreted simultaneously by both the clinician and the individual. Dr. Kathy Burgio, a behavioral psychologist, has researched extensively the use of multichannel measurement of bladder, vaginal, and rectal signals for physical therapies such as PFMT and behavior modification with BT and urge suppression strategies. Using biofeedback, the individual is able to visualize the inappropriateness of rectal and bladder pressure with simultaneous contraction of the external anal sphincter, and is able to learn to suppress the sphincter contractions.

Biofeedback therapy is also used as treatment for muscle dysfunction (abnormality). Biofeedback-assisted treatment may be helpful for muscles that have increased tension even when the patient or clinician cannot detect it. This is particularly true of the PFM because denervation damage may lead to impaired sensation. High levels of resting activity and fleeting muscle spasms may only be visualized using biofeedback instruments. A biofeedback-assisted exercise program that stabilizes the PFM can reduce or eliminate symptoms of chronic pelvic pain and vulvodynia.

Biofeedback Methods

Biofeedback therapy uses either electromyography (EMG) or manometric pressure. Electromyography graphs the electrical activity of a muscle during contraction and relaxation, and as a practical indicator of muscle activity has been defined as

• The study of electrical potentials generated by the depolarization of muscle

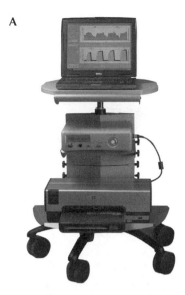

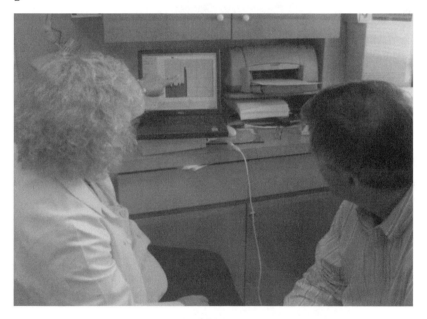

Figure 8.9A,B.   EMG biofeedback session using the Prometheus Feedback System.

- A monitor of bioelectrical activity correlating to motor unit activity; it does not measure the muscle contractility itself but rather the electrical correlate of the muscle contraction
- An indicator of the physiological activity of muscle

Electromyography measures the electrical activity of a muscle in microvolts (μV). Activity is measured through surface EMG (referred to as "sEMG")

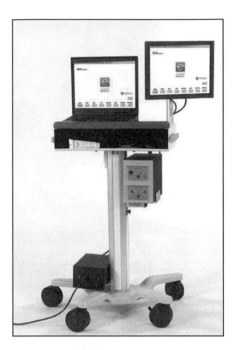

Figure 8.10. Evadri Bladder Control System. (Courtesy of Hollister, Libertyville, IL.)

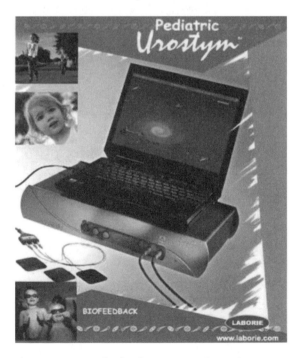

Figure 8.11. Biofeedback equipment for pediatric use. (Courtesy of Laborie Technologies, Burlington, VT.)

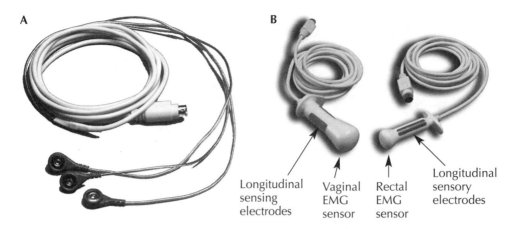

Longitudinal sensing electrodes Vaginal EMG sensor Rectal EMG sensor Longitudinal sensory electrodes

Figures 8.12. Surface skin electrodes used for EMG measurement of the pelvic floor muscles and vaginal and rectal sensors with longitudinal sensing electrodes. (Courtesy of Prometheus, Dover, NH.)

using electrodes placed on the skin (Figure 8.12A) or sensors that are inserted into the vagina or rectum. The sensing electrodes for the internal probes can either be longitudinal or circular and come in different lengths (Figure 8.12B). People may find the internal sensors uncomfortable, preferring the use of external skin electrodes. One of the authors (DKN) prefers surface EMG measurements when performing biofeedback-assisted PFMT.

Manometry is the use of an instrument to detect, assess, and record pressure. A pressure perineometer consists of a vaginal or rectal probe with a connector tube leading to a manometer (Theofrastous et al., 2002). The pressure changes can be measured in centimeters of water (cm H_2O) or millimeters of mercury (mm Hg). Depending on the sophistication of the equipment, the pressure changes may be shown on a dial, a digital readout, a bar chart, or a graphical representation. Different types of probes—air filled, water filled, individually made, and mass produced—have been developed, and manometry can be performed by inserting sensors into the vagina or the rectum (Figure 8.13).

Dr. Arnold Kegel first used the term *perineometer* for an intravaginal pressure gauge that demonstrated changes in pressure, observed on a manometer gauge, caused by the contraction of the PFM (Figure 8.14). He developed this instrument for both diagnosis and nonsurgical treatment for women with SUI and PFM relaxation. Although manometers and pressure sensors are available with certain clinical systems and have been used in several clinical trials, they are primarily used for treatment of rectal dysfunction, not for treatment of UI or OAB. Manometry is the only method of measuring internal sphincter resting tone in the anal canal. The internal anal sphincter is responsible for approximately 70%–80% of the resting tone in the anal canal. Measurement of the resting tone therefore provides an assessment of the internal anal sphincter function.

The advantage of EMG over manometric pressure is that, provided the machinery is of sufficient sophistication with adequate filtering, EMG apparatus

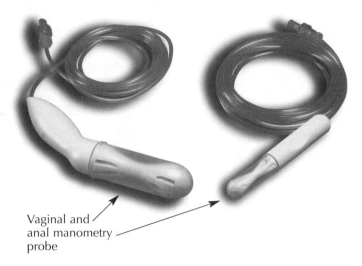

Vaginal and
anal manometry
probe

Figure 8.13.   Vaginal and rectal sensors. (Courtesy of Prometheus, Dover, NH.)

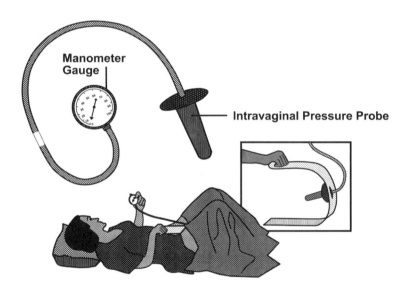

Figure 8.14.   Dr. Arnold Kegel's intravaginal perineometer. In the 1940s, a gauze strip was recommended to hold the Kegel perineometer in place so that the woman would not have to touch her genitalia. (Courtesy of Robin Noel.)

can engage the use of the newer types of electrodes that are lightweight and designed to stay in place, hence allowing more functional positions during assessment and treatment (Newman, 2003). Muscle training that utilizes EMG biofeedback may improve the effectiveness of the muscle relaxation efforts while strengthening weak PFM, thus reducing pain.

Measurement Parameters

To determine outcome of PFMEs, the two most important indices, which can be recorded by EMG or manometry, are the peak muscle contraction value (strength) and the average muscle contraction (endurance). They and several other indices are described as follows:

- *Strength*—recorded as the peak maximum pressure (the highest wave-forms) and the ability to sustain or hold the contraction.

- *Contractibility*—the rate of the original rise of the muscle contraction.

- *Power*—the ability of the muscle to "contract–relax" as quickly and strongly as possible, until the muscle fatigues; these are often called "quick flicks."

- *Endurance*—the time (up to 10 seconds) that the maximum muscle contraction can be maintained or repeated before a reduction in power of 50% or more is detected. In other words, the muscle contraction is timed until the muscle fatigues. Comparing subsequent contractions to an initial or baseline level of muscle strength can determine a muscle endurance index.

- *Repetitions*—the number of repetitions (up to 10) of the muscle contraction of equal force that can be achieved. At least a 5-second muscle relaxation period should be used between each contraction, because easily fatigable muscles need a chance to recover, without permitting excessive rest periods for strong muscles.

- *Fatigue*—failure to maintain the required or expected force of the PFM contraction for more than one or two times in succession.

EMG Measurement of Lower Urinary Tract Dysfunction

Four methods of EMG measurements have been used in the investigation of lower urinary tract dysfunction:

- Surface electrodes (sEMG)

  Vaginal sensor

  Anal or rectal sensor or plug electrode

  Adhesive skin electrodes

- Needle electrodes

  Vaginal and anal sensors are designed to provide accurate detection of EMG muscle activity. When using an internal sensor, only a small amount of water-soluble lubricant (e.g., K-Y jelly) should be used on the tip of the sensor to facilitate insertion. Too much lubricant may

- Coat the sensing surfaces

- Cause inaccurate measurements

- Cause the sensor to be expelled on muscle contraction

Before inserting the rectal sensor, the anal canal is dilated with a lubricated index finger as the sensor is introduced into the canal with the other hand. After insertion, a few minutes are allowed for the surrounding tissue to adapt before taking a resting baseline muscle measure. If the rectum is full of stool, it may be difficult or impossible to advance the rectal sensor.

When the levator ani muscle is in spasm, passage of the sensors may be uncomfortable and not feasible. Instead, skin surface electrodes are used to perform an EMG. In addition, the use of vaginal or rectal sensors is contraindicated in the following cases:

- Active infection or genital disease
- Severe pelvic pain that causes discomfort with insertion of the sensor
- Pregnancy
- Recent (within last 6 months) pelvic or rectal surgery
- Untreated atrophic vaginitis
- Dyspareunia
- Menstruation
- Painful hemorrhoids

In these cases, the use of skin surface electrodes should be considered. Surface skin electrodes are relatively noninvasive and well tolerated. They give quantitative information about muscle activity rather than data for qualitative analysis. The authors use skin electrodes with elderly women with vaginal atrophy. The first choice of electrode placement is at the 3 and 9 o'clock positions on either side of the anus (Figure 8.15). Electrodes should be placed close to the anus without touching another sensor or without sensors overlapping. Prior to electrode placement, assess for the presence of the following:

- *Hair*—To ensure an adequate electrode adhesive connection to the skin, hair around the anus may have to be trimmed or clipped. Do not shave the hair because shaving may cause irritation.
- *Scars*—Electrodes should not be placed over scars.
- *Hemorrhoids*—Clinical judgment must be used when deciding if the electrode can be positioned over a hemorrhoid. If the client has inflamed or large external hemorrhoids, alternate placement of electrodes can be at either the 10 and 4 o'clock or the 8 and 2 o'clock positions on either side of the anus.
- *Irritation or perineal dermatitis*—Electrodes should not be placed over areas of nonhealthy skin.

Needle electrodes are used during some urodynamic testing protocols and by neurologists to assess basic EMG characteristics of striated muscle.

The baseline and all follow-up EMG recordings should include two sets of measurements:

- First Set:

    Maximum or "short/quick" muscle contractions of 2-second duration.

    Resting muscle activity of 2-second duration.

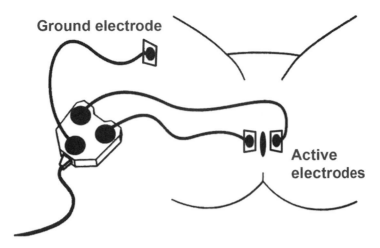

Ground electrode

Active electrodes

Figure 8.15.   Placement of surface skin electrodes at 3 and 9 o'clock on either side of the anus.

- Second Set:

    Sustained or "long" muscle contractions (5, 10, or 30 seconds). The clinician should not go directly from 3- to 10-second muscle contractions but increase in increments of 5 seconds as the individual's ability warrants.

    Resting muscle activity of 5-second duration or for the same length of time as muscle contraction.

    The ability to relax one's pelvic muscle following a contraction is of most importance if one is to gain control and coordination of these muscles.

Monitoring for Accessory Muscle Recruitment

When an additional muscle group is contracting at the same time as the PFM, it is called "recruitment." A common error in contracting the PFM is simultaneous contraction (called co-contraction) of the abdominal, gluteal, or hip adductor muscles. This may mask the strength of the PFM contraction and cause bladder neck and urethral descent (Bø, 2004a). Abdominal contraction increases intra-abdominal pressure that mechanically elevates bladder pressure, so it is important to measure concurrent use of abdominal contraction. Monitoring for accessory muscle recruitment during initial biofeedback and subsequent visits is necessary until recruitment stops, and should be considered in all individuals receiving PFMT. Signs indicating undesirable recruitment of these muscles include

- Holding of breath

- Tensing of stomach muscles

- Tensing of arms, legs, or both

- Lifting of heels off the floor

- Curling toes under

- Lifting up off of the chair (contracting gluteal muscles) or exam table

Treatment of PFM Dysfunction

There are two primary types of PFM dysfunction. *Low-tone* dysfunction is the clinical finding of an impaired ability to isolate and contract the pelvic floor muscles in the presence of weak and atrophic PFM. Ideally, the individual will gain the ability to recognize the difference between relaxation and contraction.

High-tone dysfunction refers to the clinical condition of hypertonic, spastic PFM with resultant impairment of muscle isolation, contraction, and relaxation. A high resting tone baseline with high variability and occasional spasms may be seen in people with chronic pelvic pain syndromes. In some cases, this excessive, elevated resting tone may be created unconsciously. Therapeutic exercise is important in the management of pelvic pain because often the patient has a reduced level of activity related to the prolonged nature of his or her pain. Rehabilitating the PFM can be central in resolving pain when muscle spasm is present. Using PFMT in patients with high tone to enhance muscle relaxation is referred to as "down training." Teaching a muscle to relax is often more difficult than teaching it how to contract ("up training") because the sensation of relaxation is weak.

Biofeedback Graphs

We perform EMG biofeedback–assisted PFMT in individuals with all types of UI, urgency, frequency, pelvic pain, and levator ani spasm. Figure 8.16A–E shows graphs from Diane Newman's Prometheus EMG system that provide examples of various muscle patterns seen during such training.

ADHERENCE TO BEHAVIORAL TREATMENT PROGRAMS

Improvement of symptoms with behavioral treatment is gradual and may take many months, leading to noncompliance or a lack of adherence to prescribed programs in many individuals. The clinician's greatest challenge when providing behavioral treatment is how to motivate the individuals he or she treats. As with most behavioral interventions, the relationship between the clinician and the patient being treated is very important to the success of behavioral or conservative treatments. Motivation and active participation also play a big part in the patient's success. It has been shown that incontinent women have diverse goals for incontinence treatment; in some cases, they may desire an improvement in urine leakage rather than continence (Sale &

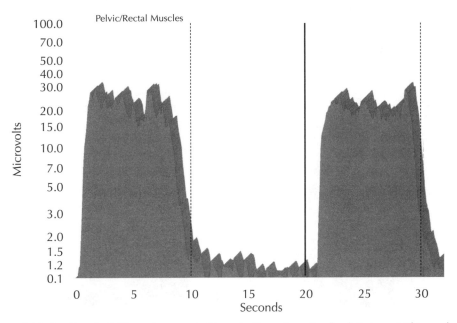

Figure 8.16. A. Sample EMG graphs generated from the Prometheus Feedback System. *A,* This graph depicts PFM contractions by use of active skin surface electrodes around the anus at 9 and 3 o'clock positions with the ground lead placed on a bony prominence (e.g., iliac crest). The waveform is measured in microvolts (µV). This graph indicates the ability to sustain muscle contractions for 10 seconds with significant muscle strength, bulk, and endurance. Maximum voluntary contraction was 29.9 µV (average 16.6 µV), with relaxation averaging 1.14 µV.

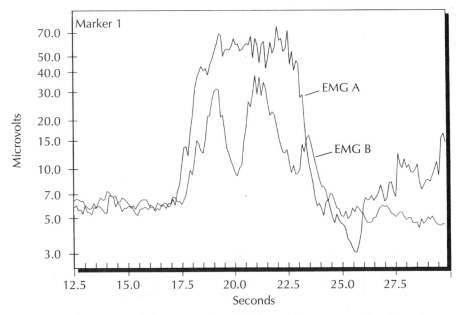

Figure 8.16. B. This EMG graph depicts two channels. Channel A measures PFM activity using a vaginal probe. Channel B measures abdominal activity through two active skin surface electrodes placed 1 inch apart just below the umbilicus, with a ground electrode on a bony prominence. This graph shows "co-contractions": both the pelvic floor and abdominal (accessory) muscles are being contracted simultaneously. The signal from the abdominal channel begins to increase in amplitude when the PFM are contracted. This reading indicates poor muscle isolation because the PFM are not isolated from the accessory abdominal muscle, as well as an inability to adequately relax muscles after pelvic muscle contraction, causing an increased resting level.

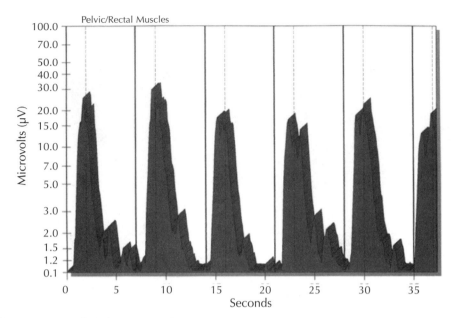

Figure 8.16. *C.* This EMG graph indicates the ability to perform quick (2- to 3-second) contractions ("flicks"). Average muscle contraction was 9.29 µV. Delayed ability or latency in returning the muscle to relaxation after each PFM contraction caused an increased resting level of 3.9 µV. The latency is the length of time from when the person was told to relax to the time the EMG measures return to baseline. The return to relaxation should occur within 1 second. In time this individual will be able to improve return to relaxation.

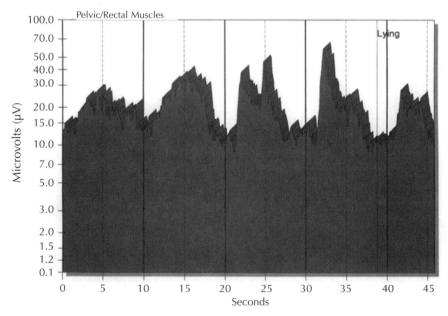

Figure 8.16. *D.* This EMG graph indicates the inability to relax the PFM, commonly referred to as levator ani spasm. This condition is commonly seen in patients with pelvic pain, or painful bladder syndrome. The tone of the muscle is considered to be elevated when resting level is above 3.0 µV. Average muscle contraction was 20.9 µV and relaxation was 16.7 µV. There was very little differentiation between contraction and relaxation.

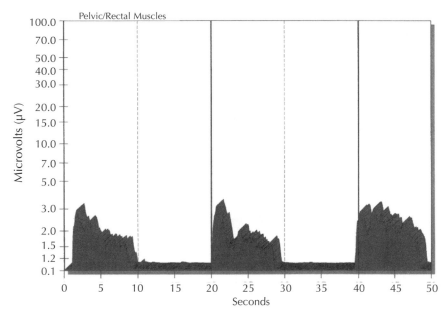

Figure 8.16. *E.* This EMG graph indicates the ability to make an initial PFM contraction, but the person is unable to sustain it. Many times this is referred to as "unstable" or weak PFM contraction. Average muscle contraction was 1.72 µV and relaxation was 0.53 µV. This graph shows good relaxation but overall weak PFM.

Wyman, 1994). Even though teaching people, particularly women, to strengthen the PFM as part of a comprehensive behavior program has been demonstrated to be effective in 50%–60% of women with UI and OAB, many women are not interested in performing these exercises. Even after being taught these interventions, there is the additional problem that many find too burdensome the daily exercises necessary to increase muscle strength and control and thus do not adhere to or comply with a prescribed program. As a result, the self-reported compliance rate for this therapy can be moderate to high, depending on the method (group vs. individual instruction) or the patient's expectations of the treatment (Palmer, 2004; Sampselle et al., 2005). This can be frustrating to clinicians who provide these treatments, because poor outcome may be secondary to noncompliance and out of their control.

To improve treatment compliance, the clinician must monitor the individual's progress on a regular basis, so follow-up visits are important. The clinician should provide praise and encouragement where appropriate. The use of a signed agreement or "contract" with the individual stating personal outcome goals can be helpful in motivating him or her to adhere to the program, and it also outlines expectations. Because forgetting to do PFMEs is a common excuse for noncompliance, any aid that can be used to remind the patient would be helpful. Ip (2004) gave men a "Continence Magnet" that provided instructions on performing these exercises and was a visible reminder because it could be hung on a refrigerator.

EFFICACY OF BEHAVIORAL
OR CONSERVATIVE TREATMENTS—THE EVIDENCE

There is sufficient evidence-based research to support the effectiveness of conservative or behavioral interventions, and this evidence has grown since the first edition of this book (Wilson et al., 2005). Several randomized, controlled trials and systematic reviews have confirmed that PFMT is an effective treatment for SUI and mixed UI, especially when compared to usual care. Cure and improvement rates are reported to be between 56% and 70% (Hay-Smith et al., 2006; Wilson et al., 2005). There has been increasing information on the use of these interventions in certain populations (e.g., pregnant women, men after prostatectomy). There is also new available research on prevention of UI using PFMT. The basic debate regarding efficacy of PFMT involves the added benefit of adjunct techniques such as biofeedback using EMG, or other methods such as pelvic floor electrical stimulation. Another concern is that most research on these interventions included testing multiple therapies in combination (e.g., BT + PFMT and biofeedback; lifestyle change + BT + PFMT and biofeedback), so difficulty arises concerning whether any single intervention is the cause of the outcome. The Third International Consultation on Incontinence committee on "Adult Conservative Management" has labeled behavioral treatment as conservative treatment, defined as any treatment that does not require drugs or surgery (Wilson et al., 2005). They have labeled combinations of behavior therapies as "Conservative Management Packages," noting Level 1 evidence (good-quality research) indicating very good efficacy. They also noted that these are low-cost and low-risk interventions. A recent extensive review of randomized controlled trials indicated that "moderate levels of evidence suggest that pelvic floor muscle training and bladder training resolved urinary incontinence in women" (Shamliyan, Kane, Wyman, & Wilt, 2008, p. 11).

Research in both men and women with UI and OAB is extensive, detailing the efficacy of the use of biofeedback-assisted behavior therapy with PFMT. However, debate continues over the use of adjuncts such as biofeedback therapy. The consensus is that conservative therapy combining lifestyle changes, toileting or BT programs, and PFMT with or without biofeedback is most effective when provided by a clinician who specializes in the area of pelvic floor dysfunction (see Chapter 13). Clinician-supervised PFMT with biofeedback is thought to provide the most favorable long-term results, and many multidisciplinary pelvic floor dysfunction or "continence" centers provide these services (Dougherty et al., 2002; Newman, 2006). Dougherty et al. (2002) instituted a behavior management for continence program provided by nurse practitioners for women living in rural counties in Florida. This program was a stepped intervention: 1) self-monitoring, 2) BT, and 3) biofeedback-assisted PFMEs. This program had the greatest impact on urine loss; at the 2-year follow-up, the severity of incontinence in the intervention group had decreased by 61%, whereas the severity in the control group had increased by 84%.

There has also been research noting the success of these interventions in frail older adults residing in their homes (Colling et al., 2003). Augmenting drug therapy with a supervised BT program is considered to yield the best outcomes in the treatment of UUI and OAB. The authors have attempted to review the current research on these different "packages," highlighting the research that has been published since the first edition of this book. The research on the use of lifestyle changes can be found in Chapter 7, and the outcomes of toileting, PV, and BT can be found earlier in this chapter.

Behavior Therapy

Taken together, the randomized controlled trial evidence for the efficacy of PFMT is strong. Typically more than 75% of studies reported improvement of UI symptoms at levels that exceeded 50% (Sampselle, 2003). Research is extensive detailing the efficacy of the use of biofeedback-assisted behavior therapy for PFMT that included BT and lifestyle changes. The 1996 clinical practice guideline *Urinary Incontinence in Adults* (Fantl et al., 1996) outlined the research that demonstrated that PFMT is indicated for people with SUI and can reduce urgency and prevent UUI. PFM reeducation has proved to be effective in women with sphincter deficiency and detrusor instability.

Use of PFMT for Prevention of Childbirth-Related Incontinence

Three systematic reviews on the prevention of UI in postnatal women provide persuasive evidence demonstrating the protective effect of PFMT (primarily with biofeedback) practiced in relation to pregnancy and childbirth (Harvey, 2003; Hay-Smith, Herbison, & Mørkved, 2002; Wilson et al., 2005). Several carefully controlled randomized trials have shown significantly lower incidence of UI up to 6 months postpartum (Mørkved et al., 2003). Dr. Carolyn Sampselle, nurse researcher at the University of Michigan, has studied the effect of PFMT on women before, during, and after childbirth (Sampselle et al., 1998; Sampselle, Palmer, Boyington, O'Dell, & Wooldridge, 2004). Her research has shown that, if nulliparous women are taught PFMT at 20 weeks' gestation, they are less likely to experience UI at 6 weeks and 6 months postpartum. Reilly et al. (2002) found that women demonstrated less UI 3 months after childbirth if they participated in supervised PFMT prenatally. Mørkved et al. (2003) randomized nulligravid women to either supervised PFMT or routine care. The supervised group were 39% less likely to report UI at 3 months postpartum than were those women who received routine care. Results in this study showed that PFMT during pregnancy prevented UI in 1 in 6 women during pregnancy and 1 in 8 women after delivery. Moreover, the effectiveness of PFMT in preventing childbirth-related UI, in conjunction with the noninvasive nature of this self-care strategy, makes it a logical focus for UI prevention efforts among women during the period of childbearing. However, a systematic review of unassisted PFMT following childbirth indicated that long-term compliance may be a problem (Wagg & Bunn, 2007).

Clinical recommendations are that women experiencing UI during pregnancy and in the postpartum period should be encouraged to participate in a PFMT program and should be advised to practice PFMEs antenatally and postnatally. Also, PFMT programs should be multifaceted, with a number of components (e.g., digital muscle assessment to determine that the woman can perform a PFM contraction, visits with a health care professional), rather than supplying printed information only.

PFMT in Men

SUI in men is common initially after prostate surgery (radical prostatectomy). In 1998, urologist Judd Moul published data showing that PFMT after prostatectomy may assist men in decreasing UI. Since then there has been some promising research to show the benefit of this intervention pre- and postsurgery (Burgio et al., 2006; Cornel, de Wit, & Witjes, 2005; Filocamo et al., 2005; Manassero et al., 2007). A study of men with UI following radical prostate surgery showed that 88% of the treatment group achieved continence in 3 months using PFMEs, compared to 56% of the control group (Van Kampen et al., 2000). Hunter, Moore, Cody, and Glazener (2004) concluded that there may be some benefit in offering biofeedback-assisted PFMT early in the postoperative period, immediately following removal of the catheter, because it may promote an earlier return to continence. Burgio et al. (2006) conducted a randomized controlled study in 125 men who were scheduled for radical prostatectomy. The men in the treatment group received a single preoperative session of biofeedback-assisted PFMT and had a significantly decreased severity of postoperative incontinence and time to continence. A recent review of randomized trials has concluded that men receiving biofeedback-assisted PFMT were more likely to achieve continence or have no continual urine leakage than those with no training within 1–2 months after radical prostatectomy (MacDonald, Fink, Huckabay, Monga, & Wilt, 2007). The authors have collaborated in the design of a postprostatectomy protocol, detailed in Figure 8.17, that includes an EMG biofeedback–assisted program instituted in the early postoperative period.

Behavioral Intervention in Older Adults

There has also been some research using these treatments in older adults (Burgio et al., 1998; Engberg et al., 2002). Tannebaum, Bachand, Dubeau, and Kuchel (2001) conducted a study of 52 women ages 65–98 years (average age 80 years) using lifestyle change and PFMT treatment, based on the individual's or caregiver's preference. Forty-five women (86%) were available for follow-up 6 months after their final visit to the clinic (45% with UUI, 33% with mixed UI and SUI, and 22% with other incontinence symptoms, including impaired bladder emptying). Of these 45 women, 30% reported being cured, 30% reported improvement, 20% were the same, and 20% were worse. Significant reductions in incontinence symptoms were achieved regardless of advanced

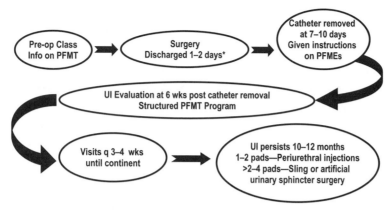

Figure 8.17. Postprostatectomy UI protocol, including an EMG biofeedback–assisted program, instituted in the early postoperative period.

age, type of UI, or type of treatment. All women with worsening symptoms reported noncompliance with treatment recommendations at the time of the follow-up interview. Perrin, Dauphinée, Corcos, Hanley, and Kuchel (2005) conducted a small ($n = 10$) sample uncontrolled study in women older than 75 who underwent six biofeedback-assisted behavioral treatment sessions. Results indicated a decrease in the number of UI and urgency episodes.

Combination Behavior Therapy

Combining BT and PFMT in a Behavioral Protocol for Prevention of UI

Diokno et al. (2004) studied the preventive effect on continent older women of a behavioral protocol of PFMT and BT in an initial group session with individualized follow-up sessions. There were 359 subjects (treatment group, $n = 164$; control group, $n = 195$), with an age range from 55 to 80 years. The treatment group underwent a group teaching session (taught by a urologist [Ananias Diokno] and a nurse [Carolyn Sampselle]) consisting of a 2-hour program with handouts and slides that included basic information on UI, details of BT and PFMT, effect of UI on lifestyle, and guidance on how to comply with the program. The women were guided through a session on how to perform PFMEs and given an audiotape that cued these exercises. They then underwent individual sessions to evaluate and ensure proper exercise technique. At the end of 12 months, women who learned the behavioral protocol were twice as likely to remain continent compared with the control group.

Behavioral Treatment with and without Biofeedback

The added benefit of biofeedback to PFMT has not been well shown. The most often quoted study was conducted by Burgio and colleagues (2002). Women ($n = 222$) who had UUI were randomized to the following groups:

Group 1 received behavioral training that consisted of BT and PFMT with biofeedback. In addition to a PFMT home program, they had four clinic visits at 2-week intervals with trained nurse practitioners.

Group 2 received behavioral training without biofeedback but with digital PFM assessment with information on muscle isolation and correct identification, and were given a home program of PFMT.

Group 3 was given a 20-page self-administered booklet that included an 8-week step-by-step program, with self-help instructions on BT and PFMT.

Results indicated that the outcomes of the three groups were not significantly different. Group 1 had a 63.1% reduction in frequency of UI episodes, group 2 had a 69.4% reduction in frequency of UI episodes, and group 3 had a 58.6% reduction in frequency of UI episodes. However, individuals' perceptions of treatment were significantly better for groups 1 and 2 because the group receiving the self-help booklet reported the lowest satisfaction.

Behavior Therapy Combined with Drug Therapy

One of the drawbacks of behavioral training is that, although most people see improvement in symptoms, most do not achieve full freedom from incontinence episodes; in fact, on average, only 20%–30% will become dry. One strategy to enhance outcomes is to combine behavioral training with drug therapy, because some data suggest that these approaches work through different mechanisms. There is evidence that drug therapy increases bladder capacity, whereas results with behavior therapy can be achieved without urodynamic changes.

As noted earlier in this chapter, there is some research to show the benefit of combination drug therapy and a toileting program in LTC residents. This research is even more extensive in community-dwelling individuals (primarily women), in whom combination therapy is the recommendation for first-line therapy in this group. Burgio, Locher, and Goode (2000) examined the effects of combined treatments on 197 women who were 55 years of age or older with UUI or urge-dominant mixed incontinence. They were randomly assigned to receive, over an 8-week period, four sessions of behavioral training with biofeedback, immediate-release oxybutynin (2.5–5.0 mg 3 times a day), or a placebo control condition. In this trial, behavioral training reduced incontinence episodes significantly more than drug treatment (mean 80.7% vs. 68.5%, respectively), and both were significantly more effective than placebo. Participant satisfaction and perceptions of improvement were higher for behavioral treatment.

Goode et al. (2002) compared biofeedback-assisted behavioral training to medical treatment (oxybutynin chloride, individually titrated) in a group of 105 older women (mean age 67 years) with SUI, UUI, or mixed UI. Behavioral training achieved an 82.3% reduction in frequency of incontinence accidents, compared with a 78.3% reduction achieved in the drug treatment group and a 51.5% reduction in the control group (no treatment).

Burgio and colleagues (2000) wanted to determine the effects of the addition of either behavioral training or drug therapy. In a conditional crossover-design study, women who initially were treated with 8 weeks of behavioral training or oxybutynin (immediate release) and were not satisfied with their results or were not completely dry were offered the option to add the other treatment to their existing therapy. In both groups, the combination treatment improved outcomes. Women initially receiving behavioral training had a 57.5% reduction in incontinence episodes; with combined treatment, this increased to 88.5%. Similarly, women initially treated with oxybutynin had a 73% reduction in incontinence episodes; with the combination, this increased to 84%. For both groups, the difference between monotherapy and combined therapy was significant.

The results of another study reported that combination therapy of duloxetine and PFMT was more efficacious in reducing SUI episodes (in women) than either therapy alone (Ghoniem et al., 2005).

USING WEIGHTS TO STRENGTHEN PFM

Vaginal weights (often called vaginal cones) are another example of a biofeedback technique that educates women on contraction of the PFM. They have been most successful in woman with SUI. They are often used as part of a structured resistive PFME program. Theoretically, when the weight is placed in the vagina, it provides sensory feedback and prompts a PFM contraction to keep it from slipping out. Maintaining the muscle contraction required to hold the weight in the vagina strengthens pelvic muscles. General PFMEs should be practiced in addition to the use of weights. There are also commercially available intravaginal resistive devices that can be used at home to aid in strengthening the PFM.

Vaginal weights are designed for one-person use, and careful washing and drying between uses will ensure the necessary cleanliness. These weights are generally accepted by women of all ages. Their use is contraindicated during menstruation and infection. The weights are either made of plastic or made of metal that is placed in a plastic casing (Figure 8.18). They are shaped like a cone and come in increasing weights. Each weight has a nylon string attached through the end of the outer plastic case to help remove it. The rounded portion is inserted first. The woman should assume a semisquatting position or stand with one foot on a chair to facilitate insertion. It is advisable to wear underwear while using the weights.

The user is instructed to insert the lightest weight into the vagina, in the position of a tampon. It should be inserted so that it cannot be felt protruding from the opening of the vagina. The woman then practices holding that weight in by contracting the PFMs; this exercise is done for up to 15 minutes twice per day. When the woman can successfully hold this cone, she is told

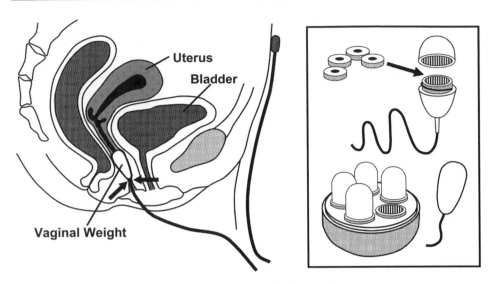

Figure 8.18.   Type of vaginal weight (cone). (Courtesy of Robin Noel).

to switch to a heavier one. The weights are worn while standing up or walking, and the exercise should be done twice per day. If a woman keeps the weight in place, she knows that she is using her pelvic muscles correctly. To increase the exercise value of these weights, the woman is instructed to practice retaining the weight during coughing, jumping, or any stress-provoking act that causes incontinence.

The perceived advantages of vaginal weight training are that it involves less teaching time, can be self-taught, may be motivational, and can be used with minimal supervision. There is strong evidence that indicates it is an effective treatment for SUI in pre- and postmenopausal women (Wilson et al., 2005). However, the evidence is inconclusive regarding the superiority of vaginal weight training over PFMEs alone or pelvic floor electrical stimulation. Furthermore, there appears to be no added benefit to the use of vaginal weight training with PFMEs (Herbison, Plevnik, & Mantle, 2002). Although vaginal weight training may take less instructional time in terms of office practice, it may be less acceptable to some women than PFMT alone. Reasons for not using vaginal weights are aesthetic dislike, unpleasantness, discomfort, difficulty of insertion, or bleeding (Wyman, 2003).

PELVIC FLOOR ELECTRICAL STIMULATION

Discovered in 1963 when an electrode was first implanted into the periurethral muscles, pelvic floor electrical stimulation (PFES) or neuromuscular electrical stimulation involves the application of low-grade electrical stimulation to the PFM. PFES has a twofold action: contraction of the PFM and inhibition of unwanted detrusor contractions. Electrical stimulation can activate inhibitory nerve fibers, causing reflex inhibition of the detrusor muscle and thereby preventing bladder overactivity. There is also an effect on the striated PFM, causing hypertrophy of the muscles by recruiting the PFM fast-twitch fibers. PFES for incontinence is thought to work by stimulating the pudendal nerve afferents, with the efferents causing the striated pelvic muscle to contract. It is believed that the striated muscle action inhibits inappropriate detrusor activity. Nonimplantable devices can be applied to the legs, vagina, anus, and PFM to treat SUI, UUI, mixed UI, and OAB. Implantable stimulation (neuromodulation) (see Chapter 12) is applied to sacral nerve roots. PFES is used as an adjunct treatment to

- Assist with identification and isolation of PFM

- Increase PFM strength

- Decrease unwanted or uninhibited detrusor (bladder) muscle contraction

- Assist with normalizing PFM relaxation

Efficacy with vaginal PFES is about 50% (Amaro, Gameiro, Kawano, & Padovani, 2006; Wilson et al., 2005). The ICI has noted that there is no extra benefit in adding PFES to PFMT (Wilson et al., 2005).

The delivery of the electric current to the tissues is via an electrode placed on the surface of the skin (called "transcutaneous electrical stimulation," where skin electrodes are placed suprapubic, perineum, or anus) or by vaginal or rectal sensors, and the technique is used in conjunction with biofeedback. Electrical stimulation can be performed in the clinician's office or may be prescribed as a home program using a battery-operated home unit (Figure 8.19). The home program consists of using the portable stimulator for 15 minutes twice a day for several weeks to months, although the length of time and number of treatments are highly variable. Several units are available. It is recommended that the patient perform PFES initially in the side-lying position until he or she becomes comfortable changing to the seated position. However, with the wide variations in stimulation parameters, including time, intensity, and frequency of sessions, it is difficult to make comparisons across studies.

Given the equivocal results, the benefit of PFES in SUI, UUI, and mixed UI in women remains controversial (Wilson et al., 2005). Goode and colleagues (2003) conducted a trial in women with SUI, randomizing them to three groups: behavioral training, behavioral training plus PFES, and a self-help booklet. Treatment with PFES did not increase effectiveness of behavioral training. McClurg, Ashe, Marshall, and Lowe-Strong (2006) found the combination of biofeedback-assisted behavioral training and PFES to be more effective than biofeedback-assisted behavioral training alone in women ($n = 30$) with multiple sclerosis and UI and OAB symptoms.

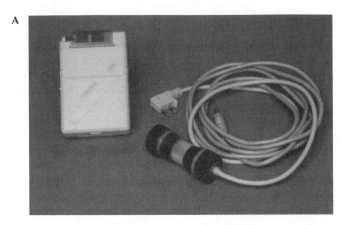

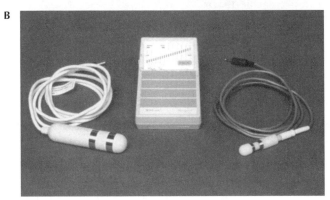

Figure 8.19. *A.* Minnova pelvic floor electrical stimulation home unit. (Courtesy of Empi, St. Paul, MN.) *B,* InCare Microgyn Plus home electrical stimulation unit with vaginal and rectal sensors. (Courtesy of Hollister, Libertyville, IL.)

Key Parameters of PFES

The parameters of most stimulation units include the amplitude of the current intensity, the ramping of impulses, the pulse frequency rate, and the on/off timing. These are defined as follows:

1. *Amplitude* is the intensity of the electric current. The amplitude (Amp) should be individualized and must be sufficient to cause the patient's anus to contract reflexively, or create an "anal wink." The current reaching the muscle is nontherapeutic if there is not an anal wink.

2. *Ramping* is the ability of the electric current to reach the muscle either quickly or slowly. The more gradually the current rises to the preset amplitude or threshold level, the more comfortable the PFES may feel to the individual. Likewise, the more aggressive the ramp-up, or the more vertical the ramping-up signal, the more likely a patient may experience discomfort. The typical setting for most PFES units is 0.5 ramps, with the

ramp-down being automatically set as the ramp-up is set. If the patient complains of discomfort at these settings, it is advisable to adjust the ramping as opposed to adjusting the amplitude.

3. The *frequency rate* (pulses per second [pps]) refers to the number of pulses that are generated per unit of time (seconds). The optimal frequency of PFES is determined by how quickly the impulses pass through the nerve being targeted (conduction velocity). The pps frequency rate is contingent on the diagnosis:

    Stress = 50 pps
    Urge = 13 pps

4. *On/off time* is also known as the duty cycle. "On" time is the amount of time that the muscle is exposed to the electric current. "Off" time is the amount of time when there is no electric current to the muscle, allowing it to recover. The ratio of "on" time to "off" time (duty cycle ratio) that allows the muscle to recover is determined by the clinician using the following guidelines:

    a. At no time should the ratio of exposure to the electric current to non-exposure be more than 1:1; in other words, time off should never be less than time on.

    b. In many cases, a 1:2 ratio, 1 being time on and 2 being time off, will be the most appropriate (e.g., 5 seconds on, 10 seconds off). This is especially true in the beginning stages of therapy when the individual has very weak muscle strength or when a frequency of 35 Hz or more is selected. This will minimize muscle fatigue.

There are no adverse side effects to electrical stimulation of the PFM, but PFES is contraindicated in the following situations:

*   Complete denervation of the pelvic floor (PFM will not respond)
*   Dementia
*   Demand cardiac pacemaker
*   Unstable or serious cardiac arrhythmia
*   Pregnancy or planning/attempting pregnancy
*   Rectal bleeding
*   Active infection (urinary tract/vaginal)
*   Unstable seizure disorder
*   Swollen, painful hemorrhoids
*   Presence of vaginal vault prolapse
*   Pelvic surgery in the past 6 months

Use of PFES in Specific Populations

People with SUI

PFES of the pudendal nerve at a relatively high frequency can cause a PFM contraction through a pudendal nerve reflex loop. The majority of the nerve fibers that supply the muscle of the urethra operate at relatively high frequencies of 50–100 Hz. This is the rationale for the use of 50 Hz or 50 pps in PFES. It causes

- A direct motor response to the muscle (limited)

- A reflex widespread contraction of the PFM

    PFES improves the function of the urethral and levator ani muscle groups. These include the smooth muscle and striated muscle types. It is postulated that stimulation in people with SUI

- Increases the proportion of fast-twitch fibers

- Increases the number and strength of slow-twitch fibers, improving resting urethral closure

- Improves recruitment of PFM fibers when doing voluntary muscle contractions

    If a patient with SUI initially experiences increased urine leakage on receiving PFES, it may be due to muscle fatigue. To decrease muscle fatigue:

- Reduce the amount of time or session length of PFES.

- Select a less aggressive duty cycle (on/off time) ratio: instead of 1:1, select 1:2.

- Do not reduce intensity because, in order to achieve a therapeutic effect, the intensity level must elicit a muscle contraction.

People with UUI

Bladder inhibition occurs through a pudendal nerve–to–pelvic nerve (afferent–efferent) reflex and a pudendal nerve–to–hypogastric nerve reflex. The application of electric current to the PFM produces a reflex muscle contraction without any effort on the part of the individual. This muscle contraction, produced by PFES, is a useful addition to PFMEs in the rehabilitation of weakened pelvic floor muscles and is very beneficial for both men and women who are unable to contract these muscles on command, because it leads to an improved comprehension of the activity of the muscles and subsequently better active contraction. The pudendal nerve–to–pelvic nerve reflex inhibits bladder contractions. Frequencies of 15 Hz or less induce bladder inhibition via the pudendal nerve–to–hypogastric nerve reflex. Nerves that innervate the bladder (sacral afferent sensory nerves) tend to be composed of poorly myelinated C fibers. These fibers conduct at a slow rate. This is the rationale for using the frequency rate of 13 Hz or 13 pps for UUI.

PFES probably decreases detrusor overactivity in the following manner:

• Stimulation of the reflex systems, which influence the urethra and the PFM during detrusor contractions

• Improved reflex inhibition of the bladder as a result of stronger PFM

• Reorganization or reeducation of neural pathways that provide central or peripheral control

Many clinical studies have reported a "carryover effect" of PFES in the treatment of UUI for up to 5 years. Some individuals see an increase in urine leakage for the first week as a result of increased sensory input. This usually resolves itself.

People with Chronic Pelvic Pain Syndrome

Pain relief occurs at selected frequencies of PFES. This technique is used to produce rhythmic contraction and relaxation of the PFM, which may reduce muscle spasm and trigger points by fatiguing the muscle and restoring a more normal pattern of muscle activity. The repeated contractions may also help to disperse products of inflammation caused by chronic muscle spasm. PFES may give immediate reduction in the level of pain early in treatment, allowing the patient to participate more fully in the treatment program, and giving hope that treatment will be effective.

TIBIAL NERVE STIMULATION

Posterior tibial nerve stimulation (PTNS) is another type of stimulation used primarily in women with UI or other voiding dysfunctions. The posterior tibial nerve contains L4–S3 nerve fibers and originates from the same sacral nerve root of the spinal cord that innervates the bladder. PTNS was first invented by Dr. Marshall Stoller and was first known as the "SANS" protocol.

The procedure involves locating the posterior tibial nerve above the medial malleolus and inserting a 34-gauge, percutaneous solid needle several inches (Figure 8.20). A ground surface electrode is placed over the ipsilateral calcaneus. The needle is connected to a low-voltage stimulator. Stimulation of the nerve results in a sensory response causing a tickling sensation in the sole of the big toe and a motor response causing plantar flexion of the big toe and fanning of the remaining toes. If the big toe bends downward with stimulation, the needle's placement is ideal. The treatment protocol includes weekly 30-minute visits for 12 weeks. Outcomes for PTNS are difficult to determine because there are few studies with only small numbers of subjects, and the studies are uncontrolled and have no long term follow-up (Vandoninck et al., 2003). Preliminary data show a 50% reduction in UI episodes and around a 25% reduction in urinary frequency.

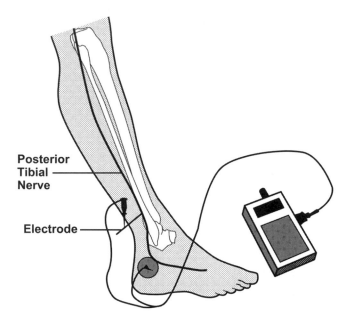

Figure 8.20.   Posterior tibial nerve stimulation for urgency and frequency symptoms using the Urgent PC Neuromodulation System. (Courtesy of Robin Noel.)

ACUPUNCTURE

Adapted from traditional Chinese medicine, acupuncture revolves around the concept of *qi* as the body's vital energy, with the idea that disruption in the flow of *qi* through the body is responsible for illness or a problem in the body's functioning. These areas of disruption are located and then stimulated with needles. One method of acupuncture treatment for UI involves two specific acupuncture pressure points on the body—*cilioa,* located over the sacrum, and *huiyang,* located over the coccyx—that regulate and activate the *qi* of the kidney and bladder. Needles are placed bilaterally in the inner legs, outer knee fold, low back, and mid-line at the lower abdomen and left in place from a few seconds to 20 minutes. Following insertion, needles are often stimulated manually or by a battery-powered electrical apparatus. Needling sensations vary but can include aching, pressure, soreness, fullness, distention, numbness, tingling, and local warm or cool sensations. Very few side effects have been reported. Treatments are usually weekly for 6–12 weeks.

The Western view of acupuncture for use in UI is that it may modulate nervous system activity by modifying abnormal afferent impulses from the bladder to the spinal cord. A few small, uncontrolled studies have supported acupuncture as a successful treatment for UI and OAB (Emmons & Otto, 2005). Success (20%) or improvement (20%) has been achieved in small groups of women. Acupuncture appears to be well tolerated and may be a viable future option for treatment (O'Dell & McGee, 2006). However, randomized, controlled studies are needed (Wilson et al., 2005).

REFERENCES

Amaro, J.L., Gamiero, M.O., Kawano, P.R., & Padovani, C.R. (2006). Intravaginal electrical stimulation: A randomized, double-blind study on the treatment of mixed urinary incontinence. *Acta Obstetricia et Gynecologica Scandinavica, 85,* 619–622.

Ashton-Miller, J.A., Howard, D., & DeLancey, J.O. (2001). The functional anatomy of the female pelvic floor and stress continence control system. *Scandinavian Journal of Urology and Nephrology: Supplementum, 207,* 1–7.

Bø, K. (2004a). Pelvic floor muscle training is effective in treatment of female stress urinary incontinence, but how does it work? *International Urogynecology Journal and Pelvic Floor Dysfunction, 15,* 76–84.

Bø, K. (2004b). Urinary incontinence, pelvic floor dysfunction, exercise and sport. *Sports Medicine, 34,* 451–464.

Bø, K., & Sherburn, M. (2005). Evaluation of female pelvic-floor muscle function and strength. *Physical Therapy, 85,* 269–282.

Bø, K., & Stien, R. (1994). Needle EMG registration of striated urethral wall and pelvic floor muscle activity patterns during cough, Valsalva, abdominal, hip adductor, and gluteal muscles contractions in nulliparous healthy females. *Neurourology and Urodynamics, 13,* 35–41.

Borello-France, D.F., Zyczynski, H.M., Downey, P.A., Rause, C.R., & Wister, J.A. (2006). Effect of pelvic-floor muscle exercise position on continence and quality-of-life outcomes in women with stress urinary incontinence. *Physical Therapy, 86,* 974–986.

Burgio, K., Goode, P.S., Locher, J.L., Umlauf, M.G., Roth, D.L., Richter, H.E., et al. (2002). Behavioral training with and without biofeedback in the treatment of urge incontinence in older women. *JAMA, 288,* 2293–2299.

Burgio, K., Goode, P.S., Urban, D.A., Umlauf, M.G., Locher, J.L., Bueschen, A., et al. (2006). Preoperative biofeedback assisted behavioral training to decrease post-prostatectomy incontinence: A randomized, controlled trial. *Journal of Urology, 175,* 196–201.

Burgio, K.L., Locher, J.L., & Goode, P.S. (2000). Combined behavioral and drug therapy for urge incontinence in older women. *Journal of the American Geriatrics Society, 48,* 370–374.

Burgio, K.L., Locher, J.L., Goode, P.S., Hardin, J.M., McDowell, B.J., Dombrowski, M., et al. (1998). Behavioral vs. drug treatment for urge urinary incontinence in older women: A randomized controlled trial. *JAMA, 280,* 1995–2000.

Centers for Medicare & Medicaid Services. (2005). *State Operations Manual, Appendix PP— Guidance to Surveyors for Long-Term Care Facilities, Tag F315, §483.25(d) Urinary Incontinence* (Rev. 8, Issued: 06-28-05, Effective: 06-28-05, Implementation: 06-28-05) (pp. 184–219). Retrieved November 11, 2007, from http://www.cms.hhs.gov/transmittals/downloads/R8SOM.pdf

Chiarelli, P., Murphy, B., & Cockburn, J. (2003). Women's knowledge, practices, and intentions regarding correct pelvic floor exercises. *Neurourology and Urodynamics, 22,* 246–249.

Choi, H., Palmer, M.H., & Park, J. (2007). Meta-analysis of pelvic floor muscle training: Randomized controlled trials in incontinent women. *Nursing Research, 56,* 226–234.

Colling, J., Ouslander, J., Hadley, B.J., Eisch, J., & Campbell, E. (1992). The effects of patterned urge response toileting (PURT) on urinary incontinence among nursing home residents. *Journal of the American Geriatrics Society, 40,* 135–141.

Colling, J., Owen, T.R., McCreedy, M., & Newman, D. (2003).The effect of a continence program on frail community dwelling elderly persons. *Urologic Nursing, 23,* 117–122, 127–131.

Cornel, E.B., de Wit, R., & Witjes, J.A. (2005). Evaluation of early pelvic floor physiotherapy on the duration and degree of urinary incontinence after radical retropubic prostatectomy in a non-teaching hospital. *World Journal of Urology, 23,* 353–355.

DeLancey, J.O., Sampselle, C.M., & Punch, M.R. (1993). Kegel dyspareunia: Levator ani myalgia caused by overexertion. *Obstetrics and Gynecology, 82*(4 Pt. 2 Suppl.), 658–659.

Diokno, A.C., Sampselle, C.M., Herzog, A.R., Raghunathan, T.E., Hines, S., Messer, K.L., et al. (2004). Prevention of urinary incontinence by behavioral modification program: A randomized, controlled trial among older women in the community. *Journal of Urology, 171,* 1165–1171.

Dougherty, M.C., Dwyer, J.W., Pendergast, J.F., Boyington, A.R., Tomlinson, B.U., Coward, R.T., et al. (2002). A randomized trial of behavioral management for continence with older rural women. *Research in Nursing and Health, 25,* 3–13.

Emmons, S.L., & Otto, L. (2005). Acupuncture for overactive bladder: A randomized controlled trial. *Obstetrics and Gynecology, 106,* 138–143.

Engberg, S.J., Sereika, S.M., McDowell, B.J., Weber, E., & Brodak, I. (2002). Effectiveness of prompted voiding in treating urinary incontinence in cognitively impaired homebound older adults. *Journal of Wound, Ostomy, and Continence Nursing, 29,* 252–265.

Eustice, S., Roe, B., & Paterson, J. (2002). Prompted voiding for the management of urinary incontinence in adults. Cochrane Incontinence Group. *Cochrane Database of Systematic Reviews,* (2), CD002113.

Fantl, J., Newman, D., Colling, J., DeLancey, J.O.L., Keeys, C., Loughery, R., et al. for the Urinary Incontinence in Adults Guideline Update Panel. (1996). *Urinary incontinence in adults: Acute and chronic management. Clinical practice guideline No. 2: Update* (AHCPR Publication No. 96-0692). Rockville, MD: Agency for Health Care and Policy Research.

Fantl, J.A., Wyman, J.F., McClish, D.K., Harkins, S.W., Elswick, R.K., Taylor, J.R., et al. (1991). Efficacy of bladder training in older women with urinary incontinence. *JAMA, 265,* 609–613.

Filocamo, M.T., Li Marzi, V., Del Popolo, G., Cecconi, F., Marzocco, M., Tosto, A., et al. (2005). Effectiveness of early pelvic floor rehabilitation treatment for post-prostatectomy incontinence. *European Urology, 48,* 734–738.

Fine, P., Burgio, K., Borello-France, D., Richter, H., Whitehead, W., Weber, W., et al., for the Pelvic Floor Disorders Network. (2007). Teaching and practicing of pelvic floor muscle exercises in primiparous women during pregnancy and the postpartum period. *American Journal of Obstetrics and Gynecology, 197,* 107.e1–107.e5.

Fonda, D., DuBeau, C.E., Harari, D., Ouslander, J.G., Palmer, M., & Roe, B. (2005). Incontinence in the frail elderly. In P. Abrams, L. Cardozo, S. Khoury, & A. Wein (Eds.), *Incontinence: Proceedings from the Third International Consultation on Incontinence* (pp. 1163–1239). Plymouth, UK: Health Publications, Ltd.

Ghoniem, G.M., Van Leeuwen, J.S., Elser, D.M., Freeman, R.M., Zhao, Y.D., Yalcin, I., et al., for the Duloxetine/Pelvic Floor Muscle Training Clinical Trial Group. (2005). A randomized controlled trial of duloxetine alone, pelvic floor muscle training alone, combined treatment and no active treatment in women with stress urinary incontinence. *Journal of Urology, 173,* 1647–1653.

Goode, P.S., Burgio, K.L., Locher, J.L., Roth, D.L., Umlauf, M.G., Richter, H.E., et al. (2003). Effect of behavioral training with or without pelvic floor electrical stimulation on stress incontinence in women: A randomized controlled trial. *JAMA, 290,* 345–352.

Goode, P.S., Burgio, K.L., Locher, J.L., Umlauf, M.G., Lloyd, L.K., & Roth, D.L. (2002). Urodynamic changes associated with behavioral and drug treatment of urge incontinence in older women. *Journal of the American Geriatrics Society, 50,* 808–816.

Harvey, M.A. (2003). Pelvic floor exercises during and after pregnancy: A systematic review of their role in preventing pelvic floor dysfunction. *Journal of Obstetrics and Gynaecology Canada, 25,* 487–498.

Hay-Smith, J., Herbison, P., & Mørkved, S. (2002). Physical therapies for prevention of urinary and faecal incontinence in adults. *Cochrane Database of Systematic Reviews,* (2), CD003191.

Hay-Smith, E.J.C., Bø, K., Berghmans, L.C.M., Hendriks, H.J.M., de Bie, R.A., & van Waalwijk van Doom, E.S.C. (2006). Pelvic floor muscle training for urinary incontinence in women. *Cochrane Database of Systematic Reviews,* (1), CD001407.

Hay-Smith, E.J.C., & Dumoulin, C. (2006). Pelvic floor muscle training versus no treatment, or inactive control treatments, for urinary incontinence in women. *Cochrane Database of Systematic Reviews,* (1), CD005654.

Herbison, P., Plevnik, S., & Mantle, J. (2002). Weighted vaginal cones for urinary incontinence *Cochrane Database of Systematic Reviews,* (1), CD002114.

Hines, S.H., Seng, J.S., Messer, K.L., Raghunathan, T.E., Diokno, A.C., & Sampselle, C.M. (2007). Adherence to a behavioral program to prevent incontinence. *Western Journal of Nursing Research, 29*(1), 36–56.

Hunter, K.F., Moore, K.N., Cody, D.J., & Glazener, C.M. (2004). Conservative management for postprostatectomy urinary incontinence. *Cochrane Database of Systematic Reviews,* (2), CD001843.

Ip, V. (2004). Evaluation of a patient education tool to reduce the incidence of incontinence post-prostate surgery. *Urologic Nursing, 24,* 401–407.

Jeffcoate, T.N.A., & Francis, W.J.A. (1966). Urinary incontinence in the female. *American Journal of Obstetrics and Gynecology, 94,* 604–618.

Kegel, A.H. (1948). Progressive resistance exercise in the functional restoration of the perineal muscles. *American Journal of Obstetrics & Gynecology, 56*(2): 238–248.

Lekan-Rutledge, D. (2000). Diffusion of innovation: A model for implementation of prompted voiding in long-term care settings. *Journal of Gerontological Nursing, 26*(4), 25–33.

Lekan-Rutledge, D., & Colling, J. (2003, March). Urinary incontinence in the frail elderly: Even when it's too late to prevent a problem, you still slow its progress. *American Journal of Nursing, Supplement,* pp. 36–40.

MacDonald, R., Fink, H.A., Huckabay, C., Monga, M., & Wilt, T.J. (2007). Pelvic floor muscle training to improve urinary incontinence after radical prostatectomy: a systematic review of effectiveness. *BJU International, 100,* 76–81.

Manassero, F., Traversi, C., Ales, V., Pistolesi, D., Panicucci, E., Valent, F., et al. (2007). Contribution of early intensive prolonged pelvic floor exercises on urinary continence recovery after bladder neck–sparing radical prostatectomy: Results of a prospective controlled randomized trial. *Neurourology and Urodynamics, 26,* 985–989.

Mattiasson, A., Blaakaer, J., Hoye, K., & Wein, A.J., for the Tolterodine Scandinavian Study Group. (2003). Simplified bladder training augments the effectiveness of tolterodine in patients with an overactive bladder. *BJU International, 91,* 54–60.

Messelink, B., Benson, T., Berghmans, B., Bø, K., Corcos, J., Fowler, C., et al. (2005). Standardization of terminology of pelvic floor muscle function and dysfunction: Report from the Pelvic Floor Clinical Assessment Group of the International Continence Society. *Neurourology and Urodynamics, 24,* 374–380.

McClurg, D., Ashe, R.G., Marshall, K., & Lowe-Strong, A.S. (2006). Comparison of pelvic floor muscle training, electromyography, biofeedback and neuromuscular electrical stimulation for bladder dysfunction in people with multiple sclerosis: A randomized pilot study. *Neurourology and Urodynamics, 25,* 337–348.

Miller, J., Ashton-Miller, J.A., & DeLancey, J.O.L. (1996). The Knack: Use of precisely timed pelvic muscle exercise contraction can reduce leakage in SUI. *Neurourology and Urodynamics, 15,* 302–393.

Miller, J.M. (2002). Criteria for therapeutic use of pelvic floor muscle training in women. *Journal of Wound, Ostomy, and Continence Nursing, 29,* 301–311.

Miller, J.M., Ashton-Miller, J.A., & DeLancey, J.O.L. (1998). A pelvic muscle contraction can reduce cough-related urine loss in selected women with mild stress urinary incontinence. *Journal of the American Geriatrics Society, 46,* 870–874.

Miller, J.M., Perucchini, D., Carchidi, L., DeLancey, J.O.L., & Ashton-Miller, J.A. (2001). Pelvic floor muscle contraction during a cough and decreased vesical neck mobility. *Obstetrics and Gynecology, 97,* 255–260.

Miller, J.M., Sampselle, C., Ashton-Miller, J., Hong, G.R., DeLancey, J.O. (2008). Clarification and confirmation of the Knack maneuver: The effect of volitional pelvic floor muscle contraction to preempt expected stress incontinence. *International Urogynecology Journal and Pelvic Floor Dysfunction, 19,* 773–782.

Mørkved, S., Bø, K., & Fjørtoft, T. (2002). Effect of adding biofeedback to pelvic floor muscle training to treat urodynamic stress incontinence. *Obstetrics and Gynecology, 100,* 730–739.

Mørkved, S., Bø, K., Schei, B., & Salvesen, K.A. (2003). Pelvic floor muscle training during pregnancy to prevent urinary incontinence: A single-blind randomized controlled trial. *Obstetrics and Gynecology, 101,* 313–319.

Moul, J.W. (1998). Pelvic muscle rehabilitation in males following prostatectomy. *Urologic Nursing, 18,* 296–300.

National Alliance for Caregiving and AARP. (2004). Caregiving in the United States. Retrieved September 2008, from http://www.caregiving.org/data/04finalreport.pdf. Funded by MetLife Foundation.

Newman, D.K. (2003). *Clinical manual—pelvic muscle rehabilitation* (pp. 89–98). Prometheus, Inc.

Newman, D.K. (2004). Lifestyle interventions. In A.P. Bourcier, E.J. McGuire, & P. Abrams (Eds.), *Pelvic floor disorders* (pp. 269–276). Philadelphia: Elsevier Saunders.

Newman, D.K. (2005a). Behavioral treatments. In S.P. Vasavada, R. Appell, P.K. Sand, & S. Raz (Eds.), *Female urology, urogynecology, and voiding dysfunction* (pp. 233–266). New York: Marcel Dekker.

Newman, D.K. (2005b). *Bladder and bowel rehabilitation program.* Philadelphia: SCA Personal Products.

Newman, D.K. (2006). The roles of the continence nurse specialists. In L. Cardozo & D. Staskin (Eds.), *Textbook of female urology and urogynecology* (2nd ed., pp. 91–98). Abingdon, UK: Informa Healthcare.

Newman, D.K. (2007a). Conservative therapy for incontinence. In H.B. Goldman & S.P. Vasavada (Eds.), *Female urology: A practical clinical guide* (pp. 63–79). Totowa, NY: Humana.

Newman, D.K. (2007b). *Program of excellence in extended care.* Bothell, WA: Verathon Corporation.

Newman, D.K., Gaines, T., & Snare, E. (2005). Innovation in bladder assessment: Use of technology in extended care. *Journal of Gerontological Nursing, 31*(12), 33–41.

Newman, D.K., & Wein, A.J. (2004). *Overcoming overactive bladder* (p. 92). Los Angeles: New Harbinger.

O'Dell, K.K., & McGee, S. (2006). Acupuncture for urinary urgency in women over 50: What is the evidence? *Urologic Nursing, 26,* 23–29.

Ostaszkiewicz, J., Johnston, L., & Roe, B. (2004a). Habit retraining for the management of urinary incontinence in adults. *Cochrane Database of Systematic Reviews,* (2), CD002801.

Ostaszkiewicz, J., Johnston, L., & Roe, B. (2004b). Timed voiding for the management of urinary incontinence in adults. *Cochrane Database of Systematic Reviews,* (1), CD002802.

Ostaszkiewicz, J., Roe, B., & Johnston, L. (2005). Effects of timed voiding for the management of urinary incontinence in adults: Systematic review. *Journal of Advanced Nursing, 52,* 420–431.

Ouslander, J.G., Griffiths, P.C., McConnell, E., Riolo, L., Kutner, M., & Schnelle, J. (2005). Functional incidental training: A randomized, controlled, crossover trial in Veterans Affairs nursing homes. *Journal of the American Geriatrics Society, 53,* 1091–1100.

Ouslander, J.G., Maloney, C., Grasela, T.H., Rogers, L., & Walawander, C.A. (2001). Implementation of a nursing home urinary incontinence management program with and without tolterodine. *Journal of the American Medical Directors Association, 2,* 207–214.

Ouslander, J.G., Schnelle, J.F., Uman, G., Fingold, S., Nigam, J.G., Tuico, E., et al. (1995). Predictors of successful prompted voiding among incontinent nursing home residents. *JAMA, 273,* 1366–1370.

Palmer, M.H. (2004). Use of health behavior change theories to guide urinary incontinence research. *Nursing Research, 53*(6 Suppl.), S49–S55.

Peschers, U.M., Gingelmaier, A., Jundt, K., Leib, B., & Dimpfl, T. (2001). Evaluation of pelvic floor muscle strength using four different techniques. *International Urogynecology Journal and Pelvic Floor Dysfunction, 12,* 27–30.

Perrin, L., Dauphinée, S.W., Corcos, J., Hanley, J.A., & Kuchel, G.A. (2005). Pelvic floor muscle training with biofeedback and bladder training in elderly women: A feasibility study. *Journal of Wound, Ostomy, and Continence Nursing, 32,*186–199.

Reilly, E.T., Freeman, R.M., Waterfield, M.R., Waterfield, A.E., Steggles, P., & Pedlar, F. (2002). Prevention of postpartum stress incontinence in primigravidae with increased bladder neck mobility: A randomized controlled trial of antenatal pelvic floor exercises. *BJOG, 109,* 68–76.

Roe, B., Milne, J., Ostaszkiewicz, J., & Wallace, S. (2007). Systematic reviews of bladder training and voiding programmes in adults: A synopsis of findings on theory and methods using metastudy techniques. *Journal of Advanced Nursing, 57,* 3–14.

Roe, B., Ostaszkiewicz, J., Milne, J., & Wallace, S. (2007). Systematic reviews of bladder training and voiding programmes in adults: A synopsis of findings from data analysis and outcomes using metastudy techniques. *Journal of Advanced Nursing, 57,* 15–31.

Roe, B., Williams, K., & Palmer, M. (2003). Bladder training for urinary incontinence in adults. Cochrane Incontinence Group. *Cochrane Database of Systematic Reviews, (4),* CD001308.

Sale, P.G., & Wyman, J.F. (1994). Achievement of goals associated with bladder training by older incontinent women. *Applied Nursing Research, 7*(2), 93–96.

Sampselle, C.M. (2003, March). Behavioral interventions in young and middle-age women: Simple interventions to combat a complex problem. *American Journal of Nursing, Supplement,* pp. 9–19.

Sampselle, C.M., & DeLancey, J. (1992). The urine stream interruption test and pelvic muscle function. *Nursing Research, 41,* 73–77.

Sampselle, C.M., Messer, K.L., Seng, J.S., Raghunathan, T.E., Hines, S.H., & Diokno, A.C. (2005). Learning outcomes of a group behavioral modification program to prevent urinary incontinence. *International Urogynecology Journal and Pelvic Floor Dysfunction, 16,* 441–446.

Sampselle, C.M., Miller, J.M., Mims, B.L., Delancey, J.O.L., Ashton-Miller, J.A., & Antonakos, C.L. (1998). Effect of pelvic muscle exercise on transient incontinence during pregnancy and after birth. *Obstetrics and Gynecology, 91,* 406–412.

Sampselle, C.M., Palmer, M.H., Boyington, A.R., O'Dell, K.K., & Wooldridge, L. (2004). Prevention of urinary incontinence in adults: Population-based strategies [Review]. *Nursing Research, 53*(6 Suppl):S61–S67.

Sapsford, R.R., Hodges, P.W., Richardson, C.A., Cooper, D.H., Markwell, S.J., & Jull, G.A. (2001). Co-activation of the abdominal and pelvic floor muscles during voluntary exercises. *Neurourology and Urodynamics, 20,* 31–42.

Schnelle, J.F., Alessi, C., Simmons, S.F., Al-Samarrai, N.R., Beck, J.C., & Ouslander, J.G. (2002). Translating clinical research into practice: A randomized trial of exercise and incontinence care with nursing home residents. *Journal of the American Geriatrics Society, 50,* 1476–1483.

Shamliyan, T.A., Kane, R.L., Wyman, J., & Wilt, T.J. (2008). Systematic review: Randomized, controlled trials of nonsurgical treatments for urinary incontinence in women. *Annals of Internal Medicine, 148,* 1–15.

Siu, L.S., Chang, A.M., Yip, S.K., & Chang, A.M. (2003). Compliance with a pelvic muscle exercise program as a causal predictor of urinary stress incontinence amongst Chinese women. *Neurourology and Urodynamics, 22,* 659–663.

Subak, L.L., Quesenberry, C.P., Posner, S.F., Cattolica, E., & Soghikian, K. (2002). The effect of behavioral therapy on urinary incontinence: A randomized controlled trial. *Obstetrics and Gynecology, 100,* 72–78.

Tadic, S.D., Zdaniuk, B., Griffiths, D., Rosenberg, L., Schäfer, W., & Resnick, N.M. (2007). Effect of biofeedback on psychological burden and symptoms in older women with urge urinary incontinence. *Journal of the American Geriatrics Society, 55,* 2010–2015.

Tannenbaum, C., Bachand, G., Dubeau, C.E., & Kuchel, G.A. (2001). Experience of an incontinence clinic for older women: No apparent age limit for potential physical and psychological benefits. *Journal of Women's Health, 10,* 751–756.

Theofrastous, J.P., Wyman, J.F., Bump, R.C., McClish, D.K., Elser, D.M., Bland, D.R., et al. (2002). Effects of pelvic floor muscle training on strength and predictors of response in the treatment of urinary incontinence in women. *Neurourology and Urodynamics, 21,* 486–490.

Vandoninck, V., van Balken, M.R., Finazzi Agr, E., Petta, F., Micali, F., Heesakkers, J.P., et al. (2003). Posterior tibial nerve stimulation in the treatment of idiopathic nonobstructive dysfunction. *Urology, 61,* 567–572.

van Houten, P., Achterberg, W., & Ribbe, M. (2007). Urinary incontinence in disabled elderly women: A randomized clinical trial on the effect of training mobility and toileting skills to achieve independent toileting. *Gerontology, 53,* 205–210.

Van Kampen, M., De Weerdt, W., Van Poppel, H., DeRidder, D., Feys, H., & Baert, L. (2000). Effect of pelvic-floor re-education on duration and degree of incontinence after radical prostatectomy: A randomised controlled trial. *Lancet, 355,* 98–102.

Wagg, A., & Bunn, F. (2007). Unassisted pelvic floor exercises for postnatal women: A systematic review. *Journal of Advanced Nursing, 58,* 407–417.

Wallace, S., Roe, B., Williams, K., & Palmer, M. (2004). Bladder training for urinary incontinence in adults. *Cochrane Database of Systematic Reviews,* (1), CD001308.

Wilson, P.D., Berghamns, B., Hagen, S., Hay-Smith, J., Moore, K., Nygaard, I., et al. (2005). Adult conservative management. In P. Abrams, L. Cardozo, S. Khoury, & A. Wein (Eds.), *Incontinence: Proceedings from the Third International Consultation on Incontinence* (pp. 855–964). Plymouth, UK: Health Publications, Ltd.

Wyman, J.F. (2003, March). Treatment of urinary incontinence in men and older women. *American Journal of Nursing, Supplement,* pp. 26–35

Wyman, J.F. (2005). Behavioral interventions for the patient with overactive bladder. *Journal of Wound, Ostomy, and Continence Nursing, 32,* S11–S15.

Wyman, J.F. (2007). Bladder training and overactive bladder. In K. Bø, B. Berghmans, S. Mørkved, & M. Van Kampen (Eds.), *Evidence-Based Physical Therapy for the Pelvic Floor* (pp. 208–218). Philadelphia, PA: Elsevier.

Wyman, J.F., & Fantl, J.A. (1991). Bladder training in ambulatory care management of urinary incontinence. *Urologic Nursing, 11*(3), 11–17.

Yap, P., & Tan, D. (2006). Urinary incontinence in dementia—a practical approach. *Australian Family Physician, 35,* 237–241.

9

Drug Therapy for Incontinence and Overactive Bladder

Urinary incontinence (UI) can often be treated with drug therapy according to the type of incontinence and severity of the symptoms. Patients with overactive bladder (OAB) and mixed UI may be treated with antimuscarinics, drugs that block the action of acetylcholine (ACh) at sites in the bladder by interfering with the attachment of ACh to its receptor sites in the smooth muscle and probably the urothelium as well (see Chapter 3). For patients with sphincter-related incontinence (stress UI) there are no currently approved agents in the United States that increase urethral closure. Postmenopausal urogenital atrophy may benefit from the use of transvaginal estrogen therapy. Unfortunately, there is little drug therapy for the underactive detrusor, although a trial of drugs that activate ACh receptors may be worthwhile.

The goal of drug therapy is to reduce or even eliminate the number of UI and OAB symptoms through "independent continence" by following prescribed drug protocols. This type of treatment may also be classified as "dependent" continence if staff in a long-term care (LTC) facility or a caregiver in the home administers the medication. To achieve optimal effectiveness, drug therapy should always be combined with behavior modification (see Chapters 7 and 8), with the specific type dependent on the type of incontinence (see Chapter 4) and the patient's history, comorbid conditions, and cognitive and mobility status (see Chapter 6).

This chapter outlines currently available drug therapy for people with all types of UI and OAB, noting the efficacy, safety concerns, and adverse effect or side effect profiles of each drug and the use of these drugs in specific populations.

DRUG THERAPY FOR OVERACTIVE BLADDER AND URGE OR MIXED INCONTINENCE

Drug therapy for OAB with UI (referred to as *OAB wet* or OAB–detrusor over-activity [DO]) or without UI (referred to as *OAB dry*) has seen the most changes since the first edition of this book. Pharmacological management of OAB traditionally focuses on modulation of muscarinic receptors, so-called antimuscarinic or anticholinergic therapy. There are many competitors for drug treatment in the OAB market. Only the antimuscarinics have achieved "proof of principle," which means that they have actually been shown to be effective and that effectiveness has been accepted by the U.S. Food and Drug Administration (FDA). There are many tantalizing possibilities that will obviously be developed in the future. Although muscarinic receptors are important in controlling detrusor function, they are not solely responsible for the symptoms of OAB (Wein & Rackley, 2006), and thus the therapy is less than perfect. In many trials on OAB-DO, there has been a high placebo response such that meaningful differences between placebo and active drug have been questioned by some. However, most experts and many clinicans believe that drug effects in individual patients may be both distinct and useful and improve quality of life in affected individuals.

The Third International Consultation on Incontinence, held in 2004, assessed drugs used for treatment of incontinence. The assessment criteria were based on the Oxford System guidelines, and the drugs included are given in Box 9.1.

Currently, five main antimuscarinic agents are approved by the FDA for treatment of the OAB syndrome. Alphabetically, they are darifenacin, oxybutynin, solifenacin, tolterodine, and trospium. Appendix Table 9.1 lists these drugs, their usual doses, side effects, and treatment considerations. A sixth drug, fesoterodine, a relative of tolerodine, may be available soon (Chapple, van Kerrebroeck, et al., 2007; Nitti et al., 2007). Antimuscarinic agents are now thought to act during the filling/storage phases of the micturition cycle by inhibiting afferent (sensory) input from the bladder, as well as directly on the smooth muscle to decrease contractility. These drugs are reviewed in this chapter alphabetically.

Tricyclic antidepressants, such as imipramine, have also been used with mixed results. Other agents that have been tried for OAB include duloxetine, alpha$_1$-adrenergic receptor antagonists, prostaglandin synthase inhibitors, potassium channel openers, prostaglandins, and selective and nonselective inhibitors of cyclooxygenase. Many of these compounds are still in the development phase. Medications that act on beta$_3$-adrenergic receptors in the detrusor muscle or that inhibit bladder afferent nerve transmission are being studied, so new drugs are on the horizon (Chapple, Yamanishi, & Chess-Williams, 2002; Wein & Rackley, 2006).

Box 9.1   Assessment of drugs used in the treatment of voiding dysfunction[a]

	Level of evidence	Recommendation
Antimuscarinic Drugs		
Tolterodine	1	A
Trospium	1	A
Solifenacin	1	A
Darifenacin	1	A
Propantheline	2	B
Drugs with Mixed Actions		
Oxybutynin	1	A
Flavoxate	2	D
Antidepressants		
Imipramine	3	C
β-adrenergic receptor agonists	3	C
Other Drugs		
Botulinum toxin[b]	2	B (see Chapter 12)
Estrogen[c]	2	C
Desmopressin[d]	1	A

International Consultation on Incontinence Assessments, 2004; Oxford Guidelines (modified)
Levels of Evidence
Level 1: Systematic reviews, meta-analyses, good-quality randomized controlled clinical trials
Level 2: Randomized controlled clinical trials, good-quality prospective cohort studies
Level 3: Case–control studies, case series
Level 4: Expert opinion

Grades of Recommendation
Grade A: Based on level 1 evidence (highly recommended)
Grade B: Consistent level 2 or 3 evidence (recommended)
Grade C: Level 4 studies or "majority evidence" (optional)
Grade D: Evidence inconsistent or inconclusive (no recommendation possible)

Adapted from Andersson, K.E., Appell, R.A., Cardozo, L., Chapple, C., Drutz, H., Fourcroy, J., et al. (2005). Pharmacological treatment of urinary incontinence. In P. Abrams, L. Cardozo, S. Khoury, & A. Wein (Eds.), *Incontinence: Proceedings from the Third International Consultation on Incontinence* (pp. 809–854). Plymouth, UK: Health Publications Ltd.
[a]Assessments according to the International Consultation on Incontinence Assessments, 2004; Oxford Guidelines (modified).
[b]Injection.
[c]Transvaginal.
[d]Nocturia.

Anticholinergic–Antimuscarinic Agents

Efficacy Versus Tolerability

In patients with involuntary bladder contractions, antimuscarinic agents will generally increase the volume of urine required to stimulate the first involuntary bladder contraction, decrease the amplitude of that contraction, and increase bladder capacity. Individuals will often report increased "control" and having "more time" to get to the bathroom after 2–3 weeks of drug therapy. However, because these drugs block cholinergic (parasympathetic) activity at muscarinic sites, they may have numerous and varied anticholinergic side effects. Also, some believe that their success may diminish with long-term use. Most research on these drugs has involved primarily women with OAB and urgency or mixed UI, so there may be limitations in applying them to the general population. Data analyses, however, seem to show equal efficacy in men. Several (oxybutynin, solifenacin, darifenacin) are available in two different doses, allowing for flexible dosing; individuals can start at the lower dose and titrate up to a higher dose if needed. Dose titration may or may not be viewed as an advantage by certain clinicians.

Antimuscarinics block the stimulation of postganglionic parasympathetic muscarinic cholinergic receptor sites on bladder smooth muscle and in the urothelium and thereby inhibit bladder contractions produced by neural or electrical stimulation (Andersson, 2004). Their activity involves an inhibitory action on the sensory side of the bladder innervation as well, and the net result is a decrease in urgency, frequency, and urgency UI episodes. In 1996, the Agency for Health Care Policy and Research (now the Agency for Healthcare Research and Quality) recommended anticholinergics as first-line therapy for urgency UI with OAB (Fantl et al., 1996). Since the release of this guideline, several new agents have been introduced. All of these drugs have received excellent ratings (Level 1, Grade A) by the International Consultation on Incontinence (Andersson et al., 2005) (see Box 9.1). These Oxford System ratings indicate that, in well-performed, randomized, controlled trials, the agents have demonstrated efficacy in the treatment of OAB and have acceptable side effect profiles. These drugs have similar efficacy in clinical trials and are associated with a significant decrease in symptoms and a 70%–80% median reduction in episodes of urgency UI (Andersson et al., 2005; Hay-Smith, Herbison, Ellis, & Morris, 2005; Herbison, Hay-Smith, Ellis, & Moore, 2003; Nabi, Cody, Ellis, Herbison, & Hay-Smith, 2006; Wein & Rackley, 2006). However, a placebo response range of 33%–56% has been reported in these studies. This effect is believed to be the result of increased self-awareness through Bladder Diaries, a form of behavior modification, interactions with a health care provider, and a strong motivation to improve. Although anticholinergics comprise first-line pharmacological therapy, to maximize their effectiveness with urgency and frequency, drug therapy must *always* be combined with behavioral treatments, as described in Chapter 8 (Burgio, Locher, & Goode, 2000; Burgio et al., 1998; Wein, 2001). Combining bladder training and drug therapy has been shown to be more effective than drug therapy alone in several studies (Mattiasson, Blaakaer, Hoye, & Wein, 2003; Song, Park, Heo, Lee, & Choo, 2006).

Using a drug that allows flexible dosing and changing the delivery of the drug may also improve outcomes. Historically, the tolerability and safety concerns that have accompanied antimuscarinic therapy (primarily immediate-release [IR] oxybutynin) have limited their use in the treatment of OAB, especially because this condition normally requires long-term treatment. The problem with antimuscarinic therapy is that it lacks bladder receptor selectivity, often resulting in common antimuscarinic side effects (see section on adverse side effects later in the chapter). The use of the newer medications (e.g., transdermal oxybutynin and extended-release [ER] formulations of darifenacin, oxybutynin, solifenacin, tolterodine ER, and trospium) seems to result in fewer side effects and safety concerns, and has greatly improved the management of this condition. Also, drugs are now available as an ER formulation, which works over a 24-hour period. Oxybutynin and tolterodine have IR preparations as well (shorter time to onset of action and shorter duration of action). The ER formulations of these drugs are preferred because this minimizes the peaks (highs) and troughs (lows) of drug blood concentration, allowing 24-hour drug delivery. A third formulation is a transdermal delivery system (TDS) or skin patch, which provides a steady release of drug over several days (Nitti et al., 2006).

When choosing an antimuscarinic agent, it is important to consider efficacy data that are specific for an individual's symptoms. When selecting any drug for UI and OAB, the clinician must also weigh efficacy versus tolerability (Newman & Wein, 2004), because the agent should have efficacy and safety profiles that are appropriate and acceptable. Individual response to antimuscarinic drugs is variable. It may therefore be necessary to try several agents, begin at the lowest dose recommended, and titrate dosages to achieve an optimal therapeutic response (Andersson & Wein, 2007; Staskin & MacDiarmid, 2006). The following case study is an example of a common presentation of a woman with OAB in clinical practice.

Emily is a 59-year-old woman who presents with urinary frequency as often as every 1–2 hours. Daytime frequency is worse in the morning, following intake of three large cups of coffee. She experiences strong urinary urgency when going into "cold rooms" or when she hears running water. She reports that urgency is so intense that at times she will "lose control" and leak small to moderate amounts of urine when rushing to the bathroom. These episodes occur several times a week. She denies incontinence with physical activities (e.g., coughing, sneezing, laughing, exercise). She uses at least three or four pantiliners or perineal pads a day to feel more secure, especially when traveling from her home. Her urgency is the most bothersome symptom because it is sudden and unpredictable. Emily denies hesitancy, dysuria, or change in urinary stream. She feels that, because she voids so often, she is completely emptying her bladder. Her 1-day "diary" indicated 12 incontinence episodes in a 24-hour period. Emily has occasional problems with constipation and can have significant straining for defecation. She tries to counter constipation with increased dietary fiber. Her medical history includes mild hypertension. Emily is postmenopausal; her last menstrual period was 1 year ago. She underwent a vaginal hysterectomy 10 years ago for uncontrolled bleeding. Current medications include multivitamins and hydrochlorothiazide 20 mg daily.

Mechanism of Antimuscarinic Action

The urinary bladder is controlled through a complex interaction between the central and peripheral nervous systems, with local regulatory factors also playing a role (see Chapter 3). The mechanisms of bladder function and dysfunction are as follows (Andersson, 2002; Andersson, 2004; Wein & Rackley, 2006):

- Mechanical and chemical interactions take place through the extensive afferent and efferent innervation of the urinary bladder, both within the detrusor muscle and in and directly below the urothelium, involving nerve fibers in a control mechanism for sensory feedback, as well as the initiation of micturition.

- Neurogenic dysfunction can be the result of changes in the structure or function of the nervous supply to the bladder or in the central control areas of the brain and central nervous system (CNS), causing decreased inhibition of the micturition reflex that occurs in certain neurological diseases (e.g., spinal cord injury following a cerebrovascular accident, multiple sclerosis).

- Myogenic dysfunction can result from structural or functional changes within the bladder muscle layers, such as patchy denervation or infiltration of smooth muscle by elastin and collagen. Changes in the electrical coupling between muscle cells may lead to uncontrolled spread of the muscle contraction over the whole bladder, resulting in sensations of urgency and even UI.

- Activation of stretch-sensitive neurons that mediate the sensation of urgency may also contribute to the symptoms of OAB as a result of localized spontaneous contractions of smooth muscle known as *micromotions*.

Potentially, drugs used to treat these conditions could do so by affecting the central and/or peripheral neural control pathways or the detrusor muscle itself (Wein, 2001). Detrusor muscle overactivity may be treated with antimuscarinics because of their ability to decrease afferent impulses and to inhibit cholinergic-induced bladder smooth muscle activation. This treatment increases the bladder volume necessary to initiate the sensation of urgency and to stimulate a detrusor contraction, while decreasing the strength of an involuntary contraction and increasing the total bladder capacity.

Role of Muscarinic Receptors. In the bladder, ACh released from cholinergic (parasympathetic) nerve terminals acts on a subtype of cholinergic receptor, the muscarinic or M receptor. Acetylcholine stimulates the muscarinic receptors in the detrusor that cause the bladder to contract. There are five subtypes of muscarinic receptors, M_1-M_5 (Abrams et al., 2006; Andersson, 2004) (Table 9.1). M_2 and M_3 receptors predominate in bladder smooth muscle. Although M_2 receptors are present in greater numbers in the bladder, M_3 receptors are considered more important in bladder contraction (Scarpero &

Table 9.1 Muscarinic receptors: location and functions

Receptor	Location	Functions
M_1	Brain, cerebral cortex, hippocampus Salivary glands, sympathetic ganglia	Memory and cognitive function Increases salivary secretion (mucus) Gastric acid secretion
M_2	Smooth muscle Heart, cardiac muscle	Bladder smooth muscle contraction Maintains normal heart rate Gastric sphincter tone
M_3	Smooth muscle Salivary and parotid glands Gastrointestinal tract Eye	Salivary and tear production, bowel motility, and visual accommodation Bladder contraction Increases salivary secretion (mucus) Bowel motility
M_4	Brain stem	Unknown
M_5	Brain Ciliary muscle (eye)	Other central nervous system—unknown Decreases visual accommodation

Dmochowski, 2003). The M_3 subtype is generally believed to be primarily responsible for the involuntary bladder contractions seen in DO, as well as the emptying contraction during normal voiding. There is a growing literature that suggests that M_2 receptors may be involved as well (Chapple, 2000; Chess-Williams, Chapple, Yamanishi, Yasuda, & Sellers, 2001; Ouslander, 2004; Taylor, 2005; Wang, Luthin, & Ruggieri, 1995; Wein, 2001). Some hypothesize that M_2 receptors may assume a greater role with aging and in obstruction and neurological lower urinary tract dysfunction (Ouslander, 2004). As M_2 receptors are involved in heart rate regulation, a drug that has a higher receptor profile for blocking these M_2 receptors could theoretically lead to a higher incidence of increased heart rate, which may or may not prove to be important.

Whether a drug gains access to the CNS through the blood–brain barrier (BBB) depends on the drug's molecular weight, its lipophilicity, and its charge. According to those characteristics, oxybutinin will be the drug most likely to cross the BBB. A quaternary amine drug (e.g., trospium) does not cross lipid barriers like the BBB very well, so in a normal individual, it should not cross the BBB. However, circumstances such as aging, diabetes, and stress may affect the ability of a drug to cross the BBB. Once the drug gets into the CNS or crosses the BBB, what it does there depends upon its blocking activities with respect to the M_1 receptor, which is thought to be the cognition receptor. A drug that is higher in M_1 blockade capability and crosses the BBB will have a

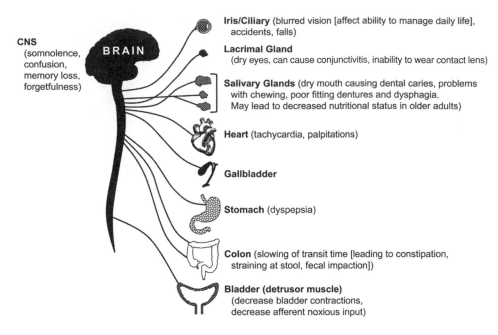

Iris/Ciliary (blurred vision [affect ability to manage daily life], accidents, falls)

Lacrimal Gland (dry eyes, can cause conjunctivitis, inability to wear contact lens)

Salivary Glands (dry mouth causing dental caries, problems with chewing, poor fitting dentures and dysphagia. May lead to decreased nutritional status in older adults)

Heart (tachycardia, palpitations)

Gallbladder

Stomach (dyspepsia)

Colon (slowing of transit time [leading to constipation, straining at stool, fecal impaction])

Bladder (detrusor muscle) (decrease bladder contractions, decrease afferent noxious input)

CNS (somnolence, confusion, memory loss, forgetfulness)

BRAIN

Figure 9.1. Distribution sites for antimuscarinics. CNS = central nervous system. (Courtesy of Robin Noel; adapted from Abrams and Wein [1998].)

higher potential for cognitive dysfunction. M_3 receptors are also active in salivary gland functioning and intestinal motility, and blockade can lead to dry mouth and constipation (Abrams & Wein, 1998; Wein, 2001) (Figure 9.1).

In and around smooth muscle, M_2 and M_3 receptors may be associated with either afferent (sensory) or efferent (motor) fibers (Andersson, 2004) (Figure 9.2). In the mucosa or epithelium, they may be associated with afferent fibers. Alpha-adrenergic receptors predominate in the bladder dome, trigone, and bladder base and may play a role in OAB, but there is little evidence that they are involved in normal bladder control (Wein, 2001). Beta-adrenergic receptors may be involved in bladder smooth muscle relaxation during filling/storage (Andersson, 2002; Wein, 2001).

The ideal agent for the treatment of OAB would be uroselective—that is, the antimuscarinic effects would be exerted on the bladder with minimal effects elsewhere in the body. Such uroselectivity would decrease adverse effects and increase drug tolerability, which should in turn increase compliance with the drug treatment. Some antimuscarinic agents affect primarily M_3 receptors to a greater degree, some affect primarily both M_3 and M_1 receptors, and, in some cases, there is no selectivity for any particular muscarinic receptor (Wein, 2001). There are many issues with antimuscarinic drugs and there are many competing claims based on differences in the molecular structure, the receptor selectivity or nonselectivity, and the properties that theoretically make one drug, at least on paper, more apt to gain entrance to the CNS than another (Andersson & Wein, 2007). The receptor profiles of the different an-

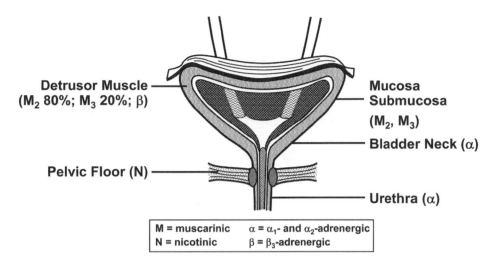

Figure 9.2.   Description of cholinergic and adrenergic receptors in the lower urinary tract. (Courtesy of Robin Noel; adapted from Andersson [2004], Chapple [2000], and Wein [2001].)

timuscarinic drugs may or may not be important in determining their efficacy, tolerability, and safety. Basically the drugs break down into three classes:

1. Drugs that are relatively balanced receptor blockers, meaning that they have relatively equal blockade characteristics for M_3 and M_2 receptors (e.g., tolterodine and trospium)

2. Drugs that are relatively selective (relatively because no drug is truly selective) for M_3 and M_1 receptors (e.g., oxybutynin and solifenacin)

3. Drugs that are relatively selective for M_3 receptors (e.g., darifenacin)

It must be noted that whether this means there is an advantage in terms of efficacy for one group over another, and whether this confers a disadvantage in terms of particular side effects and tolerability, is yet to be definitively proven, although it seems that the drugs that have a strong M_3 blockade activity are associated with a greater incidence of dry mouth and constipation, especially with higher doses.

Other receptors may have a role in mediating the contraction and relaxation of smooth muscle in the urethra and bladder (see Figure 9.2). A number of neurotransmitters are involved in the storage and voiding phases of micturition and may contribute to the symptoms of OAB (Andersson & Wein, 2007; Ouslander, 2004). A few of these neurotransmitters are listed here:

• Glutamate is known to have excitatory effects in CNS pathways controlling the lower urinary tract.

• Norepinephrine relaxes smooth muscle in the bladder body (dome) via beta-adrenergic receptors and contracts smooth muscle in the bladder base via alpha-adrenergic receptors.

- Nitric oxide causes relaxation of the bladder base and inhibits peripheral afferents.

- Bradykinin, angiotensin, tachykinins, leukotrienes, adenosine, and prostanoids cause contraction of the bladder smooth muscle.

- Serotonin, through a variety of receptors centrally and peripherally, can act to inhibit or activate micturition.

- Dopaminergic (dopamine) pathways can have both inhibitory and facilitatory effects on voiding.

- Capsaicin-sensitive afferent nerve fibers, vanilloid receptors, and second-order neurons, following activation of afferent neurons in the dorsal horn of the spinal cord in bladder function and dysfunction, may play a role also.

Review of Available Antimuscarinic Drugs

> After reviewing Emily's 3-day voiding diary, it was recommended that Emily decrease her caffeine intake. Additional recommendations included behavior therapy of bladder training and urge suppression techniques and pelvic floor muscle exercises, combined with antimuscarinic therapy. Emily was opposed to medications, so she began behavioral treatment. After 6 weeks, Emily reported that, if she practiced the urge suppression techniques, she would have a decrease in urgency and she was now only using two incontinence pads, but she felt she was only 50% better. She was still fearful of traveling to places where the location of bathrooms was unknown. She expressed frustration because she felt her bladder "was controlling my life." The clinician discussed the benefits of adding antimuscarinic medication.

The following is a review of the current antimuscarinic drugs. Appendix Table 9.1 provides specifics on usual dose, side effects, and treatment considerations. Table 9.2 lists the pharmocodynamics of these drugs, including peak plasma levels and serum half life. Appendix Table 9.2 reviews drug efficacy based on product information, and Appendix Table 9.3 lists the side effects of each drug and placebo. The drugs are listed alphabetically.

Darifenacin (Enablex [Novartis, Proctor & Gamble]).   Darifenacin hydrobromide is a relatively selective M_3 muscarinic receptor antagonist that has demonstrated efficacy in clinical trials in patients with OAB and incontinence without CNS or cardiovascular side effects (Haab, 2005). Among the approved muscarinic receptor antagonists, darifenacin has the greatest affinity for the M_3 receptor subtype (Steers, 2006). It is available in flexible dosing of 7.5 mg and 15 mg, administered once daily with liquid, and can be taken with or without food. To allow once-daily administration, thus increasing convenience, the active ingredient has been embedded in an insoluble matrix that leaks out as it

Table 9.2   Antimuscarinic pharmacodynamics[a]

| Drug | Pharmacodynamics | |
	Peak plasma level	Elimination half-life
Darifenacin	7 hours	13–19 hours
Oxybutynin IR	1 hour	2–3 hours
Oxybutynin ER	4–6 hours	13 hours
Oxybutynin TDS	10 hours with continuous use	7–8 hours after patch is removed
Tolterodine IR	0.5–2 hours	2.4 hours with multiple dosing
Tolterodine ER	2–6 hours	5-Hydroxymethyl metabolite: 8.8 hours
		Tolterodine: 7 hours
Trospium IR	5–6 hours	20 hours
Trospium XR	4–5 hours	35 hours
Solifenacin	3–8 hours	45–68 hours

Key: ER = extended-release; GI = gastrointestinal; IR = immediate-release; NA = not applicable; TDS = transdermal delivery system.

[a]Obtained from drug product information: Detrol LA, Ditropan XL, Enablex, Oxytrol, Sanctura, Sanctura IR, VESIcare.

traverses the intestine. Darifenacin is metabolized by the liver and is absorbed in the gastrointestinal (GI) tract. Its use is not recommended for patients with severe hepatic impairment, a prohibition that perhaps should apply to the other drugs in this class that are metabolized by cytochrome P-450 (CYP) isoenzymes. Darifenacin is reported to have greater selectivity for the M_3 receptors on the bladder than those on the salivary gland.

FDA approval of darifenacin was based on efficacy from four pivotal studies and safety data from studies in which more than 7,000 subjects (mean age = 58 years) were treated with varying doses (Chapple, 2004; Haab, Stewart, & Dwyer, 2004; Steers, Corcos, Foote, & Kralidis, 2005; Zinner et al., 2005). Chapple et al. (2005) analyzed three phase III studies and found that after 12 weeks of treatment both doses of darifenacin achieved a significantly greater reduction in the median number of incontinence episodes per week. The median change in weekly incontinence episodes from baseline was −8.8 for 7.5 mg darifenacin (−68.4%, 335 patients) and −10.6 for 15 mg darifenacin (−76.8%, 330 patients) against placebo (−53.8% for 7.5 mg and −58.3 for 15 mg). There were significant dose-response trends for which 7.5 and 15 mg darifenacin were evaluated. There was also a significant improvement in other diary variables compared with placebo, including decreases in the number of significant leaks (i.e., number of incontinence episodes that resulted in a change of clothing or pads), voiding frequency, and the number/severity of urgency episodes as well as increased bladder capacity. The proportion of patients who achieved a ≥ 70% reduction in incontinence episodes from baseline was 48% for 7.5 mg and 57% for 15 mg darifenacin, compared with only 33% and 39% of patients in the corresponding placebo groups.

Dry mouth occurred in 20% of people treated with darifenacin 7.5 mg and 35% of those treated with darifenacin 15 mg; CNS and cardiovascular safety was comparable to that of placebo. Constipation occurred in 15% of subjects receiving 7.5 mg and 21% of those receiving 15 mg. However, despite side effects, discontinuation rates were low (7.5 mg, 0.6%; 15 mg, 2.1%; placebo 0.3%). Subanalyses of these data found similar efficacy and safety in older adults (age ≥ 65 years), along with improvement in nocturia.

Oxybutynin (Ditropan, generic).   Oxybutynin chloride has been used for the management of DO for over 30 years (Diokno & Ingber, 2006) and is one of the most commonly used antimuscarinic preparations. Oxybutynin is available in IR, ER, and TDS formulations. The FDA approved oxybutynin in 1975 for the treatment of "uninhibited and reflex neurogenic bladders" and for the treatment of enuresis, and in 1992 for the treatment of "detrusor instability." Off-label use has been described, with intravesical use in individuals with severe OAB. Oxybutynin offers flexibility because of its extensive array of formulations and doses (5, 10, and 15 mg). The drug is approved for adults and children 6 years and older. At this time, oxybutynin is the only antimuscarinic drug approved by the FDA for pediatric use.

Oxybutynin is said to have a "mixed" drug action because it has antispasmodic and local anesthetic actions in the laboratory setting, as well as antimuscarinic properties. Whether the antispasmodic and local anesthetic properties contribute to the clinical efficacy is a matter of debate (Diokno & Ingber, 2006). Oxybutynin is reported to result in increased bladder capacity and decreased "spasticity," thereby reducing urgency, frequency, and incontinence. It may have higher affinity for parotid gland receptors than for receptors in the bladder, which may be the reason it is associated with a higher incidence of dry mouth compared with other anticholinergics (Diokno & Ingber, 2006).

Oxybutynin IR.   The pharmacokinetics of oxybutynin IR provide an explanation for the tolerability issues experienced by the majority of patients treated with this formulation. On ingestion, oxybutynin IR is rapidly absorbed in the small intestine, reaching maximum plasma concentrations within approximately 1 hour (Yarker, Goa, & Fitton, 1995). Because of this rapid absorption, many patients take oxybutynin IR episodically, on an as-needed (PRN) basis to facilitate participating in certain activities (e.g., prior to going to the movies, before playing tennis). However, there has never been a study showing that PRN use of an IR form of any of these drugs is effective. The problem is that the onset of peak action is probably about 2–3 hours and it takes a while for the drug to achieve maximum effect, even with the IR form, so it is unclear how PRN use would be effective unless taken well in advance.

Oxybutynin is metabolized by the CYP isoenzyme 3A4 in the gut and in the liver to its active metabolite *N*-desethyloxybutynin (N-DEO) and to phenylcyclohexylglycolic acid, which is inactive. Oxybutynin IR is susceptible to extensive first-pass metabolism in the gut, yielding high serum concentrations of the metabolite N-DEO. N-DEO circulates at concentrations approximately 4–10 times that of the parent oxybutynin compound (Zobrist, Quan, Thomas, Stanworth, & Sanders, 2003). This metabolite is thought to be responsible for the majority of the side effects.

In early placebo-controlled studies, the oral IR formulation of oxybutynin demonstrated efficacy in reducing symptoms of OAB, such as urinary urgency and urgency UI, in 55%–70% of subjects (Yarker et al., 1995). Although effective, the major drawback of oxybutynin IR was its side effects, which are often severe enough to cause as many as 61%–78% of people receiving high doses of medication to stop taking it. Side effects can be reduced by decreasing the dose. Other attempts to minimize the side effects of oxybutynin have included intravesically administered doses in people with catheters, use of TDS or skin patches (Oxytrol), and the development of an ER formulation (Ditropan XL).

Oxybutynin ER (Ditropan XL [Ortho-McNeil]). Oxybutynin ER is the sustained-release formulation of oxybutynin. The ER form is approved for OAB in adults and children 6 years or older and is available in 5-, 10-, and 15-mg tablets. It has a controlled-release delivery system called an osmotic drug delivery system (OROS), delaying absorption until the drug reaches the large intestine rather than the stomach, thus providing a slower, prolonged uptake and less liver metabolism. OROS technology involves an osmotically active component behind the drug reservoir that "pushes" oxybutynin through a small, laser-drilled opening. As the pill passes through the aqueous environment in the GI tract, the osmotic push element drives the delivery of oxybutynin. With slower uptake of the drug, the ratio of oxybutynin to N-DEO is considerably lower for the oxybutynin ER formulation than for the oxybutynin IR formulation, and serum concentrations of N-DEO are lower following oral administration of oxybutynin ER than the IR formulation. This is believed to be the reason that fewer side effects are seen with the ER formulation versus the older generic or IR versions of the drug. However, both oxybutynin IR and to a lesser degree ER are still associated with GI and CNS side effects.

Oxybutynin ER taken once daily has efficacy comparable to the IR formulation (taken 3 times daily) at the same total daily dosage (MacDiarmid, Anderson, Armstrong, & Dmochowski, 2005). Oxybutynin ER has been compared to the IR formulation in several studies (Anderson et al., 1999; Gleason, Susset, White, Munoz, & Sand, 1999; Versi, Appell, Mobley, Patton, & Saltzstein, 2000). Studies that evaluated oxybutynin ER have demonstrated effective reductions in the symptoms of OAB; for example, it has produced an 83% decrease in urgency UI, similar to the reduction seen with oxybutynin IR. However, compared to the IR formulation, decreases in reports of dry mouth and other anticholinergic adverse effects were modest. Oxybutynin should be used with caution in elderly patients because of possible cognitive side effects, probably owing to its lipophilicity (makes it more apt to cross the BBB) and receptor blockade profile (primarily M_3–M_1).

Oxybutynin TDS (Oxytrol [Watson Pharma]).   The skin is becoming more common as an approach to deliver drugs, with skin patches now available to treat menopause, provide birth control, control hypertension, decrease angina, and deliver nicotine, and with skin gels available to treat estrogen and testosterone deficiency. Now there is drug delivery of oxybutynin using a TDS, or skin patch (Oxytrol), and in 2009 a gel (oxybutynin chloride topical gel) may be available. At a dose of 3.9 mg/day, one patch (39 cm^2 = 36 mg of oxybutynin) is applied twice weekly (every 3–4 days) (Cartwright & Cardozo, 2007). The drug is delivered through the skin, avoiding extensive gastric and hepatic first-pass metabolism. This results in a significant reduction in circulating levels of the primary active metabolite, N-DEO. High concentrations of N-DEO are thought to provoke the high incidence of anticholinergic side effects that have been observed following oral administration of oxybutynin (Zobrist et al., 2003). Because TDS oxybutynin bypasses GI and hepatic metabolism, the formation of N-DEO is reduced, even when compared with oxybutynin ER (Davila, Starkman, & Dmochowski, 2006). This correlates with quantifiable reductions in N-DEO–associated adverse effects, as demonstrated in clinical trials (Davila, Daugherty, & Sanders, 2001; Dmochowski, Sand, et al., 2003). Also, by avoiding first-pass metabolism, less drug is required to obtain effective blood concentrations. This form of oxybutynin also provides steady-state and continuous drug delivery with each application, minimizing the drug peak-to-trough fluctuations in plasma concentrations that occur with oral administration (Zobrist, Schmid, Feick, Quan, & Sanders, 2001).

Oxybutynin TDS (Oxytrol) has been compared to the oxybutynin IR formulation and to tolterodine (see Appendix Table 9.2), its efficacy being similar to that of oral antimuscarinic agents, but with an incidence of anticholinergic adverse effects comparable to placebo (Davila et al., 2001; Dmochowski, Sand, et al., 2003; Dmochowski et al., 2002, 2005). Randomized, placebo-controlled studies established the safety and efficacy of oxybutynin TDS in reducing the number of incontinence episodes, decreasing urinary frequency, and increasing voided volume in individuals with OAB (Dmochowski, Sand, et al., 2003; Dmochowski et al., 2002, 2005). Secondary end points from those studies also revealed significant improvements in quality of life (QoL) for people treated with oxybutynin TDS, relative to placebo.

Oxytrol is a clear, matrix patch, not easily detected on exposed skin. The active ingredient, oxybutynin, is dissolved in the thin layer of adhesive, delivering the medicine slowly and constantly for the 3 or 4 days that the patch is worn. The TDS patch is applied twice weekly to intact, clean skin of either the abdomen, hip, or buttock. Other areas of the skin can be used for patch application. Cutting the oxybutynin matrix patch in half will not alter the drug delivery rate but will lower the total delivered dose; the unused half can be stored up to 7 days. The manufacturer does not recommend cutting the patch. To ensure compliance, patients are instructed to change the patch on the same two days each week. Skin patch disadvantages include local irritation such as pruritus and erythema, with nearly 9% of study subjects thinking that the reactions were severe enough to cause them to withdraw from the study (Dmochowski, Sand, et al., 2003). This problem may be alleviated if an oxybutynin gel receives FDA approval.

Elevated skin temperature, heat, moisture, and the integrity of the patch can affect the absorption of the medication. Rotation of the application site (at least 1 week between applications to the same site) is important for avoiding skin reactions (Davila et al., 2001). Also, the drug may not be absorbed as well through adipose tissue (e.g., the skin of the abdomen in a person with large abdominal girth). The manufacturer provides explicit user information on applying and removing the patch. As noted, oxybutynin TDS has shown dry mouth and constipation rates similar to placebo.

Oxybutynin Intravesical. Intravesical delivery (delivery directly into the bladder) of oxybutynin has also been investigated as a means of bypassing first-pass metabolism and reducing the adverse effects associated with the metabolite of oxybutynin (Dmochowski, 2005). A solution is compounded by crushing 5-mg tablets of oxybutynin and dissolving them in 60 mL of distilled water. This solution is then instilled in the bladder using a catheter. This method is a consideration for patients with neurogenic causes of bladder DO, such as multiple sclerosis or myelodysplasia, in whom indwelling or intermittent catheters are used to treat urinary dysfunction.

Solifenacin (VESIcare [Astellas, GlaxoSmithKline]). Solifenacin succinate is a muscarinic receptor antagonist that primarily blocks M_3 and M_1 receptors and may have more selectivity for M_3 receptors in the bladder. Solifenacin, at a daily dose of 5 mg or 10 mg, is an effective and well-tolerated treatment option in patients who have OAB. Solifenacin increases functional bladder capacity and decreases urgency, frequency, and incontinence. In animal models, solifenacin has demonstrated selectivity for muscarinic receptors in the bladder over those in the salivary glands, which may account for a lower incidence of dry mouth and constipation reported in the clinical trials.

Solifenacin 5 mg or 10 mg has been shown to decrease daily incontinence episodes, voids per day, urgency episodes, and nocturia and to increase bladder capacity (Abrams & Swift, 2005; Cardozo, Lisec, et al., 2004). A 12-week study of solifenacin 5 mg and 10 mg ($n = 578$) and tolterodine ER 4 mg ($n = 599$) was done in subjects with OAB symptoms (Chapple, Martinez-Garcia, et al., 2005). Subjects receiving solifenacin were permitted to adjust dosing. Flexible dosing with solifenacin was more effective than fixed dosing with tolterodine for most of the measured outcomes, with 74% of solifenacin patients experiencing a mean reduction of at least 50% in incontinence episodes by the end of the study, compared with 67% of subjects receiving tolterodine. Side effects were generally mild to moderate, and discontinuation because of adverse effects was infrequent (3.5% of solifenacin subjects and 3.0% of tolterodine subjects).

Dry mouth rates increase with increasing doses of solifenacin. Cardozo, Lisec, and colleagues (2004) reported overall rates of 2.3% in the placebo group, 7.7% in subjects receiving 5 mg of solifenacin, and 23.1% of those receiving 10 mg.

Tolterodine (Detrol, Detrol LA [Pfizer]).   Tolterodine tartrate is a nonselective muscarinic receptor antagonist. In 1998, tolterodine was developed specifically to treat OAB symptoms of urgency, frequency, and urgency UI and became the second antimuscarinic drug approved by the FDA. Tolterodine appears to be more selective than oxybutynin for bladder rather than salivary gland muscarinic receptors in certain laboratory animals. Tolterodine is available in a twice-daily 1-mg and 2-mg IR formulation (Detrol) and in a convenient once-daily 2-mg and 4-mg ER formulation (Detrol LA). Tolterodine ER is a capsule containing identical beads each of which has an insoluble core surrounded by a prolonged-release layer composed of 85% ethyl cellulose. Tolterodine slowly dissolves through this semipermeable polymer, with each bead providing a prolonged release of the compound over the 24-hour administration interval. A small amount of the bead is insoluble and exits the body through the stool. The ER formulation of tolterodine was developed to improve tolerability and to simplify administration with a single-daily-dose regimen.

Tolterodine is a tertiary amine that is metabolized (broken down) in the liver to an active metabolite (5-hydroxymethyl) that is mediated by the CYP isoenzyme 2D6. The incidence of dry mouth with tolterodine IR is lower than that with oxybutynin ER.

Actual comparisons of tolterodine IR and tolterodine ER showed that the ER formulation was more effective in reducing mean incontinence episodes (ER 71% vs. IR 60%) and in increasing mean voided volume, but with more favorable tolerability (van Kerrebroeck, Kreder, Jonas, Zinner, & Wein, 2001). The ER formulation of tolterodine (Detrol LA), at a dosage of 4 mg daily, provided significant improvements in the symptoms of OAB in women and was 18% more effective than the IR formulation in a comparative study (Chancellor et al., 2000). Studies show that fewer patients taking tolterodine suffer from dry mouth and other GI side effects when compared with oxybutynin IR at a presumably equal dose (i.e., 5 mg 3 times per day).

Trospium (Sanctura, Sanctura XR [Allergan]).   Trospium chloride has been available in Europe for 25 years and was approved in the United States early in 2004 at a 20-mg twice-daily dose. In contrast to the other available agents, which are negatively charged tertiary amines, trospium chloride is a positively charged (hydrophilic) quaternary amine, which should prevent it from crossing the BBB and also slows its absorption from the GI tract (Staskin, 2006). Therefore, trospium chloride is thought to have a low potential for CNS side effects. Trospium chloride is minimally metabolized by the CYP system, and because it does not compete for CYP3A4 or CYP2D6, its potential for drug–drug interactions is limited. As with other quaternary amines, trospium chloride has low bioavailability, so it should be taken on an empty stomach because the bioavailability is decreased by 70%–80% if taken with a high-fat meal. The recommendation to administer on an empty stomach may be a potential disadvantage in terms of compliance (Rovner, 2004).

Trospium (20-mg twice-daily dose) significantly reduces the frequency and severity of urgency, urinary leakage, voids per day, and nocturnal awakenings (Madersbacher et al., 1995; Rudy, Cline, Harris, Goldberg, & Dmochowski, 2006; Zinner et al., 2004). U.S.-based studies attempted to determine subjects' perception of urgency by using a validated Indevus Urgency Severity Scale (Nixon et al., 2005). This scale notes that subjects may feel a very strong urge to urinate and at other times feel a milder urge before onset of a toilet void. They are asked to rate this feeling by circling 0, 1, 2, or 3, which are defined as: (0) None, no urgency; (1) Mild, awareness of urgency, but *easily tolerated* and the person can continue with usual activity or tasks; (2) Moderate, enough urgency discomfort that it *interferes with or shortens* usual activity or tasks; and (3) Severe, extreme urgency discomfort that abruptly *stops all* activity or tasks. Reduction of urgency based on this scale was seen with trospium (Zinner et al., 2004), and onset of the clinical effect with this drug was seen within 7 days (Rudy et al., 2006). Also, subject discontinuation rates in these studies were similar to placebo, which indicates a well-tolerated drug. Researchers reported decreased daytime and nighttime symptoms, improved QoL, and good tolerability in subjects given trospium compared with placebo (Zinner et al., 2004). Commonly reported side effects are outlined in Appendix Table 9.3 (Zinner, 2005).

Trospium ER (Sanctura ER), a 60-mg once-daily dose, was released in 2008. Staskin, Sand, Zinner, and Dmochowski (2007) published results of a 12-week multicenter, parallel, double-blind, placebo-controlled trial of this new ER dose of trospium. Subjects, who were prescribed trospium once daily ($n = 298$), experienced an average decrease from 4.4 urgency UI episodes per day at baseline to 1.6 episodes per day at week 12. Daily frequency decreased from 12.8 voids per day at baseline to fewer than 10 voids per day at week 12. This study analyzed "normalization" (subjects with no urgency UI episodes and a daily void frequency of 8 times or fewer), in which twice as many subjects treated with trospium achieved normalization at week 12 compared with those given placebo (20.5% vs. 11.3%). The most common adverse effects were dry mouth (trospium 8.7% vs. placebo 3%) and constipation (trospium 9.4% vs. placebo 1.3%).

Fesoterodine: A Forthcoming Medication for OAB.

Fesoterodine has been approved for treatment of OAB symptoms in Europe and will doubtless be submitted for review in the United States. Fesoterodine is a prodrug, meaning that it is rapidly converted to DD01, the active metabolite of tolterodine. It is also dose flexible (4 mg and 8 mg) and has a tighter range of serum concentration than tolterodine.

Two studies have shown efficacy versus placebo in subjects taking fesoterodine 4 and 8 mg (Chapple, van Kerrebroeck, et al., 2007; Nitti et al., 2007). A more pronounced effect was observed with fesoterodine 8 mg, especially regarding urgency UI episodes and increased volume voided per micturition. Side effects of fesoterodine are similar to those seen with the previously discussed medications, and are increased with the 8-mg versus the 4-mg dose.

Drug Comparisons: Efficacy and Tolerability

There are very few head-to-head (comparing one antimuscarinic medication to another) clinical trials comparing the efficacy and tolerability of the different antimuscarinic drugs (Rosenberg, Newman, Tallman, & Page, 2007). Also, many of these studies have not included a placebo group.

The OPERA (*O*veractive Bladder: *P*erformance of *E*xtended-*R*elease *A*gents) study compared the ER formulations of both oxybutynin 10 mg/day and tolterodine 4 mg/day for a period of 12 weeks in 790 women (Diokno et al., 2003). The two agents showed similar efficacy in reducing weekly episodes of urgency UI, but oxybutynin was significantly more effective in decreasing micturition frequency. Nearly one quarter of women (23%) taking oxybutynin reported no episodes of UI, compared with 16.8% of those using tolterodine. The incidence of dry mouth was higher in the oxybutynin group (30% vs. 22%), but tolerability was otherwise comparable (Diokno et al., 2003).

The efficacy and safety of oxybutynin TDS 3.9 mg/day compared with tolterodine ER 4 mg/day were studied in subjects with urgency or mixed UI who had previously been successfully treated (Dmochowski, Sand, et al., 2003). Both agents significantly reduced the number of daily incontinence episodes, increased the average voided volume, and improved QoL—all primary end points of the study. However, it should be noted that the oxybutynin skin patch had a higher incidence of skin irritations (22.3%), which were not seen with the oral agents. The most common adverse effects for the oxybutynin patch were application site reactions, including localized pruritus (14% vs. 4.3% placebo) and erythema (8.3% vs. 1.7% placebo). There was a slightly higher incidence of anticholinergic effects, including dry mouth, in subjects receiving tolterodine (7.3%) versus those using the oxybutynin skin patch (4.1%).

Solifenacin in a 5-mg or 10-mg dose was compared with tolterodine ER 4 mg daily in a flexible dosing trial called STAR (*S*olifenacin and *T*olterodine as an *A*ctive Comparator in a *R*andomized Trial) (Chapple, Martinez-Garcia, et al., 2005). This was a "noninferiority" trial. Solifenacin was found to be slightly more effective than tolterodine in all outcomes. A subanalysis of this study was performed on outcomes of subjects who remained on solifenacin 5 mg and tolterodine 4 mg (Chapple, Fianu-Jonsson, et al., 2007). After 4 weeks of active treatment, there were improvements (only the difference in UI episodes was statistically significant) in all OAB symptoms, including urgency, frequency (primary endpoint), incontinence, and nocturia. In both groups,

52% of solifenacin patients and 49% of tolterodine ER patients in the full analysis population chose to continue as previously and did not request a dose increase. Subjects treated with solifenacin 5 mg experienced mean improvements in all OAB symptoms, that were greater than those experienced by patients randomized to tolterodine ER 4 mg. For OAB symptoms of frequency (associated with volume voided per micturition), urgency, and nocturia, the mean results for the solifenacin group were an improvement of 16%–19% greater than the mean for tolterodine ER 4 mg. For incontinence and pad use, the differences were considerably more, ranging from 34% to 51%, and were statistically significant. At 4 weeks, the incidence of dry mouth was 18.2% in the solifenacin 5 mg group and 14.5% in the tolterodine ER 4 mg group. Both solifenacin 5 mg and tolterodine ER 4 mg were well tolerated; the incidence of constipation was 3.0% and 1.2% and that of blurred vision 0.2% and 1.2% for the solifenacin 5 mg and tolterodine ER 4 mg groups, respectively.

Community-Based Studies

An important outcome of drug therapy is the impact on QoL. Research has been conducted in clinical "real-life" settings to determine the effect of the use of antimuscarinic medication on an individual's daily life. We have reviewed a few of these studies, as they have applicability to everyday clinical practice.

The *Antimuscarinic Clinical Effectiveness Trial* (ACET) used a global measure of efficacy called the Patient Perception of Bladder Condition (PPBC), shown in Chapter 6 (Sussman & Garely, 2002). The PPBC is a subjective, validated, single-item visual analogue scale that asks subjects to rate their bladder condition on a 6-point scale from 1 (no problems at all) to 6 (many severe problems) used as the primary end point (Coyne, Matza, Kopp, & Abrams, 2006). This scale is being used in other OAB research and is a simple scale that can be used in clinical practice. This study involved the use of two doses of oxybutynin ER (5 mg or 10 mg) and two doses of tolterodine ER (2 mg or 4 mg) in two separate trials. Greater perceived improvement occurred in the 4-mg tolterodine ER group over the 10-mg oxybutynin ER group.

Another community-based study involved the efficacy of tolterodine ER 4 mg daily (Elinoff et al., 2006; Roberts et al., 2006). In a study labeled IMPACT (*IM*provement in *P*atients *A*ccessing Symptomatic *C*ontrol with *T*olterodine), the most bothersome OAB symptoms were studied. Among incontinent subjects who were evaluated in a primary care setting ($n = 772$), the most bothersome OAB symptoms were daytime frequency (28%), urinary incontinence (urge UI; 27%), nocturnal frequency (26%), and urgency (19%); among continent subjects ($n = 91$), they were daytime frequency (47%), nocturnal frequency (42%), and urgency (10%). Improvement in bladder condition was experienced by 78.8% of the "intent-to-treat" population and by 86.2% of the urgency group, 78.5% of the nocturnal frequency group, 78.0% of the daytime frequency group, and 74.6% of the urgency UI group. In the IMPACT trial, more men than women reported urgency, daytime frequency, and nocturnal frequency as most bothersome, and more women than men reported urgency UI as most bothersome. It was surprising that urgency UI was not the most bothersome OAB symptom noted by subjects in this study. Subjects had high treatment expectations, with most expecting considerable symptom relief and some expecting complete relief. Clinicians should take patient expectations into account when discussing anticipated treatment benefits; individuals whose expectations are met may be more likely to adhere to the treatment regimen. Expectations should be discussed and unrealistic ones adjusted.

A more recent study is one that looked at change in QoL as the primary outcome measure (Sand et al., 2007). Called the *M*ulticenter *A*ssessment of *TR*ansdermal Therapy *I*n Overactive Bladder with O*X*ybutynin TDS (MATRIX), this study evaluated a community-dwelling adult population with OAB during treatment with oxybutynin TDS. All subjects received Oxytrol (3.9 mg/day, twice-weekly patch application) for up to 6 months. Study sites were randomized 1:1, within investigator medical specialty, to receive user behavior education materials (educational intervention) or standard user instructions (ordinary care) along with a supply of the drug. The additional education materials included an educational booklet, OAB newsletters, dosing reminders, calendar reminder stickers, and a Bladder Diary (not used for data collection). In addition to completing all baseline questionnaires, subjects also provided a global assessment of OAB severity using the PPBC. The primary end point was the change in QoL. Improvements were seen across all areas of the symptom severity domain; the greatest changes occurred among the most bothersome symptoms, with more than 40% of subjects reporting improvements in frequency, nocturia, urgency, and urgency UI. The greatest proportion of subjects' improvements in individual item responses were observed in the role limitations domain (household tasks, 41.5%; activities outside the home, 42.0%), incontinence impact domain (41.3%), physical limitations domain (physical activities, 39.2%; ability to travel, 39.0%), and sleep/energy domain (sleep, 38.4%; feeling tired, 34.4%).

Considerations When Choosing an OAB Drug

Clinicians have many antimuscarinic preparations to choose from but, when it comes to drug choice, there is no "best" drug for OAB "wet" or OAB "dry." As mentioned, all can have bothersome systemic antimuscarinic side effects. Appendix Table 9.1 discusses treatment considerations for these drugs, and this section provides a more detailed review of these considerations.

Chemical Structure.   Antimuscarinic agents differ primarily in whether their chemical structure is a tertiary or quaternary amine. The tertiary amines (oxybutynin, tolterodine, darifenacin, solifenacin) have three carbon groups on the nitrogen atom, whereas the quaternary amines (trospium) have four carbon groups on the nitrogen atom. The tertiary amines are generally well absorbed and readily distributed throughout the body. Quaternary amines, by being more polar, have lower GI absorption and must be taken on an empty stomach.

The tertiary amines utilized for OAB treatment are metabolized by the CYP system. CYP isoenzymes, such as CYP3A4 and CYP2D6, are found in the liver (and other tissues) and are the major catalysts of drug metabolic reactions. The greatest number of drug–drug interactions involve this isoenzyme system. In some cases, one or more of coadministered agents can compete for the same isoenzyme. In other cases, a specific drug can induce or inhibit the level of a specific isoenzyme, up-regulating (increasing) or down-regulating (decreasing) the number of available receptors, and thereby altering the ability to metabolize drugs that are substrates for that CYP isoenzyme (Chancellor & de Miguel, 2007). The CYP2D6 isoenzyme metabolizes most antidepressants, including selective serotonin reuptake inhibitors and many tricyclic antidepressants; beta blockers; antiarrhythmics; and antipsychotics. Fluoxetine, a very commonly prescribed antidepressant, is a potent inhibitor of CYP2D6 and can significantly increase tolterodine concentrations.

Whereas most drugs indicated for OAB—tolterodine, darifenacin, solifenacin, and oxybutynin—are extensively metabolized by the CYP system, trospium is not. Trospium is eliminated mostly as unchanged drug, suggesting that it has lower potential for drug–drug interactions. It may therefore represent a safer treatment option for OAB, from the standpoint of drug–drug interactions, in older adults who are taking multiple medications (polypharmacy).

Drug Excretion. Excretion of the antimuscarinic drugs may make a difference in symptoms. Many of the tertiary amines undergo extensive hepatic metabolism, so that the urine then contains 1% or less of the parent compound for oxybutynin, tolterodine, and darifenacin, and approximately 15% for solifenacin (Andersson, 2002). Trospium ER is poorly absorbed (10%) and metabolized in the kidneys, and approximately 60% of the absorbed compound is excreted unchanged in the urine. Because the tertiary amines are metabolized in both the liver and kidneys, the recommended dose in patients with impaired hepatic or renal function may need to be reduced. For example, the recommended doses for Detrol (2 mg/day) or Detrol LA (4 mg/day) may be reduced to 1 mg/day and 2 mg/day, respectively. In patients with reduced renal creatinine clearance, trospium IR 20 mg may be prescribed once a day.

Drug Molecular Characteristics. The molecular weight, lipophilicity, and charge of the drug molecule may also be important in the activity of a drug. If a drug is hydrophilic (lipophobic), with a large molecular size and positive charge (e.g., trospium), it may have difficulty in crossing lipid cell membranes, thereby limiting GI absorption and bioavailability. These same properties also would limit transit across the BBB. If the drug is lipophilic (hydrophobic), with a small molecular size, a neutral charge, and low polarity, it has decreased solubility in crossing the water layer adjacent to the cell, and thus can more readily cross the BBB. Such compounds also tend to be reabsorbed in the glomerulus, slowing the rate of elimination from the body (Staskin, 2005). However, a lipophilic drug is better suited for transdermal delivery.

Darifenacin, oxybutynin, solifenacin, and tolterodine have characteristics that allow for drug passage into the brain, including high lipophilicity, low molecular weight, and a low to moderate number of positively charged molecules. As a result, these compounds are able to pass through the BBB, with the potential of inducing CNS adverse effects. Darifenacin appears to be an exception to this, perhaps because it has less affinity for the brain muscarinic (M_1) receptor, thought to be the cognition receptor. Conversely, trospium has low lipophilicity, high-molecular-weight molecules, and a high positive charge that should prevent its entry into the brain (Todorova, Vonderheid-Guth, & Dimpfel, 2001). Some believe that the BBB is altered (increased permeability) in certain conditions (e.g., aging, stress).

Drug Delivery.   The term *pill burden* is generally considered a function of the number of pills required each day for therapy. However, a comprehensive definition of *pill burden* also encompasses the difficulty patients have in taking prescribed doses because of other factors, such as frequency of pill ingestion, pill size, pill form (capsule vs. tablet), and method of ingestion. In LTC facilities, medication distribution is a resource-consuming task. In such settings, decreasing staff pill burden with a twice-weekly transdermal formulation (Oxytrol) may be appropriate.

Compliance with Drug Therapy.   Compliance is a problem for many patients, and the clinician should assess the ability of an individual to adhere to a recommended drug therapy prior to prescribing a specific OAB drug. Age and comorbidity are associated with lower adherence to medications (Balkrishnan, Bhosle, Camacho, & Anderson, 2006). The route of drug delivery (e.g., skin patch or gel versus a pill) may also affect compliance, because nicotine and estrogen skin patches have been shown to have increased treatment compliance (Potts & Lobo, 2005).

Financial considerations are an additional factor in compliance. The monthly cost of the prescribed dosage is comparable across all these medications. However, with the advent of Medicare Part D drug coverage, some of the newer agents are not covered. Coverage by state Medicaid programs depends on the individual state plan. Many insurers who have prescription drug plans may not have a particular antimuscarinic drug in their "formulary" of covered drugs, or may require that the person fail on the generic, less expensive, and less well-tolerated agent (e.g., oxybutynin IR) before he or she is allowed to use a newer drug in a particular class. This places an added burden and frustration on the clinician and the patient. Patients may not be willing or able to pay "out of pocket" for OAB treatments, but will purchase absorbent products, often at double the cost of drug therapy per month. We have encountered many patients with severe UI who will spend upward of $200 per month on absorbent products but will discontinue a prescribed OAB medication because of unwillingness to pay even a $20 copayment. Clinicians may need to initiate a dialogue about drug cost prior to prescribing an anticholinergic medication.

Antimuscarinic Use in Specific Populations

Older Adults. Antimuscarinics are often underutilized in older adults despite the marked increase in the prevalence of urgency UI and OAB in this age group. Although efficacy has been demonstrated in adult populations, few studies have reported results specifically on antimuscarinic (e.g., darifenacin, oxybutynin TDS, tolterodine) use in the older adult population (Foote, Glavind, Kralidis, & Wyndaele, 2005; Malone-Lee, Shaffu, Anand, & Powell, 2001; Sand et al., 2007; Zinner, Mattiasson, & Stanton, 2002). Sand et al. (2007) conducted a community-based trial looking at a drug "safety" population embedded in the larger study ($N = 2,878$). The safety group included 1,366 participants (47.5%) who were 65 years or older and 699 subjects 75 years or older. Adverse effects possibly related to treatment were reported by 28.8% of elderly participants; none of these effects was serious. The most common treatment-related adverse effect was application skin site reaction (13.3%). Treatment-related antimuscarinic adverse effects were infrequently reported: dry mouth, 33 participants (2.4%); constipation, 30 participants (2.2%); and other adverse effects, 1% of participants or less.

Although drug absorption does not generally change with aging, drug distribution may change, depending on water content and muscle mass. Such a change would result in greater distribution of drugs that are fat soluble. Drug metabolism can also change. Because there is a reduction of renal function with aging, drugs that are cleared by the kidneys may have to be reduced in dosage. Oral oxybutynin IR can have a significant increase in plasma concentration in "frail" elderly adults, compared with healthy elderly control subjects, which may suggest that a lower dose should be used for the older adult population that has significant comorbidity.

Another explanation for the apparent underuse of antimuscarinics in the elderly population is the frequency of adverse effects due to "anticholinergic load" (the cumulative effect of taking multiple medications that have anticholinergic side effects). There are 600 known anticholinergic medications. The elderly individual has increased vulnerability to anticholinergic side effects and toxicity as related to

- Slower metabolism and elimination of drug

- Possible increased permeability in the BBB that can occur with aging

- Changes in the number and distribution of muscarinic receptors that occur with aging and dementing disorders

- Age-related deficits in neurotransmission

- Use of multiple anticholinergics, resulting in additive total anticholinergic burden

- Other individual differences

The possibility of drug–drug interactions is an important consideration with any medication, and particularly important in this group because older adults are more likely to be using multiple medications. The average number of medications per person is 6.5 (4.5 prescribed plus 2 over the counter) in this age group. Also, this group is more likely to be taking other anticholinergic medications, and this anticholinergic load may potentiate the number and severity of side effects (Scheife & Takeda, 2005). The older adult often has co-morbid conditions (e.g., Parkinson's disease, type 2 diabetes) that may exaggerate anticholinergic effects on cognitive function (Kay et al., 2005). In many older adults, OAB drug effects on cognition may go undetected. Little is known about the cognitive effects of these drugs on older adults because few well-conducted studies exist. Most studies are not placebo controlled, and have not used clinically relevant cognitive assessments, especially in elderly subjects.

Oxybutynin (oral) and tolterodine have both been associated in case reports with cognitive adverse effects and effects on sleep architecture and quality. There have been case reports on the adverse effect of tolterodine in older adults with dementia (Edwards & O'Connor, 2002). An early placebo-controlled study showed significant deficits on cognitive function tests in healthy older volunteers taking oxybutynin IR (Katz et al., 1998). Case studies reported impaired immediate learning and impaired delayed recall after use of tolterodine (Malavuad, Bagheri, Senard, & Sarramon, 1999; Tsao & Heilman, 2003; Womack & Heilman, 2003). Confusion and hallucinations are listed as potential adverse effects in the prescribing information for the OAB drugs tolterodine, oxybutynin, and trospium (Williams & Staudenmeier, 2004). Oxybutynin TDS has not been reported to cause cognitive changes and is often considered the OAB treatment of choice in the older individual (Saltzstein, 2005). Darifenacin does not appear to be associated with cognitive adverse effects. In a study of healthy subjects 60 years of age and older, darifenacin had no significant effects on memory (Name–Face Association Test—delayed recall) when compared to high doses of oxybutynin ER, which showed memory deterioration (Kay et al., 2006). A study of 129 older volunteers taking both dosing levels of darifenacin showed no significant effect across primary cognitive function tests (see Chapter 6).

Several trials in community-dwelling elderly populations have compared tolterodine and oxybutynin and have found comparable effectiveness in treating OAB. A study of tolterodine comparing younger (mean age 51 years) and older (mean age 74 years) individuals showed that tolterodine works as well in older patients as in younger patients. A study of LTC residents that added short-acting oxybutynin to a prompted voiding protocol helped about a third of the residents who were not responding to prompted voiding alone. These studies are reviewed in Chapter 8.

Patients with Dementia. The cholinesterase inhibitors—donepezil (Aricept), rivastigmine (Exelon), and galantamine (Razadyne)—are medications prescribed for dementia. Because of their effect on the autonomic nervous system, it is possible for them to cause or exacerbate urgency UI (Gill et al., 2005).

Adding to this complexity is the fact that new-onset or worsening dementia can also cause UI. Many clinicians, especially those working in LTC facilities, attribute new-onset urgency UI to worsening dementia when in fact it is caused by the dementia drug therapy. Many have voiced concerns about the use of antimuscarinic OAB medications in patients taking cholinergic medications such as cholinesterase inhibitors because they have opposing actions (Carnahan, Lund, Perry, & Chrischilles, 2004; Roe, Anderson, & Spivack, 2002; Sink, 2008). These drugs mimic the action of ACh. In theory, concurrent use of anticholinergic drugs may dilute the benefits of the cholinesterase inhibitors (Gill et al., 2005). Such concomitant use has been shown to occur in about one third of cases (Carnahan et al., 2004). Clinicians treating both conditions may consider switching the individual to memantine (Namenda), since the mode of action of this drug is independent of ACh and acetylcholinesterase. However, one must be mindful that this type of drug may be less effective for certain types of dementia. In any case, clinicians should not ignore UI in a person with dementia but, instead, consider treatment and closely monitor the person for adverse effects on cognitive function (Jewart, Green, Lu, Cellar, & Tune, 2005).

Residents in LTC Facilities.   In the LTC setting (e.g., skilled nursing facilities), OAB medications are rarely prescribed despite UI and OAB prevalence of over 50%. A study of 33,301 nursing facility residents found that an average of 6.7 medications were ordered per resident, with 27% of residents taking 9 or more medications (Tobias & Sey, 2001). Narayanan, Cerulli, Kahler, and Ouslander (2007) noted that only a small portion (7%) of nursing home residents with mobility and cognitive function receives drug therapy for UI. Most incontinence specialists believe this reflects an unmet need for treating UI and OAB in this population.

When prescribing in this population, the clinician must exercise caution. The Beers Criteria for assessment of inappropriate medications in patients 65 years of age and older were developed in 1997, updated in 2003, and adopted by the Centers for Medicare & Medicaid Services (CMS) in July 1999 for elderly-resident nursing facility regulation purposes (Flick et al., 2003). On the list of medications likely to cause adverse effects because of concomitant illness were oxybutynin IR, tolterodine IR, and flavoxate. The CMS has since issued the Tag F329 surveyor guidance *Unnecessary Drugs* for use in LTC facilities (CMS, 2006). In this guidance, the CMS noted that medications are an integral part of the care provided to residents of nursing facilities, and that proper medication selection and prescribing, including dose, duration, and type of medication(s), may help stabilize or improve a resident's outcome, QoL, and functional capacity. The CMS recommended that, as part of medication management, it is important for LTC staff, medical directors, nurse practitioners, and pharmacists to consider nonpharmacological approaches to OAB and incontinence (e.g., toileting or bladder training programs). This guideline emphasizes that the facility must monitor the resident for the effects and potential adverse consequences of the medication regimen. The document lists the anticholinergic medications as having adverse effects but does not say that these medications are contraindicated. If such drugs are prescribed, assessments of the effects of the medication on the individual's UI, as well as on lower urinary tract symptoms, should be done periodically. Also, drug therapy is most appropriate in residents who are in either an active toileting or on independent bladder training program (CMS, 2005). Monitoring should be done after 2–3 months to see if the resident is benefiting from drug therapy.

Men with Benign Prostatic Hyperplasia.   Few studies have investigated men who have OAB as a result of benign prostatic hyperplasia (BPH) (Dmochowski, Abrams, Marschall-Kehrel, Wang, & Guan, 2007). The following case presentation is often seen in clinical practice.

> *Michael is a 68-year-old lawyer, presenting with a 2-year history of urgency and frequency that has gradually worsened over the past 6 months. Frequency includes nocturnal episodes of three to four times per night. He denies incontinence. Nocturia is the most bothersome symptom because Michael is unable to sleep more than 3 hours. As a practicing lawyer, increased frequency can be a problem for him because of court duties and the continual need to leave the courtroom because of urgency. Nocturia also adversely affects his work because he experiences increased fatigue by late afternoon. He has been taking alfuzosin and dutasteride for 3 years as treatment for BPH. Initially, these medications decreased his nocturia, but it reoccurred after 6 months. He has a strong urinary stream and feels that he has complete bladder emptying. He was unable to identify events that may "trigger" symptoms. Michael attempted to modify his diet and has eliminated caffeinated products. Recordings in a 3-day Bladder Diary indicated voiding frequency of approximately 13 times daily and 3–4 times nightly. His prostate-specific antigen blood level has been within normal limits.*

Symptoms of OAB (urgency, frequency) may decrease somewhat with alpha blocker therapy, but less so than symptoms attributed to obstruction (hesitancy, slow stream). Men with OAB syndrome and a small residual urine volume (some say < 125 mL), who neither tolerate nor have a response to alpha blockers, may benefit from a trial of an antimuscarinic agent, provided they are carefully monitored for the development of urinary retention (Lee, Kim, & Chancellor, 2006). It is thought that these agents may offer relief for significant symptoms of frequency and urgency in such patients. Studies of men with BPH who were tested unsuccessfully with alpha blocker therapy have shown that antimuscarinic therapy (tolterodine) could significantly decrease lower urinary tract symptoms (Kaplan et al., 2006; Roehrborn et al., 2006). Many clinicians believe that antimuscarinic therapy is an option either as initial therapy in men with OAB or as additional therapy if alpha blocker and 5-alpha-reductase inhibitor treatments fail to improve symptoms in men with OAB and benign prostatic obstruction (BPO; defined in Chapter 4). Indications from this research (Kaplan et al., 2006; Roehrborn et al., 2006) are that, in men with BPO, antimuscarinics are safe and unlikely to produce urinary retention.

Individuals with Neurological Disease.   Oxybutynin was classically the drug widely used in patients who have neurogenic bladder dysfunction or neurogenic DO (see Chapter 4). Bennett et al. (2004) evaluated the efficacy and safety of high-dose oxybutynin ER in a small number of patients who had multiple sclerosis ($n = 22$), spinal cord injury ($n = 10$), and Parkinson's disease ($n = 7$). Doses were increased by 5 mg at weekly intervals to a maximum dose of 30 mg daily. Participant perception of efficacy versus side effects directed dose escalation. Within 1 week of treatment, over half of the subjects reported a decrease in frequency, episodes of nocturia, and incontinence episodes. Most (74.4%) subjects in this study requested higher doses (15 mg or greater) of oxybutynin ER; therefore, these investigators concluded that, in this population, doses of up to 30 mg may be more effective.

O'Leary et al. (2003) evaluated the effects and tolerability of oxybutynin ER on neurogenic bladder function in a small number of subjects with spinal cord injury. In a 12-week study, 10 subjects with complete or incomplete spinal cord injury were given oxybutynin ER 10 mg once daily. The primary efficacy measure, urodynamic bladder capacity, was found to increase from 274 mL at baseline to 380 mL (39% increase) at the end of the study, with the number of incontinence episodes decreasing from 13 to 6 episodes per week (54% decrease).

An 8-week, multicenter, open-label, dose titration study of oxybutynin TDS in adult subjects (mean age, 42.2; 86.4% were male) with neurogenic bladder dysfunction resulting from spinal cord injury (Newman, Kennelly, Lemack, & McIlwain, 2007) was conducted in subjects on intermittent catheterization who had UI between catheterizations. The oxybutynin TDS dose could be adjusted every 2 weeks by increasing or decreasing by one dose level (3.9 mg/day, 7.8 mg/day, 9.1 mg/day, and 11.7 mg/day). Treatment with oxybutynin TDS was associated with improved QoL and fewer urinary leakages between scheduled intermittent catheterizations in these subjects.

Children.   Oxybutynin is the only antimuscarinic medication approved for use in children in the United States. It has been used effectively for a number of years in the pediatric population (Berry, 2006). Early studies showed that oxybutynin IR significantly increased bladder capacity and decreased intravesical pressure, leading to resolution or downgrading of vesicoureteral reflux (Homsy, Nsouli, Hamburger, Laberge, & Schick, 1985). Children who have neurogenic bladder with DO have benefited greatly from the use of the drug, with success rates of 90%. Usually, oxybutynin IR had to be dosed 3 times daily in children because a more severe drop in plasma levels is seen in children (Autret et al., 1994).

More recently, Youdim and Kogan (2002) evaluated the safety and efficacy of oxybutynin ER in children who had neurogenic bladder dysfunction and in children who had urinary urgency and frequency but not neurological dysfunction. Dosage was as close to 0.3 mg/kg daily as possible. All subjects who had neurogenic bladder ($n = 11$) reported a reduction in the number of incontinence episodes between catheterizations. Of the children diagnosed with urgency, frequency, and urgency UI ($n = 11$), all reported a "cure" in daytime incontinence with oxybutynin ER. Nearly half of the subjects (48%) experienced no side effects. Of those who did, the most common side effects were dry mouth, constipation, heat intolerance, and drowsiness, occurring in 40%, 16%, 16%, and 12% of all subjects, respectively. With the increasing use of oxybutynin ER in children, issues of compliance and tolerability can be greatly minimized.

Anticholinergic–Antimuscarinic Contraindications and Adverse Side Effects

As mentioned, the problem with antimuscarinic medications, as with most medications, is that they are contraindicated in certain individuals and have certain adverse side effects (see Appendix Table 9.3). These side effects are usually minor and time limited and can be managed using simple interventions. They can be classified as issues with drug tolerability or safety. Clinicians should discuss the side effect profile with the individual when a particular drug is prescribed. Providing information such as that in the patient education tool "The Side Effects of Treatment for Overactive Bladder" (on the companion CD), developed by the University of Minnesota School of Nursing clinical practice group, Minnesota Continence Associates, is an example. Appendix Table 9.1 lists side effects, with a more detailed review provided in this section.

Contraindications.   Antimuscarinic agents should be used with caution in patients with the risk of urinary retention or gastric retention. They are contraindicated in patients with controlled narrow-angle glaucoma.

Adverse Side Effects.   An adverse side effect is an unpleasant symptom or event that is due to or associated with a medication, such as impairment or decline in an individual's mental or physical condition or functional or psychosocial status. OAB drugs have anticholinergic side effects that affect drug tolerability (dry mouth, constipation) or drug safety. Adverse effects related to antimuscarinic drug safety can include blurred vision, exacerbation of gastroesophageal reflux, cardiac changes (increased heart rate, which is an anticholinergic side effect; increased QT interval, which occurs with some of these drugs but is not related to their anticholinergic properties), urinary retention, and the likelihood of detrimental CNS effects, including somnolence, tiredness, impaired concentration, headache, confusion, dementia/memory impairment, delirium, disorientation, cognitive impairment, and sleep disturbances. With the OAB drugs, there is also the potential for harmful interactions with other prescribed drugs. These side effects are dose dependent but are clearly evident even at normal therapeutic levels. Other potential problems with this class of drugs include adverse drug reactions and interactions (e.g., drug–drug, drug–food, and drug–disease). A comparison of the OAB anticholinergic drug side effects, compared to placebo, is found in Appendix Table 9.3.

Drug Tolerability

Dry Mouth. Dry mouth is the side effect most often reported by patients taking these medications, and it increases incrementally with increasing doses of drug (Ouslander, 2004). The effects on the salivary gland are primarily the result of blockade of M_3 receptors found in the salivary gland (Abrams et al., 2006). IR formulations are more likely to cause more tolerability adverse effects than ER formulations, and oxybutynin, in general, appears to cause a higher incidence of dry mouth than the other OAB drugs (Ouslander, 2004). Dry mouth appears to increase with increasing doses of these medications. Many clinicians will instruct patients to take the medication at bedtime to minimize the side effect of dry mouth. A nighttime tolterodine ER dosing regimen was associated with a lower incidence of adverse effects, particularly dry mouth, while maintaining 24-hour efficacy (Dmochowski et al., 2007; Rackley, Weiss, Rovner, Wang, & Guan, 2006). Attempts to control dry mouth by excessive fluid intake are not advisable because this will increase urine production and excretion, which will probably exacerbate urinary frequency and incontinence. In patients who report significant dry mouth, we recommend the use of regular or sugar-free candy, lozenges, gum, or mouthwash.

There is no doubt that patients will discontinue the medication on their own if dry mouth is significant or not controllable. The clinician should try to adjust the dosage or prescribe one of the many other antimuscarinic medications.

Constipation. Another side effect, constipation, is of great concern, especially in elderly individuals. Bowel motility is dependent to a great degree on activity of the M_3 receptor, so agents with M_3 blockade capability (all the agents possess this to some extent) will decrease GI motility and constipation will occur. Darifenacin may have a greater impact on bowel regularity because M_3 receptors contribute 75% of the muscarinic effect on gut motility, and should be used with caution in patients with conditions such as severe constipation, ulcerative colitis, and myasthenia gravis. Clinicians need to perform a thorough bowel history (see Chapter 5) to identify those individuals with or who are at risk for developing constipation and institute a bowel regimen (see Chapter 5) if indicated.

Drug Safety

Cardiac Safety. The cardiac safety of OAB drugs is important, and there is a growing concern about the prolongation of the QT interval (associated with torsades de pointes, a potentially fatal ventricular arrhythmia). Factors for drug-induced torsades de pointes are female gender, bradycardia, hypokalemia, and congestive heart failure. QT interval prolongation has nothing to do with muscarinic blockade activity. It is just a characteristic of some individual drugs, and there are strict limits set by the FDA as to what constitutes cautionary QT interval prolongation. Some drugs have a statement about QT prolongation in their package insert (see Appendix Table 9.1). Obviously the danger is combining an antimuscarinic drug that causes prolongation with other drugs, already prescribed for the patient, that also cause QT prolongation.

Some also voice concern about the effect on heart rate. The M_2 receptor is the receptor that primarily controls cardiac rate activity, so a drug that has considerable M_2 blockade activity might be expected to increase heart rate. If the heart rate goes up even to a slight degree on a chronic basis, especially in older individuals with heart disease, it could constitute a cardiac risk factor. Cardiac rate increases with some of these drugs have been shown; increased cardiac mortality or morbidity has not been shown at this time.

All OAB drugs, except oxybutynin, have undergone cardiac safety studies for QT interval prolongation as part of their FDA approval process. However, darifenacin and trospium were the only antimuscarinics that did not prolong the QT/corrected QT interval in clinical studies designed to look at this variable (Serra et al., 2005). M_2 receptor antagonism can increase resting heart rate (Pietzko, Dimpfel, Schwantes, & Topfmeier, 1994; Todorova et al., 2001). Darifenacin and solifenacin have been shown not to change heart rate compared to placebo (Dmochowski & Staskin, 2005). Trospium (twice-daily dosage) has been reported to increase heart rate by 3–4 to 8 beats per minute. No changes have been reported with the once-daily preparation. Older medications such as oxybutynin and tolterodine have been used in many patients without causing cardiac problems, so they are considered to be "heart safe," but concerns remain among some clinicians.

Alteration in Sleep.   Some research has found that the antimuscarinics used for OAB may affect sleep structure and sleep quality. In one trial, Diefenbach et al. (2003) found that both oxybutynin and tolterodine impaired rapid-eye-movement (REM) sleep. However, in patients using trospium, no impairments of REM sleep were seen, as was the case for sleep patterns with placebo (Staskin & Harnett, 2004).

Skin Side Effects.   Skin side effects are seen only with transdermal products. When using oxybutynin TDS, clinicians need to educate patients about skin preparation, patch application sites, the number of patches to apply, and the need to rotate sites. The patch should be placed on a clean, dry, and smooth (skinfold-free) area of clean, dry, hairless skin that is easily accessed. It should never be applied to skin that is inflamed, is broken, or has any type of irritation. Patients should be advised to avoid use of moisturizers on the area where the patch will be applied, and instead to moisturize the area once the patch is removed. Areas of the skin that have redness or rashes or have been treated with oils, lotions, or powders that could keep the patch from sticking well should be avoided. The person should avoid the waistline area, since tight clothing may rub against the patch. The product information insert recommends use of the abdomen, hip, or buttock. It is helpful to place the patch on an area of skin that is not easily accessible in certain individuals (e.g., on the upper back in patients with dementia). The patch is placed on a different area of the skin each time and should be removed before placing a new one.

Although rare (<1%–3%), bathing, showering, or excessive sweating can result in loss of adhesion and detachment of the patch. Individuals also should avoid exposure of the patch to excessive heat because increased skin temperature may increase drug delivery via increased skin permeability and blood flow (Nitti et al., 2006).

When the patch is removed, the stratum corneum (the top layer of skin) is removed along with it. Patches should not be abruptly pulled off the skin because this causes more trauma to the stratum corneum. Moistening the patch for removal decreases stratum corneum trauma, so the clinician should suggest that the person remove the patch in the shower or when bathing. Nursing staff in LTC facilities can moisten the patch with a warm cloth for removal. Users also need instructions on removal of residual adhesive (the sticky residue) after the patch is removed. Mild soap and water, baby oil, or medical adhesive removal products can be used. Patients should not use cleaners such as alcohol, nail polish removers, or paint thinners.

Other Drugs Used for Urge Incontinence and OAB

Appendix Table 9.1 includes second-line medications that are indicated for patients with urgency UI and OAB but are not prescribed as often as the antimuscarinic drugs. A much less commonly used agent is propantheline (Pro-Banthine), a quaternary ammonium compound that has antimuscarinic and ganglionic receptor-blocking effects. Even in young patients, the drug has a high incidence of side effects, and it must be used with caution in patients with glaucoma, coronary artery disease, or prostatism. Elderly patients are especially prone to confusion, agitation, and orthostatic hypotension when taking propantheline. When using this medication, postvoid urine residuals should be monitored to avoid urinary retention.

Hyoscyamine (Cystospaz) and hyoscyamine sulfate (Levsin, Cystospaz-M) are used by some for treatment of neurogenic bladder and to control "spastic bladder." Some report that they have about the same anticholinergic actions and side effects as other drugs of this class. Flavoxate (Urispas) is a tertiary amine that, in the laboratory, has a direct "antispasmodic" effect, as well as an anticholinergic effect on the bladder smooth muscle. It is indicated for dysuria, urgency, nocturia, suprapubic pain, frequency, and UI. Research has not demonstrated the efficacy of any of these drugs (Andersson et al., 2005).

Desmopressin acetate (DDAVP), a synthetic analogue of antidiuretic hormone (vasopressin), was originally licensed to treat the polyuria of diabetes insipidus and for nocturnal enuresis in children (Asplund, 2007). It increases renal tubular reabsorption of water, resulting in decreased urine output. This drug is most often prescribed in children with bed-wetting because it can decrease urine production for 6 hours, with effectiveness up to 68% (Monda & Husmann, 1995). The greater the disorder of the vasopressin system (large nocturnal urine output), the greater the improvement seen with desmopressin. Antimuscarinic medications such as oxybutynin or tolterodine are prescribed with desmopressin in children with reduced functional bladder capacity or who have daytime incontinence (Berry, 2006). Desmopressin has also been used in women with multiple sclerosis and nighttime frequency. It can be administered orally or intranasally; it may be given nightly or as needed (e.g., on overnight trips). The onset of the medication's action is rapid, and the drug effects last at least 6 hours, with a maximum antidiuretic effect occurring 2 hours after administration (Skoog, Stokes, & Turner, 1997). Adverse effects of desmopressin can include headache and hyponatremia, a potentially serious issue, especially in the elderly.

This drug has been suggested as a treatment for adults who suffer from the OAB symptom nocturia and those with nocturnal enuresis. In a study in men, treatment with desmopressin in the evening has been proven to be effective in statistically reducing the number of early nocturnal micturition episodes and improving sleep (Mattiasson, Abrams, van Kerrebroeck, Walter, & Weiss, 2002). Van Kerrebroeck et al. (2007) conducted a placebo-controlled trial of adults ($n = 184$, with $8 > 65$ years of age) with nocturia (>2 voids/night) who received desmopressin tablets (0.1, 0.2, or 0.4 mg) during a 3-week dose titration period. Compared with placebo, oral desmopressin tablets reduced nocturnal voiding frequency (39% reduction with desmopressin vs. 15% with placebo), increased duration of the first sleep period (prolonged by 108 minutes with desmopressin vs. 41 minutes with placebo), and improved sleep quality. Hyponatremia is the only serious potential adverse effects associated with the use of desmopressin in nocturia, especially in people age 65 years or older. This drug should only be used with caution in the elderly, and with careful monitoring of blood sodium levels (Johnson, Miller, Tang, Pillon, & Ouslander, 2006).

Other Drugs Used for Mixed Incontinence and OAB

Tricyclic Antidepressants

Tricyclic antidepressants (specifically imipramine) have been used to treat patients with OAB and urgency, stress, and mixed UI. The tricyclics are thought to block the reuptake of serotonin and norepinephrine, along with having antihistamine activity and anticholinergic effects. Imipramine is believed to facilitate urinary storage by decreasing bladder contractility by a spinal cord–

inhibitory effect and to increase urethral resistance through its alpha agonist properties. Imipramine is approved by the FDA for enuresis in children but not in adults. Nevertheless, it is often prescribed to manage nocturnal enuresis in both children and adults. The mechanism of action is not well understood; the drug is believed to alter the sleep pattern, so that the person arouses more easily when the bladder becomes full. Unfortunately, no placebo-controlled clinical studies have been conducted for the use of imipramine. Gepertz and Neveus (2004) found it to be effective in 50% of children with enuresis. It has not been studied in adults.

Adverse effects of imipramine can be significant and serious and are listed in Appendix Table 9.1. Side effects may include postural hypotension and cardiac conduction disturbances in older individuals. Older patients with cardiac conduction problems should avoid treatment with this category of drugs unless the benefits outweigh the risks. Additional side effects can include dry mouth, weakness, fatigue, sedation, manic or schizophrenic behavior, parkinsonian effects (e.g., fine tremor), orthostatic hypotension, excessive sweating, orgasmic impotence, and arrhythmia.

DRUG THERAPY FOR BLADDER UNDERACTIVITY

Bethanechol (Duvoid, Urecholine) is a cholinergic agonist drug that is sometimes used to treat bladder (detrusor) underactivity in those individuals with incomplete bladder emptying, but there is little evidence to support its routine use (Table 9.3). The drug stimulates muscarinic receptors in the bladder smooth muscle and GI tract, resulting in increased bladder muscle contractions and peristalsis of the GI tract. This drug is contraindicated in patients with asthma, bradycardia, and Parkinson's disease. Its side effects include sweating and excessive salivation, which are often considered intolerable.

Table 9.3   Drug therapy for underactive bladder and incomplete bladder emptying

Drug	Usual dose	Side effects	Treatment considerations
Bethanechol (Urecholine) Cholinergic agonist	Supplied: 5-, 10-, 25-, and 50-mg tablets Dosage: 10–50 mg bid–qid or 50 mg tid or qid, on an empty stomach	Dizziness, orthostatic hypotension, tachycardia, headache, malaise, diarrhea, nausea, vomiting	• Take on empty stomach to avoid nausea. • Avoid use in person with asthma or heart disease. • Short-term use only. Never give IV or IM because of life-threatening cardiovascular and GI reactions. In elderly patients, use lowest dose possible.

Key: bid = twice daily; GI = gastrointestinal; IM = intramuscularly; IV = intravenously; qid = 4 times daily; tid = 3 times daily.

DRUG THERAPY FOR STRESS INCONTINENCE

The bladder neck and proximal urethra contain a preponderance of alpha-adrenergic receptors that, when stimulated, contribute to urethral closure in the continent person. Theoretically, manipulation of these receptors should alter outlet resistance. However, pharmacotherapy for the treatment of stress UI (SUI) has been limited because of the lack of specificity of the drugs proposed to act on these receptors. This nonspecificity contributes to the wide range of side effects and questions regarding product safety. Although some drugs have been shown to decrease the incidence or magnitude of SUI, the adverse side effects make them clinically impractical. In fact, drug therapy for SUI is considered by some to be a thing of the past. This section presents a short review of drugs used for SUI.

Alpha-Adrenergic Receptor Agonists

The alpha-adrenergic receptor agonists, as a group, have been used for patients with SUI, but efficacy is poor (Alhasso, Glazener, Pickard, & N'Dow, 2005) (Table 9.4). These drugs include ephedrine, pseudoephedrine, and phenylpropanolamine. Because urethral smooth muscle tone is mediated by norepinephrine activation of alpha receptors, the use of alpha-adrenergic receptor agonists would presumably increase the urethral smooth muscle tone, increase urethral closing pressure, and decrease incontinence. Although some of these drugs have been shown to decrease frequency and amount of UI in patients with mild to moderate SUI, their use was discontinued because of their lack of lower urinary tract specificity and the associated potential for hypertension, arrhythmias, headache, and sleep disturbance (insomnia), and potentially lethal side effects such as hemorrhagic stroke. Phenylpropanolamine, an ingredient in these drugs, has been associated with an increased risk of hemorrhagic stroke (bleeding into the brain or into tissue surrounding the brain) in women (Kernan et al., 2000); men may also be at risk. Although the risk of hemorrhagic stroke is low, the FDA recommends that patients not use any products that contain phenylpropanolamine.

Additional adverse drug reactions with alpha-adrenergic agonists are infrequent but include anxiety, agitation, dyspnea, and sweating. These agents should be used cautiously in individuals with hypertension, hyperthyroidism, cardiac arrhythmias, or angina. The adverse side effects can occur as early as 1–6 hours after drug administration and tend to occur in fewer than 10% of patients.

Duloxetine

A balanced serotonin-norephinephrine reuptake inhibitor called duloxetine has been studied for effectiveness in women with SUI. The application for

Table 9.4   Drug therapy for stress urinary incontinence[a]

Drug	Dosage	Side effects	Comments
Phenylpropanolamine[b]	Immediate release: 25–50 mg bid/tid Extended release: 75 mg bid	Tachycardia, elevated blood pressure, stomach cramping, nervousness, respiratory difficulty, dizziness. Hemorrhagic stroke in women.	Do not modify sustained-release forms to achieve dose. Components are found in OTC decongestants. Use with caution in people with hypertension, angina, hyperthyroidism, or diabetes. Combination with beta blockers or digoxin may cause dangerous drug—drug interactions.
Phenylpropanolamine/ chlorpheniramine	Ornade: 1 capsule every 12 hours (75 mg phenyl-propanolamine and 12 mg chlor-pheniramine per capsule)	Signs of overdose or serious adverse effects include headache, confusion, seizures, and hallucinations.	Sudafed and Ornade are OTC drugs. Use for UI constitutes an off-label use.
Pseudoephedrine	Sudafed: 15–30 mg tid (immediate release); 120 mg every 12–24 hours (extended release)		

Key: bid = twice daily; OTC = over-the-counter; tid = 3 times daily; UI = urinary incontinence.

[a]Not recommended by the International Consultation on Incontinence.

[b]The U.S. Food and Drug Administration is taking steps to remove phenylpropanolamine (PPA) from all drug products and has requested that all drug companies discontinue marketing products containing PPA.

approval for this use in the United States was withdrawn, but it has been approved in other countries at a dose of 40 mg twice a day for treatment of SUI. (In the United States, duloxetine [Cymbalta] in 20-, 30-, and 60-mg capsules has been approved as an antidepressant.) Duloxetine increases serotonin and norepinephrine at the sacral spinal cord (Onuf's nucleus) in the synaptic cleft, potentiating an increase in urethral rhabdosphincter contractility during bladder filling and storage via the pudendal nerve. A North American, double-blind, placebo-controlled study enrolled 683 women with a weekly incontinence episode frequency of 7 or greater (Dmochowski, Miklos, et al., 2003). Each subject received either placebo or 80 mg of duloxetine daily for

12 consecutive weeks. In this study, among the treatment group, 51% experienced a 50%–100% decrease in incontinence episode frequency compared with 34% of those on placebo. However, a review voiced concerns that these effects may not be sustainable (Mariappan, Alhasso, Ballantyne, Grant, & N'Dow, 2007).

The most common side effect is nausea, occurring in approximately 22% of women, followed by fatigue, insomnia, and dry mouth in approximately 15%, 14%, and 12%, respectively. Other reports have suggested that duloxetine may increase blood pressure; the clinical significance of this effect has yet to be determined. The duloxetine label in the United States includes a black box warning regarding suicidal tendencies during early use, a class label requirement mandated by the FDA.

USE OF ESTROGEN

The lower urinary tract and pelvis are full of estrogen receptors. Estrogen receptors have been identified in the vagina, vestibule, distal urethra, trigone of the bladder, and pelvic floor muscles (Ballagh, 2005). Some experts have proposed that estrogen increases urethral blood flow, alpha-adrenergic receptor sensitivity, sympathetic nerve density in the pelvis, and urethral cellular maturation and prevents bladder contractions. Menopausal and postmenopausal women experience a decrease of the hormone estrogen, causing a loss of urogenital secretions and vaginal elasticity. The loss of estrogen may lead to not only vaginal, but also urogenital complaints, including UI, urgency, and frequency. Declining estrogen also causes a shift in vaginal bacterial flora, with a decrease in the normal lactobacilli responsible for maintaining an acid pH, sometimes accompanied by a concomitant overgrowth of enteric bacteria, particularly *Escherichia coli*. The change in the ecology of the urogenital environment can also complicate or contribute to urinary tract infections (UTIs), pelvic organ prolapse, UI, and OAB (see Chapters 4 and 11). Lower estrogen levels cause thinning and irritation of the bladder trigone, which may be associated with symptoms of bladder overactivity (Cardozo, Lose, McClish, & Versi, 2004).

Although estrogen replacement therapy, orally or transvaginally, has been a controversial drug therapy in women with UI and/or OAB (Palmer & Newman, 2007; U.S. Preventive Services Task Force, 2005), some clinicians and researchers believe there are urogenital benefits associated with estrogen use, especially when applied vaginally for atrophic vaginitis, UTIs, and OAB (Cardozo, Lose, McClish, Versi, & de Koning Gans, 2001; Maloney, 2002). Many incontinence experts, routinely prescribe transvaginal estradiol products in women with urogenital atrophy identified on pelvic examination and in women who complain of OAB symptoms of urgency and frequency. The dosage and duration are rarely considered and discussed in a formal manner.

Oral Estrogen

The oral mode of delivery of estrogen is controversial. Despite the relationship between hypoestrogenization and lower urinary tract symptoms, estrogen may be helpful in irritative OAB symptoms such as urgency and frequency, but studies do not support the use of oral (systemic) estrogen for SUI (DuBeau, 2005; Hendix et al., 2005). Oral estradiol/progesterone products are not recommended for the treatment of any type of UI or OAB. Hendix et al. (2005) examined estrogen's effects in 27,347 women between 50 and 79 years of age. Their findings revealed that continent women taking oral conjugated equine estrogen (CEE) alone or estrogen with progestin (medroxyprogesterone acetate [MPA]) developed UI at a statistically significantly higher rate than did continent women taking a placebo. In addition, preexisting UI worsened in women on CEE alone or those on CEE and MPA compared with those taking a placebo.

Transvaginal Estrogen

In the absence of vasomotor and other systemic symptoms of menopause, the current standard of practice recommends that vaginal complaints related to hypoestrogenism be treated with transvaginal or topical estrogen (Table 9.5). Although there is very little evidence-based research on the efficacy of transvaginal estrogens, they are widely used in clinical practice for symptoms of urogenital atrophy and urgency and frequency (Palmer & Newman, 2007). Many clinicians believe that low-dose, intravaginal estrogen may restore urethral mucosal coaptation, improve local vascularity, and increase urethral tone and resistance to outflow. Topical or systemic estrogens are believed to thicken the urethral mucosa, perhaps via increased vascularity of the tissue, allowing for a better apposition and seal of the urethra. Estrogens are also thought to increase the number of neuroreceptors, but further research is needed to confirm this hypothesis. It is believed that, when there is a vaginal response to estrogen, there will be a similar response in the urethral and bladder mucosa (Carson, Chaikin, Haney, & Staskin, 2000). With adequate treatment, symptoms of urogenital atrophy remit in a few days to several weeks, but the intracellular response takes longer.

A second theoretical basis for the use of transvaginal estrogen is recolonization of the vaginal vault by lactobacilli, restoration of an acid vaginal pH, and restoration of normal vaginal flora (Maloney & Oliver, 2001). Studies have shown that estrogen therapy can protect women from bacteriuria and UTIs (Cardozo et al., 2001; Maloney, 1997). In elderly women with diagnosed atrophic vaginitis, low-dose vaginal conjugated estrogen cream applied to urogenital tissues either intravaginally or externally for 6 weeks was found to reduce vaginal pH. Local application of estrogen may also prevent UTIs, especially in elderly women with recurrent infections (Maloney, 1998).

Table 9.5   Estrogen hormone preparations[a]

Agent	Usual dose	Side effects	Treatment considerations
Conjugated estrogens/ estradiol vaginal cream	Estradiol vaginal cream topically (Premarin: conjugated estrogens 0.625 mg/g; Estrace: estradiol 0.01%) Insert 2- to 4-g (marked on applicator) dose intravaginally daily at bedtime for 2 weeks, then gradually reduce to ½ initial dose for 2 weeks, followed by maintenance dose of 1 g 1–3 times/wk	Vaginal dryness and discomfort, breast tenderness/enlargement, vaginal bleeding, nausea vomiting	Contraindicated in women with history of blood clots or breast or uterine cancer. Monitor women with intact uterus for signs of endometrial cancer. If applicator causes discomfort during insertion, insert using gloved finger.
Estradiol vaginal tablets	2.5-mcg estradiol intravaginal tablets (Vagifem) Insert 25-mcg tablet daily at bedtime for 2 weeks, then 1 tablet twice weekly.	Vaginal spotting, allergic reactions, headache, abdominal pain	Low dose of estrogen so not absorbed systemically. If applicator causes discomfort during insertion, insert tablet using gloved finger.
Estrogen vaginal ring	2-mg estradiol intravaginal ring (Estring) delivering 7.5 mcg/24 hours for a period of 90 days. Insert ring deeply into upper ⅓ of vaginal vault.	Headache, leukorrhea, back pain, vaginal discomfort, vaginal bleeding, abdominal pain	Releases a steady, low dose of estrogen that is absorbed into the vaginal tissues over a period of 3 months.

[a]Topical preparations are indicated for the treatment of atrophic vaginitis and urogenital atrophy.

Side Effects

Vaginal delivery of estrogen bypasses the GI tract and has minimal impact on lipids, globulins, and clotting and fibrinolytic factors (Ballagh, 2005). The risks of estrogen, however, appear to be dose dependent, and administration of high doses of estrogen through the vaginal route can result in high systemic levels and risks similar to those seen with oral administration. Estrogen preparations all carry a black box warning on their label contraindicating their use in women with cardiovascular disease, breast cancer, endometrial cancer, venous thromboembolic events, and stroke, and in geriatric patients because of a risk of dementia. Side effects and other adverse events include the following (http://www.nlm.nih.gov/medlineplus/druginfo/medmaster/a682922. html#side-effects):

• Breast pain or tenderness

• Nausea, vomiting, reflux, gallstones

• Weight gain or loss

• Leg cramps

• Nervousness, depression

• Dizziness

• Hair loss, or unwanted hair growth

• Spotty darkening of the skin on the face

• Vaginal discharge

• Change in sexual desire

It normally takes 4–6 weeks to see the full effects of estrogen therapy.

Transvaginal Estrogen Products

In the past, very high doses of vaginal estrogens were administered transvaginally, often delivering amounts as high as oral treatment. The trend has been toward marked reductions in dose and, after an initial regimen of daily treatment, changing to less frequent administration once tissue integrity has been restored. The most common forms of local estrogen therapy are estradiol and conjugated estrogen vaginal creams. A fingertip-sized amount of estradiol cream (Estrace, Premarin), which weighs about 1 g, contains 0.01% (0.1 mg or 100 mcg) of estradiol. Vaginal cream has some disadvantages. The applicators that come with the tube of cream can abrade or lacerate atrophic tissues. Accurate dosing is difficult because the user must measure and then insert the cream, so the actual amount that is applied varies considerably. Some cream inevitably leaks out or is absorbed by clothing. Techniques to obviate these problems are manifold. Many clinicians instruct the individual to squeeze 1 inch of cream onto the index finger (usually from the tip to the first knuckle) and insert the finger into the vagina, rotating it to apply the cream. Women complain that the cream is "messy" and leaves a residue on the vulva and undergarments, and necessitates deferring coitus.

Other low-dose estrogen delivery systems include an estradiol vaginal ring (Estring) and vaginal tablets (Vagifem). The ring is soft, slightly opaque, and flexible and is inserted into the upper part of the vagina like a contraceptive diaphragm would be. The vaginal ring releases a steady, low dose of estrogen that is absorbed into the vaginal tissues over a period of 3 months. The estradiol release rate is determined by the silicone ring and is constant at 7.5 mg/24 hours for a period of 90 days (Casper & Petri, 1999). It normally takes 2–3 weeks after insertion to feel the full effects of the ring. Estradiol vaginal tablets are small, white, film-coated, hydrophilic tablets containing 25 mg of estradiol. The tablet is contained in a disposable single-use applicator used for insertion of the tablet into the vagina. A gel layer forms when the tablet comes in contact with the vagina. The estradiol is released from this gel layer. The recommended regimen for use is a 14-day induction phase in which 1 tablet is inserted each day, with a maintenance phase of 1 tablet twice weekly thereafter. The weekly dose during the maintenance phase of treatment—50 mcg (approximately 7 mcg/day)—is similar to that with the ring.

CONCLUSION

Drug therapy is a treatment option for patients with urgency UI, OAB, and mixed symptoms. There are no currently approved drugs for SUI, and transvaginal estrogen should be used with caution. A combination of behavior modification and antimuscarinic therapy (in 2008) will provide substantial relief and improved QoL for many OAB patients, but the combination does not represent a "cure." Short-term compliance (1 year) with these drugs in an unselected population has been relatively poor. In choosing a drug, each clinician must make his or her own decisions about the data and claims regarding the various agents, understanding what may be theoretical claims versus real advantages and what special circumstances and concomitant medication use may have to be considered regarding an individual patient. This chapter has attempted to outline those considerations. Finally, clinicians should be careful when comparing one drug to another on the basis of published data in different studies or promotional material, claiming to compare a particular aspect of one drug's efficacy, tolerability, or safety to that of another.

Appendix Table 9.1 Drug therapy for overactive bladder and urinary incontinence[a]

Drug	Usual dose	Side effects	Treatment considerations
Antimuscarinic–Anticholinergic: Effects are usually seen within 2–3 weeks			
Darifenacin (Enablex) Tertiary amine Relative selective M_3 antagonist	Supplied: 7.5-mg ER (white-colored) tablet and 15-mg ER (peach-colored) tablet Dosage: 7.5 daily up to 15 mg daily	Dry mouth, constipation, dyspepsia, abdominal pain	• Daily doses should not exceed 7.5 mg when coadministered with potent CYP3A4 inhibitors (e.g., ketoconazole, itraconazole, clarithromycin, ritonivir, nelfinavir, and nefazadone. • No dosing adjustments when coadministered with moderate CYP3A4 inhibitors (e.g., erythromycin, fluconazole, diltiazem, verapamil). • Use with caution in combination with flecainide, thioridazine, and tricyclic antidepressants because of their metabolism by CYP2D6 and narrow therapeutic window. • Should not be prescribed in individuals taking warfarin (Coumadin). • Decrease dose (should not exceed 7.5 mg/day) in person with moderate hepatic impairment; not recommended for people with severe hepatic impairment. • Should not be chewed, divided, or crushed. FDA Pregnancy Category: C
Oxybutynin IR (Ditropan, generic) Tertiary amine Relative selective M_1/M_3 antagonist Some calcium antagonist properties	Supplied: 5-mg IR tablets, 5-mg/5 mL syrup Dosage: 2.5–5.0 mg bid–tid, up to qid	Dry mouth, blurred vision, constipation, increased intraocular pressure, gastro-esophageal reflux, delirium or confusion, cardiac disturbance	• IR formulation is not recommended in nursing home residents. • No formal recommendations in person with hepatic impairment, but drug has extensive hepatic elimination. • Caution when coadministered with potent CYP3A4 inhibitors (e.g., ketoconazole, itraconazole, clarithromycin, ritonivir, nelfinavir, nefazadone, flecainide, thioridazine). FDA Pregnancy Category: B
Oxybutynin ER (Ditropan XL)	Supplied: 5-mg (pale yellow), 10-mg (pink), and 15-mg (gray) ER tablets Dosage: 5–30 mg daily orally		• Do not crush, chew, or break ER tablets. • Long-acting (ER) preparations have fewer side effects than short-acting (IR) preparations. • ER shell may be excreted in the stool.

(continued)

Appendix Table 9.1 (*continued*)

Drug	Usual dose	Side effects	Treatment considerations
Antimuscarinic–Anticholinergic: Effects are usually seen within 2–3 weeks			
Oxybutynin transdermal (skin patch) (Oxytrol)	Supplied: 3.9 mg (one patch) Matrix patch with 3 layers Dosage: apply every 3–4 days, to abdomen, buttocks, or hip.	Dry mouth (low) and application site reactions such as pruritis, erythema, vesicles, and macules	• Apply to clean, intact skin. • Must rotate application sites. • Apply to clean skin; avoid application over hair. • Moisten patch for removal to minimize skin irritation.
Solifenacin (VESIcare) Tertiary amine Relative selective M_3/M_1 antagonist	Supplied: 5-mg ER (yellow) tablet and 10-mg ER (red) tablet Dosage: 5–10 mg daily	Blurred vision, dry mouth, constipation, heat prostration	• Daily doses should not exceed 5 mg when coadministered with potent CYP3A4 inhibitors (e.g., ketoconazole, itraconazole, clarithromycin, ritonivir, nelfinavir, nefazadone, flecainide, thioridazine). • Decrease dose (5 mg) in patient with moderate hepatic or severe renal impairment. • Do not give to patients with severe hepatic impairment. • There is a risk of prolonged QT interval and potential serious cardiac arrhythmias if combined with other drugs that prolong QT interval. FDA Pregnancy Category: C
Tolterodine IR (Detrol IR) Tertiary amine Balanced muscarinic receptor antagonist	Supplied: 1-mg and 2-mg IR tablets Dosage: 1–2 mg bid	Dry mouth, dyspepsia, headache, constipation, somnolence, and xerophthalmia	• The long-acting and short-acting preparations have similar efficacy. • Lowest dose possible (2 mg daily recommended) should be used in people with severe liver or renal impairment. • Reduce dose (1 mg bid or 2 mg LA) when coadministered with potent CYP3A4 inhibitors (e.g., ketoconazole, itraconazole, clarithromycin, ritonivir, nelfinavir, nefazadone, flecainide, thioridazine).
Tolterodine ER (Detrol LA)	Supplied: 2-mg (blue-green capsule) and 4-mg ER tablets (blue capsule) Dosage: 2–4 mg daily		• Do not crush, chew, or break ER tablets. • There is a risk of prolonged QT interval and potential serious cardiac arrhythmias if combined with other drugs that prolong QT interval. FDA Pregnancy Category: C

Drug	Supplied/Dosage	Side Effects	Comments
Trospium (Sanctura, Sanctura XR) Quaternary amine Balanced muscarinic receptor antagonist	Supplied: 20-mg (Sanctura), 60-mg tablets (Sanctura XR) Dosage: 60 mg daily or 20 mg bid 1 hour before meal or on an empty stomach.	Dry mouth, constipation, headache, dyspepsia, flatulence	• Quaternary ammonium compound that should minimally cross the blood–brain barrier. • If renal impairment is present (CrCl < 30 mL/min), a once-a-day dose of 20 mg hs is recommended. • Do not crush, chew, or break capsule. FDA Pregnancy Category: C

Less Commonly Used Drugs

Drug	Supplied/Dosage	Side Effects	Comments
Propantheline (Pro-Banthine)	Dosage: 15 mg bid, with maximum dose 30 mg qid	Blurred vision, confusion, agitation, orthostatic hypotension	• High incidence of side effects, especially in older adults. • Use with caution in people with glaucoma, CAD, or prostatism.
Hyoscyamine (Cytospaz)	Dosage: 0.15 mg (tablets) Preferred dose in older adults: 0.125–0.25 mg tid–qid	Tachycardia, heart palpitations, ataxia, dizziness, drowsiness, headache, insomnia, nervousness, dry mouth, constipation, blurred vision	• Decreased effect with antacids • Should be taken before meals • Doses should not exceed 1.5 mg within 24 hours. • Increased toxicity with amantidine, antihistamines, antimuscarinics, haloperidol, phenothiazines, tricyclic antidepressants, and MAO inhibitors
L-hyoscyamine (Anaspaz, Cystospaz, Cystospaz-M, Gastrosed, Levbid, Levsin, Levsin Drops, Levsin SL, Levsinex, Timecaps, NuLev)	Supplied: 0.375 mg ER capsules, 0.375 mg ER tablets Dosage: 0.375 to 0.75 mg qid 8–12 hrs Supplied: 0.125 mg/5 ml elixir (Levsin, Levsin drops); 0.125 mg/ml oral spray (Levsin, Levsin drops); 0.125 mg orally disintegrating; 0.125 mg, 0.15 mg tablets; 0.125 mg SL tablets Dosage: 0.125 to 0.25 mg oral or spray SL tid or qid before meals and hs. Maximum of 1.5 mg/24 hrs		
Flavoxate hydrochloride IR (Urispas) "Antispasmodic"	Supplied: 100 mg tablets (round, white film-coated) Dosage: 100–200 mg tid–qid	GI upset, anticholinergic effects as noted earlier	• Reduce dosage on improvement. • Use cautiously in patients with suspected glaucoma. FDA Pregnancy Category: B

(continued)

349

Appendix Table 9.1 *(continued)*

Drug	Usual dose	Side effects	Treatment considerations

Less Commonly Used Drugs

Drug	Usual dose	Side effects	Treatment considerations
Desmopressin acetate (DDAVP) Antidiuretic hormone	Supplied: 0.1-mg and 0.2-mg scored tablets 100-mcg/mL (5-mL) intranasal spray (delivers 10 mcg/mL) Dosage: *Adults:* 10–40 mg intranasally hs, 0.1–0.4 mg orally hs. *Children:* 0.2 mg hs, 10–40 mcg intranasally once/day	Headache, nausea, nasal congestion, rhinitis, flushing, abdominal cramps, hyponatremia, water retention	• Avoid use in patients with dependent edema. • Start with low dose in elderly. A test period of several days at low dose can determine if medication will be effective. • Use with caution in older adults; monitor sodium before and within 3–4 days of treatment. • Evening and nighttime fluids should be restricted. • Serum sodium should be monitored in elderly.
Imipramine (Tofranil) Tricyclic antidepressant Tertiary amine	Supplied: 10-mg, 25-mg, and 50-mg tablets Dosage: 25 mg qid to maximum dose of 75 mg daily Single dose of 25–50 mg hs for nocturia.	Cardiovascular side effects, including orthostatic hypotension, dizziness, insomnia, bradycardia, and ventricular dysrhythmias, as well as weakness, fatigue, nausea, vomiting, dry mouth	• FDA has approved for enuresis in children, but not in adults. • Can cause cardiac bundle-branch block. • Because of sedation effects, it is often given at bedtime for nocturia. • Use caution if prescribed to older adults and people with depression. • An overdose of imipramine can be lethal, so safety precautions must be discussed.

Key: bid = twice daily; CAD = coronary artery disease; CrCl = creatinine clearance; CYP = cytochrome P-450; ER = extended-release; FDA = U.S. Food and Drug Administration; GI = gastrointestinal; hs = at bedtime; IM = intramuscularly; IR = immediate-release; IV = intravenously; LA = extended-release formulation; PRN = as needed; qid = 4 times daily; SL = sublingual; tid = 3 times daily; XL = extended-release formulation.

[a]Obtained from drug product information: Detrol LA, Ditropan XL, Enablex, Oxytrol, Sanctura, Sanctura IR, VESIcare.

As of July 30, 2008, the following events have been noted in worldwide post-marketing experience:

Darifenacin
General: hypersensitivity reactions, including angioedema
Central Nervous: confusion and hallucinations
Cardiovascular: palpitations

Oxybutynin (Ditropan)
Psychiatric Disorders: psychotic disorder, agitation, hallucinations
Nervous System Disorders: convulsions
Eye Disorders: cycloplegia, mydriasis
Cardiac Disorders: tachycardia
Gastrointestinal Disorders: decreased gastrointestinal motility
Skin and Subcutaneous Tissue Disorders: rash, decreased sweating
Renal and Urinary Disorders: impotence
Reproductive System and Breast Disorders: suppression of lactation

Oxytrol
Central: dizziness

Solifenacin
General: hypersensitivity reactions, including angioedema, rash, pruritis, and urticaria

Central Nervous: confusion and hallucinations
Cardiovascular: QT prolongation, torsade de pointes.

Tolterodine
General: anaphylactoid reactions, including angioedema
Cardiovascular: tachycardia, palpitations, peripheral edema
Gastrointestinal: diarrhea
Central/Peripheral Nervous: confusion, disorientation, memory impairment, hallucinations. Reports of aggravation of symptoms of dementia (e.g., confusion, disorientation, delusion) have been reported after tolterodine therapy was initiated in patients taking cholinesterase inhibitors for the treatment of dementia

Trospium (20 mg bid)
General: rash
Gastrointestinal: gastritis
Cardiovascular: palpitations, supraventricular tachycardia, chest pain, syncope, "hypertensive crisis"
Imunological: Stevents-Johnson syndrome, anaphylactic reaction
Nervous System: vision abnormal, hallucinations and derlirium
Musculoskeletal: rhabdomyolysis

Appendix Table 9.2 OAB drug efficacy[a]

	Number of incontinence episodes/week (treatment group/placebo) Reduction in UI		Frequency/24 hours (treatment group/placebo) Decrease in frequency	
Darifenacin				
Study 1 (Change in median)	7.5 mg Baseline: 16.3/16.6 After treatment: −9.0/−7.6	15 mg Baseline: 17.0/16.6 After treatment: −10.4/−7.6	7.5 mg Baseline: 10.1/10.1 After treatment: −1.6/−0.8	15 mg Baseline: 10.1/10.1 After treatment: −1.7/−0.8
Study 2 (Change in median)	7.5 mg Baseline: 14.0/16.1 After treatment: −8.1/−5.9	15 mg Baseline: 17.3/16.1 After treatment: −10.4/−5.9	7.5 mg Baseline: 10.3/10.1 After treatment: −1.7/−1.1	15 mg Baseline: 11.0/10.1 After treatment: −1.9/−1.1
Dose Titration Study (Change in median)	7.5 mg/15 mg Baseline: 16.0/14.0 After treatment: −8.2/−6.0		7.5 mg/15 mg Baseline: 9.9/10.4 After treatment: −1.9/−1.0	
Oxybutynin				
Oxybutynin ER Fixed-Dose Escalation Study	Baseline: 15.9/20.9 After treatment: −15.8/−7.6			
Oxybutynin TDS 3.9 mg (Mean change from baseline, Study 1)	Baseline: 34.3/37.7 After treatment: 21.0/19.2		Baseline: 11.8/12.3 After treatment: 2.2/1.6	
Solifenacin				
Study 905-CL-015 5 mg/24 hr (Change in mean)	Baseline: 2.6/2.7 After treatment: 1.4/0.8		Baseline: 12.1/12.2 After treatment: 2.2/1.2	
Study 905-CL-015 10 mg/24 hr (Change in mean)	Baseline: 2.6/2.7 After treatment: 1.5/0.8		Baseline: 12.3/12.2 After treatment: 2.6/1.2	
Study 905-CL-018 5 mg/24 hr (Change in mean)	Baseline: 2.6/3.2 After treatment: 1.6/1.3		Baseline: 12.1/12.3 After treatment: 2.4/1.7	

(continued)

Appendix Table 9.2 *(continued)*

	Number of incontinence episodes/week (treatment group/placebo)	Frequency/24 hours (treatment group/placebo)
	Reduction in UI	Decrease in frequency
Study 905-CL-018 10 mg/24 hr (Change in mean)	Baseline: 2.8/3.2 After treatment: 1.6/1.3	Baseline: 12.1/12.3 After treatment: 2.9/1.7
Study 905-CL-013 10 mg/24 hr (Change in mean)	Baseline: 3.1/3.0 After treatment: 2.0/1.1	Baseline: 12.1/11.5 After treatment: 2.9/1.5
Study 905-CL-014 10 mg/24 hr (Change in mean)	Baseline: 2.9/2.9 After treatment: 2.0/1.2	Baseline: 11.5/11.8 After treatment: 2.4/1.3
Tolterodine ER 4 mg at 12 weeks (Change in mean)	Baseline: 22.1/23.3 After treatment: 11.8/6.9	Baseline: 10.9/11.3 After treatment: 1.8/1.2
Trospium IR 20 mg bid Study 1 (Mean change from baseline to end treatment)	Baseline: 27.3/30.1 After treatment: 15.4/13.9	Baseline: 12.7/12.9 After treatment: 2.4/1.3
20 mg bid Study 2 (Mean change from baseline to end treatment)	Baseline: 26.9/27.3 After treatment: 16.1/12.1	Baseline: 12.9/13.2 After treatment: 2.7/1.8
Trospium ER 60 mg Study 1 (Change in mean)	Baseline: 28.8/29.0 After treatment: 13.0/8.7	Baseline: 12.8/12.7 After treatment: 1.7/1.2
60 mg Study 2 (Change in mean)	Baseline: 28.2/28.3 After treatment: 11.9/7.3	Baseline: 12.8/12.9 After treatment: 1.4/1.2

Key: bid = twice daily; ER = extended-release; GI = gastrointestinal; IR = immediate-release; TDS = transdermal delivery system.

[a]Obtained from drug product information: Detrol LA, Ditropan XL, Enablex, Oxytrol, Sanctura, Sanctura IR, VESIcare.

Appendix Table 9.3 OAB drug side effect profile[a]

Drug	Dry mouth	GI	Vision	CNS	Urinary	Other	Skin (application site)
Darifenacin					Side Effects (drug/placebo)		
7.5 mg (reported in at least 2% of patients)	20.2%/8.2%	Constipation: 14.8%/6.2% Diarrhea: 2.1%/1.8% Dyspepsia: 2.7%/2.62% Nausea: 2.7%/1.5% Abdominal pain: 2.4%/0.5%	Dry eyes: 1.5%/0.5%	Dizziness: 0.9%/1.3%	UTI: 4.7%/2.6%	Asthenia: 1.5%/1.3%	NA
15 mg (reported in at least 2% of patients)	35.3%/8.2%	Constipation: 21.3%/6.2% Diarrhea: 0.9%/1.8% Dyspepsia: 8.4/2.62% Nausea: 1.5%/1.5% Abdominal pain: 3.9%/0.5%	Dry eyes: 2.1%/0.5%	Dizziness: 2.1%/1.3%	UTI: 4.5%/2.6%	Asthenia: 2.7%/1.3%	NA
Oxybutynin ER[b]							
5–30 mg (reported in at least 5% of patients)	60.8%	Constipation: 13% Diarrhea: 9.1% Nausea: 8.9% Dyspepsia: 6.3%	Blurred vision: 7.7% Dry eyes: 6.1%	Somnolence: 11.9% Dizziness: 6.3%	UTI: 5.1%	Headache: 9.8% Asthenia: 6.8% Pain: 6.8% Rhinitis: 5.6%	NA
10 mg (% of corresponding AEs in 2 fixed dose studies)	29.3%	Constipation 6.6% Diarrhea: 7.8% Nausea: 2.4% Dyspepsia: 4.9%	Blurred vision: 1.6% Dry eyes: 3.1%	Somnolence: 2.1% Dizziness: 4.2%	UTI: 5.2%	Headache: 6.4% Asthenia: 3.0% Pain: 3.8% Rhinitis: 1.7%	NA
5–30 mg (reported in at least 1% of patients)	61%	Constipation: 13% Diarrhea: 9% Nausea: 9% Dyspepsia: 7%	Blurred vision: 8% Dry eyes: 6%	Somnolence: 12% Dizziness: 6%	UTI: 5%	Headache: 10% Asthenia: 7% Pain: 7% Rhinitis: 6%	NA

(continued)

Appendix Table 9.3   *(continued)*

			Side Effects (drug/placebo)				
Drug	Dry mouth	GI	Vision	CNS	Urinary	Other	Skin (application site)
10 mg (reported in at least 1% of patients of studies 1 & 2)	29%	Constipation: 7% Diarrhea: 7% Nausea: 2% Dyspepsia: 5%	Blurred vision: 1% Dry eyes: 3%	Somnolence: 2% Dizziness: 4%	UTI: 5%	Headache: 6% Asthenia: 3% Pain: 4% Rhinitis: 2%	NA
Oxybutynin TDS 3.9 mg Study 1	9.6%/8.3%	Diarrhea: 3.2%/2.3%			Dysuria: 2.4%/0%		Pruritis: 16.8%/6.1% Vesicles: 3.2%/0% Erythema: 5.6%/2.3%
3.9 mg Study 2	4.1%/1.4%	Constipation: 3.3%/0%	Abnormal vision: 2.5%/0%				Pruritis: 14.0%/4.3% Erythema: 8.3%/1.7% Rash: 3.3%/0.9% Macules: 2.5%/0%
Solifenacin 5 mg qid (reported in at least 1% or more of patients for combined pivotal studies)	10.9%/4.2%	Constipation: 5.4%/2.9% Dyspepsia: 1.4%/1.0% Nausea: 1.7%/2.0% Abdominal pain, upper: 1.9%/1.0% Vomiting NOS: 0.2%/0.9%	Blurred vision: 3.8%/1.8% Dry eyes NOS: 0.3%/0.6%	Dizziness: 1.9%/1.8% Depression: 1.2%/0.8%	UTI: 2.8%/2.8% Urinary retention: 0%/0.6%	Influenza: 2.2%/1.3% Pharyngitis NOS: 0.3%/1.0% Fatigue: 1.0%/1.1% Lower limb edema: 0.3%/0.7% Cough: 0.2%/0.2% Hypertension NOS: 1.4%/0.6% placebo	NA

Drug/Dose		GI	Ophthalmic	CNS/Psychiatric	GU	Systemic/Other	
10 mg qid (reported in at least 1% or more of patients for combined pivotal studies)	10.9%/27.6% 4.2%	Constipation: 13.4%/2.9% Dyspepsia: 3.9%/1.0% Nausea: 3.3%/2.0% Abdominal pain, upper: 1.2%/1.0% Vomiting NOS: 1.1%/0.9%	Blurred vision: 4.8%/1.8% Dry eyes NOS: 1.6% 0.6%	Dizziness: 1.8%/1.8% Depression: 0.8%/0.8%	UTI: 4.8%/2.8% Urinary retention: 1.4%/0.6%	Influenza: 0.9%/1.3% Pharyngitis: NOS 1.1%/1.0% Fatigue: 2.1%/1.1% Lower limb edema: 1.1%/0.7% Cough: 1.1%/0.2% Hypertension NOS: 0.5%/0.6%	NA
Tolterodine ER 4 mg qid	23%/8%	Constipation: 6%/4% Dyspepsia: 3%/1% Abdominal pain: 3%/2%	Xerophthalmia: 3%/2% Vision abnormalities: 1%/0%	Somnolence: 3%/2% Anxiety: 3%/0% Dizziness: 2%/1%	Dysuria: 1%/0%	Headache: 6%/4% Fatigue: 6%/1% Sinusitis: 2%/1%	NA
Trospium IR 20 mg bid (reported in at least 1% of patients of studies 1 & 2)	20.1%/5.8%	Constipation: 9.6%/4.6% Constipation, aggravated: 1.4%/0.8% Dyspepsia: 1.2%/0.3% Flatulence: 1.2%/0.8% Abdominal pain, upper: 1.2%/1.5%	Dry eyes: 1.2%/0.3%	Headache: 4.2%/2.0%	Urinary retention: 1.2%/0.3%	Fatigue: 1.9%/1.4%	NA
Trospium XR 60 mg qid (reported in at least 1% of patients)	10.7%/3.7%	Constipation: 8.5%/1.5% Constipation, aggravated: 1.2%/0.5% Flatulence: 1.6%/0.5% Nausea: 1.4%/0.3% Abdominal distension: 1.0%/0.3%	Dry eyes: 1.63%/0.2%	None	UTI: 1.25%/0.9%	Nasal dryness: 1.0%/0%	NA
60 mg qid (reported in at least 1% of patients)	11.1%/3.7%	Constipation: 9.0%/1.7% Nausea: 1.2%/0.7%			UTI: 7.3%/4.9%	Nasopharyngitis: 2.9%/1.7%	NA

Key: ER = extended-release; GI = gastrointestinal; IR = immediate-release; NA = not applicable; NOS = not otherwise specified; TDS = transdermal delivery system; qid = 4 times daily; bid = 2 times daily; UTI = urinary tract infection.

[a]Obtained from drug product information: Detrol LA, Ditropan XL, Enablex, Oxytrol, Sanctura, Sanctura IR, VESIcare.

[b]Placebo rates not reported.

355

REFERENCES

Abrams, P., Andersson, K.E., Buccafusco, J.J., Chapple, C., de Groat, W.C., Fryer, A.D., et al. (2006). Muscarinic receptors: Their distribution and function in body systems, and the implications for treating overactive bladder. *British Journal of Pharmacology, 148,* 565–578.

Abrams, P., & Swift, S. (2005). Solifenacin is effective for the treatment of OAB dry patients: A pooled analysis. *European Urology, 48,* 483–487.

Abrams, P., & Wein, A.J. (1998). *The overactive bladder: A widespread but treatable condition* (p. 50). Stockholm: Eric Sparre Medical AB.

Alhasso, A., Glazener, C.M.A., Pickard, R., & N'Dow, J. (2005). Adrenergic drugs for urinary incontinence in adults [Review]. *Cochrane Database of Systematic Reviews, (3),* CD001842.

Anderson, R.U., Mobley, D., Blank, B., Saltzstein, D., Susset, J., Brown, J.S., for the OROS Oxybutynin Study Group. (1999). Once daily controlled versus immediate release oxybutynin chloride for urge incontinence. *Journal of Urology, 161,* 1809–1812.

Andersson, K.E. (2002). Bladder activation: Afferent mechanisms. *Urology, 59,* (Suppl. 5A), 43–50.

Andersson, K.E. (2004). Antimuscarinics for treatment of overactive bladder. *Lancet Neurology, 3,* 46–53.

Andersson, K.E., Appell, R.A., Cardozo, L., Chapple, C., Drutz, H., Fourcroy, J., et al. (2005). Pharmacological treatment of urinary incontinence. In P. Abrams, L. Cardozo, S. Khoury, & A. Wein (Eds.), *Incontinence: Proceedings from the Third International Consultation on Incontinence* (pp. 809–854). Plymouth, UK: Health Publications Ltd.

Andersson, K.E., & Wein, A.J. (2007). Pharmacologic management of storage and emptying failure. In A.J. Wein, L.R. Kavoussi, A.C. Novick, A.W. Partin, & C.A. Peters (Eds.), *Campbell's urology* (9th ed., pp. 2091–2123). Philadelphia: Elsevier Saunders.

Asplund, R. (2007). Pharmacotherapy for nocturia in the elderly patient. *Drugs & Aging, 24*(4), 325–343.

Autret E., Jonville A., Dutertre J., Bertiere, M.C., Robert, M., Averous, M., et al. (1994). Plasma levels of oxybutynin chloride in children. *European Journal of Clinical Pharmacology, 46,* 83–85.

Balkrishnan, R., Bhosle, M.J., Camacho, F.T., & Anderson, R.T. (2006). Predictors of medication adherence and associated health care costs in an older population with overactive bladder syndrome: A longitudinal cohort study. *Journal of Urology, 175,* (3 Pt. 1), 1067–1071.

Ballagh, S. (2005). Vaginal hormone therapy for urogenital and menopausal symptoms. *Seminars in Reproductive Medicine, 23*(2), 126–140.

Bennett, N., O'Leary, M., Patel, A.S., Xavier, M., Erickson, J.R., & Chancellor, M.B. (2004). Can higher doses of oxybutynin improve efficacy in neurogenic bladder? *Journal of Urology, 171*(2 Pt. 1), 749–751.

Berry, A.K. (2006). Helping children with nocturnal enuresis: The wait-and-see approach may not be in anyone's best interest. *American Journal of Nursing, 106*(8), 58–65.

Burgio, K., Locher, J., Goode, P., Hardin, M., McDowell, B., Dombrowski, M., et al. (1998). Behavioral vs. drug treatment for urge urinary incontinence in older women. *JAMA, 280,* 1995–1999.

Burgio, K.L., Locher, J.L., & Goode, P.S. (2000). Combined behavioral and drug therapy for urge incontinence in older women. *Journal of the American Geriatrics Society, 48,* 370–374.

Cardozo, L., Lisec, M., Millard, R., van Vierssen Trip, O., Kuzmin, I., Drogendijk, T.E., et al. (2004). Randomized, double-blind placebo controlled trial of the once daily antimuscarinic agent solifenacin succinate in patients with overactive bladder. *Journal of Urology, 172,* (5 Pt. 1), 1919–1924.

Cardozo, L., Lose, G., McClish, D., & Versi, E. (2004). A systematic review of the effects of estrogens for symptoms suggestive of overactive bladder. *Acta Obstetricia et Gynecologica Scandinavica, 83,* 892–897.

Cardozo, L., Lose, G., McClish, D., Versi, E., & de Koning Gans, H. (2001). A systematic review of estrogens for recurrent urinary tract infections: Third report of the Hormones and Urogenital Therapy (HUT) committee. *International Urogynecology Journal and Pelvic Floor Dysfunction, 12,* 15–20.

Carnahan, R.M., Lund, B.C., Perry, P.J., & Chrischilles, E.A. (2004). The concurrent use of anticholinergics and cholinesterase inhibitors: Rare event or common practice? *Journal of the American Geriatrics Society, 52,* 2082–2087.

Carson, C.C., Chaikin, D., Haney, A.F., & Staskin, D.R. (2000). Urogenital consequences of estrogen deficiency. *Contemporary Urology, 12*(Suppl.), 3–12.

Cartwright, R., & Cardozo, L. (2007). Transdermal oxybutynin: Sticking to the facts. *European Urology, 51,* 907–914.

Casper, F., & Petri, E. (1999). Local treatment of urogenital atrophy with an estradiol-releasing vaginal ring: A comparative and a placebo-controlled multicenter study. Vaginal Ring Study Group. *International Urogynecology Journal and Pelvic Floor Dysfunction, 10,* 171–176.

Centers for Medicare & Medicaid Services. (2005). *State Operations Manual, Appendix PP—Guidance to Surveyors for Long-Term Care Facilities, Tag F315, §483.25(d) Urinary Incontinence* (Rev. 8, Issued: 06-28-05, Effective: 06-28-05, Implementation: 06-28-05) (pp. 184–219). Retrieved November 11, 2007, from http://www.cms.hhs.gov/transmittals/downloads/R8SOM.pdf

Centers for Medicare & Medicaid Services. (2006). *State Operations Manual, Appendix PP—Guidance to Surveyors for Long-Term Care Facilities, Tag F329, §483.25(l) Unnecessary Drugs* (Rev. 22, Issued: 12-15-06, Effective/Implementation: 12-18-06). Retrieved May 28, 2007, from http://www.cms.hhs.gov/manuals/Downloads/som107ap_pp_guidelines_ltcf.pdf

Chancellor, M., Freedman, S., Mitcheson, D., Antoci, A., Primus, G., & Wein, A. (2000). Tolterodine: An effective and well tolerated treatment for urge incontinence and bladder symptoms. *Clinical Drug Investigation, 19,* 83–91.

Chancellor, M.B., & de Miguel, F. (2007). Treatment of overactive bladder: Selective use of anticholinergic agents with low drug–drug interaction potential. *Geriatrics, 62,* 15–24.

Chapple, C., Steers, W., Norton, P., Millard, R., Kralidis, G., Glavind, K., et al. (2005). A pooled analysis of three Phase III studies to investigate the efficacy, tolerability and safety of darifenacin, a muscarinic M_3 selective receptor antagonist, in the treatment of overactive bladder. *BJU International, 95,* 993–1001.

Chapple, C., van Kerrebroeck, P., Tubaro, A., Haag-Molkenteller, C., Forst, H.T., Massow, U., et al. (2007). Clinical efficacy, safety, and tolerability of once-daily fesoterodine in subjects with overactive bladder. *European Urology, 52,* 1204–1212.

Chapple, C.R. (2000). Muscarinic receptor antagonists in the treatment of overactive bladder. *Urology, 55,* 33–46.

Chapple, C.R. (2004). Darifenacin: A novel M_3 muscarinic selective receptor for the treatment of overactive bladder. *Expert Opinion in Investigational Drugs, 13,* 1493–1500.

Chapple, C.R., Fianu-Jonsson, A., Indig, M., Khullar, V., Rosa, J., Scarpa, R.M., et al., for the STAR Study Group. (2007). Treatment outcomes in the STAR study: A subanalysis of solifenacin 5 mg and tolterodine ER 4 mg. *European Urology, 52,* 1195–1203.

Chapple, C.R., Martinez-Garcia, R., Selvaggi, L., Toozs-Hobson, P., Warnack, W., Drogendijk, T., et al. (2005). A comparison of the efficacy and tolerability of solifenacin succinate and extended release tolterodine at treating overactive bladder syndrome: Results of the STAR Trial. *European Urology, 48,* 464–470.

Chapple, C.R., Yamanishi, T., & Chess-Williams, R. (2002). Muscarinic receptor subtypes and management of overactive bladder. *Urology, 60,* 82–88.

Chess-Williams, R., Chapple, C.R., Yamanishi, T., Yasuda, K., & Sellers, D.J. (2001). The minor population of M_3 receptors mediate contraction of human detrusor muscle in vitro. *Journal of Autonomic Pharmacology, 21,* 243–248.

Coyne, K.S., Matza, L.S., Kopp, Z., & Abrams, P. (2006). The validation of the Patient Perception of Bladder Condition (PPBC): A single-item global measure for patients with overactive bladder. *European Urology, 49,* 1079–1086.

Crandall, C. (2002). Vaginal estrogen preparations: A review of safety and efficacy for vaginal atrophy. *Journal of Women's Health, 11,* 857–877.

Davila, G.W., Daugherty, C.A., & Sanders, S.W. (2001). A short-term, multicenter, randomized double-blind dose titration study of the efficacy and anticholinergic side effects of transdermal compared to immediate release oral oxybutynin treatment of patients with urge urinary incontinence. *Journal of Urology, 166,* 140–145.

Davila, G.W., Starkman, J.S., & Dmochowski, R.R. (2006). Transdermal oxybutynin for overactive bladder. *Urologic Clinics of North America, 33,* 455–463.

Detrol® LA (Tolterodine Tartrate) Prescribing Information. (2005). Retrieved February 15, 2008, from http://pfizer.com/files/products/uspi_detrol_la.pdf

Diefenbach K, Donath F, Maurer A, Quispe Bravo, S., Wernecke, K.D., Schwantes, U., et al. (2003). Randomised, double-blind study of the effects of oxybutynin, tolterodine, trospium chloride and placebo on sleep in healthy young volunteers. *Clinical Drug Investigation, 23,* 395–404.

Diokno, A., & Ingber, M. (2006). Oxybutynin in detrusor overactivity. *Urologic Clinics of North America, 33,* 439–445.

Diokno, A.C., Appell, R.A., Sand, P.K., Dmochowski, R.R., Gburek, B.M., Klimberg, I.W., et al. for the OPERA Study Group. (2003). Prospective, randomized, double-blind study of the efficacy and tolerability of the extended-release formulations of oxybutynin and tolterodine for overactive bladder: Results of the OPERA Trial. *Mayo Clinic Proceedings, 78,* 687–695.

Ditropan® XL (Oxybutynin Chloride) Prescribing Information. (2004). Retrieved March 9, 2008, from http://www.janssen-ortho.com/JOI/pdf_files/Ditropan_E.pdf

Dmochowski, R., Abrams, P., Marschall-Kehrel, D., Wang, J.T., & Guan, Z. (2007). Efficacy and tolerability of tolterodine extended release in male and female patients with overactive bladder. *European Urology, 51,* 1054–1064.

Dmochowski, R., & Staskin, D.R. (2005). The Q-T interval and antimuscarinic drugs. *Current Urology Reports, 6,* 405–409.

Dmochowski, R.R. (2005). Improving the tolerability of anticholinergic agents in the treatment of overactive bladder. *Drug Safety, 28,* 584–600.

Dmochowski, R.R., Davila, G.W., Zinner, N.R., Gittleman, M.C., Saltzstein, D.R., Lyttle, S., et al. for the Transdermal Oxybutynin Study Group. (2002). Efficacy and safety of transdermal oxybutynin in patients with urge and mixed urinary incontinence. *Journal of Urology, 168,* 580–586.

Dmochowski, R.R., Miklos, J.R., Norton, P.A., Zinner, N.R., Yalcin, I., Bump, R.C., for the Duloxetine Urinary Incontinence Group. (2003). Duloxetine versus placebo for the treatment of North American women with stress urinary continence. *Journal of Urology, 170*(4 Pt. 1), 1259–1263.

Dmochowski, R.R., Nitti, V., Staskin, D., Luber, K., Appell, R., & Davila, G.W. (2005). Transdermal oxybutynin in the treatment of adults with overactive bladder: Combined results of two randomized clinical trials. *World Journal of Urology, 23,* 263–270.

Dmochowski, R.R., Sand, P.K., Zinner, N.R., Gittelman, M.C., Davila, G.W., Sanders, S.W., for the Transdermal Oxybutynin Study Group. (2003). Comparative efficacy and safety of transdermal oxybutynin and oral tolterodine versus placebo in previously treated patients with urge and mixed urinary incontinence. *Urology, 62,* 237–242.

DuBeau, C. (2005). Estrogen treatment for urinary incontinence: Never, now, or in the future? *JAMA, 293,* 998–1001.

Edwards, K.R., & O'Connor, J.T. (2002). Risk of delirium with concomitant use of tolterodine and acetylcholinesterase inhibitors. *Journal of the American Geriatrics Society, 50,* 1165–1166.

Elinoff, V., Bavendam, T., Glasser, D.B., Carlsson, M., Eyland, N., & Roberts, R. (2006). Symptom-specific efficacy of tolterodine extended release in patients with overactive bladder: The IMPACT trial. *International Journal of Clinical Practice, 60,* 745–751.

Enablex® (Darifenacin) Prescribing Information. (2006). Retrieved February 15, 2008, from http://www.pharma.us.novartis.com/product/pi/pdf/enablex.pdf

Fantl, J., Newman, D., Colling, J., DeLancey, J.O.L., Keeys, C., Loughery, R., et al. for the Urinary Incontinence in Adults Guideline Update Panel. (1996). *Urinary incontinence in adults: Acute and chronic management. Clinical practice guideline No. 2: Update* (AHCPR Publication No. 96-0692). Rockville, MD: Agency for Health Care and Policy Research.

Flick, D., Cooper, J., Wade, W., Waller, J., Maclean, J., & Beers, M. (2003). Updating the Beers Criteria for potentially inappropriate medication use in older adults. *Archives of Internal Medicine, 163,* 2716–2724.

Foote, J., Glavind, K., Kralidis, G., & Wyndaele, J.J. (2005). Treatment of overactive bladder in the older patient: Pooled analysis of three Phase III studies of darifenacin, an M_3 selective receptor antagonist. *European Urology, 48,* 471–477.

Gepertz, S. & Neveus, T. (2004). Imipramine for therapy resistant enuresis: A retrospective evaluation. *Journal of Urology, 171*(6 Pt. 2), 2607–2610.

Gill, SS., Mamsani, M., Naglie, G., Streiner, DL., Bronskill, SE., Kopp, A., et al. (2005). A prescribing cascade involving cholinesterase inhibitors and anticholinergic drugs. *Archives of Internal Medicine, 165,* 808–813.

Gleason, D.M., Susset, J., White, C., Munoz, D.R., Sand, P.K., for the Ditropan XL Study Group. (1999). Evaluation of a new once-daily formulation of oxybutynin for the treatment of urinary urge incontinence. *Urology, 54,* 420–423.

Haab, F. (2005). Darifenacin in the treatment of overactive bladder. *Drugs of Today, 41,* 441–452.

Haab, F., Stewart, L., & Dwyer, P. (2004). Darifenacin, an M_3 selective receptor antagonist, is an effective and well-tolerated once-daily treatment for overactive bladder. *European Urology, 45,* 420–429.

Hay-Smith, J., Herbison, P., Ellis, G., & Morris, A. (2005). Which anticholinergic drug for overactive bladder symptoms in adults [Review]. *Cochrane Database of Systematic Reviews,* (3), CD005429.

Hendix, S., Cochrane, B., Nygaard, I., Handa, V., Barnabei, V., Iglesia, C., et al. (2005). Effects of estrogen with and without progestin on urinary incontinence. *JAMA, 293,* 935–984.

Herbison, P., Hay-Smith, J., Ellis, G., & Moore, K. (2003). Effectiveness of anticholinergic drugs compared with placebo in the treatment of overactive bladder: Systematic review. *BMJ, 326,* 841–844.

Homsy, Y., Nsouli, I., Hamburger, B., Laberge, I., & Schick, E. (1985). Effects of oxybutynin on vesicoureteral reflux in children. *Journal of Urology, 134,* 1168–1171.

Jewart, R.D., Green, J., Lu, C.J., Cellar, J., & Tune, L.E. (2005). Cognitive, behavioral, and physiological changes in Alzheimer disease patients as a function of incontinence medications. *American Journal of Geriatric Psychiatry, 13,* 324–328.

Johnson, T.M. 2nd, Miller, M., Tang, T., Pillon, D.J., & Ouslander, J.G. (2006). Oral ddAVP for nighttime urinary incontinence in characterized nursing home residents: A pilot study. *Journal of the American Medical Directors Association, 7,* 6–11.

Kaplan, S.A., Roehrborn, C.G., Rovner, E.S., Carlsson, M., Bavendam, T., & Guan, Z. (2006). Tolterodine and tamsulosin for treatment of men with lower urinary tract symptoms and overactive bladder: A randomized controlled trial. *JAMA, 296,* 2319–2328.

Katz, I.R., Sands, L.P., Bilker, W., DiFilippo, S., Boyce, A., & D'Angelo, K. (1998). Identification of medications that cause cognitive impairment in older people: The case of oxybutynin chloride. *Journal of the American Geriatrics Society, 46,* 8–13.

Kay, G., Crook, T., Rekeda, L., Lima, R., Ebinger, U., Arguinzoniz, M., et al. (2006). Differential effects of the antimuscarinic agents darifenacin and oxybutynin ER on memory in older subjects. *European Urology, 50,* 317–326.

Kay, G.G., Abou-Donia, M.B., Messer, W.S. Jr., Murphy, D.G., Tsao, J.W., & Ouslander, J.G. (2005). Antimuscarinic drugs for overactive bladder and their potential effects on cognitive function in older patients. *Journal of the American Geriatrics Society, 53,* 2195–2201.

Kernan, W.N., Viscoli, C.M., Brass, L.M., Broderick, J.P., Brett, T., Feldman, E., et al. (2000). Phenylpropanolamine and the risk of hemorrhagic stroke. *New England Journal of Medicine, 343,* 1826–1832.

Lee, J.Y., Kim, D.K., & Chancellor, M.B. (2006). When to use antimuscarinics in men who have lower urinary tract symptoms. *Urologic Clinics of North America, 33,* 531–537.

Lose, G., Lalos, O., Freeman, R.M., & van Kerrebroeck, P., for the Nocturia Study Group. (2003). Efficacy of desmopressin (Minirin) in the treatment of nocturia: A double-blind placebo-controlled study in women. *American Journal of Obstetrics and Gynecology, 189,* 1106–1113.

MacDiarmid, S.A., Anderson, R.U., Armstrong, R.B., & Dmochowski, R.R. (2005). Efficacy and safety of extended release oxybutynin for the treatment of urge incontinence: An analysis of data from 3 flexible dosing studies. *Journal of Urology, 174,* 1301–1305.

Madersbacher, H., Stohrer, M., Richter, R., Burgdorfer, H., Hachen, H.J., & Murtz, G. (1995). Trospium chloride versus oxybutynin: A randomized, double-blind, multicentre trial in the treatment of detrusor hyper-reflexia. *British Journal of Urology, 75,* 452–456.

Malavaud, B., Bagheri, H., Senard, J.M., & Sarramon, J.P. (1999). Visual hallucinations at the onset of tolterodine treatment in a patient with a high-level spinal cord injury. *BJU International, 84,* 1109.

Malone-Lee, J, Shaffu, B, Anand, C, & Powell, C. (2001). Tolterodine: superior tolerability than and comparable efficacy to oxybutynin in individuals 50 years old or older with overactive bladder: a randomized controlled trial. *Journal of Urology, 165,* 1452–1456.

Maloney, C. (1997). Estrogen in urinary incontinence treatment: An anatomic and physiologic approach. *Urologic Nursing, 17,* 88–91.

Maloney, C. (1998). Hormone replacement therapy in female nursing home residents with recurrent urinary tract infection. *Annals of Long-Term Care, 6*(3), 77–82.

Maloney, C. (2002). Estrogen & recurrent UTI in postmenopausal women. *American Journal of Nursing, 102*(8), 44–52.

Maloney, C., & Oliver, M.L. (2001). Effect of local conjugated estrogens on vaginal pH in elderly women. *Journal of the American Medical Directors Association, 2,* 51–55.

Mariappan, P., Alhasso, A., Ballantyne, Z., Grant, A., & N'Dow, J. (2007). Duloxetine, a serotonin and noradrenaline reuptake inhibitor (SNRI) for the treatment of stress urinary incontinence: A systematic review. *European Urology, 51,* 67–74.

Mattiasson, A., Abrams, P., van Kerrebroeck, P., Walter, S., & Weiss, J. (2002). Efficacy of desmopressin in the treatment of nocturia: A double-blind placebo-controlled study in men. *BJU International, 89,* 855–862.

Mattiasson, A., Blaakaer, J., Hoye, K., Wein, A.J., for the Tolterodine Scandinavian Study Group. (2003). Simplified bladder training augments the effectiveness of tolterodine in patients with an overactive bladder. *BJU International, 91,* 54–60.

Monda, J.M., & Husmann, D.A. (1995). Primary nocturnal enuresis: A comparison among observation, imipramine, desmopressin acetate and bed-wetting alarm systems. *Journal of Urology, 154*(2 Pt. 2), 745–748.

Nabi, G., Cody, J.D., Ellis, G., Herbison, P., & Hay-Smith, J. (2006). Anticholinergic drugs versus placebo for overactive bladder syndrome in adults. *Cochrane Database of Systematic Reviews,* (4), CD003781.

Narayanan, S., Cerulli, A., Kahler, K.H., & Ouslander, J.G. (2007). Is drug therapy for urinary incontinence used optimally in long-term care facilities? *Journal of the American Medical Directors Association, 8,* 98–104.

Newman, D.K., Kennelly, M.J., Lemack, G.E., & McIlwain, M. (2007). Transdermal treatment for neurogenic bladder: Patient safety and quality of life. *Journal of Wound, Ostomy, and Continence Nursing, 34*(3 Suppl.), S64.

Newman, D.K. & Wein, A.J. (2004). *Overcoming overactive bladder* (pp. 103–114). Los Angeles: New Harbinger.

Nitti, V.W., Dmochowski, R., Sand, P.K., Forst, H.T., Haag-Molkenteller, C., Massow, U., et al. (2007). Efficacy, safety and tolerability of fesoterodine for overactive bladder syndrome. *Journal of Urology, 178,* 2488–2494.

Nitti, V.W., Sanders, S., Staskin, D.R., Dmochowski, R.R., Sand, P.K., McDiarmind, S., et al. (2006). Transdermal delivery of drugs for urologic applications: Basic principles and applications. *Urology, 67,* 657–664.

Nixon, A., Colman, S., Sabounjian, L., Sandage, B., Schwiderski, U.E., Staskin, D.R., et al. (2005). A validated patient reported measure of urinary urgency severity in overactive bladder for use in clinical trials. *Journal of Urology, 174,* 604–607.

O'Leary, M., Erickson, J.R., Smith, C.P., McDermott, C., Horton, J., & Chancellor, M.B. (2003). Effect of controlled-release oxybutynin on neurogenic bladder function in spinal cord injury. *Journal of Spinal Cord Medicine, 26,* 159–162.

Ouslander, J.G. (2004). Management of overactive bladder. *New England Journal of Medicine, 350,* 786–799.

Oxytrol Prescribing Information. Retrieved February 15, 2008, from http://pi.watson.com/data_stream.asp?product_group=1295&p=pi&language=E

Palmer, M.H., & Newman, D.K. (2007). Urinary incontinence and estrogen. *American Journal of Nursing, 107*(3), 35–36, 37.

Pietzko, A., Dimpfel, W., Schwantes, U., & Topfmeier, P. (1994). Influences of trospium chloride and oxybutynin on quantitative EEG in healthy volunteers. *European Journal of Clinical Pharmacology, 47,* 337–343.

Potts, R.O., & Lobo, R.A. (2005). Transdermal drug delivery: Clinical considerations for the obstetrician-gynecologist. *Obstetrics and Gynecology, 105,* 953–961.

Rackley, R., Weiss, J.P., Rovner, E.S., Wang, J.T., & Guan, Z. (2006). Nighttime dosing with tolterodine reduces overactive bladder-related nocturnal micturitions in patients with overactive bladder and nocturia. *Urology, 67,* 731–736.

Roberts, R., Bavendam, T., Glasser, D.B., Carlsson, M., Eyland, N., & Elinoff, V. (2006). Tolterodine extended release improves patient-reported outcomes in overactive bladder: Results from the IMPACT trial. *International Journal of Clinical Practice, 60,* 752–758.

Roe, C.M., Anderson, M.J., & Spivack, B. (2002). Use of anticholinergic medications by older adults with dementia. *Journal of the American Geriatrics Society, 50,* 836–842.

Roehrborn, C.G., Abrams, P., Rovner, E.S., Kaplan, S.A., Herschorn, S., & Guan, Z. (2006). Efficacy and tolerability of tolterodine extended-release in men with overactive bladder and urgency urinary incontinence. *BJU International, 97,* 1003–1006.

Rosenberg, M.T., Newman, D.K., Tallman, C., & Page, S.A. (2007). Overactive bladder: Recognition requires vigilance for symptoms. *Cleveland Clinic Journal of Medicine, 74,* (Suppl. 1), S23–S29.

Rovner, E.S. (2004). Trospium chloride in the management of overactive bladder. *Drugs, 64,* 2433–2446.

Rudy, D., Cline, K., Harris, R., Goldberg, K., & Dmochowski, R. (2006). Multicenter Phase III trial studying trospium chloride in patients with overactive bladder. *Journal of Urology, 67,* 275–280.

Saltzstein, L. (2005). Management of overactive bladder in a difficult-to-treat patient with a transdermal formulation of oxybutynin. *Urologic Nursing, 25,* 260–262.

Sanctura XR™ (Trospium) Prescribing Information. (2006). Retrieved March 9, 2008, from http://www.sancturaxr.com/HCP/prescribing.html

Sand, P., Zinner, N., Newman, D., Lucente, V., Dmochowski, R., Kelleher, C., et al. (2007). Oxybutynin transdermal system improves the quality of life in adults with overactive bladder: A multicentre, community-based, randomized study. *BJU International, 99,* 836–844.

Scarpero, H.M., & Dmochowski, R.R. (2003). Muscarinic receptors: What we know. *Current Urology Reports, 4,* 421–428.

Scheife, R., & Takeda, M. (2005). Central nervous system safety of anticholinergic drugs for the treatment of overactive bladder in the elderly. *Clinical Therapeutics, 27,* 144–153.

Serra, D.B., Affrime, M.B., Bedigian, M.P., Greig, G., Milosavljev, S., Skerjanel, A., et al. (2005). QT and QTc interval with standard and supra-therapeutic doses of darifenacin, a muscarinic M$_3$ selective receptor antagonist for the treatment of overactive bladder. *Journal of Clinical Pharmacology, 45,* 1038–1047.

Sink, K.M., Thomas J. III, Xu, H., Craig, B., Kritchevsky, S., & Sands, L.P. (2008). Dual use of bladder anticholinergics and cholinesterase inhibitors: Long-term functional and cognitive outcomes. *Journal of the American Geriatrics Society, 56*(5), 847–853.

Skoog, S.J., Stokes, A., & Turner, K.L. (1997). Oral desmopressin: A randomized double blind placebo controlled study of effectiveness in children with primary nocturnal enuresis. *Journal of Urology, 158* (3 Pt. 2), 1035–1040.

Song, C., Park, J.T., Heo, K.O., Lee, K.S., & Choo, M.S. (2006). Effects of bladder training and/or tolterodine in female patients with overactive bladder syndrome: A prospective, randomized study. *Journal of Korean Medical Science, 21,* 1060–1063.

Staskin, D., Sand, P., Zinner, N., Dmochowski, R., for the Trospium Study Group. (2007). Once daily trospium chloride is effective and well tolerated for the treatment of overactive bladder: Results from a multicenter Phase III trial. *Journal of Urology, 178,* (3 Pt. 1), 978–983.

Staskin, D.R. (2005). Overactive bladder in the elderly: A guide to pharmacological management. *Drugs and Aging, 22,* 1015–1028.

Staskin, D.R. (2006). Trospium chloride: Distinct among other anticholinergic agents available for the treatment of overactive bladder. *Urologic Clinics of North America, 33,* 465–473.

Staskin, D.R., & Harnett, M.D. (2004). Effect of trospium chloride on somnolence and sleepiness in patients with overactive bladder. *Current Urology Reports, 5,* 423–426.

Staskin, D.R., & MacDiarmid, S.A. (2006). Pharmacologic management of overactive bladder: Practical options for the primary care physician. *American Journal of Medicine, 119,* 245–285.

Staskin, D.R., Rosenberg, M.T., Dahl, N.V., Polishuk, P.V., & Zinner, N.R. (2008). Effects of oxybutynin transdermal system on health-related quality of life and safety in men with overactive bladder and prostate conditions. *International Journal of Clinical Practice, 62,* 27–38.

Steers, W., Corcos, J., Foote, J., & Kralidis, G. (2005). An investigation of dose titration with darifenacin, an M$_3$-selective receptor antagonist. *BJU International, 95,* 580–586.

Steers, W.D. (2006). Darifenacin: Pharmacology and clinical usage. *Urologic Clinics of North America, 33,* 475–482.

Sussman, D., & Garely, A. (2002). Treatment of overactive bladder with once-daily extended-release tolterodine or oxybutynin: The Antimuscarinic Clinical Effectiveness Trial (ACET). *Current Medical Research and Opinion, 18,* 177–184.

Taylor, P. (2005). Pharmacologic management of overactive bladder. *Journal of Wound, Ostomy, and Continence Nursing, 32*(Suppl. 1), S16–S24.

Tobias, D.E., & Sey, M. (2001). General and psychotherapeutic medication use in 328 nursing facilities: A year 2000 national survey. *The Consultant Pharmacist, 15,* 34–42.

Todorova, A., Vonderheid-Guth, B., & Dimpfel, W. (2001). Effects of tolterodine, trospium chloride, and oxybutynin on the central nervous system. *Journal of Clinical Pharmacology, 41,* 636–644.

Tsao, J.W., & Heilman, K.M. (2003). Transient memory impairment and hallucinations associated with tolterodine use. *New England Journal of Medicine, 349,* 2274–2275.

U.S. Preventive Services Task Force. (2005). *Hormone therapy for the prevention of chronic conditions in postmenopausal women: Recommendation statement.* Retrieved April 30, 2006, from http://www.ahrq.gov/clinic/uspstf05/ht/htpostmenrs.htm

Van Kerrebroeck, P., Kreder, K., Jonas, U., Zinner, N., Wein, A., for the Tolterodine Study Group. (2001). Tolterodine once-daily: Superior efficacy and tolerability in the treatment of the overactive bladder. *Urology, 57,* 414–421.

Van Kerrebroeck, P., Rezapour, M., Cortesse, A., Thüroff, J., Riis, A., & Nørgaard, J.P. (2007). Desmopressin in the treatment of nocturia: A double-blind, placebo-controlled study. *European Urology, 52,* 221–229.

Versi, E., Appell, R., Mobley, D., Patton, W., & Saltzstein, D. (2000). Dry mouth with conventional and controlled-release oxybutynin in urinary incontinence. The Ditropan XL Study Group. *Obstetrics and Gynecology, 95,* 718–721.

VESIcare® (Solifenacin Succinate) Prescribing Information. (2004). Retrieved from http://www.astellas.us/docs/vesicare.pdf

Wang, P., Luthin, G.R., & Ruggieri, M.R. (1995). Muscarinic acetylcholine receptor subtypes mediating urinary bladder contractility and coupling in GTP binding proteins. *Journal of Pharmacology and Experimental Therapeutics, 273,* 959–966.

Wein, A.J. (2001). Pharmacological agents for the treatment of urinary incontinence due to overactive bladder. *Expert Opinion on Investigational Drugs, 10,* 65–83.

Wein, A.J., & Rackley, R.R. (2006). Overactive bladder: A better understanding of pathophysiology, diagnosis and management. *Journal of Urology, 175,* S5–S10.

Williams, S.G., & Staudenmeier, J. (2004). Hallucinations with tolterodine. *Psychiatric Services, 55,* 1318–1319.

Womack, K.B., & Heilman, K.M. (2003). Tolterodine and memory: Dry but forgetful. *Archives of Neurology, 60,* 771–773.

Yarker, Y.E., Goa, K.L., & Fitton, A. (1995). Oxybutynin: A review of its pharmacodynamic and pharmacokinetic properties, and its therapeutic use in detrusor instability. *Drugs and Aging, 6,* 243–262.

Youdim, K., & Kogan, B.A. (2002). Preliminary study of the safety and efficacy of extended-release oxybutynin in children. *Urology, 59,* 428–432.

Yu, Y.F., Nichol, M.B., Yu, A.P., & Ahn, J. (2005). Persistence and adherence of medications for chronic overactive bladder/urinary incontinence in the California Medicaid program. *Value in Health, 8,* 495–505.

Zinner, N., Gittelman, M., Harris, R., Susset, J., Kanelos, A., Auerbach, S., for the Trospium Study Group. (2004). Trospium chloride improves overactive bladder symptoms: A multicenter Phase III trial. *Journal of Urology, 171,* 2311–2315.

Zinner, N., Susset, J., Gittelman, M., Arguinzoniz, M., Rekeda, L., & Haab, F. (2005). Efficacy, tolerability and safety of darifenacin, an M$_3$ selective receptor antagonist: An investigation of warning time in patients with OAB. *International Journal of Clinical Practice, 60,* 119–126.

Zinner, N.R. (2005). Trospium chloride: An anticholinergic quaternary ammonium compound for the treatment of overactive bladder. *Expert Opinion on Pharmacotherapy, 6,* 1409–1420.

Zinner, N.R., Mattiasson, A., & Stanton, S.L. (2002). Efficacy, safety, and tolerability of extended-release once-daily tolterodine treatment for overactive bladder in older versus younger patients. *Journal of the American Geriatrics Society, 50,* 799–807.

Zobrist, R.H., Quan, D., Thomas, H.M., Stanworth, S., & Sanders, S.W. (2003). Pharmacokinetics and metabolism of transdermal oxybutynin: In vitro and in vivo performance of a novel delivery system. *Pharmaceutical Research, 20,* 103–109.

Zobrist, R.H., Schmid, B., Feick, A., Quan, D., & Sanders, S.W. (2001). Pharmacokinetics of the *R*- and *S*-enantiomers of oxybutynin and *N*-desethyloxybutynin following oral and transdermal administration of the racemate in healthy volunteers. *Pharmaceutical Research, 18,* 1029–1034.

10

Urinary Collection and Management Products

Incontinence products for both urinary incontinence (UI) and fecal incontinence can be effective as primary management for patients with UI and their caregivers. These products contain urine leakage, maintain skin integrity, conceal the problem, and maintain and in some cases improve quality of life (Newman, Fader, & Bliss, 2004). There are incontinence products and devices to

- *Contain or manage* incontinence, such as toilet substitutes (e.g., commodes and urinals), absorbent products, catheters, and urinary and anal tubes and pouches

- *Prevent* urine and/or fecal leakage with urethral occlusion or inserts, anal plugs, intravaginal devices (see Chapter 11), and penile compression devices

- *Treat* incontinence, with artificial sphincters, implantable nerve stimulators, enuresis alarms, and pelvic floor muscle stimulators (see Chapters 8 and 12)

Each year, millions of Americans—primarily older adults in acute care hospitals, extended care facilities, and their homes—use urinary collection devices (often referred to as containment devices) or occlusive devices (Newman, 2004; Newman et al., 2004). In nursing homes, absorbent products and, to a lesser degree, indwelling catheters are the primary management system for "containing" UI. Roger et al. (2008) conducted a retrospective cohort study to evaluate the types of urinary collection devices used by long-term skilled nursing facilities (SNF) residents in California, Florida, Michigan, New York, and Texas. All residents (n = 57,302) who were newly admitted to these SNFs in 2003 (100% sample) were followed for one year. Of the 57,302 patients, 69% of whom were female, 7,242 (12.6%) were using an indwelling catheter at admission. This declined to 4.5% at year one. The use of an indwelling catheter was 5.4% in this population at the 3-month assessment, 4.7% at the 6-month assessment, and 4.3% at the 9-month assessment. A disturbing finding was that fewer than 1% of patients used intermittent or external catheterization at admission or at year one. Overall, the use of incontinence pads or briefs was the most common urinary collection strategy. A majority (56.1%) of residents were using these at admission, and 57.8% were using these products at year one. Indwelling and external catheters, toileting substitutes, and absorbent products are used to contain or collect urine as part of the management of UI. Other products such as penile compression devices and urethral inserts are used to prevent urine leakage. Information on devices for containment of feces is found in Chapter 5. The objective in using these products is either for the person to remain as dry as possible or to prevent urine leakage while preserving dignity and quality of life. Their role in managing urine leakage is viewed by clinicians and caregivers as an essential adjunct of treatment for many patients with UI. Patients who use containment devices are classified as having "contained continence" (being "socially" continent) and are managed by the most appropriate product technology (Cottenden et al., 2005). This chapter reviews the use of many of these products, but many more are available.

OVERVIEW

Incontinence products and devices are effective as primary management in those individuals who 1) are unable to achieve the desired effects from interventions, 2) have advanced dementia and are cognitively unable to respond to standard treatment, or 3) are bedridden or frail and are not candidates for other treatments (Newman et al., 2004). These products also relieve caregiver burden and act as a supplement to bladder rehabilitation programs for those individuals undergoing treatment. Many of these products—particularly catheters, urethral inserts, penile compression devices, and drainage bags—qualify for reimbursement under most insurance carriers. Appendix Table 10.1 is a list of codes currently used for billing these products.

Even though these products are an integral part of the nursing care of patients with urinary dysfunction, there is little or no research in the United States on their long-term use. Currently, continence care for patients with chronic intractable UI is often based on personal opinion, manufacturers' claims, folklore, convenience of the caregiver, or cost of the products (Fantl et al., 1996). Both health care providers and device users erroneously believe that these products and devices undergo U.S. Food and Drug Administration (FDA) approval for safety and efficacy. However, Box 10.1 outlines the FDA process for device review, and it is evident that most incontinence products do not need a formal evaluation. In Great Britain, government-funded, multicenter evaluations of urinary collection devices have provided research-based evidence for product selection (Fader, Cottenden, & Brooks, 2001).

Prior to choosing a product or device described in this chapter, individuals need to undergo an evaluation as described in Chapter 6. Key elements of assessment include type and severity of UI or bladder dysfunction, cognition, dexterity, eyesight, lifestyle, laundry facilities, mobility, ability to perform activities of daily living, and personal preferences and priorities of both the individual and, where applicable, the caregiver (Cottenden et al., 2005).

Box 10.1   Product Classification and Approval in the United States*

The Food and Drug Administration (FDA) Center for Devices and Radiological Health (CDRH) determines the efficacy and safety of devices that are designated for medical use. FDA classification of a device is determined by the amount of regulation necessary to provide a reasonable assurance of safety and effectiveness. The FDA must classify devices into one of three regulatory classes: class I, II, or III. Because the Medical Device Amendments did not exist until 1976, it was necessary to grandfather all existing medical devices unless they presented an unreasonable risk to public health. Most of these "older" devices were classified as I and II, with a few classified as III. Typically those devices classified as III were high-risk devices, but in some cases this classification was the result of the lack of safety and effectiveness data.

Class I and II Devices

By definition, class I devices are those that only require general controls (i.e., adequate labeling, registration, and listing) to assure their safety and effectiveness. There are no significant safety issues or performance issues that require extensive review by the FDA. Class I devices now are all exempt, so that they no longer need to submit any information directly to the FDA.

Class II devices are those devices that require not only general controls but "special controls," which include performance testing or labeling specific to the device that is necessary to assure its safety and effectiveness. More technically, the special controls assure that the device is as safe and as effective as what is already on the market. Sling material used for surgery (see Chapter 12) is classified as a class II device. Some class II devices are now exempt from FDA notification.

Class I and II devices, unless exempt, require Premarket Notification, which is also known as a "510k" (§ 510(k) of the Food, Drug and Cosmetics Act) and requires only that the manufacturer demonstrate "substantial equivalence to another device." The FDA attempts to determine how similar and how different the device is to something already on the market (legally). On occasion, the FDA may ask for clinical data, but the majority of the time it is only "bench data" from the manufacturer rather than data from clinical studies.

Class III Devices

Class III devices require Premarket Approval (PMA) and for the most part require clinical studies. These are often novel devices or devices that are not currently on the market as class I or II. Under PMA regulations, the manufacturer must demonstrate a reasonable assurance of safety and effectiveness. Under this classification, the FDA can require more rigorous data, whereas under 510k it is harder to do so unless there is a specific concern. Devices in this class undergo an approval process that includes a review by an FDA Advisory Panel.

Classification of Products and Devices Used for Incontinence

• Class 1 (exempt): penile compression devices, catheter holders or anchor devices, external catheters, external urethral occlusion devices, urinals, and commodes

• Class II: indwelling catheters, pessaries, intermittent/straight catheters, and implanted electrical stimulator (Interstim)

• Class III: artificial sphincters (urinary and fecal), urethral inserts, anal plugs, sling materials, enuresis alarms, urinary drainage bags, and external pelvic floor muscle stimulators

    The FDA does require that all medical devices containing latex be identified by including a latex warning statement on the product label.

*http://www.accessdata.fda.gov/scripts/cdrh/cfdocs/cfCFR/CFRSearch.cfm?CFRPart=876

ABSORBENT INCONTINENCE PRODUCTS

Absorbent incontinence products (referred to worldwide as "body-worn" products) are the most common method of incontinence containment and management used by nurses (e.g., registered nurses, licensed practical nurses, and nursing aides) (Newman, 2004). Absorbent products include innovative perineal pads or pantiliners for slight leakage, undergarments and protective underwear, traditional diaper-style products (called adult briefs) for moderate to heavy leakage, and guards and drip collection pouches for men (Figure 10.1). There are also underpads of differing sizes and absorbency for bed and furniture protection. All of these products absorb or contain urine and are either disposable (single-use) or reusable (washable). Advantages of the use of absorbent products to manage UI include the ability to

- Soak up or contain urine
- Preserve the person's dignity and comfort
- Provide protection for clothes, furniture, bedding, and floors

Absorbent products can be a useful and rational way to manage incontinence, and nurses routinely make the decision about their use (Palese et al., 2007). However, few absorbent products have been subjected to user and clinician evaluation that has been published in the medical literature. Nurses are the primary researchers in this area of continence care (Clarke-O'Neill, Pet-

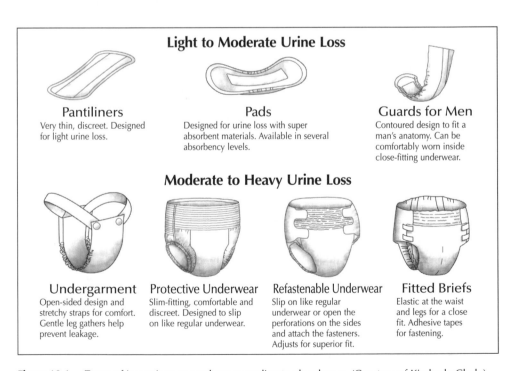

Light to Moderate Urine Loss

Pantiliners
Very thin, discreet. Designed for light urine loss.

Pads
Designed for urine loss with super absorbent materials. Available in several absorbency levels.

Guards for Men
Contoured design to fit a man's anatomy. Can be comfortably worn inside close-fitting underwear.

Moderate to Heavy Urine Loss

Undergarment
Open-sided design and stretchy straps for comfort. Gentle leg gathers help prevent leakage.

Protective Underwear
Slim-fitting, comfortable and discreet. Designed to slip on like regular underwear.

Refastenable Underwear
Slip on like regular underwear or open the perforations on the sides and attach the fasteners. Adjusts for superior fit.

Fitted Briefs
Elastic at the waist and legs for a close fit. Adhesive tapes for fastening.

Figure 10.1.   Types of incontinence products according to absorbency. (Courtesy of Kimberly Clark.)

tersson, Fader, Cottenden, & Brooks, 2004; Dunn, Kowanko, Paterson, & Pretty, 2002; Fader, Macaulay, Pettersson, Brooks, & Cottenden, 2006). However, the applicability of some of this research to clinical practice in the United States is poor because many of the products studied are not available in the United States. Absorbent incontinence products are considered a hygiene product in the United States and are sold in retail stores. In many other countries they are considered a medical product and distributed by government-run health systems. When faced with choosing or recommending a product, the clinician often has little information about product performance on which to base a choice (Fader, Cottenden, & Brooks, 2001). This may lead to misuse or overuse because it has been reported that 99% of nursing home residents wore absorbent products (Watson, Brink, Zimmer, & Mayer, 2003). Table 10.1 gives recommendations for use of absorbent products based on current evidence.

> Dave D. is an 82-year-old man who has been bedridden for the past 5 years. He is cared for by his daughter, Becky. Dave has urgency incontinence and often urinates without any warning. His daughter finds him wet before she can offer him the urinal. Becky managed her father's problem by wrapping blue pads around his penis and placing several blue pads underneath him on the bed. Lately his visiting nurse has noted an ever-increasing red area on his scrotum. She suggested a condom catheter, but Becky could never get the device to stay on, because her father's penis was retracted. The visiting nurse fears that the reddened area on Dave's buttocks will progress to a bedsore and has suggested more aggressive management of his incontinence. She advised Becky to wash her father's perineum, penis, scrotum, and buttocks with a perineal cleanser, and to apply a skin moisture barrier product after washing, in the morning. The nurse also suggested that Becky use cloth underpads and an incontinence product with super-absorbent material to manage her father's incontinence. Since starting this program, Dave's skin has improved dramatically.

Absorbent incontinence products have made UI much more manageable for most patients; however, early dependency on absorbent pads, especially in frail, older adults with chronic illness, may be a deterrent to continence, giving the wearer a false sense of security and acceptance of the condition. In long-term care (LTC) settings, product selection is an administrative or corporate decision that is often influenced by cost as opposed to quality and effectiveness. Absorbent products account for significant costs to acute and LTC facilities. In nursing facilities, incontinence costs are the third highest resident care costs. However, the use of absorbent products may remove the motivation to seek evaluation and treatment for UI. In addition, improper use of absorbent products contributes to skin breakdown and infection. To avoid these problems, adult briefs (informally referred to as "diapers" in many LTC settings) and pads should be changed frequently to limit a person's exposure to the wet garment and eliminate buildup of moisture and odor.

Table 10.1 Absorbent products: evidence-based recommendations

Products	Recommendations
Reusables versus disposables	• There is no clear evidence for making choices based on cost or environment issues. • In considering washables vs. reusables, factor in the outlay costs/commitment risks and laundry issues. • Consider a mix of washables and disposables depending on the situation. • Reusable products for moderate to heavy urinary incontinence may not be as effective as disposable products.
Pads for light incontinence	• For light urine leakage, use disposable inserts (pantiliners). • Select disposables with superabsorbent polymer (SAP) over those without. • Poor research base for male products. • Poor research base for fecal or for fecal plus urinary (double) incontinence. • More evidence is needed to compare performance and cost-effectiveness of different disposable and reusable pad-pant designs.
Products for heavy incontinence	• Select disposables with SAP over those without. • Use mesh pants with disposable inserts. • For very heavy incontinence, use disposable diaper-style products rather than inserts. • Some children with disabilities benefit from "pull-ups" rather than diapers (but diapers are better for night). • In general, avoid reusables. • More evidence is needed to compare performance and cost-effectiveness of different disposable and reusable designs.
Underpads	• Disposable underpads (without body-worn product) are not generally recommended. • Washable underpads can be effective for use alone or as backup to body-worn products. • More evidence needed to determine best products for nighttime use (body-worn product versus underpad).

Adapted from Cottenden et al. (2005).

Absorbent Product Design

The design of most absorbent products is fairly uniform, with some variation to conform to the gender of the user. The type of absorbent fiber is different depending on the fluid it is to absorb or contain: blood, urine, or chlorinated water. The number, size, and arrangement of these fibers are factors in the absorption capacity. As feminine hygiene products are designed to absorb menstrual blood, absorbent incontinence products are designed specifically to absorb and contain urine. These products are not interchangeable. These products are designed so that the surface area that is against the perineum collects the urine and transmits it to an absorbent inner core. The urine-holding capacity of absorbent incontinence products is not standardized, and the quality and materials used in these products vary widely. There is also debate as to whether disposable products are more skin-friendly and more absorbent when compared to reusable or washable products (Cottenden, Fader, Pettersson, & Brooks, 2003).

It would be helpful to have product performance tests that include assessment of three areas:

1. Re-wet value, which measures the product's ability to retain moisture under pressure. The re-wet value indicates the amount of fluid against the patients' skin after incontinence occurs. A lower re-wet value reflects product dryness.

2. Rate of acquisition, which measures how quickly an absorbent product acquires a given volume of fluid, because products that acquire fluid quickly may have less leakage.

3. Total absorbent capacity, which measures how much fluid a product can absorb. This may determine the differences between light, moderate, and heavy absorbency.

A recent advance in absorbent incontinence disposable products has been the addition of a superabsorbent polymer (SAP) to the fluff that significantly increases the total amount of fluid that can be absorbed. The polymer is a hydrocolloid material, typically a cross-linked polyacrylate, that is embedded within this layer as a powder (Edlich, Winters, Long, & Gubler, 2006). Upon the addition of a liquid, it converts to a gel particle swollen with fluid but retains its original shape and remains undissolved. The gel improves the pad's absorption capacity, minimizes urine leakage, and is pH balanced to control odor. These products keep the urine away from the perineal skin. Currently, SAPs can absorb up to 70 times their original weight in urine and swell to an average particle size of 1–2 mm. This absorbent inner core allows the urine to spread throughout the entire pad, facilitating absorption capacity while preventing urine leakage. Most of these products have a plastic layer for added protection. There is less skin breakdown and urine leakage in patients using disposable products with absorbing properties (Runeman, 2008). However, despite the technology, the clinician and the individual must remember that every absorbent product has a saturation point, depending on the frequency of urine loss, the quantity of urine loss, and the changing schedule (Brazzelli, Shirran, & Vale, 2002; Fader, Cottenden, & Getliffe, 2007).

Washable and reusable incontinence products are available in different styles and designs for men and women (Figure 10.2). Reusables are made of cloth material with a rayon or polyester fiber core (Clarke-O'Neill et al., 2002). The size and stated absorbency of the pad components vary, but most products are suitable for light incontinence. Reusable pants with an integral pad are designed to provide an alternative to disposable pads for small amounts of urine leakage. Reusable pants look like regular underwear but have an absorbent pad sewn into the crotch to absorb any leakage. An advantage over disposable pads is that the pad portion is fixed in position so that it cannot shift during use.

Washable or absorbent reusable products may be an attractive option for managing incontinence, especially because many patients believe they are environmentally friendly, and they are often considered to be more economical because they can be washed and reused many times. However, the energy, resources, effort, inconvenience, and cost associated with washing and drying these products, and the high initial cost to purchasers, must be considered (Dunn et al., 2002).

Types of Absorbent Incontinence Products

The most commonly used absorbent incontinence products are reviewed in this section.

Perineal Pads   Perineal pads, shields, inserts, or liners are for light to moderate incontinence. These are most appropriate for patients with light to mod-

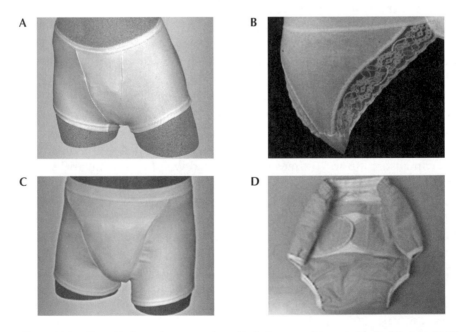

Figure 10.2.   Reusable incontinence products. (*A, B,* Courtesy of Augusta Medical Systems LLC.)

erate urine leakage and are preferred for their discreetness (Baker & Norton, 1996; Fader et al., 2007). Disposable perineal pads are attached to underwear or panties with an adhesive strip and have side gathers for fit (Figure 10.3A). Some are designed with a wide front or back for larger volumes of leakage or to fit the body more snugly. Shaped perineal pads with elastic edges conform closely to the body and may leak less than rectangular pads. These pads are similar in design to feminine hygiene pads but provide more effective protection. Reusable pads are usually designed more simply (Figure 10.3B).

Drip-Collecting Pouch   For men, a "guard" or leaf-shaped pad is available. Many men find this type of design and shape to be more comfortable and discreet (Fader et al., 2006) (Figure 10.4A). These products have an adhesive strip that attaches to male brief-style underwear. They may be more difficult to use with boxer shorts, which are favored by elderly men. Another product for men is a pouch- or sock-like product ("drip collector") in which the penis is placed in the pouch (Figure 10.4B).

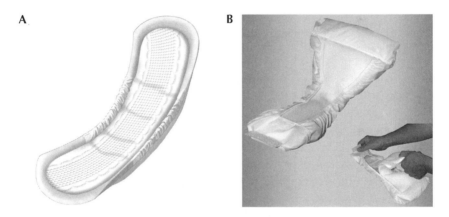

Figure 10.3.   *A,* TENA Serenity disposable perineal pad. (Courtesy of SCA Personal Products.) *B,* Wunderpad reusuable perineal pad (Courtesy of Afex.)

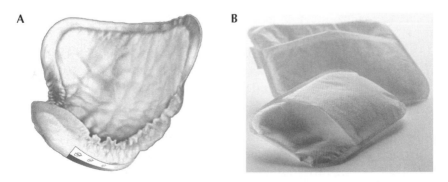

Figure 10.4.   *A,* Male TENA product. (Courtesy of SCA Personal Products.) *B,* Male drip collector pouches. (Courtesy of Coloplast.)

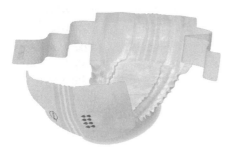

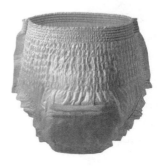

Figure 10.5. TENA Flex refastenable undergarment. (Courtesy of SCA Personal Products.)

Figure 10.6. TENA protective underwear. (Courtesy of SCA Personal Products.)

Undergarments   Undergarments are large form-fitting pads that extend to the waist and are held in place by elastic side straps using Velcro or buttons. Most have a soft, breathable outer cover for a clean, comfortable feeling. The button-type undergarment may be more difficult for older adults with arthritis. A new type of undergarment is one that fastens around the waist before the front is pulled into position and secured (Figure 10.5). This can be applied while the person is standing. These are sometimes referred to as "T-shaped" undergarments.

Protective Underwear   Protective underwear is a disposable product similar to cloth underwear in that it has an elasticized waist with added absorbent protection (Figure 10.6). These originated from the "pull-ups" used for children. We find protective underwear to be the most popular product used by both men and women in our practice. This type of product should be considered in patients with dementia who "pull off their diaper."

Adult Brief   The adult brief (similar to a child's diaper) is used for moderate to severe UI and in patients with both fecal incontinence and UI (Figure 10.7). The brief usually has an elasticized waist and self-adhesive tabs that can be refastened. This allows for use by an individual who is primarily bedridden. Many have a built-in wetness indicator, which is one of the reasons they are the product of choice in the LTC environment (Figure 10.7B).

Pad-and-Pant System   Pad-and-pant systems can be a combination of cloth (reusable) pants (mesh or knit) and disposable pads (Figure 10.8). They are useful for those patients with moderate UI and allow for self-toileting in those who are more independent.

Homemade Products   Many patients invent their own method of protection to minimize expense. These homemade products may include washcloths, paper towels, undershirts, and, most frequently, tissues. In some cases, patients place these items in their own underwear or in a disposable product

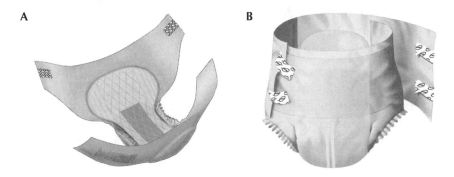

Figure 10.7.   *A*, Adult brief with curved cut (Courtesy of Tyco Kendall). *B*, Adult brief (TENA) with wetness indicator. (Courtesy of SCA Personal Products.)

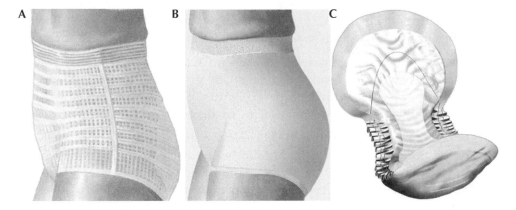

Figure 10.8.   Pad-and-pant incontinence products. *A*, mesh pant; *B*, knit pant; *C*, disposable pad insert. (Courtesy of SCA Personal Products.)

such as an undergarment. They will usually throw away the self-made product as it becomes saturated.

Product Selection

Selecting the most appropriate product is difficult because there is little research comparing absorbent products. At present, product selection is done by the consumer through trial and error and depends on budgetary constraints and/or availability in the practice setting. Clinicians and caregivers need to be aware of the characteristics of and indications for available products so they can counsel individuals on proper use. Two principles should be considered:

- Select the most appropriate product designed for ease in self-toileting in those individuals who are "independently" continent, but who need some protection for occasional urine leakage.

- Select a product that is designed to contain urinary leakage in those patients who are not capable of maintaining continence independently or through regular toileting or other measures.

Personal preferences in products may vary. Studies have shown that pad usage preference varies for women with stress UI and other types of UI. Women still chose a small, discreet pad such as a pantiliner despite the need to change the product more frequently. It is estimated that as many as 30% of all feminine hygiene pads are used by young women who have slight UI. Mc-Clish, Wyman, Sale, Camp, and Earle (1999) reported that 77% of women who enrolled in a clinical trial for UI used a protective perineal pad at least once per week. This study also showed that women used lower-cost products such as menstrual pads rather than specific incontinence pads. One clinical study looked at usage of perineal pads in women with stress UI (Thornburn, Fader, Dean, Brooks, & Cottenden, 1997). The study found that the most popular time for putting pads on was in the morning. Mean wear time was 6.6 hours.

Considerations when choosing an absorbent product include the following:

1. The best product should be selected on the basis of comfort, ease of application/removal, and containment of urine and control of odor. It should be discreet, which means it does not "show" under clothing, is not bulky, and does not cause "noise" or rustle when the person moves.

2. Correct sizing and product type are important. The one-size-fits-all and one-product-for-all mentality should be avoided, especially when choosing a product for a resident in a nursing home. Sizing of the product may be related to product type and to specific measurements (e.g., weight, waist size, thigh diameter). The type of UI and the amount of urine leakage should be considered as follows:

    a. If the quantity of urine is slight or small, then light or thin perineal pads or pantiliners that attach to underwear will be adequate. This type of product will allow for easy removal when the person is attempting to urinate.

    b. If urine leakage is severe, constant, or both, then a superabsorbent, larger product is needed. In these situations, many clinicians and caregivers choose wrap-around brief products. These products may be excellent at containing large amounts of urine leakage, but they can deter the person from self-toileting because they are difficult to remove and reapply. Protective underwear or a pant-and-pad system may be more appropriate because these products are similar to underwear.

    c. If nighttime leakage is a problem, both bed pads and body-worn products may be necessary. More evidence is needed to determine the best products for nighttime use, but a protocol of "open air" (lying on an underpad without a brief or undergarment) during the night is not recommended. This type of nighttime urine containment was advocated because it was believed that "open air" promoted air circulation, but that was before the new SAP technology was available.

3. Handling and disposal of the soiled product should be done in a sanitary manner. A product should not be flushed down the toilet. The individual or caregiver should wash the hands after handling soiled absorbent products.

4. Costs should be considered with the understanding that cheaper products do not necessarily save money. If a product quickly becomes saturated because of poor absorbency, it may need to be changed more frequently, leading to greater use of pads, higher replacement or laundry costs, or both.

Products for Bed and Furniture Protection

Underpads are absorbent, sheet-like products that are placed on top of the bed or other furniture to contain urine for both comfort to the person and protection of the furniture and bedding. The basic structure of an underpad consists of three layers: a fluid-impermeable backing sheet against the bed, a fluid-permeable top layer to contain and conceal the underlying absorbent core while also directly contacting the person's body, and an inner absorbent core to rapidly contain moisture and disseminate it throughout the entire pad. The backing sheet is composed of a strong film or hydrophobic material, usually a polyolefin, rendering this side an effective barrier and reinforcing the product as a whole. A low coefficient of friction is preferable to allow the underpad to shift easily with movements (Edlich et al., 2006).

PERINEAL SKIN CARE

Skin problems associated with incontinence can range from irritation (dermatitis) to pressure ulcers (Centers for Medicare & Medicaid Services [CMS], 2004) (Table 10.2). Perineal skin breakdown (referred to as incontinence-associated dermatitis [IAD]) and erythema are directly related to exposure to urine and feces (Bliss, Zehner, Savik, Thayer, & Smith, 2006). A common site for pressure ulcer formation is the sacral area, which is problematic in patients with incontinence. Maintaining intact skin can be a common incontinence nursing care problem in individuals whose urine leakage is being managed by incontinence products (Hanson et al., 2006). The role that incontinence plays in the development of pressure ulcers is not yet adequately defined in terms of a clearly recognized and statistically significant clinically documented association. However, uncontrolled or poorly managed incontinence can predispose patients to skin irritation and IAD, and subsequently lead to the formation and inhibition of the healing of pressure ulcers (Gray et al., 2007).

Table 10.2 Common perineal skin conditions

Skin condition	Definition	Presentation	Treatment
Erythema	Inflammatory response caused by dilation of the superficial capillaries and increased vascular permeability.	Occurs as a red, macular rash that may be sensitive and tight. Edema may be present.	• Depends on underlying cause, but reduction of perineal moisture by decreasing perineal skin exposure to urine and feces is important.
Maceration	Superficial softening of the skin from overhydration as a result of prolonged or excessive exposure to moisture, which causes separation of the skin tissues and denudation.	Appearance is white and soggy in texture. Areas that are prone to macerate include perineal skin, abdominal and breast folds, tube insertion sites, between toes and fingers, and skin surrounding wound sites.	• Moisture barriers, absorbent dressings, or both should be used on all areas at risk for maceration and on maceration that occurs around wound edges. • An aqueous formulation with dimethicone is better than petrolatum and dimethicone as a moisturizer. • Petrolatum is superior to dimethicone and zinc oxide in preventing skin maceration (Hoggarth, Waring, Alexander, Greenwood, & Callaghan, 2005).
Intertrigo	Partial-thickness skin loss that occurs on opposing skin surfaces as a result of friction and maceration (Lekan-Rutledge, 2006).	Appears as an erythema with erosions. Common sites include groin skinfolds and the skin between the buttocks.	• Avoid aggressive perineal cleansing and friction.
Irritant or perineal dermatitis	Inflammatory process caused by direct damage to the water–protein–lipid matrix of the skin (Gray, 2004a).	Erythema or reddened skin (in white-skinned person) or skin darker than surrounding skin (in dark-skinned person) that rapidly progresses to blistering, erosion, and exudates (Gray, 2004a). The dermatitis more typically presents as intense erythema, scaling, itching, papules, weeping, and eruptions. Chronic perineal dermatitis can lead to thickening of the skin (called lichenification) and scarring, which further compromises the ability of the skin to serve as a barrier, resulting in conditions (e.g., excoriation) that expose the dermis.	• Containment devices such as absorbent products or external condom catheters can trap moisture against perineal skin, increasing the risk for breakdown. Containment devices such as internal devices or external pouches can prevent prolonged perianal exposure to liquid stool (Newman, Fader, & Bliss, 2004). • Zinc oxide is superior to petrolatum and dimethicone in protecting against irritants (Hoggarth et al., 2005).

Pruritis ani	Inflammation of the peri-anal area.	• Good perineal hygiene program. Avoid soaps, creams, and scratching. Patients should clean themselves using a moistened towelette and avoid excessive drying (Newman, 2007c).
	Pruritis ani will cause intense perianal itching and chronic scratching, causing linear lesions (Gray, Ratliff, & Donavan, 2002). This condition is directly related to perineal hygiene that includes overzealous wiping or cleansing of the anal area. It can also occur as a generalized pruritis in patients with systemic diseases such as liver or renal failure.	
	May be misdiagnosed as irritant dermatitis.	
Candidiasis (also known as moniliasis or yeast dermatitis)	Secondary epidermal in-fection with the fungus *Candida*, most com-monly *C. albicans*.	• Treatment includes use of antifungal products (e.g., Aloe Vesta Antifungal ointment, Critic-Aid Clear Moisture Barrier with Antifungal, Baza Antifungal Cream, DermaFungal, Micro-Guard Antifungal Cream & Powder, Secura Antifungal, Mitrazol Powder). Creams and ointments should be used sparingly because they can trap moisture.
	Risk factors include im-munosuppression, dia-betes mellitus, obesity, and long-term antibi-otic therapy (Evans & Gray, 2003).	• Reduce or eliminate moisture buildup and use a breathable incontinence product that contains absorbing properties (Newman, 2002, 2004; Newman et al., 2004).
	Characterized by bright to dull red central areas with peripheral red, round vesicles, referred to as "satellite lesions." These lesions can become macules if the vesicles are damaged by friction during containment product changes or movement.	• Current evidence-based research for treating *Candida* in clinical practice recommends dusting skinfolds with moisture-absorbing powders, and avoidance of dusting powders such as talc, because they tend to "cake" and further aggravate the infection (Evans & Gray, 2003).
	In dark skin, the central area may appear as more darkened skin (Bryant, 2000). It has an erythematous base that may itch or burn. Spread of the lesion is inhibited when it reaches dry skin.	• Avoid use of antifungal creams in ostomy patients because they may interfere between the ostomy appliance and seal. It is recommended that a powder be applied sparingly in these patients.

(continued)

Table 10.2 *(continued)*

Skin condition	Definition	Presentation	Treatment
Bacterial infections with common organisms, including coagulase-positive staphylococci (*Staphylococcus aureus*), coagulase-negative staphylococci, and gram-negative bacteria (*Escherichia coli*) common in patients with fecal incontinence	Secondary infection from microorganisms that irritate and inflame the skin.	Reddened, scaling areas of skin irritation that often resemble fungal infection. These types of perineal skin irritations are most common in moist areas such as skinfolds.	• Usually treated with systemic antibiotics. Topical antibiotic solutions may be used in certain cases; however, an antimicrobial ingredient in a skin cleanser will not provide adequate treatment for a bacterial infection (Gray et al., 2002).
Pressure ulcer	Localized areas of tissue necrosis that develop when soft tissue is compressed between a bony prominence and an external surface for a prolonged period of time.	Stage I—Observable pressure-related alteration of intact skin. Stage II—Partial-thickness skin loss involving epidermis, dermis, or both. Stage III—Full-thickness skin loss involving damage to or necrosis of subcutaneous tissue that may extend down to, but not through, underlying fascia. Stage IV—Full-thickness skin loss with extensive destruction, tissue necrosis, or damage from muscular fascia to bone.	• Avoid the four main factors that are implicated in causing pressure ulcers: pressure, shear, friction, and moisture.

Adapted from Newman, Preston, and Salazar (2007).

Development of Skin Problems

Several factors cause perineal skin problems and IAD (Box 10.2). The perineum (particularly the scrotal area) is the most absorptive area of the skin, and it has a high moisture content that is sensitive to moisture barriers and toxins. The perineal skin does not tolerate being wet for long periods of time, and wetness destroys the natural barriers for the skin's protection against destructive agents such as urine (CMS, 2005). The skin is slightly acidic, with a pH of 5.5 (range of 4–6). One of the most important components is often referred to as the "protective acid mantle" of the skin. The skin's acidic environment is a major factor in helping to prevent the invasion of the skin by bacteria, yeast, and fungi. An alkaline pH adversely affects the skin, promoting the loss of normal skin integrity.

Both urine and feces contain substances that may irritate the epidermis and may make the skin more susceptible to breakdown. Continued exposure to urine is a direct factor in skin breakdown. When skin is subjected to moisture from urine in combination with fecal matter, further skin trauma results. Bacteria in the stool cause the urea (from the urine) to break down into ammonia. In the person whose skin is already compromised by exposure to urine and feces, the resulting increase in skin pH (into the alkaline range) can be particularly devastating (Thompson, Langemo, Anderson, Hanson, & Hunter, 2005).

Furthermore, the presence of excessive skin surface moisture can contribute to growth of bacteria that can lead to skin breakdown and infection. Waste from UI can overhydrate the skin and promote the growth of microorganisms such as *Candida albicans,* resulting in candidiasis or yeast dermatitis (Figure 10.9A). Moisture may also make skin more susceptible to damage from friction and shear during repositioning. Friction can cause skin abrasion to

---

Box 10.2   Factors affecting perineal skin

- **Excessive perineal moisture** from perspiration, urine, and feces causes skin saturation and maceration. When this occurs, skin cannot act as a barrier to water, chemicals, pathogens, and the chemical components of urine and feces. This encourages growth of bacteria and fungi. This risk of infection is higher in patients with fecal incontinence, because of the skin's exposure to gastrointestinal flora (*Escherichia coli*) and digestive enzymes.

- **Friction** is caused by rubbing against a device, clothing, or bed. Shearing often occurs with friction and can contribute to pressure injury or ulceration.

- **Increased skin pH** can promote a more alkaline skin environment, raising the risk of dermatitis and bacterial colonization.

- **Colonization with microorganisms** can lead to bacterial overgrowth, which causes cutaneous infections. The most common organisms are *Candida albicans* from the gastrointestinal tract and *Staphylococcus* from the perineal skin.

Adapted from Newman, Preston, and Salazar (2007).

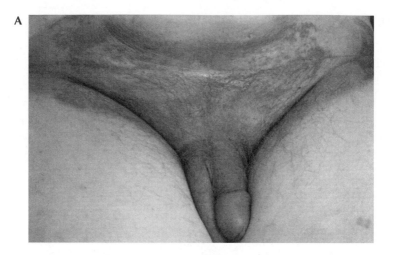

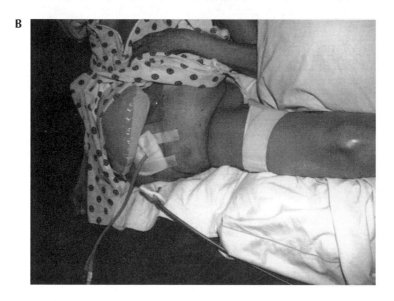

Figure 10.9.   *A,* Incontinence-related candidiasis. *B,* Hemipelvectomy resulting from incontinence-related pressure ulcers.

occur. Wet skin is more easily abraded by movement of skin against an object such as cloth, plastic in leg gathers, or tape fasteners on adult briefs. Tape cuts are commonly seen in obese adults who are wearing a tight-fitting incontinence brief. Potential sources of excessive moisture on the skin include

- UI

- Fecal incontinence

- Too frequent washes

- Nonabsorbent or poorly ventilated padding on the skin
- Skin occlusion

Research has shown that diarrhea or fecal incontinence may pose an even greater threat to skin integrity than UI, most likely because of digestive acids and enzymes in the feces that irritate and erode the epidermis. At least 60% of dry stool contains bacteria, which cause destruction of the skin cellular defense necessitating preventive perineal skin care. Prolonged exposure to urine and feces, moisture, and friction combine to macerate, abrade, and blister the skin over the buttocks and sacrum. All of these factors work in concert to cause skin irritation, breakdown, and further skin problems. This is a self-perpetuating cycle of events that can predispose the skin to pressure ulcer formation (Newman, Preston, & Salazar, 2007), which can have severe consequences (Figure 10.9B).

Skin Care Products

Proper use of soaps, skin products, topical antimicrobials (agents that inhibit the growth of germs), gentle pH-balanced cleansers, and appropriate barrier products, as well as effective use of incontinence pads, is important in skin care management (Gray, Ratliff, & Donavan, 2002) (Appendix Table 10.2 and Figure 10.10). One must also consider the impact skin care products may have on efficacy of absorbent products. Petrolatum-based skin protectants are often used both prophylactically and as a treatment for incontinence dermatitis. However, there may be an incompatibility between petrolatum-based skin protectants and absorbent products such as adult briefs, causing increased skin irritation (Zehrer, Newman, Grove, & Lutz, 2005).

Perineal Cleansers

Despite the availability of skin care products designed specifically to prevent skin breakdown, cleansing with soap and water, often applied with a washcloth, has traditionally been thought of as a "gold standard" for skin hygiene and continues to be the most widely used skin care regimen in LTC facilities. This is true despite the fact that there is research to show that a soap-and-water regimen alone is the least effective in preventing skin breakdown when compared with moisture barriers and no-rinse incontinence cleansers (Subbannayyn, Bhat, Junu, Shetty, & Jisho, 2006). Bar soaps can be especially harmful because the residue created by soap stored in a moist soap dish may harbor bacteria, and the same bar of soap may be used on multiple patients, contributing to the spread of bacteria. Also, bar soaps used with washcloths can be very irritating, can cause increased friction, and may remove oils from the skin, reducing the skin's barrier properties. Soap removes the skin's natural lipids; it also decreases natural lubricants, which leads to increased epidermal

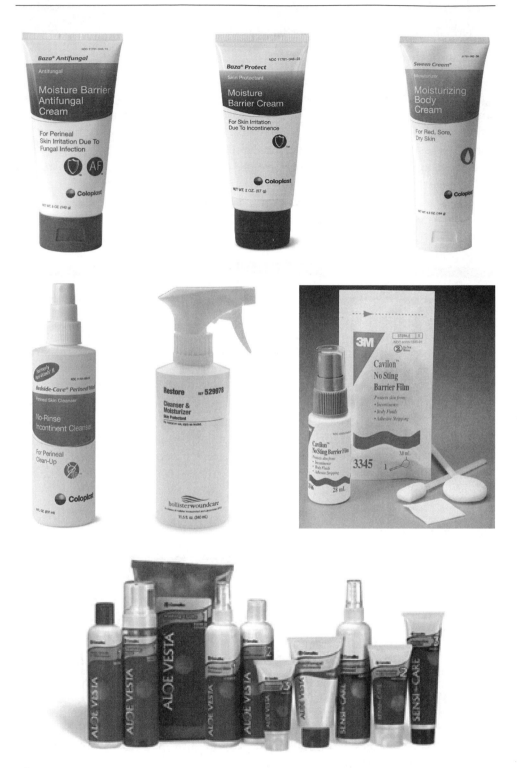

Figure 10.10.   Bathing and skin care products. (Courtesy of Coloplast, Hollister, 3M, and ConvaTec.)

water loss (measured as water vapor diffusing to the environment through the epidermis). It is associated with problems such as increased skin pH, dry skin from dehydration, contact dermatitis, and eczema (Newman et al., 2007). Although it is easier to dispense proper amounts of soap in liquid form, liquid soap can also be harmful.

Because frequent washing with soap and water can dehydrate the skin, the use of a perineal rinse may be indicated, and use of bar soaps, harsh cleansers, and solvents should be avoided. Skin dryness or dehydration is especially a problem in older adults (Hodgkinson, Nay, & Wilson, 2007). The use of disposable wipes or washcloths rather than toilet tissue may be more beneficial to the perineal skin. No-rinse perineal cleansers are more convenient and time saving, and are preferred over the popular bar soaps because the cleansing agents and antiseptics used in these formulations are gentler to the skin than those used in bar soaps (Warshaw, Nix, Kula, & Markon, 2002). Perineal cleansers are liquid solutions that remove bacteria or effluent. These cleansers also effectively remove urine and feces without personal discomfort because they can help emulsify and loosen stool and urine. In addition, no-rinse perineal cleansers are pH balanced for the skin, whereas bar soaps are almost always in the alkaline range. Some perineal cleansers are also formulated with topical antimicrobials that may decrease the bacteria on the skin.

Fragrances and alcohol and alkaline agents should be avoided when choosing a cleanser. Alcohol and alkaline agents should be avoided because they can be irritants and sensitizers, especially if skin integrity is compromised.

Moisturizers

To preserve the moisture in the skin by either sealing in existing moisture or adding moisture to the skin, moisturizers should be used. Loss of moisture from the stratum corneum (top layer of the skin) causes dryness, increasing the risk for skin breakdown. Topical moisturizers replace lost lipids from the skin. Ingredients can increase water content and elasticity and improve desquamation by hydrating the stratum corneum. The best time to moisturize the skin is during and after bathing so as to trap water next to the skin. However, overall clinical effectiveness is short lived because of quick shedding along with the desquamating corneocytes. Therefore, moisturizers should be applied on a daily basis to attain the maximum benefit.

Product types include lotions, creams, pastes, and ointments (Loden, 2005). Pastes are created by adding powder to an ointment, and do not need to be removed each time an area is washed. An aqueous formulation with dimethicone is better than petrolatum and dimethicone as a moisturizer. Petrolatum is superior to dimethicone and zinc oxide in preventing skin maceration. Zinc oxide is superior to petrolatum and dimethicone in protecting against irritants (Hoggarth, Waring, Alexander, Greenwood, & Callaghan, 2005).

Barrier Products

Barrier products protect the skin from contact with moisture and decrease friction from absorbent products (Gray, 2004a). However, if the skin barrier product is easily removed with water during cleansing of an area, then it is not likely to provide a durable barrier to urine and feces. Barrier skin products can be differentiated into two general types: one works by forming a film on the skin after evaporation of a solvent (spray or applied with an applicator) and the other, such as ointments and creams, forms a hydrophobic, physical barrier. Clear, solvent-based, film-forming skin protectants are an even better alternative than creams, ointments, and pastes. Film-forming skin protectants are acrylate-based copolymers that quickly evaporate when applied to the skin, leaving the copolymer behind to form a protective film. This clear film allows for air flow but is impervious to external moisture and skin irritants.

Barrier products containing topical antifungal agents are available in ointments, powders, and creams. Some topical antifungals with anti-*Candida* activity are available as over-the-counter products (e.g., clotrimazole, miconazole). Topical antifungal cream should be applied after each incontinence episode in individuals with perineal candidiasis and continued until any erythema is completely resolved. Other barrier products should not be used when using antifungals.

Perineal Skin Care Management

Careful and close attention to skin care reduces the occurrence of skin breakdown in patients with incontinence. The key to preventing skin problems is to keep the perineal skin clean and dry. It is important for the caregiver to carefully select the appropriate absorbent product, preferably one that minimizes the possibility of IAD. It has been shown that products designed to absorb moisture and present a quick-drying surface to the skin (e.g., absorbent incontinence products with SAP) keep the skin drier and are associated with a significantly lower incidence of skin rashes than cloth products. The length of time an individual wears an adult brief should be limited because these products have a tight, permeable covering that can lead to perineal dermatitis.

All individuals who have UI and wear absorbent products or use external or internal catheters to manage their UI need a perineal skin care program. The following is an example of a program for perineal skin care (Newman, 2006b):

1. Put on gloves and remove soiled perineal pad or absorbent product, if indicated.

2. Inspect the skin of the groin, buttocks, coccyx, rectal area, scrotum/perineum, genitalia, and upper thighs carefully every day. Assessment of the skin includes separation of skinfolds and wrinkles, looking for presence of rash, irritation, or skin breakdown. Assess perineal skin for

signs of dermatitis, erythema, swelling, oozing, vesiculation, crusting, and scaling.

3. Always wash the skin after any urine or bowel incontinence episode. Cleanse skin thoroughly with a mild soap (e.g., Dove), a no-rinse cleanser, or premoistened, alcohol-free towelettes in the following manner:

   a. Woman—Position on the bed, supine with legs apart and knees flexed. Clean the genitalia with a washcloth or wipes using a downward motion from the pubis (front) to the anus (back), using a different section of the washcloth or discarding wipes after each stroke to avoid contamination.

   b. Man—Cleanse the penis with special attention to the folds of the foreskin and glans (tip) of the penis (particularly in the uncircumcised man). If the man is uncircumcised, pull back the foreskin and clean around the glans of the penis. Then, replace the foreskin back over the glans. Skin integrity is at risk in a man with scrotal edema. To reduce scrotal edema, roll up a soft towel, tape it close, and place it under the scrotum to provide elevation.

4. Provide gentle cleansing with a mild cleansing agent immediately after soiling, and avoid force and friction during cleansing. Minimal use of any soap product reduces irritation, especially in the elderly woman who has atrophic perineal changes.

5. After washing, let the skin air dry rather than rubbing with a towel to avoid irritation and skin tears.

6. Skin care for patients with urinary or bowel incontinence is as follows:

   a. With or without mild redness or chafing, use a barrier cream twice a day.

   b. With redness or minimal open, weepy skin lesions, use a barrier paste after each incontinence episode or with absorbent product changes and reapply as necessary.

   c. With fungal rash but no open areas, use an antifungal cream and cover with a barrier cream at least 3 times a day.

7. If the person is bedridden or uses a wheelchair, protect the skin from moisture. Avoid having the person sit or lie on any areas that are open or have a rash. Turn the individual frequently and support him or her in different positions by using pillows or wedges.

TOILETING SUBSTITUTES AND DEVICES

Toilet substitutes are portable devices that substitute for a regular toilet. There are two general categories: commode seats or bedside commodes, and hand-held devices such as a bedpan or urinal. These devices are appropriate when 1) there are inaccessible toilet areas, 2) doorways and bathrooms are too narrow for access (e.g., when using a walker or a wheelchair), 3) nocturnal frequency and urgency are significant problems, and 4) decreased mobility is an issue (Newman, 2004). Several hand-held, reusable urine collection containers and devices are also available that can be successfully used by patients and their caregivers as long as the proper device is identified. Current designs have changed little, and none has been specifically designed for elderly individuals who are frail or have disabilities. In the United States, these devices have received little attention as aids to containing urine.

Teaching the person to use a toileting device is an important part of rehabilitation and a valuable use of nursing staff time. The person can promote or maintain self-toileting through the independent use of these devices. However, if these devices are shared, how they are cleaned and disinfected is important because there is some evidence demonstrating that shared clinical equipment becomes contaminated with pathogens. One study found that more than 50% of commodes tested were contaminated with *Clostridium difficile* (Wilcox et al., 2003).

Types of Toileting Substitutes or Devices

Toilets

Adequacy and availability of bathroom facilities, including number of toilets, are important and are reviewed in Chapter 6. The height, location, and width of the toilet are important in all care settings. To increase height, raised toilet seats (referred to as toilet risers) that are placed over a regular toilet allow the individual to get up and down on his or her own, thus allowing for self-toileting (Figure 10.11). Seats with grab bars on either side are most often recommended to prevent falling and to aid with rising. A toilet seat that is a different color from the floor may be helpful for patients with visual impairments.

Commodes

If the person can get out of bed to urinate, a commode is a better alternative than a bedpan. Many different commodes exist that can ease toileting (Figure 10.12). A bedside commode can be placed close to the bed for easy use at night, or located on a floor of the house that does not have a bathroom. Some commodes have drop arms and adjustable heights to allow for individual needs. To minimize the odor and to make cleaning the bucket easier, water with a disinfectant should be kept in the bucket at all times. The commode can be camouflaged with an attractive cloth, or placed behind a screen. There are also wooden rather than metal commodes that can be disguised as an easy chair.

Problems with commode design include difficulties with sideways transfer, ineffective brakes causing commodes to move during transfer, and poor

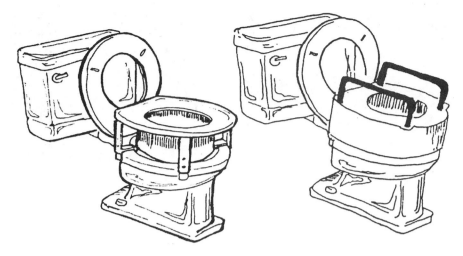

Figure 10.11.   Toilet riser and toilet riser with grab bars.

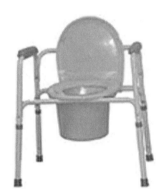

Figure 10.12.   Commode chair.
(Courtesy of AdaMed.)

trunk support (Cottenden et al., 2005). General considerations when selecting a commode include the following (Newman, 2004):

- Height and weight of the person using the commode

- Mobility and dexterity, especially if the person will need to empty and clean the commode

- Type of seat—A plastic seat with a large, soft surface area may allow even distribution of body weight

- Seats with grab bars on either side, which are most often recommended to prevent falling and to aid with rising

- Cost—Most insurers will pay for a commode only when a physician writes a letter of medical necessity

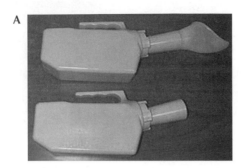 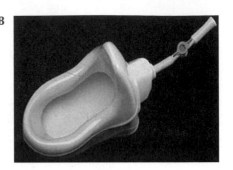

Figure 10.13.   Hand-held urinals. *A (top),* female spillproof urinal with cup. *A (bottom),* male urinal with spill-proof neck. *B,* Urinal can be attached to drainage bag.

Urinals

Urinals are usually small, lightweight, bottle-shaped containers made from plastic or metal. They usually have two different types of neck, narrow for men and wider for women. Urinals have the potential to enable elderly men and women who experience difficulty accessing a toilet to regain continence. They are useful for patients who have severe mobility restrictions, particularly when visiting places with inaccessible restrooms, when traveling, when bed-ridden, or when using a wheelchair (Newman, 2004; Newman et al., 2004). The basic design of the urinal has remained unchanged for years, although disposable plastic variants are more often used (Figure 10.13). Urinals have handles so they can be placed next to the person or hung on a bed rail, wheelchair, or walker. Rehabilitation urinals have a flat bottom so that they can be laid flat on the bed. The openings in these "rehab" urinals have a flange that extends into the urinal and does not allow backflow even when held almost upside down (Figure 10.13A). Urinals can be obtained by mail order, in retail stores, or in pharmacies.

There are difficulties with positioning the urinal, enabling drainage toward the front, and providing for sufficient volume without producing a cumbersome product (Fader, Pettersson, Dean, Brooks, & Cottenden, 1999; MacIntosh, 1998). The body of the urinal must be lower than the urine entry point because urine flows downward with gravity. For men, spill-proof urinals with large funnel openings are available to deal with a retracted penis. Urinals for women are shaped so that the opening is designed to cup or fit snugly against the perineal area and funnel the urine inside (Macaulay, et al., 2006). Most types of urinals are more likely to be successful when used in the standing or crouching position. It is very difficult to find a female urinal that can be used effectively by women with very poor mobility. In choosing a female product, the focus should be on being able to position and remove the urinal easily and feeling confident that it will contain urine without spilling. If sitting in a chair, the female patient will need to be able to move forward to position the urinal correctly. Female urinals are needed that work for difficult postures.

The following considerations are important when choosing a urinal (Fader et al., 1999; Vickerman, 2006):

- Material of the urinal—Lightweight plastic urinals are useful for patients who have difficulty lifting. Steel urinals are very heavy and cumbersome.

- Handles to hold the urinal—If grip is a problem, rubber around the handle will increase grip. An extended handle may help if wrist movement is restricted.

- Mobility, manual dexterity, and agility—These factors will dictate the ease of use in specific positions (e.g., flat in bed, side-lying, sitting in a wheelchair, standing).

- Ability to remove, empty, and clean the urinal.

- Spill-proof design—Urine should not spill during use when the urinal is removed or when being carried.

- Discreetness—Consideration should be given to size, shape, and color.

- Clothing—It can impede use of the urinal.

Bedpans

Bedpans are generally the least effective container for maximizing continence because they are difficult to position without creating excess pressure on the sacral area. Also, they do not promote correct position to aid in complete bladder emptying. The most successful bedpan is a "fracture pan," which is commonly used in the acute care setting in postsurgery patients. Often the use of a fracture pan enables women to urinate without pain, especially in the postoperative period after a fracture or hip repair. Sprinkling talcum powder or cornstarch on the bedpan will make sliding the pan under the person easier.

New Devices

New technology in the area of "toilet substitutes" includes portable, vacuum or battery-operated pump systems that draw urine into a collection bag or container (Macaulay et al., 2007). One such device available in the United States attaches the receptacle to any standard institutional bed or to a wheelchair (Figure 10.14). The individual or caregiver positions a collection cup (male or female, accordingly) under the perineum, and the pump gently drains the urine into the collection bag, eliminating odor, leakage, and possible spills. Once the individual is finished voiding, the cup is replaced, the door to the unit is closed, and the pump automatically shuts off. Visual and auditory alerts indicate when the collection bag is nearly full. Alerts can be silenced with the push of a button, and the bag can easily be emptied in less than 30 seconds. This product will need wider use to determine long-term effectiveness.

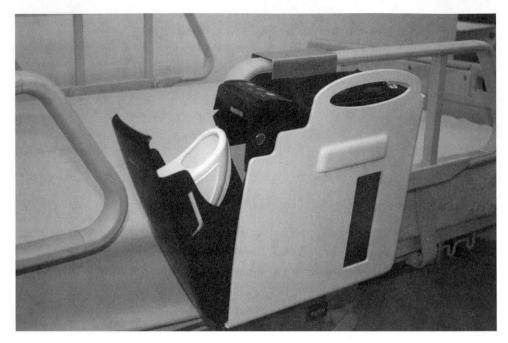

Figure 10.14.   UrAssist pump-assisted urinal. (Courtesy of Preferred Medical Devices.)

Making Toilets Accessible

In an LTC facility, the location of toilets should be clearly indicated. Poorly designed signs to designate bathrooms, or the use of terminology that residents do not understand to identify the bathroom, can be a deterrent to self-toileting. Changes in bathroom architecture can also aid in toileting. For ease in toileting, bathroom size should be at least 5 feet by 5 feet. Grab bars in the right spot and a toilet seat adapter make the toilet safer. At least one grab bar should run parallel to the floor at a height of 33 inches. Bathrooms with gravity-assisted door closer mechanisms are helpful; however, many patients cannot open bathroom doors because they cannot grasp and turn the door-knob. To remedy this, doorknobs can be replaced with lever-type devices or the door can be disabled so that it opens and closes with a push. Removing the bathroom door and using a curtain or swinging doors makes access by a wheel-chair possible.

CATHETERS

A catheter is used for two common medical problems: UI and urinary retention. To ease these conditions, the catheter is put into the bladder to drain the urine. It may stay in place for a short or long period of time depending on the type of catheter and the reason for its use. Catheters are used in several different ways:

- Inserted intermittently into the bladder (intermittent catheterization)

- Placed in the bladder on a more permanent or chronic basis (indwelling urethral or suprapubic catheterization)

- Used on the outside of the body for men (external condom catheters)

Most of the medical literature states that prevention of infection should be the primary factor when deciding which type of catheter to use for patients requiring urinary collection. Yet most professionals in clinical practice would agree that the use of catheters is governed by caregiver/individual preference, the degree of caregiver burden related to the patient's urinary problem, and ease of urinary management.

Indwelling Urinary Catheters

An indwelling urinary catheter, generally referred to as a "Foley" catheter, is a closed sterile system with a catheter and retention balloon that is inserted either through the urethra or suprapubically to allow for bladder drainage. Figure 10.15 shows inserted suprapubic and urethral catheters. They are identified as short or long term depending on the time they remain in place. Indwelling urinary catheters have been around since the third century, when reeds and metal tubes were used to treat urinary retention. More durable and flexible catheters made their appearance in the 1800s with the introduction of rubber. Dr. Frederick Foley, a 1930s urologist, designed the first true "retention" catheter when he used a rubber tube with a separate lumen used to inflate a balloon to hold the catheter in place in the bladder (Newman, 2004) (Figure 10.16). In the 1900s, catheters made of new plastic materials—silicone, Teflon coatings, and polyvinyl chloride (PVC)—were developed that caused fewer problems than latex rubber catheters. Table 10.3 lists the different types of indwelling urinary catheters.

Indwelling urethral catheters are currently being used to relieve urinary retention and to manage long-term UI. Although catheters are prescribed by urologists, patients with long-term catheters are primarily under the care and supervision of nurses. However, this type of "management" or drainage system has several medical and nursing care problems; strict indications for use are outlined in Box 10.3. Indwelling urinary catheters are recommended only for short-term use, defined as less than 30 days, but typically stay in place for 2 weeks or less. Short-term uses include management of acute urinary retention, postoperative bladder decompression, and monitoring urinary output in acutely ill patients. Long-term use, defined as greater than 30 days, is discouraged because it provides access for bacteria from a contaminated environment into a vulnerable body organ and system. As a result, catheter-associated urinary tract infection (CAUTI) is the most common type of infection acquired in hospitals and LTC facilities (Nicolle, 2005). Indwelling catheters are associated with multiple complications and side effects as well as increased morbidity and mortality. Long-term catheterization should only be used as a last resort in the person with UI.

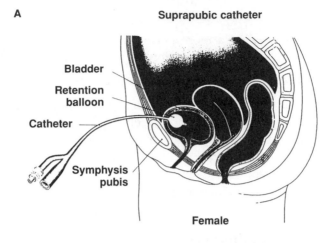

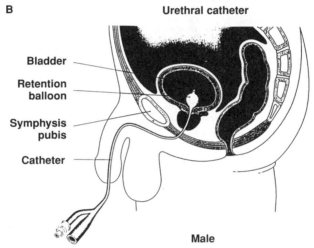

Figure 10.15. *A,* Suprapubic and *B,* urethral catheters. (Courtesy of CR Bard.)

Indications for Use

Each year, urinary catheters are inserted in more than 5 million patients in acute care hospitals and LTC facilities. Historically, indwelling catheters have been used in the chronically medically compromised elderly person. The settings in which the prevalence of long-term indwelling catheter usage is the greatest are 1) skilled nursing facilities, where they are used in residents with UI, and 2) homes where the person requires skilled nursing visits. In the home care setting, the prevalence of indwelling catheters is increasing with the increasing numbers of older adults. However, the number of "home-bound" patients who use a catheter indefinitely to manage UI or because of urinary retention has not been well documented in medical or nursing research.

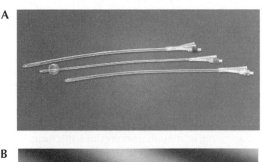

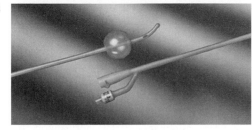

Figure 10.16. Indwelling catheters. *Top,* Silicone. (Courtesy of Rochester Medical.) *Bottom,* Latex. (Courtesy of CR Bard.)

These devices increase mortality and morbidity in both men and women. Indwelling urinary catheters are also associated with other morbid events such as delirium and with longer lengths of stay and higher costs of medical care (Roth, Lovell, Harvey, Bode, & Heinemann, 2002; Saint et al., 2000). Inappropriate catheter use has been equated to a "one-point restraint," and, as a form of restraint, catheters could be associated with discomfort, nosocomial infection, pressure ulcers, functional impairment, and death (Saint, Lipsky, & Goold, 2002). In hospitalized older medical patients without a specific medical indication, urinary catheterization was associated with a greater risk of death: 4 times as great during hospitalization and 2 times as great within 90 days after discharge (Holroyd-Leduc et al., 2007). In many cases, catheters are inserted for the convenience of the nursing staff responsible for cleaning and changing incontinent individuals. Catheters can and do have serious adverse effects. Catheters drain the bladder, but obstruct the glands in the wall of the urethra. Indwelling urethral catheters can produce urethral strictures, epididymitis, orchitis, and prostatitis in men. Inappropriate and excessive use of antimicrobial drugs in catheterized individuals leads to selection for antibiotic-resistant microorganisms and accounts for nosocomial outbreaks of infection with multidrug-resistant strains.

Indications for urinary catheter use are based on federal guidelines outlined in Box 10.3 (CMS, 2005; Fantl et al., 1996, Wong & Hooton, 1981). In a skilled nursing facility and in home care, the use of an indwelling urinary catheter is allowed on a long-term basis only when medical necessity is determined, not necessarily because the individual has a "neurogenic" diagnosis.

Table 10.3   Types of indwelling urinary catheters

Type	Characteristics
Latex (natural rubber)	Very soft, flexible catheter that is low cost.
	Latex is the base of most catheters but has an increased risk of local inflammation and hypersensitivity. The individual may develop latex allergy with long-term use, and latex allergy also can affect the caregiver or nurse. Latex has also been implicated in causing toxicity to mucosal tissue, resulting in inflammation and urethral strictures in long-term catheterization (Emr & Ryan, 2004; Smith, 2003).
	The chemical properties of latex cause it to swell as a result of absorption of body fluids, decreasing the drainage lumen and increasing the outside diameter of the catheter (Newman, 2007a). If the latex catheter is coated with Teflon, this problem is resolved. Nevertheless, latex catheters have been associated with a higher rate of encrustation, which leads to blockage of catheter eyes and impedes drainage (Hukins, 2005). Coatings such as silver, hydrogels, polytetra-fluoroethylene (PTFE), and silicone have been added.
Polytetrafluoroethylene (PTFE) or Teflon	PTFE coating on a latex core has good biological compatibility and low friction. It has a rough external texture that may cause infection and encrustation.
	Because these are Teflon-coated latex catheters, allergy remains a concern.
Silicone-coated (elastomer) latex	These catheters tend to be yellow or golden in color. The coating is chemically bonded to the inner and outer surface of the latex catheter, ensuring minimum urethral irritation and good flow. This coating provides smoothness to the latex surface and eases catheterization.
	The coating helps prevent urethral contact with the latex. The elastomer provides "elasticity" and prevents any chemical release from the latex catheter. However, these catheters should only be used short term because this coating will dissolve over time, and latex hypersensivity may still occur.

Use (and Misuse) of Indwelling Urinary Catheters

Although indwelling urinary catheters are commonly used in most clinical settings, data suggest that more than 20% of these catheters are placed without a specific medical indication and that they often remain in place without the knowledge of the patient's physician (Kunin, 2006; Saint et al., 2000). Studies of the appropriateness of use of urinary catheters indicate that 21%–38% of initial urinary catheterizations are unjustified, and one third to one half of days of continued catheterization are unjustified (Munasinghe, Yazdani, Siddique, & Hafeez, 2001). The current challenges are to develop effective methods to sensitize the minds of clinicians to avoid the routine use of indwelling catheters, remove catheters when they are no longer needed, develop alternative methods for care of incontinence, employ noninvasive methods to measure bladder function and urine output, and improve urine drainage systems.

Table 10.3   *(continued)*

Type	Characteristics
100% silicone	These catheters are clear or white in color. They are thin-walled, more rigid catheters with a wider lumen diameter because they are uncoated. Fewer problems seem to occur in long-term use because these catheters are compatible with the lining of the urethra and do not allow buildup of protein and mucus. However, this may be because all-silicone catheters have a slightly wider lumen than other coated catheters. Silicone catheters are now popular because people are developing allergies to latex catheters. The balloon loses fluid over time and tends to form creases or cuffs when deflated; this may make the catheter difficult to remove, or cause the catheter to "fall out."
Hydrogel-coated latex or lubricious (e.g., Bard Lubricath) latex	Hydrogel is a polymer that absorbs water to produce a slippery outside surface. When the catheter is inserted, the hydrogel absorbs secretions from the urethra (hydrophilic), causing the catheter to soften and be more comfortable. It produces a slippery (lubricious) outside surface that reduces friction and protects from urethral tissue damage. It resists encrustation and bacteria colonization. Catheters with hydrogel bonding may be better tolerated and preferred by the person for long-term usage. Urine leakage may be less of a problem with the hydrogel-coated than the silicone catheters.
Silver alloy, antimicrobials	Silver alloy coating decreases CAUTIs in short-term use. These catheters reduce bacterial adherence and minimize biofilm formation through their release of silver ions, which prevent bacteria from settling on the surface. Antimicrobial coatings may decrease CAUTIs.

Adapted from Edlich et al. (2000), Gray (2006), Lawrence and Turner (2005), and Newman (2007a).

Acute Care Catheter Use   In acute care hospital settings, 15%–25% of patients may have a catheter inserted sometime during their stay, usually for surgery, urine output measurement, urinary retention, or UI (Warren, 2005). Hospitals use indwelling catheters more than any other medical device. Because the most important risk factor for catheter-associated bacteriuria is duration of catheterization, most catheters in hospitalized patients are placed for only 2–4 days. Extended indwelling catheter use in older patients sustaining hip fracture who are discharged to skilled nursing facilities with a catheter in place has been associated with poorer outcomes because these individuals are at higher risk of rehospitalization for CAUTIs and sepsis (Wald, Epstein, & Kramer, 2005). Increased mortality at 30 days is seen in these individuals when compared to patients whose catheter was removed prior to discharge (Kalsi, Arya, Wilson, & Mundy, 2003). The risk of infection is associated with the method and duration

Box 10.3   Indications (medical necessity) for indwelling catheter

- Short term for acute urinary retention
  - Sudden and complete inability to void
  - Need for immediate and rapid bladder decompression
- Monitoring of intake and output
- Temporary relief of bladder outlet obstruction secondary to:
  - Enlarged prostate gland
  - Urethral stricture
  - Obstructing pelvic organ prolapse
- Chronic urethral obstruction or urinary retention and surgical interventions, or the use of intermittent catheterization has failed or is not feasible, or both
- Short term following a urological or gynecological surgical procedure
- Irreversible medical conditions are present (e.g., metastatic terminal disease, coma, end stages of other conditions)
- Presence of stage III or IV pressure ulcers that are not healing because of continual urine leakage
- Instances in which a caregiver is not present (primarily occurs in the home care setting) to provide incontinence care

Adapted from Centers for Medicare & Medicaid Services (2005), Newman (2007b), Newman, Fader, and Bliss (2004), and Wong and Hooten (1981).

of catheterization, the quality of catheter care, and host susceptibility. Around 50% of hospitalized patients catheterized longer than 7–10 days contract bacteriuria. Although frequently asymptomatic, 20%–30% of individuals with catheter-associated bacteriuria will develop symptoms of CAUTI. Many of these infections are serious and lead to significant morbidity and mortality (Saint, Lipsky, Baker, McDonald, & Ossenkop, 1999). The CMS has placed a high priority on reducing CAUTIs. On August 7, 2007, a modification was made to the Inpatient Prospective Payment System (IPPS) by the CMS that will change the reimbursement system to hospitals so they will be accountable for failing to avert preventable harms from medical care (Wald & Kramer, 2007). CAUTIs will be viewed as unacceptable harm resulting from medical care, and hospitals will be at risk for financial losses (nonpayment for additional costs) if CAUTIs occur.

A common reason for inappropriately prolonged catheter use is that physicians forget, or were never aware of, the presence of the catheter. In a multicenter evaluation, physicians at four academic medical centers were asked whether or not each patient on their service had a urinary catheter in place. Incorrect negative responses were recorded for over one third of attending physicians and more than a quarter of resident physicians (Saint et al., 2000). For inappropriately catheterized patients, the proportion of physicians unaware of the presence of a catheter was even higher (over 50% of attending physicians and over 40% of senior residents). These forgotten catheters often remain in the person until either a catheter-related complication occurs or the person's discharge is imminent (Saint et al., 2000). There is some evidence to suggest that computer management systems improve documentation and in so doing reduce the length of time catheters are in situ (Cornia, Amory, Fraser, Saint, & Lipsky, 2003). In addition, a nurse-driven protocol could be developed that allows nurses to discontinue a catheter independent of a physician's order when established criteria for catheter use are no longer met. Also, the use of portable ultrasound machines (e.g., BladderScan) should be instituted for noninvasive bladder volume assessment (Topal et al., 2005).

LTC Catheter Use   The prevalence of indwelling urinary catheter use in nursing homes has been established as 7%. It may be greater in facilities that have poor success with toileting programs because the catheter is used as a means to maintain resident dryness (Gammack, 2003). At least 40% of all infections seen in nursing homes are in the urinary tract. Of these infections, 80% are due to urinary tract catheterization and instrumentation (Nicolle, 2000, 2001). CAUTI is of major importance because of its effect on outcomes and treatment costs. The major reason for use of an indwelling catheter in LTC is incontinence or pressure ulcers. Mody, Maheshwari, Galecki, Kauffman, and Bradley (2007) noted that indications for an indwelling urinary catheter in 14 community nursing homes in southeast Michigan were for bladder retention (42%), incontinence (16%), comfort care (6%), and unspecified (34%). The urine of virtually all of these individuals was persistently colonized with multiple species of microorganisms, many resistant to most antibiotics (Mody et al., 2007). It is therefore not surprising that the urinary tract accounts for 51% of episodes of often polymicrobial bacteremia, with *Escherichia coli* (27%), *Staphylococcus aureus* (18%, with methicillin-resistant *S. aureus* [MRSA] 29% of that), and *Proteus mirabilis* (13%) the most common bacteria present (Mylotte, Tayara, & Goodnough, 2002). Urine that is cloudy and foul smelling often prompts a call from an LTC facility to the physician, with an expectation that an evaluation, if not antibiotic therapy, will be ordered. However, in the asymptomatic person, most physicians do not consider cloudy or foul-smelling urine an indication for urinalysis, culture, or antimicrobial treatment (Nicolle et al., 2005).

Although many approaches have been used to minimize CAUTI, elimination of catheter usage remains the best method. For a resident with an indwelling urinary catheter, the facility is in compliance with CMS requirements if they have 1) recognized and assessed factors affecting the resident's urinary function and identified the medical justification for the use of an indwelling urinary catheter; 2) defined and implemented pertinent interventions to try to minimize complications from an indwelling urinary catheter, and to remove it if clinically indicated; 3) monitored and evaluated the resident's response to interventions; and 4) revised the approaches as appropriate (CMS, 2005).

Home Care Catheter Use   Few research studies have looked at the use of catheters in homebound and hospice patients. A publication from the Centers for Disease Control and Prevention on characteristics of elderly home health care users in the 1994 National Home and Hospice Care Survey reported that 12% of older men and 7% of older women had an ostomy or an indwelling catheter (Day, 1996). One visiting nurse agency study noted that the presence of catheters in individuals with UI meant the continuation of skilled nursing services, home health aide services, and Medicare-covered catheter supplies (Newman, Parente, & Yuan, 1997). A more recent study indicated a 38% prevalence of indwelling catheter use in community-dwelling incontinent women (Landi et al., 2004). These subjects also had a higher mortality.

Catheter-Associated Complications

Patients with indwelling urinary catheters are at increased risk for catheter-related problems that range from simple obstruction (blockage) to serious infections, sepsis, and death (Fantl et al., 1996). The following is a review of the catheter-associated complications encountered with indwelling urinary catheters.

Bacteriuria   Bacteriuria (bacteria in the urine) usually occurs in most patients who have a catheter in place for 2–10 days (Goodsarran & Katz, 2002). A large number and a variety of types of organisms are present in the periurethral area and in the distal part of the urethra that may be introduced into the bladder at the time of catheter insertion. Other factors that increase the risk of bacteriuria include the presence of residual urine because of inadequate bladder drainage in the bladder (urine stasis promotes bacterial growth), ischemic damage to the bladder mucosa through overdistention, mechanical irritation from the presence of a catheter, and biofilm formation on the catheter intraluminal surface.

Most bacteria causing CAUTI gain access to the urinary tract either extraluminally or intraluminally. Extraluminal contamination may occur as the catheter is inserted, by contamination of the catheter from any source. Extraluminal contamination is thought also to occur by microorganisms ascending from the perineum along the surface of the catheter. Most episodes of bacteriuria in catheterized women are believed to occur through extraluminal entry of organisms. Fecal strains contaminate the perineum and urethral meatus, and then ascend to the bladder along the external surface to cause bacteriuria, catheter biofilm formation, and encrustation (Mathur, Sabbuba, Suller, Stickler, & Feneley, 2005). Intraluminal contamination occurs by ascent of bacteria from a contaminated catheter, drainage tube, or urine drainage bag (Pratt et al., 2007). Microorganisms can migrate up the catheter into the bladder within 1 to 3 days (Donlan & Costerton, 2002). At least 66% of CAUTIs result from extraluminal contamination, whereas 34% are a result of intraluminal route (Tambyah, Halvorson, & Maki, 1999). There are three catheter-associated entry points for bacteria: 1) the urethral meatus, with introduction of bacteria occurring on insertion of the catheter; 2) the junction of the catheter–bag connection, especially when a break in the closed catheter system occurs; and 3) the drainage port of the collection bag (Figure 10.17). All of these mechanisms involved in the pathogenesis of colonization and infection of the urinary tract combine to make CAUTI very difficult to prevent in individuals with urinary catheters in place for longer than 2 weeks.

Two catheter hygiene principles should be used to prevent bacteriuria: a "closed" system should be used, and the catheter should be removed as soon as possible. A systematic review suggested that sealed (e.g., taped, presealed) drainage systems contribute to preventing bacteriuria (Dunn, Pretty, Reid, & Evans, 2000). The basic components of a closed system include the catheter, a preconnected collecting tube with an attached sampling port, and a vented drainage bag with a port for drainage (Figure 10.18). Catheter-associated bacteriuria is usually asymptomatic and uncomplicated and gradually resolves in an otherwise normal urinary tract after the catheter is removed.

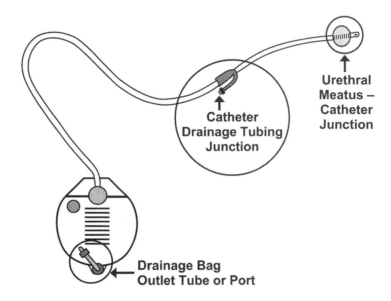

Figure 10.17.   Indwelling catheter infection entry points. (Courtesy of Robin Noel.)

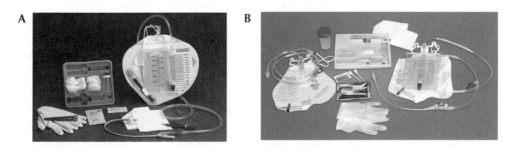

Figure 10.18.   Catheter trays with tamper-resistant seals. (Courtesy of CR Bard [A] and Rochester Medical [B].)

Catheter-Associated Urinary Tract Infections   The most severe and common catheter-associated complication, which can lead to urosepsis and septicemia, involves CAUTIs, the most common nosocomial infections in hospitals and nursing homes, comprising more than 40% of all institutionally acquired infections (Maki & Tambyah, 2001). CAUTIs are considered complicated urinary tract infections (UTIs) and are the most common complication associated with long-term catheter use. CAUTIs may occur at least twice a year in patients with long-term indwelling catheters, requiring hospitalization. They are associated with increased urosepsis, septicemia, and mortality. Catheters are a good medium for bacterial growth because bacterial biofilms (layers of organisms) adhere to the many surfaces of the catheter system (Morris, Stickler, & Mclean, 1999; Saint & Chenoweth, 2003; Saye, 2007).

CAUTI is more likely to occur in women than men; because of the shorter female urethra and because of the urethra's close proximity to the anus, bacteria have a shorter distance to travel (Saint, 2000). Most CAUTIs involve multiple organisms and resistant bacteria from catheter-associated biofilms (discussed later). These include Enterobacteriaceae other than *E. coli* (e.g., *Klebsiella, Enterobacter, Proteus,* and *Citrobacter*), *Pseudomonas aeruginosa,* enterococci and staphylococci, and *Candida.* Candiduria is especially common in individuals with prolonged urinary catheterization receiving broad-spectrum systemic antimicrobial agents. However, because of increased antibiotic use, there has been an increase in antibiotic-resistant microorganisms, particularly *P. aeruginosa* and *C. albicans,* two organisms frequently involved in device-associated nosocomial infections (Trautner & Darouiche, 2004).

A problem in hospitals and LTC facilities is infection with vancomycin-resistant *Enterococcus* (VRE) and methicillin-resistant staphylococcus aureus (MRSA). Residents in LTC facilities are believed to be especially at risk because of their exposure to patients transferred from acute care hospitals, where VRE and MRSA prevalence rates are high. If individuals with VRE are identified and isolated at the time of admission to the LTC facility, the chance of spreading VRE is low (Silverblatt et al., 2000). In addition to identification and isolation of infected individuals, staff should practice strict handwashing and Standard Precautions (single room, gowns and gloves, and additional cleansing) to prevent spread of the organism resulting from environmental contamination.

In patients with long-term indwelling urinary catheters, symptoms of catheter-related infection are often nonspecific. Symptoms of a UTI are caused by an inflammatory response of the epithelium of the urinary tract to invasion and colonization by bacteria (Gray, 2004b). Among catheterized individuals, clinical manifestations of UTI (pain, urgency, dysuria, fever, and leukocytosis) are uncommon even when bacteria or yeast is present, and are no more prevalent with positive urine culture results than with negative results (Tambyah & Maki, 2000). *Confusion or unexplained fever may be the only symptoms of catheter-related CAUTI in patients residing in nursing homes.* Similarly, diagnosing catheter-related infection in patients with spinal cord injury (SCI) may be especially challenging from history and physical examination because of frequent lack of localizing symptoms (Tambyah, 2004). Often, *the only symptom of catheter-related UTI in individuals with SCI is fever, diaphoresis, abdominal discomfort, or increased muscle spasticity* (Biering-Sørensen, Bagi, & Hoiby, 2001).

Catheter-Associated Biofilms   Once an indwelling urinary catheter is inserted, bacteria quickly develop into colonies known as biofilms (living layers) that adhere to the catheter surface and drainage bag (Pratt et al., 2007). A biofilm is a collection of microorganisms with altered phenotypes that colonize the surface of a medical device such as an indwelling urinary catheter (Talsma, 2007). Urine contains protein that adheres to and primes the catheter surface. Microorganisms bind to this protein layer and thus attach to the surface. Such bacteria are different from free-living planktonic bacteria (bacteria that float in urine). Urinary catheter biofilms may initially be composed of single organisms, but longer exposures inevitably lead to multiorganism biofilms. Bacteria in biofilms have considerable survival advantages over free-living microorganisms, being extremely resistant to antibiotic therapy. The link between biofilm and infection is that the biofilm provides a sustained reservoir for microorganisms that, after detachment, can infect the patient. These biofilms cause further problems if the bacteria (e.g., *P. mirabilis*) produce the enzyme urease (Trautner & Darouiche, 2003). The urine then becomes alkaline (increased pH), causing the production of ammonium ions, followed by crystallization of calcium and magnesium phosphate within the urine. These crystals are then incorporated into the biofilm, resulting in encrustation of the catheter over a period of time.

Several features of biofilms have important implications for the development of antimicrobial resistance in organisms growing within the biofilm. Because the presence of the biofilm inhibits antimicrobial activity, organisms within the biofilm cannot be eradicated by antimicrobial therapy alone. The urinary biofilm provides a protective environment for the microorganisms, which allows evasion of the activity of antimicrobial agents. The biofilm also allows for microbial attachment to catheter surfaces in a manner that does not allow for removal with gentle rinsing, such as irrigation (Donlan, 2001; Donlan & Costerton, 2002). Biofilms can begin to develop within the first 24 hours after catheter insertion. Biofilms have reportedly become so thick in some circumstances as to block a catheter lumen (Saint & Chenoweth, 2003). The presence of urinary catheter biofilms has important implications for antimicrobial resistance, diagnosis of UTIs, and prevention and treatment of CAUTIs.

Encrustations   Mineral deposition within the catheter biofilm causes encrustations, which are unique to biofilms formed on urinary catheters (Hukins, 2005). Encrustations are seen typically on the inner surface of the catheter and can build to block catheter flow completely. They can coat the balloon, making it hard to deflate. Once the balloon is deflated, they fall off into the bladder. Encrustation is generally associated with long-term catheterization, because it has a direct relationship with the duration of catheterization. Some patients are more prone to persistent catheter encrustation, and these patients are referred to as "blockers" as opposed to "nonblockers." As noted previously, an alkaline urinary pH is an important factor in causing catheter encrustation.

Urosepsis   Urosepsis can result from a UTI, leading to generalized sepsis, and death from severe UTIs has been reported. Mortality has been documented as more than 3 times higher in catheterized than in noncatheterized individuals.

Urethral Damage   Urethral damage occurs primarily in men because the catheter may interfere with drainage of seminal secretions. Urethral catheterization in men is associated with epididymitis, orchitis, scrotal abscess, prostatitis, and prostatic abscess. It can start at the time of insertion of the catheter but increases with long-term catheter use. Difficulty passing the catheter may mean that the catheter has encountered a urethral stricture, or has entered or created a false passage in the urethra, or that its passage is blocked by an obstructing prostate, bladder neck, or sphincter. The catheter may turn on itself and curl in the urethra. The following are common urethral complications:

1. Urethritis, or inflammation of the urethral meatus, is a major source of discomfort and contributes to a breakdown in tissue integrity. It may be due to frequent insertion of catheters or forceful catheterization against an obstruction. Urethritis may occur more frequently in patients who have latex catheters.

2. Erosion (tearing) of the urethra, primarily the urinary meatus, occurs in individuals who have had indwelling catheters for a long period of time (Figure 10.19). This erosion is usually secondary to catheter tension on the distal urethra at the meatus. The manner in which a catheter is secured should be alternated to prevent prolonged tension or pressure at an individual site (LeBlanc & Christensen, 2005).

3. Creation of a false passage can occur primarily in men with persisting urethral strictures. Men with enlargement of the prostate gland are most at risk.

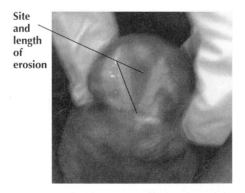

Figure 10.19.   Erosion caused by indwelling urinary catheter.

4. Urethral fistulas can develop in patients being managed long term with a urethral catheter. Such fistula formation most commonly develops in women between the bladder and the anterior vaginal wall. Many times the woman who has developed a fistula will complain of leakage and drainage from the vagina.

Other Complications   Other complications associated with indwelling catheter use include the following:

*   *Epididymitis* caused by urethral and bladder inflammation or by scrotal abscess seen in men.

*   *Hematuria* occurs in patients who have long-term catheters and is a possible sign of bladder cancer or kidney stones. Some bleeding may occur during catheter insertion, but, if the bleeding persists, urine cystology and a cystoscopy should be considered. A referral to a urologist may be indicated.

*   *Bladder stones* occur in at least 8% of patients with indwelling catheters and can form on the catheter or retention balloon (Moy & Wein, 2007). Therefore, patients with these catheters should be seen by a urologist annually. It is recommended that cystoscopy be performed to determine the environment within the bladder and the presence of stones or cancer.

*   *Bladder cancer* can occur in some patients with indwelling catheters for long periods of time (Delnay, 1999). This has been seen in SCI patients (West et al., 1999). Monitoring for bladder cancer through yearly cystoscopy and urine cytology is recommended.

*   *Pain and discomfort* can occur in addition to the morbidity and mortality caused by CAUTI. In a study at a Veterans Affairs (VA) Medical Center, 42% of catheterized patients surveyed reported that the indwelling catheter was uncomfortable, 48% complained that it was painful, and 61% noted that it restricted their activities of daily living (Saint et al., 1999). Additionally, 30% of survey respondents stated that the catheter's presence was embarrassing, and in unsolicited comments supplementing the structured questionnaires, two respondents noted that it "hurts like hell." Additionally, indwelling catheters can restrict activities and hinder rehabilitation in many individuals.

Types of Indwelling Catheters

Indwelling urinary catheters are soft, flexible tubes that have double lumens, one that allows for urine drainage by connection to a drainage bag and the other for inflation and deflation of the retention balloon (Figure 10.20). Once inflated, the balloon allows for retention of the catheter in the bladder.

Catheter Design   Catheters are fairly rigid structures. They drain the bladder, but block the urethra. The catheter should have a smooth surface with

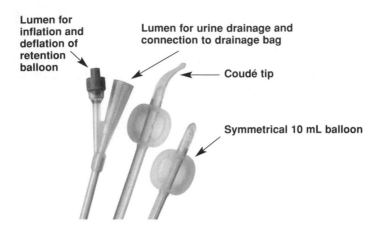

Lumen for inflation and deflation of retention balloon

Lumen for urine drainage and connection to drainage bag

Coudé tip

Symmetrical 10 mL balloon

Figure 10.20.   Indwelling silicone catheters with Coudé and straight tips. (Courtesy of Coloplast.)

two drainage eyes at the tip that allow for urine drainage. Drainage eyes are placed either laterally or opposed. Opposing drainage eyes generally facilitate better drainage. Catheter products have changed significantly in their composition, texture, and durability since the 1990s. The challenge is to produce a catheter that matches as closely as possible the normal physiological and mechanical characteristics of the voiding system (Kunin, 2006). This requires construction of a thin-walled, continuously lubricated, collapsible (conformable) catheter to protect the integrity of the urethra; a system to hold the catheter in place without a balloon; and a design to imitate the intermittent washing of the bladder with urine.

Catheter Tips   The most commonly used catheter is a straight-tipped catheter. A Coudé-tipped catheter, or Tiemann catheter, is angled upward at the tip to assist in negotiating the upward bend in the male urethra (Figure 10.20). This feature facilitates passage through the bladder neck in the presence of a slightly enlarged prostate gland (e.g., in benign prostatic hyperplasia). A whistle-tipped catheter is open at the end and allows drainage of large amounts of debris (e.g., blood clots).

Catheter Size and Length   Each catheter is sized by the outer circumference and according to a metric scale known as the French (Fr) gauge (range is 6–18 Fr), in which each French unit equals 0.33 mm in diameter. The golden rule is to use the smallest catheter size (termed *bore*), generally 14 to 16 Fr, that allows for adequate drainage. The use of large-size catheters (e.g., 18 Fr or larger) is not recommended because catheters with larger diameters can cause more erosion of the bladder neck and urethral mucosa, can cause stricture formation, and do not allow adequate drainage of periurethral gland secretions, causing a buildup of secretions that may lead to irritation and infection. Also, large catheters can cause pain and discomfort.

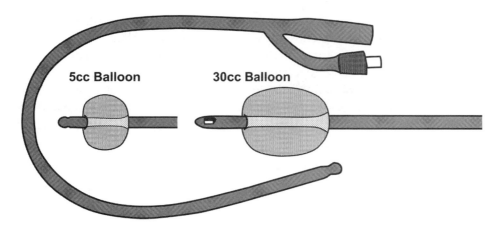

Figure 10.21.   Urine drainage with two different balloon sizes. (Courtesy of Robin Noel.)

Balloon Size   A retention balloon prevents the catheter from being expelled. The preferred balloon size may be labeled either 5 mL or 10 mL, and both are instilled with 10 mL of sterile water for inflation per manufacturer's instructions (see "Best Practices" for Indwelling Catheter Care later in the chapter). A fully inflated balloon allows the catheter tip to be located symmetrically (Figure 10.21). If a 5-mL balloon is inflated with more than 10 mL of water, irritation may occur unilaterally on the bladder wall from increased pressure of the balloon. Underfilling or overfilling may interfere with the correct positioning of the catheter tip, which may lead to irritation and trauma of the bladder wall. The catheterized bladder is in a collapsed state as a result of constant urine drainage. However, a 30-mL balloon will allow persistence of a small pool of undrained urine, so the bladder emptying is not complete. A balloon with a filled size greater than 10 mL, such as a 30-mL balloon, is not recommended because the 10-mL size keeps residual urine minimal, thus reducing the risk of infections and irritation. The use of a larger balloon size is mistakenly believed by many nurses to be a solution to catheter leakage or urine bypassing around the catheter. However, a large balloon increases the chance of contact between the balloon or catheter tip and the bladder wall, leading to bladder spasms that may cause urine to be forced out around the catheter. The 30-mL balloons are used primarily to facilitate traction on the prostate gland to stop bleeding in men after prostate surgery or to stop bleeding in women after pelvic surgery. Routine use of larger capacity balloons (30 mL) should be avoided for long-term use as they can lead to bladder neck and urethral erosion (Moy & Wein, 2007).

In men, the catheter should be passed initially to the bifurcation (the "Y" junction where the balloon arm and catheter meet) to ensure that the balloon will not be inflated in the urethra. On occasion, the balloon will fail to deflate (See Appendix Table 10.3).

Catheter Material   A wide range of catheter materials are available, and the material selected should be chosen by 1) how long the catheter will remain in place, 2) comfort, 3) presence of latex sensitivity, 4) ease of insertion and removal, and 5) ability to reduce the likelihood of complications such as urethral and bladder tissue damage, colonization of the catheter system by microorganisms, and encrustation (Newman, 2004). Catheter types (coated and uncoated) are reviewed in detail in Table 10.3 (Newman, 2007a). They include

- Silicone-coated latex catheters, which have a chemically bonded coating of silicone elastomer or Teflon that prevents urethral contact with the latex

- Teflon-coated catheters, which are thought to reduce the rate of absorption of water

- 100% silicone catheters, which are thin-walled, more rigid catheters with a larger diameter drainage lumen

- Hydrogel-coated latex catheters, which absorb water to produce a slippery outside surface

- Antimicrobial catheters (antibacterial, silver alloy)

Of note, several catheter materials have been found to lose water from an inflated balloon; 100% silicone catheters can lose as much as 50% of volume within 3 weeks. Prior to insertion, all indwelling catheters should be visually inspected for any imperfections or surface deterioration.

Problems with Latex Catheters   It is important for the clinician to be aware of the results of research on the use of certain types of indwelling catheters (Gray, 2006). There are reported increases in allergies and reactions in patients with long-term use of all urinary latex and rubber catheters. Patients who have asthma and other allergies are at increased risk for these allergies. Latex allergy can result in symptoms such as skin irritation, rashes, and blisters. Urethritis and urethral strictures can also result from latex allergies. Coatings such as silicone and polytetrafluoroethylene (PTFE) are used to coat latex catheters. Also, hydrogel coating, which remains intact when used, has demonstrated the ability to reduce the high level of cytotoxicity associated with latex catheters. However, coated latex catheters do not protect against an allergic reaction to the underlying latex because the coating wears off. Silicone- and hydrogel-coated catheters usually last longer than PTFE-coated catheters. If the person is latex sensitive, silicone catheters should be used.

Avoiding latex catheters may also decrease the incidence of encrustation. All-silicone (100%) catheters are biocompatible and are believed to have encrustation-resistant properties (see Figure 10.20). In a study of encrustation of different catheter materials, although all catheters became blocked, the all-silicone catheters took longer to become blocked than other types (Morris, Stickler, & Winters, 1997). However, this may be because all-silicone catheters have a slightly wider lumen than other coated catheters. They also may be more resistant to kinking when compared to latex-based products (Lawrence & Turner, 2005).

Bonded hydrogel-coated latex catheters may be longer lasting than silicone catheters because their hydrogel coating prevents bacterial adherence and reduces mucosal friction. Hydrogels or polymers coat the catheter, absorbing water to produce a slippery outside surface. This results in the formation of a thin film of water on the contacting surface, thus improving its smoothness and lubricity. These properties might act as potential barriers to bacterial infection and reduce the adhesion of both gram-positive and gram-negative bacteria to catheters (Ha & Cho, 2006).

Preventing Bacterial Colonization   In an attempt to prevent bacterial colonization, catheters have been coated with silver alloy or nitrofurazone, a nitrofurantoin-like drug (Johnson, Kuskowski, & Wilt, 2006). A systematic review of these catheters determined that bacteriuria can be decreased by their use in hospitalized patients (Johnson et al., 2006). Both nitrofurazone-coated and silver alloy–coated catheters seem to reduce the development of asymptomatic bacteriuria during short-term (<30 days) use. Despite their unit cost, there is a suggestion that these devices might be a cost-effective option if overall numbers of infections are significantly reduced through their use (Lee et al., 2004; Pratt et al., 2007).

Antibiotic-Coated Catheters   Antibiotic-coated catheters were found in a meta-analysis to prevent or delay bacteriuria in short-term-catheterized hospitalized patients (Johnson et al., 2006). A systematic review was inconclusive (Drekonja, Kuskowski, Wilt, & Johnson, 2008). The catheters were impregnated with an antibacterial agent that elutes from the catheter over a period of days after insertion (Figure 10.22). Two catheters impregnated with anti-infective solutions have been studied in randomized trials, one impregnated with the urinary antiseptic nitrofurazone and the other with a new broad-spectrum antimicrobial drug combination, minocycline and rifampin. Nitrofurazone is active

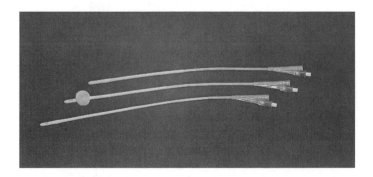

Figure 10.22.   RELEASE-NF nitrofurazone-coated silicone indwelling catheter. The coating is the color yellow. (Courtesy of Rochester Medical.)

against a broad range of gram-positive and gram-negative bacilli (Maki & Tambyah, 2001). Both catheters showed a significant reduction in bacterial CAUTIs; however, the studies were small, and the issue of selection of antimicrobial drug–resistant uropathogens was not satisfactorily resolved (Lee et al., 2004). The theoretical risk of developing antimicrobial resistance to minocycline, rifampin, or both (two agents occasionally used systemically) may limit the use of catheters coated with these antibiotics. Cost savings have yet to be demonstrated in a randomized trial with any of these devices and in any patient population.

Silver Alloy–Coated Catheters   Silver alloy–coated catheters are thought to cause less inflammation and have a bacteriostatic effect because they reduce microbacterial adherence and migration of bacteria to the bladder (Ahearn et al., 2000; Verleyen, De Ridder, Van Poppel, & Baert, 1999). Because they prevent bacterial adherence, these catheters also minimize biofilm formation through their release of silver ions that prevent bacteria from settling on the surface (Seymour, 2006). The use of a silver alloy–coated urinary catheter may reduce CAUTIs by 32%–69% if the catheter is in for a short time (< 30 days) (Brosnahan, Jull, & Tracy, 2004; Karchmer, Giannetta, Muto, Strain, & Farr, 2000; Lai & Fontecchio, 2002). However, other studies have found silver alloy–coated catheters ineffective in preventing CAUTIs (Srinivasan, Karchmer, Richards, Song, & Perl, 2006). It may be reasonable to consider short-term use of these catheters in individuals who are at highest risk for developing consequences from a UTI (Rupp et al., 2004). There appear to be few adverse effects, and microbial resistance to the active agent is unlikely. Each silver alloy–coated urinary catheter tray costs about $5.30 more than a standard, noncoated urinary catheter tray, and they provide both clinical and economic benefits in patients receiving indwelling catheterization for 2–10 days (Saint, 2001).

Catheter Changing Schedule

Usual medical practice is to change indwelling catheters every 3–4 weeks; however, this practice is based not on research, but on insurance-reimbursable allowances. Most experts believe that changing schedules should be arranged according to the user's needs. The catheter should be changed more often if obstruction occurs, if the person develops frequent infections, or if difficulty with removal of the catheter or deflation of the balloon occurs. To prevent the occurrence of catheter-related problems, clinicians should identify when problems occur and develop a changing schedule that helps to prevent their recurrence.

"BEST PRACTICES" FOR INDWELLING CATHETER CARE

Management of indwelling catheters varies according to the setting and the caregiver. Many nurses follow certain practices for catheter care and management, but there are few, if any, evidence-based guidelines (Fantl et al., 1996; Gray, 2004b; Pratt et al., 2007; Tenke et al., 2008). Tenke et al. (2008) reviewed the literature to determine guidelines on management of CAUTIs and found that written catheter care protocols are necessary but lacking. Clinicians should routinely monitor the use of indwelling catheters, suggest removal when appropriate, evaluate risk factors, determine alternatives to continuing catheterization, assist in selection of type of catheter and accessory equipment, and educate individuals and their caregivers about catheter care. The objectives of effective catheter care are to

- Prevent or minimize the complications related to catheterization

- Promote the independence, comfort, and dignity of the person

- Ensure that individuals and their caregivers are knowledgeable about and proficient in the management of long-term indwelling catheters

Problems arising from long-term indwelling catheters are described in Appendix Table 10.3 and include

- Unprescribed (inadvertent) dislodgment

- Leakage

- Obstruction or encrustation

- Catheter or balloon malfunction

- Pain and urethral discomfort

The available catheter management strategies have been developed from research conducted in the 1970s and 1980s (Fantl et al., 1996) and can prevent complications and nursing care problems (Newman, 2004). Some of the key elements to consider include 1) catheter insertion procedures, 2) care of the drainage bag, 3) maintaining catheter patency, 4) perineal care, 5) catheter irrigation, 6) fluid and hydration, 7) handwashing and glove use, and 8) patient and nursing staff education (Senese, Hendricks, Morrison, & Harris, 2006). In general, the use of oral antibiotics and urinary acidifying agents, antimicrobial bladder irrigations, antimicrobial drainage bag solutions, and topical meatal antiseptics has been studied, and it has been shown that bacteriuria and UTI can be suppressed temporarily, but resistant flora eventually appear. Best practices for catheter management follow.

Documentation of Catheter Use Is Important. Because the insertion of an indwelling catheter carries many risks for the individual, advice from best practice emphasizes the importance of documenting all procedures involving the catheter or drainage system in the person's records and providing the person with adequate information. Poor documentation will affect communication between members of the multidisciplinary team in relation to factors such as catheter used, latex allergy history, and possible complications with previous catheters. Data that must be recorded in relation to catheterization include

---

Box 10.4   Best Practices for Indwelling Catheter Care

- Document in the patient's medical record all procedures involving the catheter or drainage system.

- Remove catheter as soon as possible to reduce the risk of CAUTIs.

- Insert catheter using an aseptic technique.

- Use the smallest size catheter possible.

- Cleanse the catheter insertion site daily with soap and water or with a perineal cleanser. Use of an antiseptic is unnecessary.

- Empty the urine in the drainage bag at least every 4–6 hours to avoid migration of bacteria up the internal and external lumen of the catheter and undue tension on the catheter.

- Adequately secure and anchor the catheter to prevent urethral and bladder neck tension.

- Ensure that urine drainage is unobstructed.

- Health care workers and clinicians in institutions should observe their facility's protocols for care of catheters and drainage bags.

- Avoid routine or arbitrary catheter changing schedules in the absence of infection.

- Maintain a uniform and adequate daily fluid intake to continuously flush the urinary drainage system.

- Maintain a closed urinary drainage system to prevent introduction of bacteria into the urinary tract.

- Clamping the catheter prior to removal is unnecessary.

- Routine catheter and bladder irrigations and/or instillations are not recommended.

- Avoid routine urine cultures in the absence of infection.

- Avoid inappropriate use of antibiotics and antimicrobials.

- Maintain acidification of urine.

- Patients and caregivers should be educated about their role in preventing CAUTIs.

- Acute and long-term care staff should be educated through quality improvement programs about the selection, insertion, and management of indwelling catheters to reduce UTI incidence.

- Patients with indwelling urinary catheters should be reevaluated periodically to determine whether an alternative method of bladder drainage can be used instead.

- Patients should undergo bladder training after catheter removal to successfully regain bladder function.

---

medical necessity for use; catheter type material and size, balloon size, batch number, expiration date, and date of insertion; reason for catheterization; name of person inserting the catheter; and any problems with insertion. Core care plans and care pathways in acute and long-term care are important components to documentation (see Care Plan #8 on the companion CD).

Remove Catheter as Soon as Possible.   If a urinary catheter is necessary, it should be removed as soon as possible. Given that the rate of infection is closely related to the duration of catheterization, the high frequency of inappropriate catheterization, and the finding that physicians are often unaware of catheter presence, it is possible that an automatic urinary catheter "stop order" or reminder would be useful. Such an innovative system-wide administrative intervention, similar to an antibiotic stop order, would ideally remind physicians that a patient has an indwelling catheter, which in turn might help reduce inappropriate catheterization (Topal et al., 2005). A before-and-after crossover study conducted at a VA Medical Center using computerized order entry found that a computerized reminder system for urinary catheters may be beneficial (Cornia et al., 2003). Instituting a computerized urinary catheter order and a computer-generated stop order 72 hours after insertion can reduce the duration of catheterization by about one third (3 days) (Huang et al., 2004). Thus a computerized reminder system might reduce CAUTI by reminding the physician and nurse to reassess the patient as to continuing need.

Ensure an Aseptic Catheter Insertion Procedure.   The catheter should always be inserted using an aseptic (sterile) procedure. In acute and long-term care, sterility is usually not a problem because additional skilled staff are available to assist the nurse doing the catheterization with positioning the person and maintaining the sterile field. However, in the home care environment, where sometimes the nurse is the only other individual in the home, it may be difficult to maintain sterility, especially in women, because of inadequate lighting and positioning. In women, it is important to clearly see the perineum and urinary meatus, so the woman should lie supine with her legs bent at the knees and separated. If the catheter erroneously enters the vagina, the clinician should not remove and reuse it but leave it in the vagina as a marker and continue catheterization with a new sterile catheter. The nurse should avoid manipulation of the catheter once inserted. Once the catheter enters the bladder, a good flow of urine confirms its location and the balloon can be inflated. If there is no urine return, it is because either there is no urine in the bladder or (the most common reason) the lubricating jelly is occluding the catheter drainage eyes. The clinician may need to instill sterile water aseptically to open these eyes. Hands should be washed immediately before and after manipulating any part of the catheter system (e.g., when changing or emptying a drainage bag). The person who is performing any catheter-related task should wear disposable gloves.

Use a Small-Sized Catheter.   A small-sized (small-bore) catheter is preferred because it is likely to be better tolerated, cause less urethral irritation, and decrease occlusion of the periurethral glands. Larger catheters have been found to be associated with more catheter-related problems, in particular leakage and blockage (Toughill, 2005). If there is concern about switching from a larger to a smaller size catheter (e.g., decreasing from 18 Fr to 14 Fr), the catheter can be decreased one size at each catheter change.

Use Sterile Water for Balloon Inflation.   Manufacturers' recommendations are for the use of sterile water for inflating the catheter. Saline can crystallize and make the balloon difficult to remove, and air can allow the catheter to "float" in the bladder, preventing adequate drainage. A 10-mL filled balloon should always be used, and 10 mL of sterile water should be instilled in a 5-mL or 10 mL balloon for symmetrical inflation (see Figure 10.21). Asymmetrical inflation can cause bladder overactivity leading to catheter leakage, and can cause irritation and incomplete bladder drainage. Smaller gauge catheters with a 10-mL balloon minimize urethral trauma, mucosal irritation, and residual urine in the bladder, all factors that predispose to CAUTI. However, in adults who have recently undergone urological or gynecological surgery, larger gauge catheters and balloons (e.g., 20–24 Fr; 30 mL balloon) may be indicated to allow for the passage of blood clots. Balloon underinflation can cause catheter expulsion (falling out), occlusion of the drainage eyes, bladder neck irritation, and inadequate urine drainage.

Daily Meatal Care with an Antiseptic Is Not Necessary.   Routine or daily perianal and meatal care should exclude the use of antiseptics (e.g., povidone-iodine [Betadine] solution or ointment) or antimicrobial creams or ointments (Siroky, 2002). Rather, the catheter insertion (e.g., suprapubic) and meatal site should be cleaned with soap and water or a perineal cleanser, avoiding frequent and vigorous cleansing of the area (Pratt et al., 2007). If possible, a patient can shower to maintain meatal hygiene. Uncircumcised men should be advised to clean underneath the foreskin daily to remove smegma, which may harbor bacteria. Routine daily bathing and showering are generally all that is needed. Women should be instructed in correct perineal cleaning after bowel movements. Talcum powder should be avoided because it can become clogged around the catheter.

Frequent Drainage Bag Emptying Is Recommended.   To avoid migration of bacteria up the internal and external lumen of the catheter and to prevent undue tension on the catheter from a "heavy" drainage bag, the urine in the drainage bag should be emptied at least every 4–6 hours. To avoid cross-contamination, catheter bags from a number of patients should not be emptied into one container, nor should the same pair of gloves be used when emptying multiple drainage bags. When attaching the drainage bag to a bed or chair, the bag must be kept off the floor and the outlet tube should not be dragged. Cleaning the drainage port with an isopropyl alcohol swab before opening and after closing may reduce bacteria burden. Selecting a bag that prevents migration of bacteria through the port (anti-reflux chamber) is preferable.

Catheter Securement Is Essential.   Although nurses agree that catheter securement is important, it is not consistently part of current catheter care practice in all settings (Siegel, 2006). Anchoring and stabilizing the catheter will prevent urethral and bladder neck tension. Unanchored or unsecured catheters can lead to urethral and bladder neck erosion, as well as lineal pressure ulcers on the buttocks and thighs (Gray, Newman, Einhorn, & Reid Czarapata, 2006; Newman, 2007a; Siegel, 2006). Unsecured catheters can be stepped on and dislodged, especially when transferring a patient. Securement of the catheter also promotes unobstructed urine flow (Hanchett, 2002). The catheter should follow the natural curve of the urethra. The catheter should be anchored on the upper thigh in women and ideally to the abdomen in men. Kinks or loops in the catheter and tubing that might decrease or impede the flow of urine should be avoided. The site of attachment should be rotated every few days. Suprapubic catheters should be secured firmly to the anterior abdominal wall to prevent traction on the catheter or balloon.

The optimal type of securement or anchoring device has never been adequately studied, so nurses use all options (Newman, 2007a). The recommended and most widely used type of securement device appears to be a wide, stretchable nonadhesive cloth band that is secured to the upper thigh or abdomen with a soft Velcro closure strap (Figure 10.23). The band is latex free and has a hypoallergenic backing. This securement device can be used both around the thigh (leg band) and the abdomen (waist band). The Belly Bag (described later in this chapter) is secured to the abdomen. Users seem to prefer the nonadhesive products because they are less irritating than tape, are simple to apply, and are less expensive because they can be used for a longer period of time. Many are washable so they can be reused. In addition, these catheter straps are now more comfortable because they are wider and made of more comfortable materials. They do not cause skin irritation. They are made from soft, breathable material, so there is little to no risk of venous compression or skin occlusion (Gray et al., 2006). There are several reusable leg anchors to choose from (e.g., Bard Catheter Leg Strap; Catheter Tube Holder Strap, Posey Company; Dale Anchor Strap).

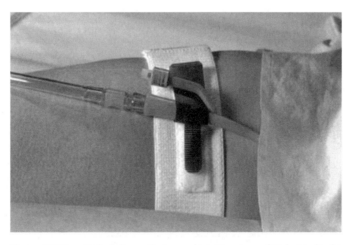

Figure 10.23.   Dale Foley catheter anchor. (Courtesy of Dale Medical.)

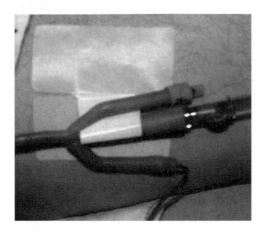

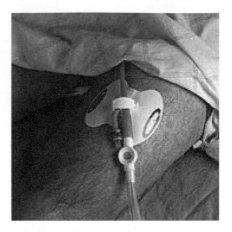

Figure 10.24.   Cath-Secure catheter anchor. (Courtesy of M.C. Johnson Co., Inc.)

Figure 10.25.   StatLock catheter anchor. (Courtesy of Venetec International.)

A commonly used adhesive catheter anchor (Figure 10.24) locks the catheter in place using wrap-around tabs that anchor it tightly to the tape using a press-on hook-and-loop fastening system so that it can be adjusted to obtain the needed tightness. The base of the anchor is a hypoallergenic tape. Another adhesive anchor was designed with the addition of a customized locking device positioned on top of an adhesive foam pad (Figure 10.25). The manufacturer describes this as a "swivel clamp" that prevents kinking and provides catheter fixation. It is recommended that the device be placed above the point of the bifurcation, proximal to the balloon inflation port.

Urine Drainage Must Be Ensured.   The collection tubing and bag should always remain below the level of the individual's bladder, but the drainage tubing should always be above the level of the collection bag. It is also recommended that urinary drainage bags be hung on an appropriate stand that prevents contact with the floor.

Additional Practices Are Necessary for Care of Catheters and Drainage Bags in Institutions.   Health care workers should observe protocols on hand hygiene and the need to use disposable gloves between catheterized patients (Tenke et al., 2008). The clinician should separate and label (name, type of excrement) graduated containers for each patient as well as each patient's drainage bag because bacteria may be transmitted by sequentially touching the emptying spouts against the same contaminated collection container. The emptying port or tap on the drainage bag should not be allowed to touch the sides of the container when emptying the bag. With multiple drainage devices for one person, drainage devices should be separated by being kept on opposite sides of the bed. In semiprivate rooms, multiple drainage devices should be kept on opposite sides of the room. If possible, catheterized patients should not share the same room to avoid transmission of bacteria (Drinka,

Stemper, Gauerke, Millerm, & Reed, 2003). If feasible, separating catheterized individuals geographically on a care unit may reduce the risk of cross-infection with multidrug-resistant nosocomial organisms such as *Serratia, Klebsiella, Pseudomonas,* and *Enterobacter.*

Routine or Arbitrary Catheter Changing Schedules Should Be Avoided. In the absence of an infection, there is no set time for changing a catheter (Gray, 2004b; Wong & Hooton, 1981). Current practice for changing catheters has been to change them every 3–4 weeks (Emr & Ryan, 2004). However, catheters should be changed according to the individual's usual pattern of catheter care and evaluation of associated catheter problems and complications rather than waiting until infection or encrustations occur. If an infection occurs frequently or obstruction is common, the catheter should be changed more often (Tenke et al., 2008). The clinician should keep a record of when catheter-related problems occur so that a proactive changing schedule can be determined. How quickly a catheter "blocks" or obstructs will determine an average catheter life span. Routine catheter changes should then be planned more often than this, whether that means changing the catheter every 4 weeks or every 4 days. In individuals who are free of catheter-related complications and have long-term catheters, changes every 3–4 weeks seem reasonable, occasionally increasing to 4–6 weeks.

Adequate Fluid Intake Is Necessary. Maintaining a uniform and adequate daily fluid intake (30 mL/kg of body weight per day) to continuously flush the system is recommended (Gray et al., 2006). The flushing action of large quantities of dilute urine will reduce the likelihood of bacteria ascending the bag and catheter. Dilute urine may also reduce the concentration of substances that precipitate the development of encrustations that lead to catheter blockage. Forcing fluids is especially difficult in older patients because aging causes a loss in the sense of thirst, so they do not know when they should be drinking. Foods that have a high liquid content may be substituted (e.g., Jell-O, popsicles, fruit, soups).

Leave the Closed System Alone! A continuously closed urinary drainage system provides a barrier to bacterial introduction into the urinary tract. Maintaining a closed system is central to the prevention of CAUTI, and should include all points of contamination, including the drain spout. The risk of infection reduces from 97% with an open system to 8%–15% when a sterile closed system is employed. Repeated disconnections of the closed system, such as unnecessary emptying of the urinary drainage bag or taking repeated urine samples, will increase the risk of CAUTI and should be avoided. Hands must be decontaminated and clean, nonsterile gloves worn before manipulation. Although the maintenance of a closed system is feasible when used short term, it may not be when the catheter is used long term, especially in a person receiving home care. The system is often disconnected to change from an overnight drainage bag to a leg bag. Staff can cause transmission of bacteria by using the same container for emptying drainage bags from multiple individuals.

Clamping the Catheter Before Removal Is Not Necessary.   Nurses have clamped catheters on patients with short-term catheters because it was believed that clamping before removal stimulates normal bladder filling and emptying and can increase the time to first void once removed. However, there is absolutely no evidence to support this practice (Fernandez & Griffiths, 2005).

Do Not Routinely Irrigate Catheter Systems.   Catheter or bladder irrigations or "washouts" of any type of solution (e.g., saline, antimicrobials, antibiotics, antiseptics) are not recommended. In the past, standard practice included catheter irrigation to "wash out" the bacteria and to dissolve blockages from encrustations; however, it has been shown that the use of such irrigation is ineffective because more organisms will gain entry to the irrigated catheters through disconnection of the system. Bladder irrigation not only is ineffective in treating UTI, but may also further disrupt the already damaged bladder epithelium, leading to further infection. Bladder irrigation with antimicrobial drug solutions not only has shown no benefit for prevention but has been associated with an increased incidence of CAUTIs caused by microorganisms resistant to the drugs in the irrigating solution.

Avoid Routine Urine Cultures.   In the absence of symptoms of an infection, routine cultures are not good practice. All individuals with long-term catheters will probably have bacteria in the bladder, and the organisms change frequently, about once or twice per month. Urine cultures should only be obtained when there is suspected clinical sepsis based on objective signs or symptoms. If a symptomatic infection does occur, the catheter should be changed *before* obtaining a specimen for cultures and prior to beginning antibiotic therapy (Raz, Schiller, & Nicolle, 2000; Simpson & Clark, 2005). This is especially important if the catheter has been in place for more than 7 days (Tenke et al., 2008). A sample of the urine that drains through the new system should be obtained because urine in the old system has organisms that may not reflect bladder urine organisms but rather "catheter" urine organisms (Shah, Cannon, Sullivan, Nemchausky, & Pachucki, 2005). The urine specimen is taken by clamping the tubing distal to the collection port for a short time to allow urine to accumulate. To maintain integrity of the sterile closed system, urine samples should be collected aseptically using a syringe to withdraw urine from the sampling port. When obtaining a urine specimen, the sampling port should be wiped with disinfectant (e.g., alcohol) before and after sampling.

Avoid Antibiotic Prophylaxis.   Bacterial colonization of the bladder and urethra (bacteriuria) is inevitable; therefore, repeated use of antibiotics and antimicrobials to prevent symptomatic UTI should be avoided (Niel-Weise & Van Den Broek, 2005). Inappropriate and excessive use of antimicrobial drugs in catheterized individuals leads to the selection of antibiotic-resistant microorganisms and accounts for nosocomial outbreaks of infection with multidrug-resistant strains. Furthermore, frequent courses of antibiotics subject catheterized individuals to possible adverse drug effects and suprainfections, such as *Clostridium difficile* colitis. The rationales for this recommendation include the following: 1) the risk of complications from asymptomatic bacteriuria is low, 2) treatment does not prevent bacteriuria from recurring, 3) treatment may lead to the presence of antimicrobial-resistant bacteria that are more challenging to treat, 4) antibiotics are costly, and 5) there are potential adverse effects associated with antibiotics. The clinician should consider treating bacteriuria if the person has an abnormal urinary tract, or will soon undergo genitourinary tract manipulation or instrumentation.

Acidification of the Urine Is Often Recommended.   In patients with repeated CAUTI and frequent biofilm formations, maintaining an acidic environment in the urine may prevent recurrence because acid urine may prevent the growth of bacteria (Morris & Stickler, 2001). The urine pH should be checked; if the pH is greater than 5, the clinician should consider acidification of urine by having the person take 1 g of ascorbic acid daily. Studies have indicated that cranberry juice (300 mL/day) may help prevent UTIs through its capacity to interfere with bacterial adherence rather than any pH-lowering tendencies. Tannins contained in cranberries interact with the tiny, hairlike protrusions on *E. coli* bacteria (the most common cause of UTIs), preventing the bacteria from adhering to the mucosal surface of the bladder. The bacteria lose their stickiness and, instead of adhering or sticking to the cells of the bladder and causing infection, get washed away in urine. Cranberry tablets (300–400 mg twice daily) may have the same benefit without calories. In a recent review, it was found that ingestion of cranberry juice or dietary supplement capsules may decrease the risk for UTI in patients in long-term and community settings, and that use of these products should be considered by clinicians and choice of the product (juice or capsules) should be individualized (Gray, 2004b).

Urine acidification also can be promoted with the use of ascorbic acid (1,000 mg daily). Another option is the combination of the oral anti-infective agent methenamine hippurate (Hiprex) with vitamin C (ascorbic acid) 1–2 g/day, which supports an acidic environment. Urine acidification occurs as a result of increased hippuric acid excretion. Hippuric acid excretion can inhibit the adherence of gram-negative and gram-positive bacteria (especially *E. coli*) to uroepithelial cells. Water does not reduce this adhesion.

Education About Catheter Care Is Essential.   Patients and their caregivers should be educated about their role in preventing CAUTIs. Research has shown that the majority of patients knew nothing about catheters before actually using one themselves, and only 43% of users stated that they received initial advice about how to care for the catheter (Roe, 1990). An educational program has been shown to reduce the frequency and severity of UTIs in persons with spinal cord injury (Cardenas, Hoffman, Kelly, & Mayo, 2004). Those patients who have catheters and their caregivers should be informed about the catheter's location, use, and subsequent management. Educating new and established catheter users about their catheter will improve their ability to cope with catheter use. The patient education tools "Care and Use of an Indwelling (Foley) Urinary Catheter" and "How to Care for Your Catheter Drainage Bag" (on the companion CD) provide information on emptying, changing, and managing the entire system. Saint et al. (2000) assessed the competency of doctors in catheterization and found considerable ignorance of practical and theoretical aspects, suggesting that doctors were inadequately taught this procedure. It has been identified in previous research that education of staff on the proper technique of insertion and care for urinary catheters is essential in improving patient care (Dumigan, Kohan, Reed, Jekel, & Fikrig, 1998).

Quality Improvement Programs for Hospital and LTC Staff Are Recommended. Education of staff concerning the selection, insertion, and management of indwelling catheters may reduce UTI incidence (Newman, 2005). The high rate of CAUTIs seen in nursing home residents has been attributed, in part, to the low level of infection control awareness and lack of knowledge of paraprofessional staff caring for the catheters. In acute care hospitals, CAUTIs have been reduced when protocols are developed that allow nurses to remove indwelling catheters without a medical order as soon as they are no longer medically necessary (Dumigan et al., 1998). This has become part of the protocol for catheter removal in the acute care hospital where the authors are employed (Hospital of the University of Pennsylvania).

Alternatives to Indwelling Urethral Catheters

Patients with indwelling catheters must be reevaluated periodically to determine whether a timed voiding trial or bladder retraining program may be effective in eliminating the need for the indwelling catheter. Many urologists recommend that suprapubic catheters be used in patients, especially men, who require chronic, long-term bladder drainage and for whom no other alternative therapy is possible. Intermittent catheterization is the safest bladder management method in terms of urological complications and should always be considered before the use of a urethral or suprapubic catheter (Weld & Dmochowski, 2000).

Bladder Retraining After Catheter Removal

Patients can successfully regain bladder function and undergo bladder training following indwelling catheter use (Newman, 2004). However, it may take as long as 6 weeks after catheter removal to determine the success of a bladder training program. Prior to catheter removal, a thorough genitourinary history and examination must be obtained (see Chapter 6). The presence of medical conditions that may precipitate urinary retention must be ascertained prior to catheter removal. The catheter removal plan should be discussed with the person's physician to determine if there are contraindications to the catheter's removal. One of the most important assessments is the person's motivation to regain bladder function. Also, caregiver involvement and agreement are imperative because many caregivers feel the person's care is easier to manage with a catheter than without. The caregiver should be informed of the benefits of catheter removal. Once the catheter is removed, the person is no longer restricted by the indwelling catheter, and is able to increase mobility and could become more independent and productive. Removing an indwelling catheter requires persistent nursing evaluation and intervention.

The following is a step-by-step approach to catheter removal:

Step 1: Patients do not need to be treated with antibiotics at the time of catheter removal. If persistent catheter-acquired bacteriuria continues 48 hours after removal, antibiotic treatment may be considered (Nicole et al., 2005). Some believe that an alpha blocker (e.g., alfuzosin or tamsulosin) increases the chances of voiding after catheter removal, especially in men. This should be initiated, if utilized, several days before catheter removal.

Step 2: Remove the catheter at a time that permits accurate recording of urine output and allows for postvoiding recatheterization if necessary. Removal of the indwelling catheter after nonurological surgery before midnight may be beneficial (Tenke et al., 2008). Clamping the catheter before removal is not necessary and can be dangerous. Clamping routines have never been shown to be helpful.

Step 3: Place the person on a timed voiding schedule or on habit training. Usually the individual is instructed to void at 2-hour intervals except during the night. The person should always void on awakening and before going to bed (see Chapter 8). If the person is uncomfortable and unable to void despite ensured privacy, maneuvers can be performed to encourage voiding, such as running water, tapping the suprapubic area, or stroking the inner thigh (see Chapter 7).

Step 4: Monitor bowel function. Fecal impaction can cause compression of the urethra and inhibition of the micturition reflex. A bowel regimen should be implemented if necessary.

Step 5: Have the person/staff/caregiver monitor the voiding pattern. Keeping a record that notes frequency, time, and amount of continent voids, as well as incontinence episodes, allows the nurse to ascertain the success of the program and identifies areas that may require further instruction. The fluid intake pattern should be monitored as well. For the first few days after catheter removal, the person should be monitored for urinary retention by checking residual urine volumes using a portable ultrasound (see Chapters 6 and 8). In patients who have a history of urinary retention, it may take days or weeks for the bladder to regain normal function. Recommendations vary, but it may be necessary to reinsert the catheter if the postvoid residual (PVR) exceeds 300–400 mL on two consecutive measurements or if the person is unable to void. If the PVR is 200 mL, the nurse should watch for delayed retention and evaluate further. If PVRs remain elevated, the person should have a urological consultation before the indwelling catheter is reinserted.

Step 6: Once the person is able to maintain a 2-hour voiding schedule, encourage him or her to delay voiding as long as possible. Bladder training and urge suppression techniques can be helpful. In addition, teaching the patient exercises to strengthen the pelvic floor muscles can decrease UI episodes (see Chapter 8).

Suprapubic Catheterization

Suprapubic catheterization typically involves the percutaneous placement of a standard urinary catheter directly into the bladder (Saint, 2001). The procedure is usually performed by a urologist, is generally performed in the operating room, and is considered minor surgery. The catheter is introduced into the bladder via an incision through the anterior abdominal wall into the bladder to permit drainage. The incision is usually placed 2 cm above the pubic bone (suprapubic) (Figure 10.26). Suprapubic catheterization has been used mainly postoperatively in patients who have undergone urological or gynecological procedures. Suprapubic catheterization is a technique used also in patients with urinary retention who have urethral damage from long-term urethral catheterization. Abrams et al. (2008) recommend that SCI patients who require continued bladder management with an indwelling urethral catheter should be switched to a suprapubic as soon as possible. Currently, it is unknown what proportion of patients who require indwelling urinary catheters receive suprapubic catheters, but their use is becoming more common. Scant long-term data are available on their use, and research is still not available that demonstrates the advantages of suprapubic compared with urethral catheters (Tenke et al., 2008). An advantage is that a suprapubic catheter does not interfere with sexual activity, as does a urethral catheter.

A suprapubic catheter may be preferable to an indwelling urethral catheter in patients who require chronic bladder drainage and for whom no other alternative therapy is possible. This type of catheter is more convenient for the patient and the caregiver. In addition, it decreases the risk of contamination with organisms from fecal material, decreases the risk of infection on a short-term basis, eliminates damage to the urethra, is more comfortable for individuals with limited mobility or who use a wheelchair, and is less cumbersome to the sexually active person. The anterior abdominal wall possesses a lower microbial load (less bacterial colonization) than the periurethal area and has a lower risk of infection (Sedor & Mulholland, 1999). In men who require long-term catheterization, suprapubic catheterization may also reduce the risk of local genitourinary complications such as meatal erosion, prostatitis, and epididymitis (Sheriff et al., 1998). Suprapubic catheters may be more

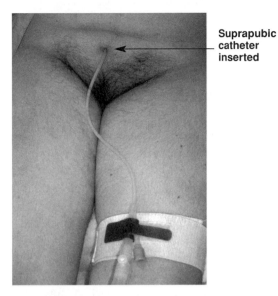

Suprapubic catheter inserted

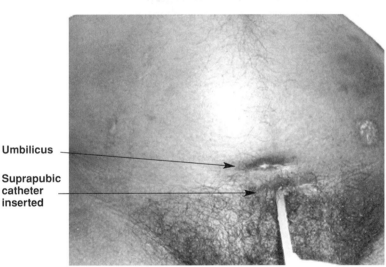

Umbilicus

Suprapubic catheter inserted

Figure 10.26. Suprapubic catheter in place.

comfortable for women using wheelchairs who find sitting on a urethral catheter uncomfortable.

Swelling at the site of insertion, bleeding, and bowel injury can occur at the time of inserting the catheter; however, these incidents are rare. Although anatomic complications such as urethral erosion and fistula formation may be fewer with suprapubic catheters, potential problems include uncontrolled urine leakage, skin erosion, hematoma, and problems with catheter reinsertion. The primary problem associated with suprapubic catheter use involves mechanical complications associated with insertion, most commonly catheter dislodgment or obstruction, and failed introduction. Overall, suprapubic catheters have a higher rate of satisfaction than indwelling urethral catheters once a tract has been established.

Care and Changing of the Suprapubic Catheter

Research is lacking in the area of long-term management and/or care of suprapubic catheters because the medical literature has only documented postsurgical, short-term use. Like urethral catheters, suprapubic catheters will have problems such as catheter leakage and blockage. In addition, difficulties exist with long-term medical and nursing management of suprapubic catheterization because of lack of knowledge and expertise on the part of health care clinicians and because of the inability of the homebound person to access medical care quickly if a problem arises.

Prevention of complications and catheter management are similar to those with indwelling urethral catheters. The safe insertion of suprapubic urinary catheters depends on trained personnel. A new suprapubic tract usually takes between 10 days and 4 weeks to become established (McMahon-Parkes, 1998). After that, the catheter should be changed. These catheters need to be changed, just like an indwelling catheter, ideally at least every 4 weeks. Evidence is not available about the frequency of catheter change and the best size of catheter to use. Some experts recommend the use of a 22–24 Fr catheter for suprapubic drainage (Linsenmeyer et al., 2006). We generally recommend a 20–22 Fr, and for the first two changes after the initial procedure, we use a guidewire to insert the catheter.

The following are some guidelines for changing a suprapubic catheter (Robinson, 2005):

- Place the person in bed and remove the cystostomy dressing (if present).

- Cleanse the abdomen around the cystostomy site with sterile water. Cleanse the cystostomy with vinegar and water to remove crusting and discharge, if necessary.

- Avoid use of an anesthetic gel (e.g., lidocaine) because absorption of the gel is likely if bleeding occurs following catheter removal.

- Assess skin surface around the cystostomy site for the presence of exudates, redness, or inflammation. If suspicious of any infection, culture the exudate.

- Instill 100 mL of sterile water through the catheter before removal to inflate the bladder and allow for easier insertion of the new catheter.

- Deflate the catheter balloon and remove the catheter. The clinician may encounter difficulty when withdrawing the catheter because it may get stuck. This may be caused by either a "cuff" that forms around the deflated balloon, making it difficult to withdraw, or spasm of the bladder. The cuff phenomenon may occur more often with 100% silicone catheters. Gently rotate the catheter and remove in an upward direction. A little force may be required for removal. Note the length of the catheter inserted. Use a guidewire-assisted catheter exchange to replace a malfunctioning catheter, or to exchange an existing catheter, only if there is no evidence of infection at the catheter site and no proven catheter-related bloodstream infection.

- Quickly cleanse the cystostomy site with sterile cotton balls and antiseptic from a sterile catheter tray.

- Insert the new catheter immediately after removal of the old catheter because the passage can begin to close within 10 minutes if insertion of a new catheter is delayed. If necessary, gentle pressure may be used. Insert the catheter gently downward toward the pelvic floor until urine flows. Inflate the balloon with sterile water.

- Attach the catheter to its closed drainage tubing and system, and anchor the catheter by securing the tubing to the lateral abdominal wall with tape. No dressing is needed if the cystostomy area is clean and dry, but some patients may feel more secure with a dressing.

- Teach the person, caregiver, or both to wash the skin area around the catheter with soap and water daily and to keep the area dry.

- Avoid the use of powder or creams around the catheter. The person can shower with this catheter in place and should not disconnect the catheter when showering.

- If the skin around the catheter gets red, swells, or opens, the person should contact the physician or nurse because this may be caused by an infection.

External Catheter Collection Systems

External catheter collection systems (ECCS) are condom-type sheaths that are placed over the penis for urine collection. External catheters are referred to as condom catheters, "Texas" catheters, penile sheaths, or external male catheters. These catheters are made from latex rubber, PVC, or silicone material. The catheters are secured to the penile shaft by a double-sided adhesive or a latex or foam strap that encircles the penis. If correctly fitted, urine should not contaminate the skin. They are connected to a urinary drainage bag by a collection tube. This system is suitable for men with moderate to severe UI and may also be used for men with urgency or frequency in circumstances in which it would be difficult to make frequent trips to restrooms. Disposable ECCS should stay in place for 24 hours, but some last up to 48 hours. Reusable ECCS should be removed every 24 hours, washed, and reapplied after cleaning the penis and allowing it to dry. Usually 35 external catheters per month are covered by most insurers. Specialty systems need documentation for medical necessity.

ECCS are an option for any man with uncontrollable UI who does not have overflow UI or a significant amount of infected residual urine. When comparing an external catheter to an indwelling catheter, the advantages include no urethral interference, no chance of urethral stricture, less incidence of bacteriuria, and less pain. However, there are few published studies comparing currently available external catheters; those studies that are available have been performed on the disposable products (Fader, Pettersson, et al., 2001). There is a need to compare the effect of different systems on the penile shaft as well as ease of use, user comfort, and improvement in catheter adherence (Newman et al., 2004). Conflicting results of the few available studies have left the role of ECCS in hospitalized patients or LTC residents unclear (Saint et al., 2006). Men at one VA Medical Center found the condom catheter more comfortable, less painful, and less restrictive of their activities. The only complaint was of urinary leakage (Saint et al., 1999). This study also indicated that nurses preferred these catheters to indwelling catheters. Saint et al. (2006) conducted a randomized, controlled trial comparing indwelling catheters with condom catheters in male inpatients. Men with ECCS had a lower incidence of bacteriuria, symptomatic UTI, or death. This protective effect was seen primarily in men who did not have dementia. An important secondary finding was that men reported that an external urinary collection device was more comfortable and less painful than an indwelling catheter.

A recent Cochrane systematic review found that no conclusions could be drawn from existing randomized or quasi-randomized controlled trials regarding when to use various types of catheters in managing individuals with a neurogenic bladder (Jamison, Maguire, & McCann, 2004). Pemberton et al. (2006) compared commonly used external catheters and found that ease of use and application with gloves were important criteria. ECCS may be associated with a lower risk of bacteriuria than indwelling catheters (Tenke et al., 2008); however, the proper role of condom catheters in hospitalized men remains unclear because many of the data are derived from men in extended care and skilled nursing facilities (Ouslander, Greengold, & Chen, 1987).

Considerations for Use

Before deciding that external catheterization is appropriate for an individual, the following assessment must be completed and the patient, the caregiver, or both should demonstrate application of the catheter.

Dexterity   If a patient has difficulty with dexterity and manipulation of small objects, the ease of application and removal of ECCS may be an issue. Identification of a caregiver or family member who will apply the catheter must be considered. In an LTC facility, staff can be taught to apply these catheters.

Size of Penis   Size of the penis (width and length or circumference and length) must be sufficient to support the catheter. With aging and prostate cancer treatments, penile length and size may decrease, causing the penis to retract, and it may be difficult to keep the ECCS from falling off. If this is the case, consideration should be given to a retracted penis pouch. There are several different sizes of external catheters with diameters ranging from 20 to

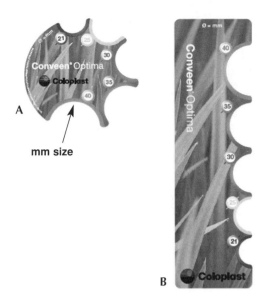

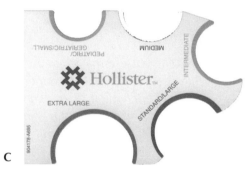

Figure 10.27. External catheter measuring guides (straight and round). Placed against shaft of penis to measure circumference. (*A, B,* Courtesy of Coloplast, *C,* Courtesy of Hollister.)

40 mm, in 5- to 10-mm increments; therefore, it is important to select the correct size. To determine the appropriate size, the clinician should use a measurement guide that is provided by all manufacturers of these products (Figure 10.27). When using the guide, the circumference of the penis should be measured when it is completely relaxed. The penis is extended by gently pulling it forward, away from the body. The measurement guide should be placed halfway down the shaft of the penis to find the closest size on the measurement guide. The clinician should note erectile function because sizing should allow for nocturnal erections.

Condition of the Skin   The penis and scrotum must be assessed for erythema (redness), open areas, and perineal dermatitis (bacteria and yeast rashes) because ECCS should be considered only in men who have intact skin. If the patient is at risk for possible skin breakdown, use of a barrier film product should be considered when applying the device. An attractive feature of silicone ECCS catheters is that they are made of clear material, allowing for monitoring of skin condition.

ECCS Size and Application

Clinicians will find that many men, like the individual described here, will use several different ECCS depending on their activity and specific need.

> *Mike A. underwent a radical prostatectomy 12 years ago and placement of an artificial urinary sphincter 5 years ago. The sphincter was removed because of an infection. Following the removal of the sphincter, Mike has had continuous UI and is having a difficult time managing the urine leakage. He has been using incontinence absorbent products; however, he plans to go on a cruise in the summer and wants a better management system. The initial recommendation was the AlphaDry Reservoir external collection device. Mike obtained this device and found it helpful, but he is concerned that it might slip off. He is interested in also using an external condom catheter attached to a drainage bag. During physical examination, Mike tried several different external condom catheters. The one that appeared to work the best for him was an adhesive type, size extra large (40 mm). He was able to apply the catheter and it was attached to a leg bag. Mike uses a skin barrier product on his penile shaft to prevent skin breakdown from the use of these condom catheters.*

The clinician should take the time to find the ECCS size that fits the individual's needs. Nothing should ever be applied to the penile shaft circumferentially (e.g., adhesive tape, string, rubber band), because this may cause pressure and ulceration, especially in a patient with diminished gluteal sensation. The catheter should be examined for tightness; fit should be snug but not constrictive. If the catheter sheath wrinkles, a smaller size should be tried. If urine leaks, the sheath can be squeezed for better seal. A medical adhesive (commonly used when applying ostomy bags) can be applied around the circumference of the penis to ensure that the catheter "sticks" to the penis. The adhesive must be dry before rolling on the catheter. A skin barrier product can be applied to the penis to protect penile skin from breakdown secondary to repetitive application and removal of an adhesive device. Mechanical damage to the penis can result from adhesives, tapes, or the shape of the catheter.

Men need to be instructed on correct application of ECCS. The patient education tool "How to Use an External 'Condom' Catheter" provides instruction for using this device (on the companion CD). External catheters are attached to the shaft of the penis by one of several different methods, depending on the system used. The different methods are described here.

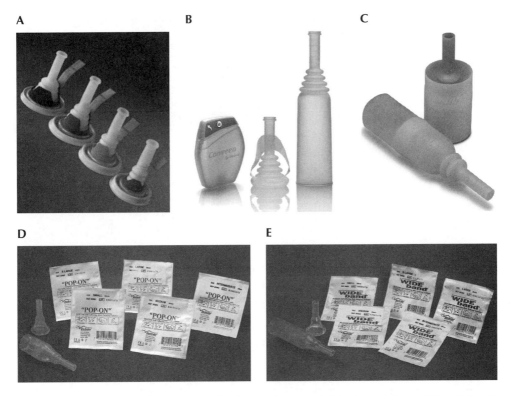

Figure 10.28. *A, B,* Self-adhesive external catheters (Courtesy of Coloplast). *C,* Latex NoTouch Sheath (Courtesy of Hollister). *D,* PopOn and *E,* Wide Band external catheters (Courtesy of Rochester Medical).

Self-Adhesive Catheters Self-adhesive (one-piece) external catheters are very popular (Figure 10.28). These are rolled over the shaft of the penis and pressed, allowing the adhesive to stick to the skin. These are preferred because they are easy to apply. New technology includes all-silicone external catheters, which cause less irritation and fewer adverse reactions and are recommended for men who have an allergy to latex (Edlich et al., 2000).

Two-Piece Systems Two-piece systems have hydrocolloid strips, separate from the sheath, that have adhesive on both sides and can be applied around the penile circumference (Figure 10.29). The catheter sheath is then rolled up and over the penis and the strips, and pressed against the strips to stick. Catheters with a circumferential band may be too restrictive for the shaft of the penis and should be used only by men who are cognitively intact and have penile sensation. These may be more difficult to apply.

Nonadhesive Catheters Nonadhesive catheters have either a Velcro strap that can be wrapped around the sheath once the sheath is applied (Figure 10.30A,B) or an inflatable retention ring securing the catheter that can be easily deflated for removal (Figure 10.30C). These catheters are supplied nonsterile and are reusable.

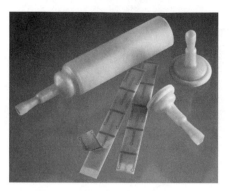

Figure 10.29. Double-sided external non-adhesive catheter with external Velcro bands. (Courtesy of Coloplast.)

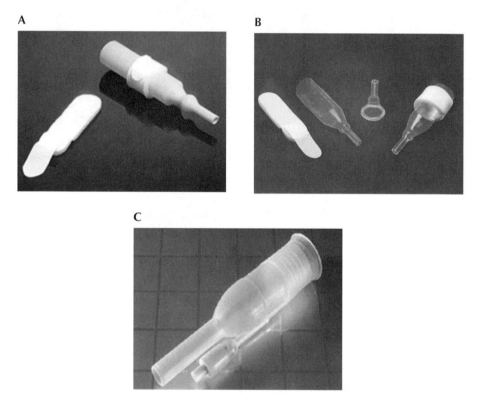

Figure 10.30. *A and B,* Nonadhesive external catheters with Velcro bands. *C,* Nonadhesive inflatable external condom catheter. (*A,* Courtesy of Coloplast; *B,* Courtesy of Rochester Medical; *C,* Courtesy of Cook Urologic.)

Applicator Catheters   Some sheaths have an applicator that assists the individual or caregiver to put the catheter on. These catheters may also be useful for patients with reduced manual dexterity (Figure 10.31).

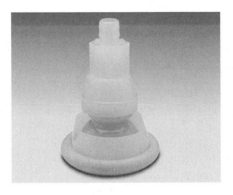
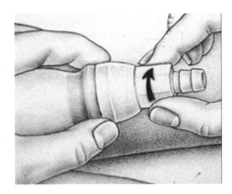

Figure 10.31. External catheter with removable tip that can be used in men with UI who also self-catheterize. (Courtesy of Hollister.)

External Continence Device An external continence device (called the Liberty Pouch) is a small, soft hydrocolloid adhesive wafer in the shape of a flower that gently seals to the tip of the penis. A "faceplate" is wrapped around the wafer to make a custom seal over the glans penis and for added security. The end of the wafer directs the flow of urine into a tube for collection in a special collection bag that can easily fit in the man's pants or shorts. It is a good product for men with a retracted or an uncircumcised penis. If present, the foreskin must be pulled back to place this device and then returned to the natural forward position over the seal (Figure 10.32).

External Pouches Current external pouches are modeled on ostomy pouches and appliances using a synthetic adhesive that secures the device to the individual (Newman et al., 2004) (Figure 10.33). Pouches are available for men with a retracted penis or with a shorter length penis or who cannot use a regular external catheter. They are also available for nonambulatory incontinent women. These pouches are one- or two-piece devices and require removal of pubic hair at the base of the penis in men and the perineum in women. The hair should be trimmed, not shaved, because shaving causes more irritation. In men, the opening in the adhesive surface should be cut to the size of the base of the penis; the pouch is then placed over the penis and adhered to the pubis with adhesive. The pouch can be connected to a drainage bag using an extension tube, or the man can empty the pouch as needed.

In women, training in device application is necessary and actual application can be time intensive, requiring shaving of the mons pubis and the use of adhesive paste to increase adherence to the perineum. A flexible plastic form-fitting "pericup" or pouch is placed over the labia. Problems with leakage persist with the pouch because of poor adherence, especially in female patients. Designs have not been significantly changed since this device was first introduced (Newman et al., 2004). The ideal device for women would be one that is easy to place and works well for women who are bedridden, who

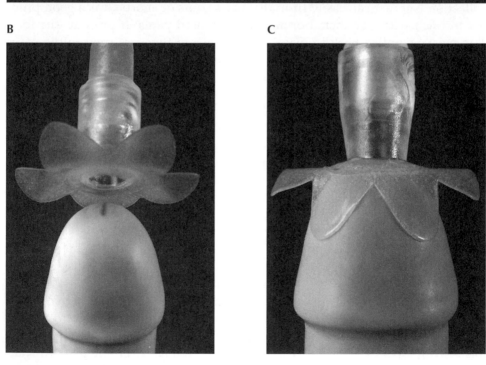

Figure 10.32. Liberty pouch self-adhesive external catheter. *A,* Components of the Liberty pouch. *B,* Centering faceplate over urinary meatus. *C,* Attaching faceplate. *D,* Smoothing petals of faceplate into place. *E,* Faceplate seal top view. *F,* Applying seal over faceplate to ensure no wrinkles. *G,* Ensuring a strong seal. (Courtesy of BioDerm.)

D

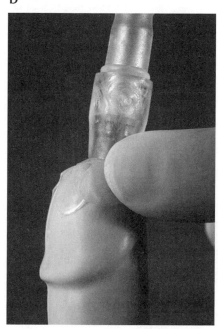

E

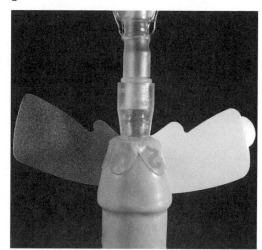

F

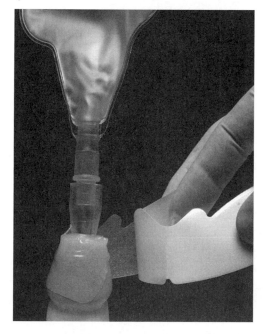

G

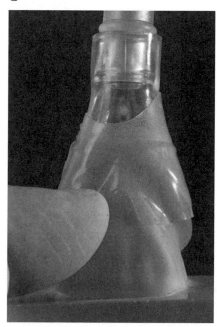

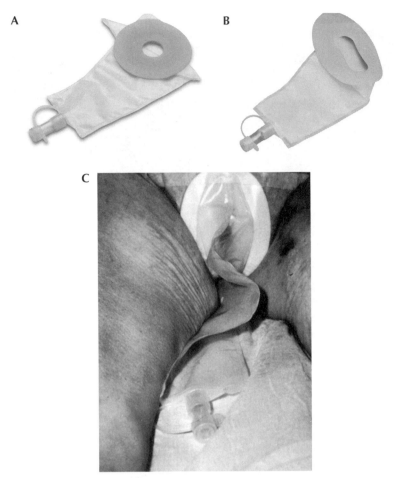

Figure 10.33. *A,B* Male and female external pouches. (Courtesy of Hollister.) *C,* Female pouch on patient.

transfer from beds to chairs, or who use wheelchairs. Unfortunately, no device has proven to be very useful for these women.

Reusable ECCSs   Reusable ECCS (sometimes referred to as "pubic pressure urinals") are body-worn and are a type of external catheter (Figure 10.34). They are only available for men and are used in those men who experience UI after prostate surgery and in aging men with intractable UI. Some men use no method of attachment and prefer a nonadhesive condom, using a foam-and-elastic reusable band fastened with Velcro to secure the catheter. There is no direct skin adhesion, and thus less chance of skin breakdown. These products use a belt (like an athletic strap) or a pant to keep them in place and to secure the drainage bag.

There is also the AlphaDry, a small discreet product that holds a small amount of urine leakage. It is a combination of a one-piece condom catheter, one-way valve, and reservoir that tucks neatly into brief-type underwear

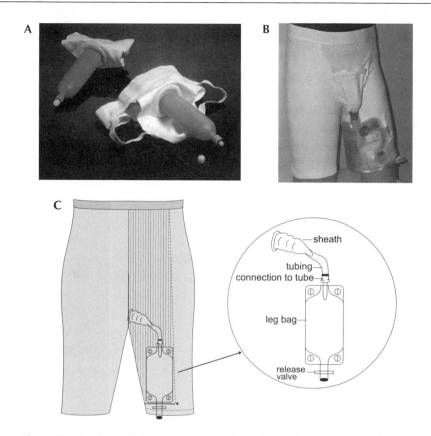

Figure 10.34.   *A,* McGuire reusable external condom catheter. (Courtesy of Coloplast.) *B,* Afex reusable external catheter system. (Courtesy of Arcus Medical.) *C,* Better Pant. (Courtesy of Uroconcepts, Inc.)

(Figure 10.35). The catheter attaches securely to the penis and urine flows directly through the one-way valve into the reservoir. The reservoir is emptied when it begins to feel heavy (usually every 2 or 3 hours).

Common Complications

Once an external catheter is applied, careful attention must be given to avoid problems such as contact dermatitis, maceration of the tip of the penis, ischemia, penile edema, and penile obstruction.

* Infection can occur but is less likely with external devices than with internal catheters (intermittent or indwelling) because they avoid instrumentation of the urethra.

* Skin breakdown (i.e., dermatitis, minor skin erosions) can occur because the skin is occluded. Clear silicone sheaths allow assessment of the skin without removing the catheter and have water and oxygen vapor transmission properties allowing the skin to breathe. If skin breakdown occurs,

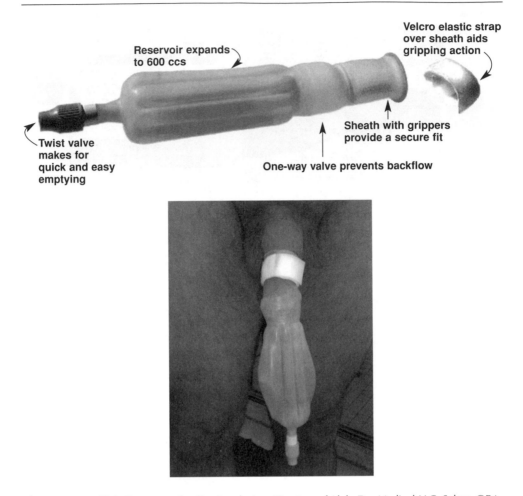

Figure 10.35.   AlphaDry external collection device. (Courtesy of AlphaDry Medical LLC, Salem, OR.)

ECCS should be removed for the skin to heal. Before returning to using the catheter, the person or caregiver should determine why the breakdown occurred (e.g., sheath too tight, sheath pulled off, tearing of the skin, possible latex allergy, UTI).

- Maceration and irritation of the skin can occur from the friction caused by an external catheter. Consideration should be given to applying a skin-barrier product prior to application of the catheter.

- Phimosis is present when the orifice of the foreskin is constricted, preventing retraction of the foreskin over the glans. This can occur as a result of over-constriction of the penis from an external device rolled over the penile shaft. Circumcision may be required.

- Constriction or strangulation of the penis can occur when using a double-sided adhesive strap to secure the condom catheter. Two types of straps are available: adhesive-coated foam straps and adhesive barrier straps. Barrier straps stretch and have the capacity to return to their original size and shape. These are the preferred type in men who retain erectile function. Foam straps are not elastic, so they will not stretch and should be used with caution.

Most of these adverse effects are the result of improper and prolonged use of these devices. These effects go unreported in men with decreased penile and scrotal sensation. Proper sizing of the condom and careful application to prevent rolling or wrinkling may reduce such events. Nurses should receive proper training on ECCS use and monitor the device frequently to avoid adverse events.

Urinary Drainage Bags

Catheters, indwelling or external, are attached to urine drainage bags that collect and store urine. Urine drainage bags fall into two main categories: 1) large-capacity bags (referred to as "overnight" or "bedside" bags; Figure 10.36A,B,D)

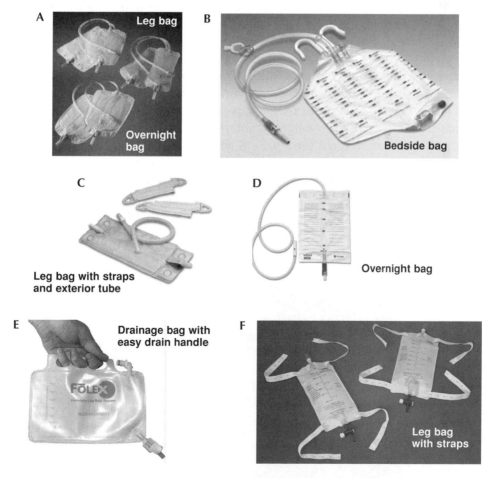

Figure 10.36.   Urinary drainage bags. (*A,* Courtesy of Coloplast; *B, C, D,* Courtesy of Hollister; *E,* Courtesy of Arcus Medical; *F,* Courtesy of Rochester Medical.)

and 2) leg bags (referred to as "body-worn" bags; Figure 10.36A,C,E,F). Most bags are made from transparent PVC or polyvinylidene fluoride, polyethylene, or latex. All bags used to connect to an indwelling urinary catheter should be sterile. Nonsterile bags are available and are mostly used for ECCS. Bags consist of a drainage tube that is connected to the catheter, a collecting bag, and a drainage port (or "tap"). There is usually a single nonreturn valve at the junction of the inlet tube and the bag that prevents reflux of urine back up the tube. Some may have a sampling port for taking urine specimens. The length of the drainage tube ranges from 4–45 cm or roughly 2–18 inches and is usually adjusted to accommodate a patient's needs. Most bags have backings that are designed to prevent or reduce plastic contact with the skin and are usually made of nonwoven material. Leg bags may have a fabric backing against the skin to reduce sweating.

Types of Urinary Drainage Bags

Large-Capacity or "Overnight" Bag   An overnight or bedside bag is usually of 1,500- or 2,000-mL capacity, with a long tube that is used for overnight drainage. The bag should be hung over the side of the bed below the level of the catheter so that the urine will flow easily and to prevent urine backflow.

Leg Bag   A bag of urine can be difficult to accommodate discreetly on the body and can present problems with appearance (bulge) and noise (urine movement) (Fader, 2003). Therefore, a leg bag is preferred for use during the day by ambulatory patients and those in rehabilitation facilities. A leg bag allows maximum freedom of movement for a patient and can be concealed easily beneath clothing. Leg bags come in different sizes (horizontal or vertical) and are made from a variety of material (vinyl, latex, and others). Capacity can range from 350 to 1,300 mL, with a 500-mL bag being the most popular. Reusable leg bags are also available (Figure 10.37). Attention should be paid to the selection of the emptying port because some patients may be able to manipulate a flip-flow port

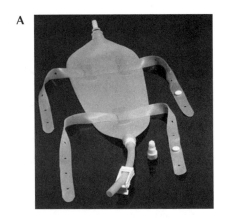
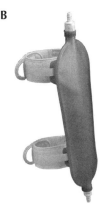

Figure 10.37.   Reusable latex leg drainage bags. (Courtesy of Coloplast.)

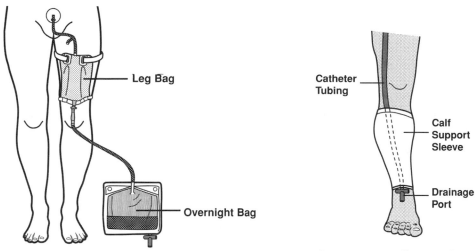

Figure 10.38. Closed catheter drainage system with leg bag attached to overnight bag. (Courtesy of Robin Noel.)

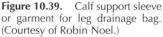

Figure 10.39. Calf support sleeve or garment for leg drainage bag. (Courtesy of Robin Noel.)

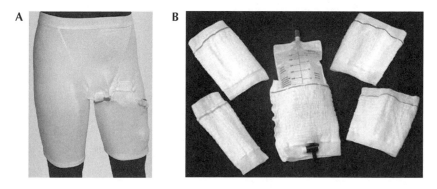

Figure 10.40. Drainage bag holders. *A,* Cloth brief. *B,* Net sleeve. (*A,* Courtesy of Arcus Medical and *B,* Rochester Medical.)

but not a sliding-type port. Two modifications, the addition of a urine sampling port in the drainage tube and a preconnected catheter/collecting tube system, seem to have advanced the design because they discourage or prevent disconnection of the system, which can predispose the user to infection (Figure 10.38). Patients like to switch to an overnight bag while asleep. To avoid repeatedly disconnecting the leg bag from the catheter, a silicone connecting tube can be attached to connect the leg bag port with the overnight bag.

More active individuals may prefer a leg bag for use at home or when away from home because these bags allow more freedom of movement. These smaller bags are more discreet because the person can attach the bag to the upper thigh or calf and conceal it under clothing. They are held in place with straps, foam, mesh, elastic straps with Velcro closures, or knitted bag holders. Holding the bag in place using a net sleeve or stocking (Figure 10.39) or cloth briefs or leg holders (Figure 10.40) eliminates the need for straps. Each strap is fixed on either side of the eyelets using buttons or Velcro. The calf is usually the easiest place on which to strap a leg bag, but women who wear skirts will need to use a thigh bag or waist belt (Newman, 2004). Straps that are too tight can restrict circulation, resulting in lesions.

Abdomen Bags   A drainage bag can also be secured on the lower abdomen. The one most often used is the Belly Bag® (Rusch), a latex-free, sterile, 1,000-mL capacity drainage bag with an easy-to-fasten waist belt and an anti-reflux valve to prevent backflow that can be worn around the abdomen under clothing (Figure 10.41). It can be used with either a urethral or a suprapubic indwelling catheter but is not recommended with ECCS. It can be purchased

A

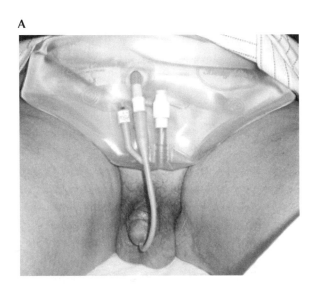

B

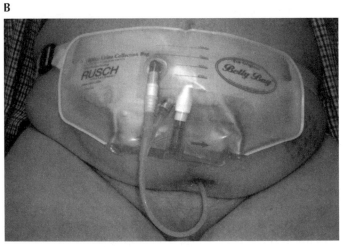

Figure 10.41.   *A,* Belly Bag® attached to indwelling urethral catheter. *B,* Belly Bag® attached to suprapubic catheter. (Courtesy of Rusch.)

with a 24-inch drain tube. Normal bladder pressure (10–25 cm H_2O) is more than enough to push urine into the bag. It has a soft backing so that it does not chafe the skin. Because it is secured on the abdomen, it eliminates the problems associated with leg and bedside bags, including inadvertent catheter extraction and leg bruising.

Considerations When Choosing a Drainage Bag

When selecting a drainage bag for a catheter system, certain factors must be considered:

- Manual dexterity of the patient and/or caregiver. Ability to manipulate the catheter, anchor the tubing, manage straps, and empty the drainage bag will need to be assessed.

- Shape and height of the user. Some thigh shapes and sizes pose a challenge to securing a leg bag.

- Clothes worn by user of a leg bag. Some bags are more discreet in shape and port design than others.

- Type of drainage port. Attention should be paid to the selection of the drainage port because the individual, the caregiver, or both may be able to manipulate a flip-flow port but not a sliding-type port (Figure 10.42). The port should be readily accessible and easily opened and closed, especially for those with limited hand function.

- Appearance and noise. A bag of urine can be quite difficult to accommodate discreetly on the body and can present problems with appearance and noise from urine movement.

- Tightness of the straps. Leg bag attachments that are too tight can restrict blood circulation.

Drainage Bag Care

A standard practice is to change drainage bags every 5–7 days, but there is little evidence to support this (Cottenden et al., 2005). A systematic review

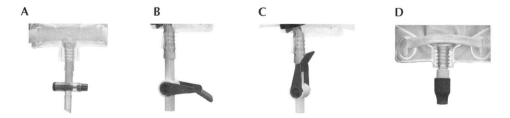

Figure 10.42.   Leg bag ports and examples of drainage spouts. *A,* T-Tap-Closed (push tap across to open). *B, C,* Fas-Tap (pull tap down to open). *D,* Twist Port (pull off cap to open). (Courtesy of Coloplast.)

suggested that adding antibiotic or antimicrobial solutions (e.g., hydrogen peroxide, silver sulfadiazine) to the bag to clean the bag and prevent the development of CAUTI has no effect on CAUTI and is not recommended (Gray, 2004b). However, it is difficult to stop individuals and caregivers from cleaning and deodorizing drainage bags. The use of a solution of household bleach with tap water (1:10 ratio) has been recommended (Nash, 2003). Others recommend a vinegar solution of 1 part vinegar to 3 parts water, although bleach has been shown to be more effective than vinegar or other solutions in urine bag decontamination. Thus the benefit of vinegar for bag decontamination is likely to be aesthetic in curtailing odor only. Dille et al. (1993) did classic research on cleansing of vinyl urinary bags and recommended the following regimen: 1) rinse bag with lukewarm water to remove any residual urine; 2) vigorously agitate clean water in the collection bag twice; and 3) pour a diluted solution of Chlorox (1:10) on drainage port, sleeve, cap, and connector. Also pour solution into the bag and vigorously agitate for 30 seconds, drain, and allow to air dry. This resulted in decreased colony counts. The bag should always be rinsed with soap and water and allowed to dry after using any disinfectant.

Purple Urine Bag Syndrome   Purple urine bag syndrome (PUBS) is the term that has been used to describe a purple discoloration of the collecting bag and tubing (Vallejo-Manzur, Mireles-Cabodevila, & Varon, 2005). It is fairly rare and is a benign condition (Robinson, 2003). The urinary catheter drainage system changes color from red or blue to violet or purple, sometimes with a differently colored tube and bag (Ribeiro, Marcelino, Marum, Fernandes, & Grilo, 2004). The etiology is still controversial, but it is believed that indigo, which is blue, and indirubin, which is red, are responsible for the colors obtained. The coloration is brought about by bacterial decomposition in the colon of tryptophan, an essential amino acid in food. By-products are absorbed, metabolized, and excreted in the urine, thus causing the color and usually a foul odor. A number of factors are involved, but not always present, in its development, including female sex, UTI, immobility, constipation, indicanuria, and alkaline urine (a common characteristic in most cases) (Tang, 2006).

Bacteriuria has been implicated in PUBS, but only a few bacterial strains that contain indoxyl phosphatase (*Providencia stuartii, Klebsiella pneumoniae, Enterobacter agglomerans*) have been reported to be capable of producing PUBS. Instead, a higher bacterial count in urine was found to be the most important of all facilitating factors in PUBS. PUBS can appear hours to days after catheterization and resolves usually after treatment of the UTI or changing of the collecting bag (Vallejo-Manzur et al., 2005). PUBS has not been demonstrated to have any implication other than the possibility of a UTI and has not been proven to cause any other problems. Clinicians dealing with patients who have indwelling bladder catheters also need to be aware of this condition because the catheter system may need more frequent changing.

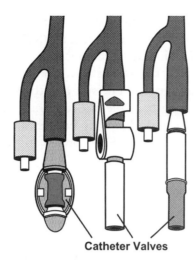

Catheter Valves

Figure 10.43. Catheter valves inserted in the urinary catheter. (Courtesy of Robin Noel.)

Use of Catheter Valves

A catheter valve (CV) is a small device similar to a drainage bag port that fits in the end of an indwelling catheter (Addison, 1999) (Figure 10.43). It has an open-and-close mechanism and is used in place of a drainage bag (Cottenden et al., 2005). Urine is stored in the bladder rather than in a bag and is drained intermittently by releasing the valve (van den Eijkel & Griffiths, 2006). CVs have been used with urethral and suprapubic catheters (e.g., Option-*vf* Valved Suprapubic Catheter). The catheter can be attached to a drainage bag at night to drain the urine while the person is asleep. It is thought that the use of a CV may maintain bladder capacity, function, and tone; decrease urethral erosion because there is no added weight from a drainage bag; and decrease migration of bacteria from drainage bags.

In some countries, such as the United Kingdom, CVs are used in place of a drainage bag (Fader et al., 1997). CVs may allow the bladder to fill and empty, mimicking the natural activity of the bladder. Patients who have intact bladder sensation can feel when the bladder needs emptying and can open the CV to release urine. It is recommended that individuals with neurologic bladder dysfunction open the CV every 3 hours to empty the bladder. This may be helpful in reestablishing voiding when removing a catheter. CVs may allow the person more independence because a drainage bag is not attached. However, there may also be an increased risk of infection with CVs because of urine stasis.

There is very little recent research on the use of CVs, especially on long-term use. German, Rowley, Stone, Kumar, and Blackford (1997) found no difference in the reported incidence of bladder spasms or discomfort and no difference in positive urine cultures when comparing the use of CVs and drainage bags in men with spinal cord injury (SCI). However, in this study there was a slightly higher incidence of nocturnal frequency and bypassing episodes. Subjects preferred to use the CV, reporting that it felt more comfortable and discreet. Many patients do not like the sensation of urine "sloshing about" when using a leg bag. We suggest that a combination of a valve during the day and an overnight bag may be the ideal solution. At this time, CVs have not been approved by the FDA for use in the United States.

Intermittent Catheterization

Intermittent catheterization (IC) is the insertion and removal of a catheter several times a day to provide bladder emptying. Catheters are inserted into the bladder via the urethra or via a stoma in patients who have undergone urinary diversion. Catheterization is performed by either sterile or clean technique. Sterile (aseptic) technique implies genital disinfection and the use of sterile catheters, gloves, and other equipment. Clean technique implies the use of disposable or cleansed reusable catheters (Abrams et al., 2002), handwashing with soap and water, and cleansing the perineum only if fecal or other wastes are present. There is no benefit to the use of an antiseptic solution for daily periurethral cleansing prior to catheterization (Webster et al., 2001). Clean intermittent catheterization (CIC) was introduced by a urologist, Dr. Jack Lapides at the University of Michigan, and has been used in the bladder management of patients with urinary retention and other voiding dysfunction for the past 30 years. CIC has proved to be the most effective and practical means of attaining a catheter-free state in the patient with SCI and chronic intractable urinary retention (Moy & Wein, 2007). Clean intermittent self-catheterization (CISC), in which catheterization is performed by the patient, has become the standard of care in this population, particularly in those patients with SCI. Woodbury, Hayes, and Askes (2008) conducted a national survey in Canada of IC practices in community dwelling people living with SCI and found that 73% of people used clean technique. When compared to the use of an indwelling catheter, this technique has resulted in improved kidney and upper urinary tract status, and improvement of continence in patients suffering from neurogenic bladder dysfunction. Also, it is considered to be less expensive and more practical for individuals because the original sterile technique was time consuming and costly.

As discussed in Chapter 3, the bladder contracts and the pelvic floor muscles relax during voiding to allow urine to pass through the urethra. Normally, after the bladder empties, a small amount of urine may remain in the bladder (called the postvoid residual [PVR]). If the person cannot urinate or empty the bladder completely, the PVR increases and can contribute to UTIs, overflow UI, and permanent damage to the bladder and kidneys. Research has shown that regular bladder emptying reduces intravesical bladder pressure and improves blood circulation in the bladder wall, making the bladder mucosa more resistant to infectious bacteria. By inserting the catheter several times during the day, episodes of bladder overdistention are avoided. In addition, the bladder wall is susceptible to bacteria that circulate in retained urine. When the bladder becomes stretched from retained urine, the capillaries become occluded, preventing the delivery of metabolic and immune substrates to the bladder wall (Heard & Buhrer, 2005). The key to avoiding UTIs is avoidance of high intravesical pressure and overdistention of the bladder, thus preserving an adequate blood supply to the bladder wall (Lapides, Diokno, Silber, & Lowe, 2002).

More than 200,000 patients in the United States have an SCI as a result of trauma, and 10,000 additional cases occur each year (Linsenmeyer et al., 2006). The majority of individuals with SCI and neurological impairment have lower urinary tract dysfunction, either UI, incomplete bladder emptying, or both (see Chapter 4). Usually the person, caregiver, or both are taught to perform IC. Long-term use of IC is preferable to indwelling urethral catheterization because of the low chance of infection and other problems. Long-term CISC is safe and well accepted. Good support and professional instruction on catheterization are necessary to obtain and maintain patient compliance. However, an early dropout rate of about 20% has been described in children and adolescents (Pohl et al., 2002).

Sterile Versus Clean Intermittent Catheterization

There remains controversy concerning the use of sterile single-use catheters or clean reusable catheters and incidence of UTIs (Getliffe, Fader, Allen, et al., 2007). There are certain patients who should perform sterile IC because of other medical conditions. For these patients and those with impaired immune systems (e.g., patients with acquired immunodeficiency syndrome, those receiving chemotherapy) and others at risk for developing UTIs, sterile technique is best. Despite research indicating equivalent efficacy of CIC and sterile IC, sterile technique is used for IC in acute care facilities and in LTC settings because of the high risk of nosocomial infections (Rainville, 1994). In cases in which a parent or caregiver is performing IC, catheterization should be performed using aseptic technique to minimize the transfer of nonindiginous skin flora to the catheterized person and avoid the possibility of cross-infection.

Debate continues, however, on the use of sterile or clean catheterization technique in clinical settings, such as the rehabilitation setting (Kovindha, Mai, & Madersbacher, 2004). CIC in the rehabilitation setting does not appear to place the person with SCI at increased risk for developing symptomatic UTI, and has significant cost- and time-saving benefits for the health care system, as well as enhancing the transition for the individual from the rehabilitation setting to the community (Linsenmeyer et al., 2006). Moore, Burt, and Voaklander (2006) compared the incidence of symptomatic UTI and asymptomatic bacteriuria in individuals with quadriplegia ($N = 36$; 16 clean IC, 20 sterile IC) admitted from the acute care neurology unit to the spinal cord rehabilitation unit. Shortly after admission to rehabilitation, subjects were randomized to either clean or sterile IC technique, using time to symptomatic UTI (pyuria plus symptoms) as the study end point. In this study, clean technique but with a single-use PVC catheter appeared safe and effective for patients with SCI in rehabilitation.

In the hospital setting, strict sterile technique is used by health care professionals. This technique is not only a time-consuming method for health care providers but also costly. In the community, patients are instructed to perform IC using a clean technique, which is less time consuming and decreases the cost of IC. However, individuals, their caregivers, and staff nurses have expressed confusion at the time of discharge over sending patients home using a technique different from the one used by nurses while the person was hospitalized (Lemke, Kasprowicz, & Worral, 2005). Simplification of the catheterization procedure may enhance the transition from rehabilitation to home.

CIC has been used in patients residing in the community; however, few data are available about the safest method in LTC facilities. A study in a VA LTC facility found no difference in frequency of UTIs between clean and sterile IC in male residents (Duffy et al., 1995).

Common Complications

Bacteriuria   Common problems that can result from IC include bacteriuria. This is seen in most long-term IC patients, but rarely leads to symptomatic UTIs. The majority of individuals usually have no symptoms and therefore should not be treated with antibiotics.

Urinary Tract Infections   Intermittent symptomatic UTIs are a common complication seen in patients using IC and are more prevalent in those who have higher residual urine volumes at the time of catheterization. Woodbury et al. (2008) noted the mean frequency of self-reported UTIs over a 12-month period was 2.6 in community dwelling people with SCI living in Canada who were performing IC and that individuals who only catheterized once per day had the highest number of infections, with 38% having five or more UTIs per year. Females had a higher incidence of UTIs than males. Also, respondents performing CISC had less UTIs than if someone else were performing the catheterization. It was interesting to note that most UTIs (78%) were managed by family physicians, with only 13% managed by urologists. This survey showed that perineal cleansing was associated with a reduced infection rate as well as that antiseptic agents (e.g., chlorhexadine) may be more effective than simply washing with soap and water. It also showed that the use of prophylactic agents, such as cranberry juice and vitamin C supplements, and increased fluid intake decreased the rate of UTI. Chronic pyelonephritis rarely develops in patients performing IC. As with indwelling catheters, the use of prophylactic antibiotics is not recommended in adults or children because use is associated with the development of resistant bacterial strains. If a clinically apparent infection occurs in these individuals, it should be treated. In patients with an internal prosthesis (pacemaker, heart valve), however, the use of prophylactic antibiotic therapy for bacteria in the urine is often recommended (Clarke, Samuel, & Boddy, 2005). There is no strict policy regarding this, however, in general the patient's specialty physician should be consulted and/or the infectious disease service about each individual patient in this category.

Urethral Damage   Urethral damage is common primarily in men and is similar in incidence to that seen in users of indwelling catheters. It is of concern because, when damage to the urethra occurs, the mucosal barrier to infections is compromised (De Ridder et al., 2005). Common urethral problems include the following:

- Rarely, *urethritis,* or inflammation of the urethral meatus, results from frequent insertion of catheters.

- *Urethral stricture* is the result of a urethral inflammatory response to repeated trauma. The risk of a urethral stricture increases with the number of years performing IC. The use of hydrophilic catheters may decrease the incidence of strictures (Perrouin-Verbe et al., 1995). Difficulty with insertion is a sign of the presence of a urethral stricture. Wyndaele and Maes (1990) conducted a 12-year follow-up of patients with SCI who were using CISC and found that urethral stricture occurred more frequently in those using CISC for more than 5 years. In addition, they found that the higher the daily frequency of catheterization, the fewer the urethral changes. This might be due to the fact that those individuals regularly performing CISC developed more skill in catheterization and therefore had less chance of urethral trauma. However, with more catheterizations the chance of urethral dilation increases. The authors thought that, over the long term, a CISC frequency of 4 times or more per day is safe for men with SCI.

- *Creation of a false passage,* primarily in men with persisting urethral strictures, may occur at the site of the external sphincter just distal to the prostate. This generally requires use of an indwelling catheter for a week or two to allow this area to heal before IC is resumed.

Other Complications of IC   Additional complications that may occur with use of IC include the following:

- *Epididymitis,* caused by urethral and bladder inflammation, is rare.

- *Scrotal abscess* is also a rare occurrence.

- *Hematuria* is common. At least 74% of patients who use uncoated catheters will experience initial bleeding when starting IC, and 28% complain of persistent urethral bleeding 3 months after starting IC (Webb, Lawson, & Neal, 1990).

- *Bladder stones* may occur in patients who perform IC over the long term. Stones have been shown to grow around introduced pubic hairs. To avoid introducing pubic hairs, patients should be instructed to trim all perineal hair.

Ways to Prevent IC-Related Problems

Recurrent UTIs   Recurrent symptomatic UTIs can be a problem for many patients performing CISC long term (Heard & Buhrer, 2005). The following may be causes:

- *Inadequate emptying at the time of catheterization.* Residual volume can be left in the bladder after catheterization. The individual must ensure adequate emptying by employing the Valsalva maneuver and a gentle Credé maneuver at the conclusion of the catheterization, before the catheter is removed.

- *Inadequate frequency of emptying.* Not emptying the bladder often enough leads to excessive bladder volumes, with long periods of urine stagnation. The combination of bacteriuria and stasis increases the risk of clinical infection. However, if the urine is "drained" regularly, bacteria are not exposed to the bladder long enough to produce symptomatic infection. Anderson (1980) found that catheterizing 6 times per day was healthier than catheterizing 3 times per day. It is recommended that total bladder emptying be done at least 4 times per day or to maintain a volume of less than 400 mL. Even a modest improvement in emptying or a modest reduction in chronic distention can produce dramatic improvement in the infection rate.

- *Inadequate fluid intake.* Inadequate intake is a companion problem to inadequate frequency of emptying. When low urine volumes are produced (<1,200 mL of urine per day), patients are less inclined to empty at desired intervals, producing urine stagnation and bladder distention.

- *Type of catheter, catheter care, and catheterization technique.* If recurrent UTIs are an issue, the clinician needs to evaluate the individual's technique and consider having the person switch to a sterile closed system or single-use catheters based on medical necessity (Box 10.5).

Excessive Fluid Intake   If the person cannot or will not adjust fluid intake appropriately for the IC schedule, he or she risks periodic or regular bladder overdistention, and possible overflow UI. Excessive intake would produce bladder volumes greater than 500 mL at one time or would be evidenced by the need to catheterize more than 6 times per day, or both. The person should be encouraged to drink regularly, taking small volumes spaced hourly between breakfast and the evening meal and reducing to sips thereafter. Large fluid intake in the evening should be discouraged so as to minimize production of excessive urine volumes during the hours of sleep.

Nocturnal Polyuria   Some patients—especially those with SCI and multiple sclerosis—may have nocturnal diuresis related to inadequate antidiuretic hormone secretion at night. Even when these individuals avoid fluid intake in the evening, they still produce large volumes of urine during the night. Even

---

Box 10.5   Medicare medical necessity and documentation requirements for intermittent catheters

---

Intermittent catheterization is covered when basic coverage criteria are met and the patient or caregiver can perform the procedure.

For each episode of covered catheterization, Medicare will cover:

• One catheter (A4351, A4352) and an individual packet of lubricant (A4332)

or

• One sterile intermittent catheter kit (A4353), if additional coverage criteria are met (1–5):

1. The patient resides in a nursing facility

2. The patient is immunosuppressed, for example (not all-inclusive):

   on a regimen of immunosuppressive drugs post-transplant
   on cancer chemotherapy
   has acquired immune deficiency syndrome (AIDS)
   has a drug-induced state, such as chronic oral corticosteroid use

3. The patient has radiologically documented vesico-ureteral reflux while on a program of intermittent catheterization

4. The patient is a spinal cord injured female with neurogenic bladder who is pregnant (for duration of pregnancy only)

5. The patient has had distinct, recurrent urinary tract infections, while on a program of sterile intermittent catheterization with A4351/A4352 and sterile lubricant A4332, twice within the 12-month period prior to the initiation of sterile intermittent catheter kits

A patient would be considered to have a urinary tract infection if he or she has a urine culture with greater than 10,000 colony forming units of a urinary pathogen **and** concurrent presence of one or more of the following signs, symptoms, or laboratory findings:

• Fever (oral temperature greater than 38° C [100.4° F])

• Systemic leukocytosis

• Change in urinary urgency, frequency, or incontinence

• Appearance of new or increase in autonomic dysreflexia (sweating, bradycardia, blood pressure elevation)

• Physical signs of prostatitis, epididymitis, orchitis

• Increased muscle spasms

• Pyuria (greater than 5 white blood cells [WBCs] per high-powered field)

Medicare Requirements for Coverage of a Coudé-Tipped Catheter

A Coudé-tipped catheter can be covered with appropriate medical necessity documentation (a medical reason why the patient cannot pass a straight-tipped catheter). A Coudé-tipped catheter is rarely covered for a woman.

---

waking several times during the night to catheterize may not be sufficient to maintain acceptable bladder volumes. If all else fails, a trial of desmopressin administration at bedtime may prevent the diuresis (see Chapter 9), but this should be administered with strict physician supervision.

Traumatic Catheterization   The individual should make every effort to gently insert a well-lubricated catheter. Bleeding and the development of strictures or false passages are associated with traumatic catheterization (Vapnek, Maynard, & Kim, 2003). Breaks in the urothelium increase the risk of infection. Difficulty passing the catheter may lead the person to avoid performing catheterization. Direct observation by the clinician to help correct faulty insertion technique may contribute to improved outcomes. An alternative catheter, such as a Coudé-tipped catheter, may ease passage. We recommend referral for urological evaluation in the event of persistent difficulty with catheter insertion.

Detrusor–Sphincter Dyssynergia   Patients with neurogenic bladder can develop a problem called detrusor–sphincter dyssynergia, in which the bladder and the external sphincter contract simultaneously (see Chapter 4). This action leads to very high pressures in the bladder, decreases the blood flow to the bladder wall, and increases the pressure in the upper urinary tract, possibly damaging the kidneys even in the absence of ureteral reflux. Patients with neurogenic bladder who use IC may need an antimuscarinic medication (see Chapter 9) to prevent dangerously high bladder pressures.

Types of Intermittent Catheters

There are several different types of intermittent catheters. Catheter surface properties may influence associated problems of IC, such as urethral complications and UTIs, as well as user satisfaction and preference. In an attempt to reduce catheter-associated bacteriuria and long-term urethral complications such as urethritis, hydrophilic-coated catheters have been introduced to the market in addition to the uncoated PVC catheters. Hedlund, Hjelmås, Jonsson, Klarskov, and Talja (2001) found clinical evidence showing that hydrophilic-coated catheters decrease urethral irritation and have a higher user satisfaction. However, there is a lack of research comparing the performance of hydrophilic-coated and uncoated catheters.

The clinician who instructs the individual usually makes the catheter choice (Newman, 2004). One of the authors (DKN) suggests at least two to three different types of catheters to the patient to try to find the preferred choice. Not all catheters are suitable for all individuals' needs and circumstances. For example, some patients may require one type of catheter for home use and another for work use.

Catheter Size and Length   Catheter sizes for IC are similar to those available for an indwelling catheter and include ranges of 6–12 Fr for children and 14–22 Fr for adults. The funnel end of the catheter is usually color coded to identify French size easily. Intermittent catheters have different lengths. Men use catheters with lengths of about 12 inches (about 40 cm) (Figure 10.44C). Women and children should ideally use shorter lengths of 6–12 inches (20–40

A

B   C

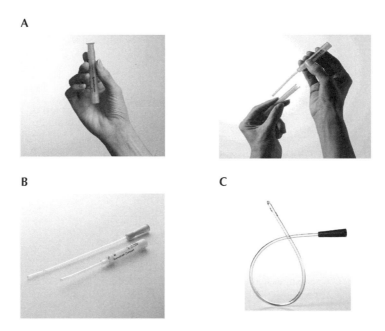

Figure 10.44. *A,* SpeediCath for women, *B,* shorter length catheters for women (5 and 7 inches), and *C,* longer length male catheter. (Courtesy of Coloplast.)

cm) because of their shorter urethral length (Figure 10.44A,B). Shorter catheters without a funnel end are available. Shorter catheters allow for more efficient drainage by reducing the risk of looping or kinking, and reduces risk of upward gradient drainage of the tube. Standard male catheters are often used by women, but care should be taken to avoid the forming of a surplus loop. Catheter tips are similar to those for indwelling catheters, such as the Coudé-tipped or curved catheters (referred to as Tiemann catheters) that have a slight curve at the tip that aids in insertion (Figure 10.45B). An additional tip design called the "olive-tipped catheter" may help a woman in identifying her urethra (Figure 10.45C). Using a Coudé-tipped or curved catheter may make it easier for men to pass the catheter past the prostate gland.

Catheter Material   IC catheters fall into two main groups (Easton, 2000):

- Those that require lubrication to be applied before insertion
- Those for which the coating provides the lubrication when water is applied

Straight Catheters   Straight catheters are silicone or rubber catheters that have two eyes at the tip that allow for urine drainage. Red-rubber catheters can be more flexible and are often recommended for patients who are performing IC on a short-term basis (e.g., following stricture dilation). Clinicians need to remember that these are latex based and that some patients find them

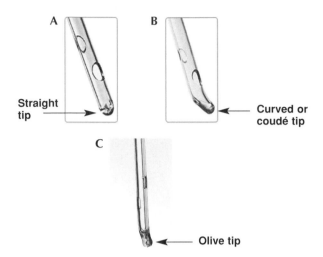

Figure 10.45.   Catheter tip configurations. *A,* Straight tip. *B,* Coudé tip (slight curve at the tip that aids in insertion, especially past prostate). *C,* Olive tip (size of small bead; catheter for women to help in identifying urinary meatus). (Courtesy of Astra Tech [A, B] and Coloplast [C].)

more difficult to insert. They also tend to become brittle with repeated use. A clear, more rigid catheter makes insertion easier.

PVC Catheters   The PVC catheter is the most commonly used catheter for IC. It is a firmer catheter with a larger internal diameter. PVC is a plastic polymer that is used in a wide array of products. Unplasticized PVC is hard and brittle at room temperature. DHEP (Di(2-ethylhexyl)phthalate) is a plasticizer (softener) that has been added to increase the flexibility of the polymer and has been added to most medical devices. DEHP in PVC and its potential harm have been debated for some time now. It is mainly a concern for PVC products that hold and store liquids that then go into the body (e.g., blood bags and feeding bags), especially liquids that contain lipids. Intermittent catheters are in the body for a short period of time and do not store liquids, so the harmful exposure is minimal (go to http://www.fda.gov/cdrh/safety/dehp.html). The material is not conducive to indwelling use but is thermosensitive and therefore becomes soft and pliable at body temperature. However, a PVC catheter should be only used for 1 week because it encrusts easily. The majority of patients use PVC catheters, using gel for lubrication (Woodbury et al., 2008).

Hydrophilic-Coated Catheters   Hydrophilic-coated catheters are similar to silicone catheters in that they have a layer of polymer coating that is bound to the catheter surface. The catheter surface consists of polyvinyl pyrrolidone (PVP) and salt, not PVC. This outer layer becomes smoother when hydrated. When soaked in water, the PVP attracts the water, and the biocompatible salt

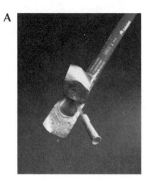
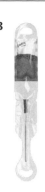

Figure 10.46. Prelubricated hydrophilic intermittent catheters. *A,* SpeediCath. (Courtesy of Coloplast.) *B,* LoFric. (Courtesy of Astra Tech.)

coating binds the water to the surface of the catheter, creating an outer layer mainly consisting of water (Giannantoni et al., 2002). This thick, slippery, smooth layer of water stays on the catheter, ensuring lubrication of the urethra in its entire length during catheter insertion and withdrawal. This outer layer has been designed to allow for easier insertion, and to minimize discomfort and reduce friction between the urethra and the catheter during IC; in addition, it may minimize the risk of urethral trauma and other complications (Fader, Moore, et al., 2001; Vapnek et al., 2003). This type of catheter is becoming very popular. A national survey in Canada noted that 15% of SCI patients used hydrophillic catheters (Woodbury et al., 2008).

PVP is a completely harmless and nonallergenic substance that has been used in the medical products and cosmetics industries since the 1930s. PVP-coated catheters may be indicated for patients who experience particular discomfort during catheterization when using gel-lubricated uncoated catheters or patients who have difficulty with other types of catheters (Diokno, Mitchell, Nash, & Kimbrough, 1995). Hydrophilic-coated catheters perform better than uncoated catheters with regard to hematuria and user preference, and certain products exert less withdrawal friction force (Stensballe, Loom, Nielsen, & Tvede, 2005). Several hydrophilic-coated catheters are available (Figure 10.46), including the SpeediCath (Coloplast A/S, Denmark and Minneapolis), which has a hydrophilic ready-to-use coating; the Advance HydroSoft Hydrophilic (Hollister Inc., Libertyville, IL), which is an uncoated silicone/PVC catheter with gel; and the LoFric (AstraTech, Sweden), a catheter with a hydrophilic coating to which water is added prior to use. Some of the available products include sterile water in the package, making it easier to activate the catheter's hydrophilic coating. New designs of hydrophilic catheters have been developed for women that are small and stored in a small case that can easily fit in a pocket or purse and can be discarded (Biering-Sørensen, Hansen, Nielsen, & Looms, 2007) (Figure 10.44A).

In clinical practice, the reduction in the number of clinically significant UTIs is the most important issue with IC, and there may be a beneficial effect regarding UTI when using hydrophilic-coated catheters (Woodbury et al., 2008). A study of patients with SCI showed that the chance of *not* developing a UTI was double in the group using a hydrophilic-coated catheter (Speedi-Cath) when compared to the PVC catheter group over a 1-year period (DeRidder et al., 2005). However, there are disadvantages to using a hydrophilic-coated catheter for IC; it is a one-time use only device because surface drying times vary by product and some become "sticky" when dry.

Closed or Self-Contained Systems   Closed or self-contained systems provide all-inclusive prelubricated catheters in a drainage bag to ensure sterile catheterization. Some contain gloves, antiseptic swabs, and a waterproof underpad (Figure 10.47). The use of this sterile system may decrease chances of UTI. These systems are often referred to as "touchless" or "no-touch" because they have a no-touch sleeve that enables the person to grip the catheter through the sleeve, avoiding the need to touch the catheter (Hudson & Murahata, 2005) (Figure 10.48A–E). These systems are usually 100% latex-free and contain a prelubricated catheter. Some have a special guide mechanism (called a protective or introducer tip) at the top of the pocket (Figure 10.48D,E). It is recommended that the catheter be advanced into the introducer tip and the tip then inserted into the distal urethra. This allows the catheter to bypass bacteria present in the first portion (15 mm) of the urethra, preventing contamination of the catheter and introduction of bacteria into the bladder. This guide provides two main benefits: it keeps the catheter straight as it is advanced, and, when squeezed, it prevents the catheter from slipping during insertion (Newman, 2004).

Some closed systems are packaged as an entire sterile kit with all equipment needed, including sterile gloves, underpad, drape, antiseptic wipe, lubricant, and catheter in a drainage bag—everything the person will need during certain situations that require aseptic catheterization (e.g., when traveling) (Figure 10.49). Some systems include a hydrophilic-coated catheter that has a sterile water pouch (LoFric Primo [AstraTech, Sweden]) that is separate from the catheter for use for hydration prior to insertion (Figure 10.47B). Some are designed to aid emptying of urine by having a narrow integrated extension sleeve that easily attaches to a toilet for urine drainage (Figure 10.48C). Many of these systems have a "finger hold" for ease with grasping the bag (Figure 10.49).

Self-contained systems are also available that provide a coating of an antibacterial agent (e.g., nitrofurazone) in the outer layer of a silicone catheter to produce local antibacterial activity.

Catheterization Schedule

The catheterization schedule should be based on the urine volume. As a general rule, catheterized volume should not exceed 400 mL. When starting IC,

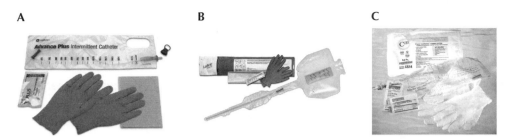

Figure 10.47.   Self-contained sterile catheter and bag systems, with all equipment needed for sterile catheterization. (Courtesy of Hollister [A], Astra Tech [B], and Cure Medical [C].)

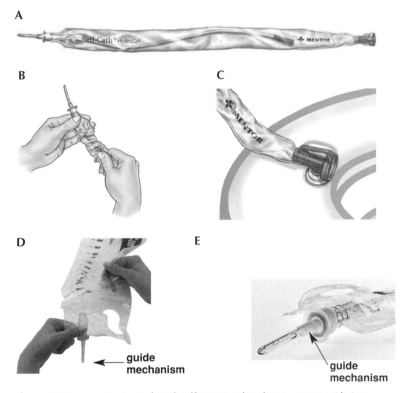

Figure 10.48.   *A, B, C,* Hydrogel self-contained catheter system with introducer guide mechanism and integrated extension sleeve with toilet attachment for urine drainage. *D, E,* InCare Advanced Plus with protective tip and guide mechanism. (Courtesy of Coloplast [A, B, C] and Hollister [D, E].)

the person, caregiver, or both should record the amount of urine drained from the bladder. If the person voids, catheterization should always be performed after voiding. Based on a person's average output, catheterization is usually done 4 times during the day. A survey of SCI community dwelling persons in Canada noted that most catheterize between 4–6 times per day regardless of type of catheter used (Woodbury et al., 2008).

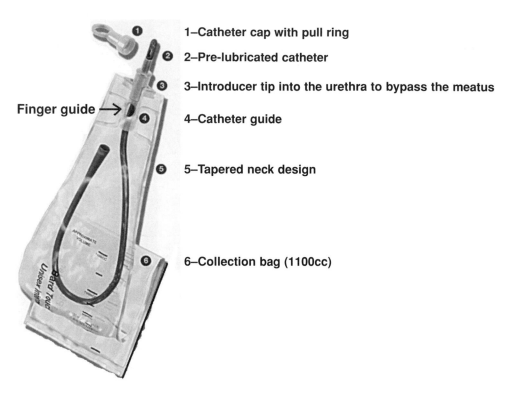

1–Catheter cap with pull ring

2–Pre-lubricated catheter

3–Introducer tip into the urethra to bypass the meatus

Finger guide ⟶

4–Catheter guide

5–Tapered neck design

6–Collection bag (1100cc)

Figure 10.49.   A closed catheter system with introducer tip. (Courtesy of CR Bard.)

Performing CISC

Age should not be a deterrent to IC because older patients with adequate cognitive function, mobility, motivation, and manual dexterity easily learn the technique of IC. A cooperative, well-motivated patient or family member and/or caregiver is a requirement. Patients who can feed themselves usually have the manual dexterity to self-catheterize.

Anatomic variations make self-catheterization difficult in women, especially if the woman is obese and unable to reach the perineum (Williams, 2005). Men with a large abdominal girth may be unable to visualize the urinary meatus or reach their penis. A man with a retracted penis will need to be taught to pull out the penis for catheter insertion or the catheter may push the retracted penis further back into the pubis. Also, it is difficult for women to perform IC in different locations and settings. Many women are taught to perform IC lying in bed and using a mirror to visualize the meatus. Most develop their own technique, but we recommend teaching women in the clinical setting using a mirror to point out structures in the perineum (the vaginal opening, clitoris, and meatus). However, a mirror is difficult to use in a toilet stall, so women are also taught IC using the "touch technique."

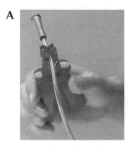 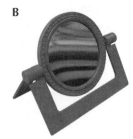 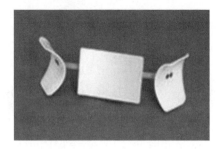

Figure 10.50. Self-catheterization aids: *A,* catheter holder and *B,* mirror. (Courtesy of Astra Tech.)

Figure 10.51. Knee spreader with mirror.

Aids such as mirrors to find the urethra and catheter handles are available that can be helpful for the person performing catheterization (Figure 10.50). In those individuals with limited dexterity, using a handle to insert catheters allows the user to hold the catheter firmly and direct it into the correct position. One aid that one of the authors (DKN) has found helpful in women who have abductor spasms or inability to separate their thighs is the knee spreader with mirror (Figure 10.51). This product is specially designed for self-catheterization. The mirror is attached with a hook and loop and may be removed as needed. The spreader provides 9 inches (23 cm) of abduction.

Teaching Self-catheterization

A knowledgeable and experienced clinician, usually a nurse, is an important component for successful self-catheterization teaching. There is a lack of uniformity and standardization in nursing practice in terms of performing self-catheterization. Initially, many patients have reservations and may be extremely reluctant to perform any procedure that involves the genitalia. They may have a fear of inability to perform catheterization. Providing an overview of anatomy with pictures or the use of an anatomic model of the perineum is very helpful. Many manufacturers provide videos (for adults and for children) that demonstrate catheterization. The nurse should assess baseline knowledge and learning ability to increase the chances for successful patient education. Most adults learn best under low to moderate stress, so teach self-catheterization in a low stress setting. The nurse should assess the patient's ability to learn the task effectively, motivation to continue with a procedure that could continue for a considerable period of time, awareness of problems associated with catheterization, and understanding of how to avoid associated problems such as UTI. An assessment of the patient's personal hygiene (handwashing and cleansing of the genitalia) is important to help avoid UTIs. A "refresher" lesson after the procedure will be more successful if there is prior knowledge to draw on. Clinicians should always provide written information to patients, caregivers, or both who have been taught to perform IC. The patient education tools "Using a Catheter—Women" and "Using a Catheter—Men" (on the companion CD) provide instruction for performing IC.

Catheter Use and Care

There are no clear guidelines about length of catheter use. The Department of Veterans Affairs (2007) recently issued guidance to clinicians on the reuse of urinary catheters for patients who use IC for bladder management. This guideline noted that urinary catheters are considered single-use devices by the FDA and that manufacturers of catheters specifically identify them as single use. The VA recommendation is that, until manufacturers specifically change labeling for urinary catheters, there is no policy interpretation that would allow the reuse of single-use urinary catheters in any setting. Therefore, clinicians who practice in the VA system are advised to follow the manufacturer's instructions for catheter use. Patients and caregivers should be told when catheters are identified for single use only. In the Pennsylvania Medicare jurisdiction, local coverage determinations for urological suppliers (L5080) were released that follows the VA recommendations but put the total catheters allowed per month at 200. Clinicians should prescribe patients with an adequate number of catheters to use a sterile catheter for each catheterization. However, most other insurers only cover four catheters per month, so most patients and clinicians reuse catheters for up to 7 days.

If reusing catheters, the cleaning of the catheter between uses is based on clinical practice. There is few data on actual patient practice. A survey of SCI persons in Canada noted that close to 80% of all individuals who reused their catheters did not disinfect them between uses (Woodbury et al., 2008). Recommended cleaning techniques include soap-and-water washing, boiling, microwave sterilization, and peroxide and povidone-iodine (Betadine) application. Rinsing and drying the catheter immediately after use is the best method for washing away any bacteria. Use of dishwashing soap or an antibacterial waterless product when catheterizing outside the home is perfectly adequate in our opinion. A home microwave oven may be used as a method to sterilize red-rubber catheters for reuse, with a recommended time of 12 minutes at full power. This technique makes aseptic IC a practical possibility. However, microwave ovens can cause catheters to melt (Bogaert et al., 2004). Patients should be encouraged to use a turntable if possible during microwave catheter sterilization.

URETHRAL INSERTS AND CLAMPS

Technological advances in the treatment of UI have been made through the development of internal and external urethral occlusive and compression devices for both men and women. Internal inserts or intraurethral devices are thin and flexible enough to insert directly into the urethra to obstruct the flow of urine into the proximal urethra. Some are single-use and disposable. They must be removed in order to urinate or opened to drain urine. External urethral devices are placed over the urinary meatus as a barrier or control pad to prevent rather than absorb urine loss. They have been developed primarily for women with mild to moderate stress UI. Internal devices have demonstrated higher efficacy (Sand et al., 1999) than external devices but have been associated with a higher incidence of complications such as urethral irritation, infection, and hematuria (Gallo et al., 1997; Staskin et al., 1996). According to one of the authors (AJW), the characteristics of an ideal occlusive or supportive device would include: 1) efficacy; 2) comfort; 3) ease of application/insertion/removal; 4) lack of interference with normal voiding; 5) lack of tissue damage; 6) lack of infection; 7) no compromise of subsequent therapy; 8) cosmetic acceptance and unobtrusive; 9) lack of interference with sexual activity. It would be nice if the device could be used continuously during the day while awake, however, many patients would be happy if the device worked well during certain activities that trigger UI symptoms (e.g., golfing, playing tennis) (Wein, 2002). Many of these devices fail because patients fear "putting something in or on me" and are concerned about discomfort or developing bleeding and/or infection. Patients also do not want to pay "out of pocket" for these devices, and insurers are unwilling to cover their repeated use. Clinicians did not recommend them to patients, as many do not understand the benefits from these devices and feel they may be harmful and will have no long-term benefit. Although many of the products developed are no longer available, especially in the United States, or are still awaiting FDA approval, it is important for the clinician who specializes in UI to understand this classification of devices. The following is a short review of these products.

Internal Urethral Inserts

Internal devices are inserted into the urethra to occlude or block urine leakage (Newman, 2006a). These have been referred to as urinary control inserts, intraurethral devices, occlusive devices, urethral inserts, and intraurethral prostheses. These devices have several common features: a meatal plate to prevent the device from migrating into the bladder, structures that enhance their retention within the urethra (e.g., inflatable balloons), and a device or mechanism to allow for an easy means of removal to permit voiding (e.g., a string) (Wein, 2002). When this category of incontinence device was introduced in the market, nurse researchers reported on results of studies in which female subjects felt that the device kept them drier, controlled odor better than other products, and gave them increased confidence during physical activities (Gallo et al., 1997). An initial design (Reliance) was catheter-like in construction and inserted by the woman into the urethra (Gallo et al., 1997; Sand et al., 1999). However, despite several clinical device trials with published results, this device is no longer available. A factor was the poor acceptance of

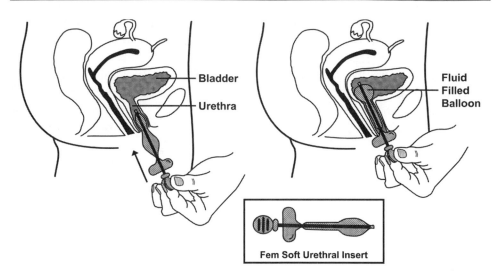

Figure 10.52.   FemSoft® urethral insert. (Courtesy of Robin Noel.)

the device by clinicians, who thought that adverse events of hematuria and UTI were unacceptable.

One of the current available devices, FemSoft® (Rochester Medical Corporation, Stewartville, MN), consists of a sterile, disposable, single-use, narrow silicone tube entirely enclosed in a soft, thin, mineral oil–filled silicone sleeve (Figure 10.52). As the insert is advanced into the urethra, fluid in the balloon is transferred toward the external retainer to facilitate passage through the urethra. Once the tip of the insert has entered the bladder, the fluid returns to fill the balloon, forming a mechanical barrier to retain urine within the bladder. To assist with insertion, the insert is supplied in a disposable applicator and with a lubricating gel. The device has a string for easy removal for normal voiding and should be removed at least once every 6 hours. It is available in three diameter sizes (16, 18, and 20 Fr) with two lengths (3.5 and 4.5 cm) for each diameter, and it is important that the insert be properly sized to the woman. The FemSoft® Insert is a prescription device and costs less than $2. Contraindications for use include the overactive bladder symptom of urgency (bladder contraction would expel the insert), primary urgency UI, active UTI, urethral stricture, and any anatomic or pathological urethral condition in which passage of a catheter is not clinically advisable.

As with most new technology, the cornerstone to successful use is patient education and available medical support, especially while the individual is learning to use the device. A 5-year ongoing, controlled multicenter study reported on 2-year follow-up in women using the FemSoft® device (Sirls et al., 2002). Statistically significant reductions in overall daily stress UI episodes were observed with the device at all follow-up intervals. Women were satisfied with ease of use of the device, comfort, and dryness, and significant improvements in quality of life were observed. Adverse events were transient

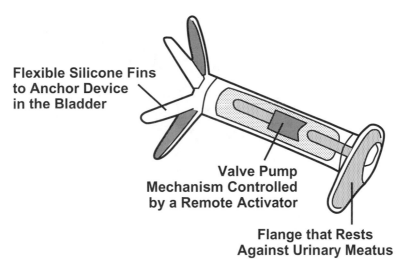

Flexible Silicone Fins to Anchor Device in the Bladder

Valve Pump Mechanism Controlled by a Remote Activator

Flange that Rests Against Urinary Meatus

Figure 10.53. InFlow intraurethral prosthesis. (Courtesy of Robin Noel.)

but included symptomatic UTI in 31.3%, mild trauma with insertion in 6.7%, hematuria in 3.3%, and migration in 1.3% of women. The authors concluded that this urethral insert should be considered as an option for the management of stress UI. Women tended to use this device episodically (e.g., when playing tennis).

Intraurethral prostheses to treat urinary retention in women and men are being developed. The management of women with chronically poorly emptying bladders is often by IC, but some women are unable to perform IC. As noted previously in this chapter, many elderly individuals are incapable of mastering the technique; arthritis, poor eyesight, mental illness, and neurological conditions (e.g., Parkinson's disease) can all make it impossible for the person to use IC.

In many cases, caregivers are not available to perform IC for the person. Many women also refuse to learn the technique. Although many experts see a need for a device that can occlude or "plug" the urethra, such devices have had a difficult time being approved by the FDA. One device currently being investigated is the InFlow™ intraurethral valve and pump (SRS Medical Systems, Inc., Billerica, MA) (Figure 10.53). The device consists of a short silicone catheter sheath of differing lengths to allow for variance in the length of the urethra. The device secures itself in the urethra by means of flexible fins that open in the bladder to maintain a position at the bladder neck and a flange at the external urinary meatus to prevent migration of the entire device into the bladder. There is an inner valve pump consisting of a magnet shaped like a turbine. The device is controlled by a remote activator that is placed over the pubic area and is magnetically coupled to the pump. Once activated, the turbine actively pumps urine out of the bladder at a rate of 6–12 mL per second until the bladder is empty. When the magnetic field is removed or reversed,

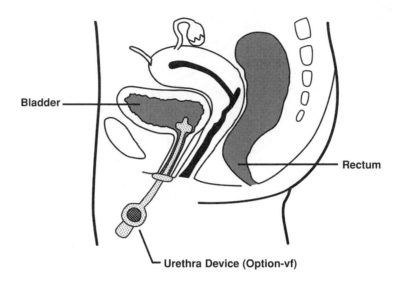

Figure 10.54.   OPTION-*vf* ™ urethral insert. (Courtesy of Robin Noel.)

the valve closes and the turbine stops spinning, maintaining continence. The device is easily inserted by a clinician and can be removed by the patient. The device is designed to be replaced every month, but successful usage to an average of 90 days has been reported, at which time the device can develop salt deposits. The prosthesis can remain in the bladder for several weeks as an alternative to IC. Adverse events include discomfort, irritation, UTI, mucous plugs, detrusor overactivity, and technical dysfunction. The lack of urethral sensations in a person with SCI may be a problem because he or she may not feel discomfort and may be unaware of local irritation or migration. The longer urethra of the man makes these devices more difficult to place and remove.

Chen et al. (2005) compared the safety, effectiveness, and user satisfaction of the InFlow versus the current standard of care (IC) for women with hypocontractile or acontractile bladder. The study was a multicenter, prospective, single-arm crossover 12-month study. A total of 273 women with a mean age of 48.9 years using IC entered the study, but only a small portion (*n* = 77) completed the InFlow treatment phase. The authors concluded that the InFlow™ catheter appears to be a viable alternative to IC in women unsatisfied with currently available treatments because they can achieve enhanced independence and quality of life with its use.

Another device is a valved urinary catheter (OPTION-*vf*™ and OPTION-*vm*™, Opticon Medical) that eliminates the need for a system of urine drainage bags and connecting tubes normally required with an indwelling urinary catheter (Figure 10.54). This insert is similar to an indwelling urinary catheter but incorporates a manually activated valve (like a catheter valve) at the end of the catheter that allows the person to store urine and to mimic normal voiding behavior. It has an adaptor so it can connect to a drainage bag. There is a valved urinary catheter for men similar in design and function to the one for women.

External Urethral Devices

An external urethral barrier or "blocking" device is placed over the urinary meatus via adhesive or suction to prevent mild to moderate stress UI in women (Newman, 2006a). The urethral barrier prevents rather than absorbs urine loss and must be removed before voiding. It has been referred to as a "continence control pad." The efficacy of one type of external device in terms of reducing urinary leakage was found to be good (Miniguard; >50% of subjects dry) by some researchers (Brubaker, Harris, Gleason, Newman, & North, 1999), whereas others have found poor reduction in urine leakage and high subject dropout rates (FemAssist) (Tincello, Adams, Bolderson, & Richmond, 2000). Adverse events include urinary meatus and vulvar irritation, possible urethrocele formation, poor adhesion, fitting difficulty, and discomfort.

The first type of external barrier device developed was a soft suction cup made of silicone (the original version was called FemAssist) that was placed externally over the urinary meatal area (Shinopulos, Dann, & Smith, 1999). Before placement, an adhesive gel was applied to the edge of the device and the central dome was squeezed to create a vacuum. The device was then placed over the meatus and the dome released to create a suction-like seal. The device was not intended as a reservoir that collected the urine during leakage. It was designed so that the suction from the device created negative pressure, which enabled coaptation of the urethral walls, thereby increasing urethral pressure (Wein, 2002). The negative pressure within the device was optimized to counteract the pressure created by activities that would usually cause stress UI in women, thereby keeping the woman dry. The device was marketed as the CapSure (Figure 10.55) (Bellin et al., 1998). It could be worn for a maximum of 4 hours, washed with soap and water, and reused. One device could be reused for 1–2 weeks.

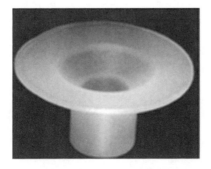

Figure 10.55. CapSure suction external urethral device. (Courtesy of CR Bard.)

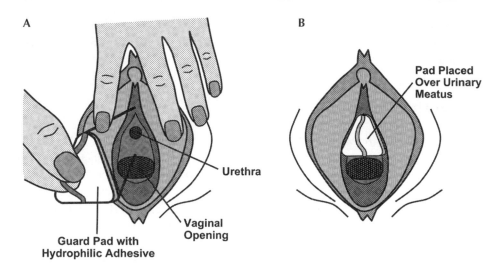

Figure 10.56.   Miniguard external urethral barrier. (Courtesy of Robin Noel.)

A second device, the urinary control pad, was a small, triangular foam pad with a layer of hydrophilic adhesive on one side (called the Miniguard). The adhesive was a hydrogel-coated material that permitted application to the intralabial epithelium (over the urinary meatus), just anterior to the vaginal introitus, without irritation or discomfort during use or removal (Figure 10.56). The device was fitted over the meatus and easily removed for voiding. It was a disposable, single-use product that would become dislodged and fall off when the woman voided. In a nationwide clinical trial, women with stress UI who used the urinary control pad were significantly drier, were less afraid of odor and embarrassment, and had an enhanced quality of life (Brubaker et al., 1999).

Studies of single-use suction devices have demonstrated significant improvements in subjective and objective (pad test) outcomes. Adverse effects have usually been transient and include vulvar and lower urinary tract irritation, vaginal irritation, and UTIs. These external urethral suction devices were removed from the market because of the belief that the constant suction on the urinary meatus may cause urethral prolapse. Currently there are no such devices available on the market in the United States. Methods to produce a leak-free occlusion while maintaining tissue perfusion and skin health are needed for women and men (Newman et al., 2004).

Penile Compression Device

A penile compression or "clamp" device is an external occlusive device that is often used by men after prostate cancer surgery to stop stress UI, or by men with continuous urine leakage. These devices mechanically compress the soft tissue of the penis by applying external urethral pressure, thus preventing any flow or leakage out of the urethra. Used correctly, penile compression devices are one method of controlling UI in certain men who are cognitively intact, have normal genital sensation, have intact penile skin, have adequate penile length, are aware of bladder filling, and have sufficient manual dexterity to open and close the device when applied at a comfortable pressure. Usually the device is placed halfway down the shaft of the penis and then tightened to compress the urethra.

These devices are either inflatable or similar to a mechanical clamp (Figure 10.57). They are reusuable. One type of device (Cunningham compression device; Davol, CR Bard) is a hinged stainless steel frame supporting two foam rubber pads, with a locking device (Figure 10.57A,B). The user places the penis between the two foam pads, which conform to fit the penis, and the hinged clamp is squeezed shut. The lower foam pad on the device has an inverted "V" shape that presses against the underside of the penis, exerting a closing pressure on the urethra, which is close to the underside of the penis. The clamping mechanism has five separate settings to control male incontinence. This permits the user to achieve the proper amount of pressure with the device to prevent urine leakage without discomfort. The device is reusable and sized by penis circumference (not length). A second type of compression device uses Velcro to close the foam pads (Baumrucker clamp) (Figure 10.57C). A third is adjustable, encircling the penis, and inflated with air to stop the flow of urine (Cook Continence Cuff) (Figure 10.57E). A fourth penile compression clamp is the ActiCuf compression pouch. This clamp has an absorbent attachment for men with stress UI (Figure 10.57D). A fifth is the C-3 penile clamp that has a contoured, cradle-like design with a Velcro elastic strap that is wrapped evenly around the penis to hold the device in position (Figure 10.57F).

Clinically, it appears that men with normal sensation are able to judge when the compression is too tight or the time too lengthy and will release the device as required. Moore et al. (2004) conducted a study to assess the safety, efficacy, comfort, and user satisfaction with three penile compression devices: the Cunningham Penile Clamp, C-3, and U-Tex. Subjects were men ($N = 12$) who had undergone prostate cancer surgery in the past 6 months. Penile Doppler ultrasonography was performed to assess circulatory impedance with and without the compression device in place. Color flow assessment was made distal to the device. The results indicated that the Cunningham device was the most efficacious and most acceptable to users, but also contributed to reduced systolic velocity in all men. None of the devices completely eliminated urine loss.

A penile clamp should be used with caution, and is only appropriate for men who have penile sensation and good manual dexterity and will comply with proper care and use of the product. There is very little research documenting effectiveness and complications of these products, and many urologists are reluctant to prescribe them. Potential complications including edema, urethral erosion, pain, and obstruction limit their use. Soft tissue damage by excess compression can occur with these clamps and thus their use is extremely risky in men with neurologic disease and sensory impairment (Wein, 2002). Skin breakdown, swelling, and strictures (scarring) can occur inside the

A

Spring Wire Loops

Ratchet Catch with Notches

Hump Side (placed on the underside of the penis)

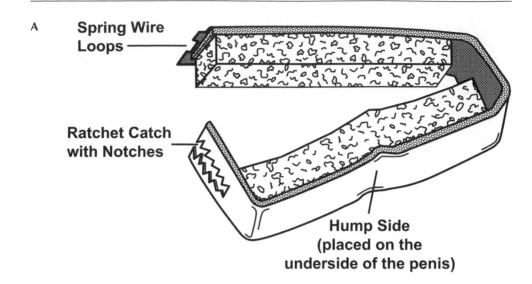

B

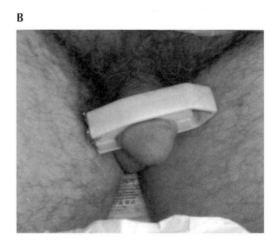

C

Velcro Strap Spring Wire Loops

Foam Pads Hump Side (placed on the underside of the penis)

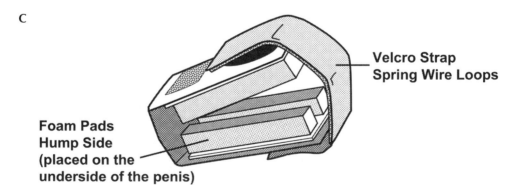

Figure 10.57.   Penile compression devices: *A,* Cunningham Penile Clamp (courtesy of Robin Noel). *B,* Cunningham Penile Clamp in place, mid-shaft (courtesy of Bard/Davol). *C,* Baumrucker clamp (courtesy of Robin Noel). *D,* ActiCuf (courtesy of GT Urological). *E,* inflatable Cook Continence Cuff (courtesy of Cook Medical). *F,* C-3 Penile Clamp (courtesy of SRS Medical).

D

E

F

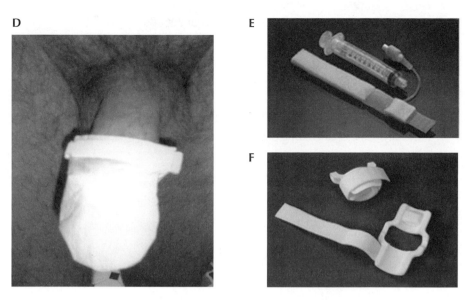

Figure 10.57   *(continued)*

urethra if a clamp is left in place too long. If used properly and released every 1–2 hours for bladder emptying, these devices can be very beneficial. Men who use a wheelchair may place a clamp over the penis when they transfer from bed to chair and vice versa. Others will keep the device on their penis loosely and only compress the device when they move from position to position. Many individuals ask if they can have a device so they can swim. Users must be told about potential complications associated with these devices and should be given written instructions on their correct use.

CONCLUSION

Patients with incontinence, family members, and clinicians are often confused about or unaware of various types of urine collection products, such as catheters, and their effectiveness in treating UI. These products are often used long term and can improve a patient's quality of life and decrease caregiver burden. Many urinary catheters, absorbent products, and collection devices are available at local pharmacies, retail stores, and medical equipment dealers or directly from manufacturers. Others require close medical supervision for initiation and follow up. Medicare and other major insurers will usually pay for only a limited monthly supply of most of these products. Most health maintenance organizations (HMOs) and managed care insurers routinely do not pay for them, but some HMOs follow Medicare guidelines for payment. Absorbent products (pads, adult briefs) sold in retail stores and through mail-order catalogs are considered personal hygiene products, and their cost is not covered by insurers.

Appendix Table 10.1   Product (HCPC) billing codes (as of 2008)

A4315	Catheter with insertion tray, drainage bag, and silicone catheter
A4326	Male external catheter
A4328	Female urinary collection pouch
A4331	Extension drainage tubing
A4332	Lubricant, sterile packet (max allowed 200 per month)
A4333	Urinary catheter anchoring device
A4334	Urinary catheter leg strap
A4338	Indwelling catheter, latex with couting (coudé)
A4340	Indwelling catheter, special
A4344	Catheter, indwelling, Foley, 2-way, silicone
A4349	Disposable male external catheter
A4351	Straight-tip intermittent urinary catheter with or without coating (max allowed 200 per month)
A4352	Coudé-tip intermittent urinary catheter with or without coating (max allowed 200 per month)
A4353	Intermittent urinary catheter with insertion supplies (max allowed 200 per month)
A4356	External urethral clamp or compression device
A4357	Bedside drainage bag
A4358	Urinary leg or abdomen bag
A4359	Urinary suspensory, without leg bag
A4365	Adhesive remover wipes
A4369	Skin barrier liquid (per ounce)
A4371	Skin barrier powder (per ounce)
A4379	Urinary plastic pouch, with faceplate
A4380	Urinary rubber pouch, with faceplate
A4381	Urinary plastic pouch, without faceplate
A4382	Urinary heavy plastic pouch, without faceplate
A4383	Urinary rubber pouch, without faceplate
A4391	Urinary pouch, with external wear barrier
A4561	Pessary, rubber, any type
A4562	Pessary, nonrubber, any type
A5105	Urinary suspensory
A5112	Urinary leg bag
A5113	Leg strap (latex)
A5114	Leg strap (foam)

Appendix Table 10.2 Review of current skin care products

Product	Description	Common ingredients	Types	Indications
Perineal cleansers	Help emulsify and loosen stool and urine and cleanse the skin.	Combination of water and a surfactant, a surface-active agent (e.g., sodium lauryl sulfate). Some perineal cleansers are also formulated with topical antimicrobials (e.g., triclosan, chlorhexidine gluconate) that may reduce odor, or decrease or limit the bacteria on the skin.	Available in both rinse and no-rinse formulas. Types include liquid, emulsion, foam, and active product impregnated in soft towelette.	Removal of irritants such as urine and feces from the surface of the perineum without compromising its acid mantle, and minimizing the loss of lipids. Products with antimicrobials should not be used for routine, daily skin care because they may damage the skin by causing irritation and altering normal skin flora.
Moisturizers	Increase water content and elasticity and improve desquamation by either trapping water in or allowing water to be drawn from the dermis into the epidermis.	**Humectants** (e.g., glycerin, *Aloe barbendensis*, PEG-10) draw water into the stratum corneum. **Emollients** (e.g., mineral oil, lanolin, PEG-80, cetyl laurate) soften skin and improve texture. **Occlusives** (petrolatum, mineral oil) prevent evaporation of water from the stratum corneum.	**Lotions**—composed of powder and held in suspension by surfactants. They have the highest water content, evaporate more quickly and therefore need to be applied frequently. Lotions are easy to apply, have a cooling effect, are nonocclusive, and do not leave a greasy film on the skin. **Creams**—either preparations of water in oil or oil in water. They are more occlusive than lotions and need to be applied frequently for maximum effectiveness. **Ointments**—mixtures of water in oil: are the most occlusive. The oil component can be either lanolin or petrolatum. It is believed that petrolatum is more effective on skin and may have a more lasting effect than either lotions or creams.	To preserve the moisture in the skin by either sealing in existing moisture or adding moisture to the skin. To lubricate and soften rough, scaly skin; to prevent cracks and fissures that can harbor bacteria; and to soothe red, inflamed skin.

(continued)

Appendix Table 10.2 *(continued)*

Product	Description	Common ingredients	Types	Indications
Barrier or skin protectants	Provide protection for "at-risk" skin and shield the skin from exposure to irritants and moisture. Moisture barriers protect the skin by coating the surface of the skin, by supplying lipids that can penetrate the intracellular spaces of the stratum corneum, or both. Liquid barrier films, often referred to as skin sealants, contain a polymer combined with a solvent, usually alcohol. When applied to the skin, the solvent evaporates, allowing the polymer to dry and form a barrier. The alcohol can be painful and irritating to skin, so its use should be avoided on compromised skin.	**Petrolatum** is a semisolid product derived from distilling off the lighter portions of petroleum. It performs better as a barrier against skin maceration and protectant against urine. It is less effective against stool, particularly liquid stool. **Dimethicone** is an oil derived from silicone. It provides a water-repellent barrier and is considered to be the barrier of the future. It is nonocclusive and compatible with the stratum corneum. Aqueous formulations containing dimethicone can perform better as a moisturizer because they are less occlusive and less greasy than petrolatum and zinc. **Zinc oxide** is a white powder with mild antiseptic and astringent properties. When mixed with a petrolatum base, it is effective against both urine and stool. However, it is greasy and difficult to remove. To remove zinc oxide paste, the person must use mineral oil and avoid excessive scrubbing.	***Moisture Barriers:*** **Creams**—water-based preparations that contain lanolin. To prevent occlusion of the stratum corneum, nonocclusive (breathable) creams are preferred. **Ointments**—thick, anhydrous semisolids that are occlusive. The oil component of ointments is typically petrolatum. Ointments tend to last longer than creams and will have a longer lasting effect. ***Liquid Barrier Films:*** **Pastes**—mixtures of an ointment with powder added for durability. A common ingredient is zinc oxide. Pastes can be difficult to remove, causing additional damage. Pastes with petrolatum are easier to remove. **Powders**—absorb excessive moisture and reduce friction and erosion. Cornstarch is preferred over talc powders. Powders should be applied as a light dusting because caking may enhance friction and erosion, especially in the area of perineal skinfolds.	Barrier skin products can be differentiated into two general types: one works by forming a film on the skin after evaporation of a solvent and the other, such as ointments and creams, forms a hydrophobic, physical barrier. Pastes are used to absorb excessive drainage and to block exposure to irritants if exudates are present in areas of perineal skin erosion. Pastes are often used to protect or treat skin that is frequently exposed to liquid stool, because these types of barrier products are more resistant to cleansing and enzymatic breakdown. Powders are often used for perianal skin care in people with fecal incontinence. A liquid film barrier should not be combined with a barrier cream or paste because these products are often incompatible. Adding an occlusive moisture barrier enhances the penetration into the liquid barrier. It is recommended that liquid barrier films be allowed to dry before applying an occlusive product.

Appendix Table 10.3   Troubleshooting common problems with long-term indwelling urinary catheterization

Problem	Causes	Intervention
Inadvertent dislodgment (catheter falling out, usually with balloon inflated)	Occurs in 41% of people with indwelling catheters. *Causes:* • Person pulling the catheter out because of confusion or discomfort; may occur in the person who does not like or want the catheter. • Secondary to catheter tension, where increased pressure and weight on the catheter cause it to dislodge. • Bladder overactivity (bladder spasms) may cause expulsion of catheter with balloon intact.	• Consider alternative urinary collection device. • Secure catheter appropriately. • Consider changing catheter more frequently. • Empty drainage bag more frequently to avoid added weight on catheter and tubing. • Assess for causes of bladder spasms, such as too-large catheter or balloon size. • Consider prescribing an antimuscarinic drug (see Chapter 9).
Leakage of urine around the catheter (referred to as "catheter bypassing")	Occurs 65% of the time and causes more catheter changes than any other reason. *Causes:* • Bladder spasms or overactivity • Infection • Obstruction, encrustation, and catheter blockage • Kinked catheter or tubing • Catheter size too large • Constipation • Secondary to an irritated bladder mucosa caused by long-term catheter use • Catheter dislodged (balloon in the urethra) • Bladder calculi	• If infection is suspected, consider treatment and subsequent acidification and dilution of urine to prevent recurrence. • Consider changing catheter more frequently. • Educate person/caregiver to regularly check tubing for kinking or twisting (e.g., place tubing over, not under, thigh). • Secure catheter. • Perform digital rectal exam to check for fecal impaction. Place person on bowel regimen or laxatives as needed (see Chapter 5). • Consider antimuscarinic drug (see Chapter 9). • Suggest yearly cystoscopy with urology consult.
Obstruction or blockage of catheter ("urine not draining")	Occurs in over 50% of people with long-term catheters. *Cause:* encrustation resulting from the collection of urease-producing organisms that build up on the catheter surface. This causes crystallization of protein, or mucous plugs. Crystalline deposits can reduce the catheter lumen, cover the balloon, and obstruct the eyes at the tip of the catheter, the lumen of the catheter, or both (Morris, Stickler, & Winters, 1997). Formation of encrustation usually occurs around the tip of the catheter, around the balloon, or within the catheter lumen.	• Make sure catheter is not kinked, twisted, or looped. • If encrustation causes occlusion of the catheter, the entire system needs to be changed. • Monitor time it takes for blockage to occur and plan catheter change prior to likely blockage. • Perform digital rectal check to determine if catheter is blocked by fecal material (impaction). • Assess for urinary tract infection. • If recurrent, consider changing to another catheter material (e.g., silicone).

(continued)

471

Problem	Causes	Intervention
Catheter/balloon malfunction	Failure of the balloon to deflate as a result of malfunction of inflation valve, or obstruction of the inflation channel by external encrustation of the balloon.	Method for deflation is controversial. Some advocate hyperinflation of the balloon (2–5 mL) to the point where it bursts, whereas others advocate the passage of a small narrow-gauge guidewire or tubular stylet into the lumen of the balloon inflation channel either to unblock it, to pop the balloon, or to permit drainage of the balloon through the stylet. Others discourage injections of air, water, or any chemical into the balloon port to rupture the balloon (Patterson, Little, Tolan, & Sweeney, 2006). Also, one can use ultrasound to localize the balloon and a percutaneous needle to pop and deflate it.
Pain and urethral discomfort	More than 50% of people find catheters painful (Saint, Lipsky, Baker, McDonald, & Ossenkop, 1999). Discomfort may be secondary to catheter's size (too large) or occlusion of periurethral glands. May be secondary to bladder spasms (overactivity).	• Decrease catheter size. Use large amounts of lubrication (e.g., K-Y jelly) at time of insertion to decrease pain and discomfort. Lubricate the urethra, not just the catheter. • Consider removal of catheter and alternative management of bladder disorder. • Consider prescribing an antimuscarinic drug.

REFERENCES

Abrams, P., Agarwal, M., Drake, M., El-Masri, W., Fulford, S., Reid, S., Singh, G., & Tophill, P. (2008). A proposed guideline for the urological management of patients with spinal cord injury. *British Journal of Urology International, 101*(8), 989–994.

Abrams, P., Cardozo, L., Fall, M., Griffiths, D., Rosier, P., Ulmsten, U., et al. (2002). The standardisation of terminology in lower urinary tract function: Report from the Standardisation Sub-Committee of the International Continence Society. *Neurourology and Urodynamics, 21*, 167–178.

Addison, R. (1999). Catheter valves: A special focus on the Bard Flip-Flo catheter. *British Journal of Nursing, 8*(9), 576–580.

Ahearn, D.G., Grace, D.T., Jennings, M.J., Borazjani, R.N., Boles, K.J., Rose, L.J., et al. (2000). Effects of hydrogel/silver coatings on in vitro adhesion to catheters of bacteria associated with urinary tract infections. *Current Microbiology, 41*, 120–125.

Anderson, R.U. (1980). Non-sterile intermittent catheterization with antibiotic prophylaxis in the acute spinal cord injured male patient. *Journal of Urology, 124*, 392–394.

Baker, J., & Norton, P. (1996). Evaluation of absorbent products for women with mild to moderate urinary incontinence. *Applied Nursing Research, 9*(1), 29–36.

Bellin, P., Smith, J., Poll, W., Bogojavlensky, S., Knoll, D., Childs, S., et al. (1998). Results of a multicenter trial of the CapSure (Re/Stor) Continence shield on women with stress urinary incontinence. *Urology, 51*, 697–706.

Biering-Sørensen, F., Bagi, P., & Hoiby, N. (2001). Urinary tract infections in patients with spinal cord lesions: Treatment and prevention. *Drugs, 61*, 1275–1287.

Biering-Sørensen, F., Hansen, H.V., Nielsen, P.N., & Looms, D. (2007). Residual urine after intermittent catheterization in females using two different catheters. *Scandinavian Journal of Urology and Nephrology, 41*, 341–345.

Bliss, D.Z., Zehner, C., Savik, K., Thayer, D., & Smith, G. (2006). Incontinence-associated skin damage in nursing home residents: A secondary analysis of a prospective multicenter study. *Ostomy/Wound Management, 52*(12), 46–55.

Bogaert, G.A., Goeman, L., De Ridder, D., Wevers, M., Ivens, J., & Schuermans, A. (2004). The physical and antimicrobial effects of microwave heating and alcohol immersion on catheters that are reused for clean intermittent catheterisation. *European Urology, 46*, 641–646.

Brazzelli, M., Shirran, E., & Vale, L. (2002). Absorbent products for containing urinary and/or fecal incontinence in adults. *Journal of Wound, Ostomy, and Continence Nursing, 29*, 45–54.

Brosnahan, J., Jull, A., & Tracy, C. (2004). Types of urethral catheters for management of short-term voiding problems in hospitalized patients. *Cochrane Database of Systematic Reviews,* (1), CD004013.

Brubaker, L., Harris, T., Gleason, D., Newman, D.K., & North, B., for the Miniguard Investigators Group. (1999). The external urethral barrier for stress incontinence: A multicenter trial of safety and efficacy. *Obstetrics and Gynecology, 93*, 932–937.

Bryant, R. (2000). Skin pathology and types of damage. In R.A. Bryant (Ed.), *Acute and chronic wounds* (pp. 125–156). St. Louis: C.V. Mosby.

Cardenas, D.D., Hoffman, J.M., Kelly, E., & Mayo, M.E. (2004). Impact of a urinary tract infection educational program in persons with spinal cord injury. *Journal of Spinal Cord Medicine, 27*, 47–54.

Centers for Medicare & Medicaid Services. (2004). *State Operations Manual, Appendix PP—Guidance to Surveyors for Long-Term Care Facilities, Tag F314, §483.25(c) Pressure Sores* (Rev. 4, Issued 11-12-2004) (pp. 129–166). Retrieved April 1, 2006, from http://cms.hhs.gov/manuals/Downloads/som107ap_pp_guidelines_ltcf.pdf

Centers for Medicare & Medicaid Services. (2005). *State Operations Manual, Appendix PP—Guidance to Surveyors for Long-Term Care Facilities, Tag F315, §483.25(d) Urinary*

Incontinence (Rev. 8, Issued: 06-28-05, Effective: 06-28-05, Implementation: 06-28-05) (pp. 184–219). Retrieved November 11, 2007, from http://www.cms.hhs.gov/transmittals/downloads/R8SOM.pdf

Chen, T.Y., Ponsot, Y., Carmel, M., Bouffard, N., Kennelly, M.J., & Tu, L.M. (2005). Multicentre study of intraurethral valve-pump catheter in women with a hypocontractile or acontractile bladder. *European Urology, 48,* 628–633.

Clarke, S.A., Samuel, M., & Boddy, S.A. (2005). Are prophylactic antibiotics necessary with clean intermittent catheterization? A randomized controlled trial. *Journal of Pediatric Surgery, 40,* 568–571.

Clarke-O'Neill, S., Pettersson, L., Fader, M., Cottenden, A., & Brooks, R. (2004). A multicenter comparative evaluation: Disposable pads for women with light incontinence. *Journal of Wound, Ostomy, and Continence Nursing, 31,* 32–42.

Clarke-O'Neill, S., Pettersson, L., Fader, M., Dean, G., Brooks, R., & Cottenden, A. (2002). A multicentre comparative evaluation: Washable pants with an integral pad for light incontinence. *Journal of Clinical Nursing, 11,* 79–89.

Cornia, P.B., Amory, J.K., Fraser, S., Saint, S., & Lipsky, B.A. (2003). Computer-based order entry decreases duration of indwelling urinary catheterization in hospitalized patients. *American Journal of Medicine, 114,* 404–407.

Cottenden, A. Bliss, D., Fader, M., Getliffe, K., Herrara, H., Paterson, J., et al. (2005). Management with continence products. In P. Abrams, L. Cardozo, A. Khoury, & A. Wein (Eds.), *Incontinence: Proceedings from the Third International Consultation on Incontinence* (pp. 149–253). Plymouth, United Kingdom: Health Publications, Ltd.

Cottenden, A.M., Fader, M.J., Pettersson, L., & Brooks, R.J. (2003). How well does ISO 11948-1 (the Rothwell method) for measuring the absorption capacity of incontinence pads in the laboratory correlate with clinical pad performance? *Medical Engineering and Physics, 25,* 603–613.

Day, A.N. (1996). *Characteristics of elderly home health care user: Data from the 1994 National Home and Hospice Care Survey.* Atlanta: Centers for Disease Control and Prevention.

Delnay, K.M., Stonehill, W.H., Goldman, H., Jukkola, A.F., & Dmochowski, R.R. (1999). Bladder histological changes associated with chronic indwelling urinary catheter. *Journal of Urology, 161*(4), 1106–1108.

Department of Veterans Affairs. (2007, December 13). *Letter on intermittent catheterization and the use of sterile catheters* (DC IL 10-2007-018). Washington, DC: Author.

De Ridder, D.J., Everaert, K., Fernández, L.G., Valero, J.V., Durán, A.B., Abrisqueta, M.L., et al. (2005). Intermittent catheterisation with hydrophilic-coated catheters (SpeediCath) reduces the risk of clinical urinary tract infection in spinal cord injured patients: A prospective randomised parallel comparative trial. *European Urology, 48,* 991–995.

Dille, C.A., Kirchhoff, K.T., Sullivan, J.J., & Larson, E. (1993). Increasing the wearing time of vinyl urinary drainage bags by decontamination with bleach. *Archives of Physical Medicine and Rehabilitation, 74*(4), 431–437.

Diokno, A.C., Mitchell, B.A., Nash, A.J., & Kimbrough, J.A. (1995). Patient satisfaction and the Lofric catheter for clean intermittent catheterization. *Journal of Urology, 153,* 349–351.

Donlan, R.M. (2001). Biofilm formation: A clinically relevant microbiological process. *Clinical Infectious Diseases, 33,* 1387–1392.

Donlan, R.M., & Costerton, J.W. (2002). Biofilms: Survival mechanisms of clinically relevant microorganisms. *Clinical Microbiology Reviews, 15,* 167–193.

Drekonja, D.M., Kuskowski, M.A., Wilt, T.J., & Johnson, J.R. (2008). Antimicrobial urinary catheters: A systematic review. *Expert Review of Medical Devices, 5*(4), 495–506.

Drinka, P.J., Stemper, M.E., Gauerke, C., Millerm, J., & Reed, K.D. (2003). Apparent transmission of two species of gram-negative rods in catheterized residents in a 50-bed nursing home unit. *Infection Control and Hospital Epidemiology, 24,* 233.

Duffy, L.M., Cleary, J., Ahern, S., Kuskowski, M.A., West, M., Wheeler, L., et al. (1995). Clean intermittent catheterization: Safe, cost-effective bladder management for male residents of VA nursing homes. *Journal of the American Geriatrics Society, 43,* 865–870.

Dumigan, D.G., Kohan, C.A., Reed, C.R., Jekel, J.F., & Fikrig, M.K. (1998). Utilizing National Nosocomial Infection Surveillance System data to improve urinary tract infection rates in three intensive-care units. Nosocomial Infection Team. *Clinical Performance and Quality Health Care, 6,* 172–178.

Dunn, S., Kowanko, I., Paterson, J., & Pretty, L. (2002). Systematic review of the effectiveness of urinary continence products. *Journal of Wound, Ostomy, and Continence Nursing, 29,* 129–142.

Dunn, S., Pretty, L., Reid, H., & Evans, D. (2000). *Management of short term indwelling urethral catheters to prevent urinary tract infections: A systematic review.* Adelaide, South Australia: The Joanna Briggs Institute for Evidence Based Nursing and Midwifery.

Dunne, W.M., Jr. (2002). Bacterial adhesion: Seen any good biofilms lately? *Clinical Microbiology Reviews, 15*(2), 155–166.

Easton, S. (2000). InstantCath from Hollister: Pre-lubricated self-catheterization. *British Journal of Nursing, 9,* 357–360.

Edlich, R.F., Bailey T., Pine, S.A., Williams, R., Rodeheaver, G.T., & Steers, W.D. (2000). Biomechanical performance of silicone and latex external condom catheters. *Journal of Long-Term Effects of Medical Implants, 10,* 291–299.

Edlich, R.F., Winters, K.L., Long, W.B. 3rd, & Gubler, K.D. (2006). Scientific basis for the selection of absorbent underpads that remain securely attached to underlying bed or chair. *Journal of Long-Term Effects of Medical Implants, 16,* 29–40.

Emr, K., & Ryan, R. (2004). Best practice for indwelling catheter in the home setting. *Home Healthcare Nurse, 22,* 820–830.

Evans, E.C., & Gray, M. (2003). What interventions are effective for the prevention and treatment of cutaneous candidiasis? *Journal of Wound, Ostomy, and Continence Nursing, 30,* 11–16.

Fader, M. (2003). Review of current technologies for urinary incontinence: Strengths and limitations. *Proceedings of the Institution of Mechanical Engineers: Part H: Journal of Engineering in Medicine, 217,* 233–241.

Fader, M., Cottenden, A., & Brooks, R. (2001). The CPE network: Creating an evidence base for continence product selection. *Journal of Wound, Ostomy, and Continence Nursing, 28,* 106–112.

Fader, M., Cottenden, A.M., & Getliffe, K. (2007). Absorbent products for light urinary incontinence in women. *Cochrane Database of Systematic Reviews,* (2), CD001406.

Fader, M., Macaulay, M., Pettersson, L., Brooks, R., & Cottenden, A. (2006). A multicentre evaluation of absorbent products for men with light urinary incontinence. *Neurourology and Urodynamics, 25,* 689–695.

Fader, M., Moore, K.N., Cottenden, A.M., Pettersson, L., Brooks, R., & Malone-Lee, J. (2001). Coated catheters for intermittent catheterization: Smooth or sticky? *BJU International, 88,* 373–377.

Fader, M., Pettersson, L., Brooks, R., Dean, G., Wells, M., Cottenden, A., et al. (1997). A multicentre comparative evaluation of catheter valves. *British Journal of Nursing, 6,* 359, 362–364, 366–367.

Fader, M., Pettersson, L., Dean, G., Brooks, R., & Cottenden, A. (1999). The selection of female urinals: Results of a multicentre evaluation. *British Journal of Nursing, 8,* 918–925.

Fader, M., Pettersson, L., Dean, G., Brooks, R., Cottenden, A.M., & Malone-Lee, J. (2001). Sheaths for urinary incontinence: A randomized crossover trial. *BJU International, 88,* 367–372.

Fantl, J., Newman, D., Colling, J., DeLancey, J.O.L., Keeys, C., Loughery, R., et al. for the Urinary Incontinence in Adults Guideline Update Panel. (1996). *Urinary incontinence in adults: Acute and chronic management. Clinical practice guideline No. 2: Update* (AHCPR Publication No. 96-0692). Rockville, MD: Agency for Health Care and Policy Research.

Fernandez, R.S., & Griffiths, R.D. (2005). Clamping short-term indwelling catheters: A systematic review of the evidence. *Journal of Wound, Ostomy, and Continence Nursing, 32,* 329–336.

Gallo, M.L., Gillette, B., Hancock, R., Pelkey, A., Rawlings, L., & Sasso, K. (1997). Quality of life improvement and the Reliance urinary control insert. *Urologic Nursing, 17,* 146–153.

Gammack, J.K. (2003). Use and management of chronic urinary catheters in long-term care: Much controversy, little consensus. *Journal of the American Medical Directors Association, 3,* 162–168.

German, K., Rowley, P., Stone, D., Kumar, U., & Blackford, H.N. (1997). A randomized cross-over study comparing the use of a catheter valve and a leg-bag in urethrally catheterized male patients. *British Journal of Urology, 79,* 96–98.

Getliffe, K., Fader, M., Allen, C., Pinar, K., & Moore, K.N. (2007). Current evidence on intermittent catheterization: Sterile single-use catheters or clean reused catheters and the incidence of UTI. *Journal of Wound, Ostomy, and Continence Nursing, 34,* 289–296.

Getliffe, K., Fader, M., Cottenden, A., Jamieson, K., & Green, N. (2007). Absorbent products for incontinence: "Treatment effects" and impact on quality of life. *Journal of Clinical Nursing, 16,* 1936–1945.

Giannantoni, A., DiStasi, S., Scivoletto, G., Virgili, G., Dolci, S., & Porena, M. (2002). Intermittent catheterization with a prelubricated catheter in spinal cord injured patients: A prospective randomized crossover study. *Journal of Urology, 166,* 130–133.

Goodsarran, V.J., & Katz, T.F. (2002). Do not go with the flow, remember indwelling catheters. *Journal of the American Geriatrics Society, 50,* 1739–1740.

Gray, M. (2004a). Preventing and managing perineal dermatitis: A shared goal for wound and continence care. *Journal of Wound, Ostomy, and Continence Nursing, 31*(1 Suppl.), S2–S9.

Gray, M. (2004b). What nursing interventions reduce the risk of symptomatic urinary tract infection in the patient with an indwelling catheter? *Journal of Wound, Ostomy, and Continence Nursing, 31,* 3–13.

Gray, M. (2006). Does the construction material affect outcomes in long-term catheterization? *Journal of Wound, Ostomy, and Continence Nursing, 33,* 116–121.

Gray, M., Bliss, D.Z., Doughty, D.B., Ermer-Seltun, J., Kennedy-Evans, K.L., & Palmer, M.H. (2007). Incontinence-associated dermatitis: A consensus. *Journal of Wound, Ostomy, and Continence Nursing, 34,* 45–54.

Gray, M., Newman, D.K., Einhorn, C.J., & Reid Czarapata, B.J. (2006). Expert review: Best practices in managing the indwelling catheter. *Perspectives,* 3–10.

Gray, M., Ratliff, C., & Donavan, A. (2002). Perineal skin care for the incontinent patient. *Advances in Skin and Wound Care, 15,* 170–178.

Ha, U.-S., & Cho, Y.-H. (2006). Catheter-associated urinary tract infections: New aspects of novel urinary catheters. *International Journal of Antimicrobial Agents, 28,* 485–490.

Hanchett, M.S. (2002). Techniques for stabilizing urinary catheters. *Home Healthcare Nurse, 20,* 185–190.

Hanson, D., Macejkovic, C., Langemo, D., Anderson, J., Thompson, P., & Hunter, S. (2006). Perineal dermatitis: A consequence of incontinence. *Advances in Skin and Wound Care, 19,* 246–250.

Heard, L., & Buhrer, R. (2005). How do we prevent UTI in prople who perform intermittent catheterization? *Rehabilitation Nursing, 30,* 44–45.

Hedlund, H., Hjelmås, K., Jonsson, O., Klarskov, P., & Talja, M. (2001). Hydrophilic versus non-coated catheters for intermittent catheterization. *Scandinavian Journal of Urology and Nephrology, 35,* 49–53.

Hodgkinson, B., Nay, R., & Wilson, J. (2007). A systematic review of topical skin care in aged care facilities. *Journal of Clinical Nursing, 16,* 129–136.

Hoggarth, A., Waring, M., Alexander, J., Greenwood, A., & Callaghan, T. (2005). A controlled, three-part trial to investigate the barrier function and skin hydration properties of six skin protectants. *Ostomy/Wound Management, 51*(12), 30–42.

Holroyd-Leduc, J.M., Sen, S., Bertenthal, D., Sands, L.P., Palmer, R.M., Kresevic, D.M., et al. (2007). The relationship of indwelling urinary catheters to death, length of hospital stay, functional decline, and nursing home admission in hospitalized older medical patients. *Journal of the American Geriatrics Society, 55,* 227–233.

Huang, W.C., Wann, S.R., Lin, S.L., Kunin, C.M., Kung, M.H., Lin, C.H., et al. (2004). Catheter-associated urinary tract infections in intensive care units can be reduced by prompting physicians to remove unnecessary catheters. *Infection Control and Hospital Epidemiology, 25,* 974–978.

Hudson, E., & Murahata, R.I. (2005). The "no-touch" method of intermittent urinary catheter insertion: Can it reduce the risk of bacteria entering the bladder? *Spinal Cord, 43,* 611–614.

Hukins, D.W. (2005). Preventing encrustation in indwelling urethral catheters. *Medical Device Technology, 16*(4), 25–27.

Jamison, J., Maguire, S., & McCann, J. (2004). Catheter policies for management of long term voiding problems in adults with neurogenic bladder disorders. *Cochrane Database of Systematic Reviews,* (2), CD004375.

Johnson, J.R., Kuskowski, M.A., & Wilt, T.J. (2006). Systematic Review: Antimicrobial urinary catheters to prevent catheter-associated urinary tract infection in hospitalized patients. *Annals of Internal Medicine, 144,* 116–126.

Kalsi, J., Arya, M., Wilson, P., & Mundy, A. (2003). Hospital-acquired urinary tract infection. *International Journal of Clinical Practice, 57,* 388–391.

Karchmer, T., Giannetta, E., Muto, C., Strain, B., & Farr, B. (2000). A randomized crossover study of silver-coated urinary catheters in hospitalized patients. *Archives of Internal Medicine, 160,* 3294–3298.

Kovindha, A., Mai, W.N.C., & Madersbacher, H. (2004). Reused silicone catheter for clean intermittent catheterization (CIC): Is it safe for spinal cord injured (SCI) men? *Spinal Cord, 42,* 638–642.

Kunin, C.M. (2006). Urinary-catheter-associated infection in the elderly. *International Journal of Antimicrobial Agents, 28*(Suppl.), S78–S81.

Lai, K.K., & Fontecchio, S.A. (2002). Use of silver-hydrogel urinary catheters on the incidence of catheter-associated urinary tract infections in hospitalized patients. *American Journal of Infection Control, 30,* 221–225.

Landi, F., Caesari, M., Onder, G., Zamboni, V., Barillaro, C., Lattanzio, F., et al. (2004). Indwelling urethral catheter and mortality in frail elderly women living in community. *Neurology and Urodynamics, 23,* 697–701.

Lapides, J., Diokno, A.C., Silber, S.M., & Lowe, B.S. (2002). Clean, intermittent self-catheterization in the treatment of urinary tract disease. 1972. *Journal of Urology, 167,* 1584–1586.

Lawrence, E.L., & Turner, I.G. (2005). Materials for urinary catheters: A review of their history and development in the UK. *Medical Engineering and Physics, 27,* 443–453.

LeBlanc, K., & Christensen, D. (2005). Addressing the challenge of providing nursing care for elderly men suffering from urethral erosion. *Journal of Wound, Ostomy, and Continence Nursing, 32* 131–134.

Lee, S.J., Kim, S.W., Cho, Y.H., Shin, W.S., Lee, S.E., Kim, C.S., et al. (2004). A comparative multicentre study on the incidence of catheter-associated urinary tract infection between nitrofurazone-coated and silicone catheters. *International Journal of Antimicrobial Agents, 24*(Suppl. 1):S65–S69.

Lekan-Rutledge, D. (2006). Management of urinary incontinence: Skin care, containment devices, catheters, absorptive products. In D.B. Doughty (Ed.), *Urinary and fecal incontinence: Current management concepts* (309–339). St. Louis: Elsevier Mosby.

Lemke, J.R., Kasprowicz, K., & Worral, P.S. (2005). Intermittent catheterization for patients with a neurogenic bladder: Sterile versus clean. Using evidence-based practice at the staff nurse level. *Journal of Nursing Care Quality, 20,* 302–306.

Linsenmeyer, T.A., Bodner, D.R., Creasey, G.H., Green, B.G., Groah, S.L., & Joseph, A., for the Consortium for Spinal Cord Medicine. (2006). Bladder management for adults with spinal cord injury: A clinical practice guideline for health-care providers. *Journal of Spinal Cord Medicine, 29,* 527–573.

Loden, M. (2005). The clinical benefit of moisturizers. *Journal of the European Academy of Dermatology and Venereology, 19,* 672–688.

Macaulay, M., Clarke-O'Neill, S., Cottenden, A., Fader, M., van den Heuvel, E., & Jowitt, F. (2006). Female urinals for women with impaired mobility. *Nursing Times, 102*(42), 42–43, 45, 47.

Macaulay, M., van den Heuvel, E., Jowitt, F., Clarke-O'Neill, S., Kardas, P., Blijham, N., et al. (2007). A noninvasive continence management system: Development and evaluation of a novel toileting device for women. *Journal of Wound, Ostomy, and Continence Nursing, 34,* 641–648.

MacIntosh, J. (1998). Realising the potential of urinals for women. *Journal of Community Nursing, 12*(8), 14–18.

Maki, D.G., & Tambyah, P.A. (2001). Engineering out the risk for infection with urinary catheters. *Emerging Infectious Diseases, 7* 342–347.

Mathur, S., Sabbuba, N.A., Suller, M.T., Stickler, D.J., & Feneley, R.C. (2005). Genotyping of urinary and fecal *Proteus mirabilis* isolates from individuals with long-term urinary catheters. *European Journal of Clinical Microbiology and Infectious Diseases, 24,* 643–644.

McClish, D.K., Wyman, J.F., Sale, P.G., Camp, J., & Earle, B. (1999). Use and costs of incontinence pads in female study volunteers. *Journal of Wound, Ostomy, and Continence Nursing, 26,* 207–213.

McMahon-Parkes, K. (1998). Management of suprapubic catheters. *Nursing Times, 94*(25), 49–51.

Mody, L., Maheshwari, S., Galecki, A., Kauffman, C.A., & Bradley, S.F. (2007). Indwelling device use and antibiotic resistance in nursing homes: Identifying a high-risk group. *Journal of the American Geriatrics Society, 55,* 1921–1926.

Moore, K.N., Burt, J., & Voaklander, D.C. (2006). Intermittent catheterization in the rehabilitation setting: A comparison of clean and sterile technique. *Clinical Rehabilitation, 20,* 461–468.

Moore, K.N., Schieman, S., Ackerman, T., Dzus, H.Y., Metcalfe, J.B., & Voaklander, D.C. (2004). Assessing comfort, safety, and patient satisfaction with three commonly used penile compression devices. *Urology, 63,* 150–154.

Morris, N.S., & Stickler, D.J. (2001). Does drinking cranberry juice produce urine inhibitory to the development of crystalline, catheter-blocking *Proteus mirabilis* biofilms? *BJU International, 88,* 192–197.

Morris, N.S., Stickler, D.J., & Mclean, R.J.C. (1999). The development of bacterial biofilms on indwelling urethral catheters. *World Journal of Urology, 17,* 345–350.

Morris, N.S., Stickler, D.J., & Winters, C. (1997). Which indwelling urethral catheters resist encrustations by *Proteus mirabilis* biofilms? *British Journal of Urology, 80,* 58–63.

Moy, L.M., & Wein, A.J. (2007). Additional therapies for storage and emptying. In A.J. Wein, L.R. Kavoussi, A.C. Novick, A.W. Partin, & C.A. Peters (Eds.), *Campbell's urology* (9th ed., pp. 2288–2304). Philadelphia: Elsevier Saunders.

Munasinghe, R.L., Yazdani, H., Siddique, M., & Hafeez, W. (2001). Appropriateness of use of indwelling urinary catheters in patients admitted to the medical service. *Infection Control and Hospital Epidemiology, 22,* 647–649.

Mylotte, J.M., Tayara, A., & Goodnough, S. (2002). Epidemiology of bloodstream infection in nursing home residents: Evaluation in a large cohort from multiple homes. *Clinical Infectious Diseases, 35,* 1484–1490.

Nash, M.A. (2003). Best practice for patient self-cleaning of urinary drainage bags. *Urologic Nursing, 23,* 334–339.

Newman, D. (2007a). The indwelling urinary catheter: Principles for best practice. *Journal of Wound, Ostomy, and Continence Nursing, 24,* 655–661.

Newman, D.K. (2002). *Managing and treating urinary incontinence* (pp. 111–127). Baltimore: Health Professions Press.

Newman, D.K. (2004). Incontinence products and devices for the elderly. *Urologic Nursing, 24,* 316–334.

Newman, D.K. (2005). *Use and care of indwelling urinary catheters, self-learning packet.* Hospital of the University of Pennsylvania CEQI Committee. Philadelphia: Hospital of the University of Pennsylvania, Department of Nursing.

Newman, D.K. (2006a). Bladder dysfunction in women: Products and devices play important role. *ADVANCE for Nurse Practitioners, 14*(5), 55–56, 58, 60–62.

Newman, D.K. (2006b). Urinary incontinence, catheters, and urinary tract infections: An overview of CMS Tag F 315. *Ostomy/Wound Management, 52*(12), 34–36, 38, 40–44.

Newman, D.K. (2007b). Nursing management: Renal and urologic problems. In S.L. Lewis, M.M. Heitkemper, S.R. Dirksen, P.G. Brien, & L. Bucher (Eds.), *Medical-surgical nursing: Assessment and management of clinical problems* (7th ed., pp. 1154–1196). St. Louis: Elsevier Mosby.

Newman, D.K. (2007c). *The skin—our first line of defense* (Educational Module). Princeton, NJ: ConvaTec.

Newman, D.K., Fader, M., & Bliss, D.Z. (2004). Managing incontinence using technology, devices and products. *Nursing Research, 53*(6 Suppl.), S42–S48.

Newman, D.K., Parente, C.A., & Yuan, J.R. (1997). Implementing the Agency for Healthcare Policy and Research urinary incontinence guidelines in a home health agency. In M.D. Harris (Ed.), *Handbook of home health care administration* (2nd ed., pp. 394–403). Gaithersburg, MD: Aspen Publishers.

Newman, D.K., Preston, A.K., & Salazar, S. (2007). Moisture control, urinary and fecal incontinence and perineal skin management. In D. Krasner, L. Rode, & D. Kane (Eds.), *Chronic wound care: A clinical source book for healthcare professionals* (4th ed., pp. 609–627). Wayne, PA: HMP Communications.

Nicolle, L.E. (2000). Urinary tract infection in long-term-care facility residents. *Clinical Infectious Diseases, 31,* 757–761.

Nicolle, L.E. (2001). The chronic indwelling catheter and urinary infection in long-term care facility residents. *Infection Control and Hospital Epidemiology, 22,* 316–321.

Nicolle, L.E. (2005). Catheter-related urinary tract infection. *Drugs and Aging, 22,* 627–639.

Nicolle, L.E., Bradley, S., Colgan, R., Rice, J.C., Schaeffer, A., & Hooton, T.M., for the Infectious Diseases Society of America; American Society of Nephrology; American Geriatric Society. (2005). Infectious Diseases Society of America guidelines for the diagnosis and treatment of asymptomatic bacteriuria in adults. *Clinical Infectious Diseases, 40,* 643–654.

Niel-Weise, B.S., & Van Den Broek, P.J. (2005). Antibiotic policies for short-term catheter bladder drainage in adults. *Cochrane Database of Systematic Reviews,* (3), CD005428.

Ouslander, J.G., Greengold, B., & Chen, S. (1987). External catheter use and urinary tract infections among incontinent male nursing home patients. *Journal of the American Geriatrics Society, 35,* 1063–1070.

Palese, A., Regattin, L., Venuti, F., Innocenti, A., Benaglio, C., Cunico, L., et al. (2007). Incontinence pad use in patients admitted to medical wards: An Italian multicenter prospective cohort study. *Journal of Wound, Ostomy, and Continence Nursing, 34,* 649–654.

Patterson, R., Little, B., Tolan, J., & Sweeney, C. (2006). How to manage a urinary catheter balloon that will not deflate. *International Urology and Nephrology, 38,* 57–61.

Pemberton, P., Brooks, A., Eriksen, C.M., Frost, S., Graham, S., Greenman, L., et al. (2006). A comparative study of two types of urinary sheath. *Nursing Times, 102*(7), 36–41.

Perrouin-Verbe, B., Labat, J.J., Richard, I., Mauduyt de la Greve, I., Buzelin, J.M., & Mathe J.F. (1995). Clean intermittent catheterization from the acute period in spinal cord injury clients: Long term evaluation of urethral and genital tolerance. *Paraplegia, 33,* 619–624.

Pohl, H.G., Bauer, S.B., Borer, J.G., Diamond, D.A., Kelly, M.D., Grant, R., et al. (2002). The outcome of voiding dysfunction managed with clean intermittent catheterization in neurologically and anatomically normal children. *BJU International, 89,* 923–927.

Pratt, R.J., Pellowe, C.M., Wilson, J.A., Loveday, H.P., Harper, P.J., Jones, S.R., et al. (2007). Epic2: National evidence-based guidelines for preventing healthcare-associated infections in NHS hospitals in England. *Journal of Hospital Infection, 65*(Suppl. 1), S1–S64.

Rainville, N.C. (1994). The current nursing procedure for intermittent urinary catheterization in rehabilitation facilities. *Rehabilitation Nursing, 19*(6), 330–333.

Raz, R., Schiller, D., & Nicolle, L.E. (2000). Chronic indwelling catheter replacement before antimicrobial therapy for symptomatic urinary tract infection. *Journal of Urology, 164,* 1254–1258.

Ribeiro, J.P., Marcelino, P., Marum, S., Fernandes, A.P., & Grilo, A. (2004). Case report: Purple urine bag syndrome. *Critical Care, 8*(3), R137.

Robinson, J. (2003). Purple urinary bag syndrome: A harmless but alarming problem. *British Journal of Community Nursing, 8,* 263–266.

Robinson, J. (2005). Suprapubic catheterization: Challenges in changing catheters. *British Journal of Community Nursing, 10,* 461–462, 464.

Roe, B.H. (1990). Study of the effects of education on patients' knowledge and acceptance of their indwelling urethral catheters. *Journal of Advanced Nursing, 18,* 223–231.

Rogers, M.A., Mody, L., Kaufman, S.R., Fries, B.E., McMahon, L.F. Jr., & Saint, S. (2008). Use of urinary collection devices in skilled nursing facilities in five states. *Journal of the American Geriatrics Society, 56*(5), 854–861.

Roth, E.J., Lovell, L., Harvey, R.L., Bode, R.K., & Heinemann, A.W. (2002). Stroke rehabilitation: Indwelling urinary catheters, enteral feeding tubes, and tracheostomies are associated with resource use and functional outcomes. *Stroke, 33,* 1845–1850.

Runeman, B. (2008). Skin interaction with absorbent hygiene products. *Clinics in Dermatology, 26*(1), 45–51.

Rupp, M.E., Fitzgerald, T., Marion, N., Helget, V., Puumala, S., Anderson, J.R., et al. (2004). Effect of silver-coated urinary catheters: Efficacy, cost-effectiveness, and antimicrobial resistance. *American Journal of Infection Control, 32,* 445–450.

Saint, S. (2000). Clinical and economic consequences of nosocomial catheter-related bacteriruria. *American Journal of Infection Control, 28,* 68–75.

Saint, S. (2001). Prevention of nosocomial urinary tract infections. In *Making health care safer: A critical analysis of patient safety practices* (Evidence Report/Technology Assessment #42, pp. 159–172). Washington, DC: Agency for Healthcare Research and Quality.

Saint, S., & Chenoweth, C.E. (2003). Biofilms and catheter-associated urinary tract infections. *Infectious Disease Clinics of North America, 17,* 411–432.

Saint, S., Kaufman, S.R., Rogers, M.A., Baker, P.D., Ossenkop, K., & Lipsky, B.A. (2006). Condom versus indwelling urinary catheters: A randomized trial. *Journal of the American Geriatrics Society, 54,* 1055–1061.

Saint, S., Lipsky, B.A., Baker, P.D., McDonald, L.L., & Ossenkop, K. (1999). Urinary catheters: What type do men and their nurses prefer? *Journal of the American Geriatrics Society, 47,* 1453–1457.

Saint, S., Lipsky, B.A., & Goold, S.D. (2002). Indwelling urinary catheters: A one-point restraint? *Annals of Internal Medicine, 137,* 125–127.

Saint, S., Wiese, J., Amory, J.K., Bernstein, M.L., Patel, U.D., Zemencuk, J.K., et al. (2000). Are physicians aware of which of their patients have indwelling urinary catheters? *American Journal of Medicine, 109,* 476–480.

Sand, P.K., Staskin, D., Miller, J., Diokno, A., Sant, G.R., Davila, G.W., et al. (1999). Effect of a urinary control insert on quality of life in incontinent women. *International Urogynecology Journal and Pelvic Floor Dysfunction, 10,* 100–105.

Saye, D.E. (2007). Recurring and antimicrobial resistant infections: Considering the potential role of biofilms in clinical practice. *Ostomy/Wound Management, 53*(4), 46–52.

Sedor, J., & Mulholland, S.G. (1999). Infections in Urology: Hospital-acquired urinary tract infections with the indwelling catheter. *Urologic Clinics of North America, 26,* 821–828.

Senese, V., Hendricks, M.B., Morrison, M., & Harris, J., for the Clinical Practice Guidelines Task Force. (2006). Clinical Practice Guidelines: Care of the patient with an indwelling catheter. *Urologic Nursing, 26,* 80–81.

Seymour, C. (2006). Audit of catheter-associated UTI using silver alloy-coated Foley catheters. *British Journal of Nursing, 15,* 598–603.

Shah, P.S., Cannon, J.P., Sullivan, C.L., Nemchausky, B., & Pachucki, C.T. (2005). Controlling antimicrobial use and decreasing microbiological laboratory tests for urinary tract infections in spinal-cord-injury patients with chronic indwelling catheters. *American Journal of Health-System Pharmacy, 62,* 74–77.

Sheriff, M.K.M., Foley, S., McFarlane, J., Nauth-Miser, R., Craggs, M., & Shah, P.J.R. (1998). Long-term suprapubic catheterisation: Clinical outcome and satisfaction survey. *Spinal Cord, 36,* 171–176.

Shinopulos, N.M., Dann, J.A., & Smith, J.J. (1999). Patient selection and education for use of the CapSure™ (Re/Stor) Continence Shield. *Urologic Nursing, 19,* 135–140.

Siegel, T.J. (2006). Do registered nurses perceive the anchoring of indwelling urinary catheters as a necessary aspect of nursing care? A pilot study. *Journal of Wound, Ostomy, and Continence Nursing, 33,* 140–144.

Silverblatt, F.J., Tibert, C., Mikolich, D., Blazek-D'Arezzo, J., Alves, J., Tack, M., et al. (2000). Preventing the spread of vancomycin-resistant enterococci in a long term care facility. *Journal of the American Geriatrics Society, 48,* 1211–1215.

Simpson, C., & Clark, A.P. (2005). Nosocomial UTI: Are we treating the catheter or the patient? *Clinical Nurse Specialist, 19*(4), 175–179.

Sirls, L.T., Foote, J.E., Kaufman, J.M., Lightner, D.J., Miller, J.L., Moseley, W.G., et al. (2002). Long-term results of the FemSoft urethral insert for the management of female stress urinary incontinence. *International Urogynecology Journal and Pelvic Floor Dysfunction, 13,* 88–95.

Siroky, M.G. (2002). Pathogenesis of bacteriuria and infection in the spinal cord injured patient. *American Journal of Medicine, 113*(Suppl. 1A), 67S–79S.

Smith, J.M. (2003). Indwelling catheter management: From habit-based to evidence-based practice. *Ostomy/Wound Management, 49*(12), 34–45.

Srinivasan, A., Karchmer, T., Richards, A., Song, X., & Perl, T.M. (2006). A prospective trial of a novel, silicone-based, silver-coated Foley catheter for the prevention of nosocomial urinary tract infections. *Infection Control and Hospital Epidemiology, 27,* 38–43.

Staskin, D., Bavendam, T., Miller, J., Davila, G.W., Diokno, A., Knapp, P., et al. (1996). Effectiveness of a urinary control insert in the management of stress urinary incontinence: Early results of a multicenter study. *Urology, 47,* 629–636.

Stensballe, J., Loom, D., Nielsen, P.N., & Tvede, M. (2005). Hydrophilic-coated catheters for intermittent catheterisation reduce urethral microtrauma: A prospective, randomised, participant-blinded, crossover study of three different types of catheters. *European Urology, 48,* 978–983.

Subbannayyn, K., Bhat, G.K., Junu, V.G., Shetty, S., & Jisho, M.G. (2006). Can soaps act as fomites in hospitals? *Journal of Hospital Infection, 62,* 245.

Talsma, S.S. (2007). Biofilms on medical devices. *Home Healthcare Nurse, 25*(9), 589–594.

Tambyah, P.A. (2004). Catheter-associated urinary tract infections: Diagnosis and prophylaxis. *International Journal of Antimicrobial Agents, 24*(Suppl. 1), S44–S48.

Tambyah, P.A., Halvorson, K.T., & Maki, D.G. (1999). A prospective study of pathogenesis of catheter-associated urinary tract infections. *Mayo Clinic Proceedings, 74*(2), 131–136.

Tambyah, P.A., & Maki, D.G. (2000). Catheter-associated urinary tract infection is rarely symptomatic: A prospective study of 1,497 catheterized patients. *Archives of Internal Medicine, 160,* 678–682.

Tang, M.W.S. (2006). Purple urine bag syndrome in geriatric patients. *Journal of the American Geriatrics Society, 54,* 3610–3611.

Tenke, P., Kovacs, B., Bjerklund Johansen, T.E., Matsumoto, T., Tambyah, P.A., & Naber, K.G. (2008). European and Asian guidelines on management and prevention of catheter-associated urinary tract infections. *International Journal of Antimicrobial Agents, 31*(Suppl. 1), S68–S78.

Thompson, P., Langemo, D., Anderson, J., Hanson, D., & Hunter, S. (2005). Skin care protocols for pressure ulcers and incontinence in long-term care: A quasi-experimental study. *Advances in Skin and Wound Care, 18,* 423.

Thornburn, P., Fader, M., Dean, G., Brooks, R., & Cottenden, A. (1997). Improving the performance of small incontinence pads: A study of "wet comfort." *Journal of Wound, Ostomy, and Continence Nursing, 24,* 219–225.

Tincello, D.G., Adams, E.J., Bolderson, J., & Richmond, D.H. (2000). A urinary control device for management of female stress incontinence. *Obstetrics and Gynecology, 95,* 417–420.

Topal, J., Conklin, S., Camp, K., Morris, V., Balcezak, T., & Herbert, P. (2005). Prevention of nosocomial catheter-associated urinary tract infections through computerized feedback to physicians and a nurse-directed protocol. *American Journal of Medical Quality, 20,* 121–126.

Toughill, E. (2005). Indwelling urinary catheters: Common mechanical and pathogenic problems. *American Journal of Nursing, 105*(5), 35–37.

Trautner, B.W., & Darouiche, R.O. (2003). Role of biofilm in catheter-associated urinary tract infection. *American Journal of Infection Control, 32,* 177–183.

Trautner, B.W., & Darouiche, R.O. (2004). Catheter-associated infections. *Archives of Internal Medicine, 164,* 842–850.

Vallejo-Manzur, F., Mireles-Cabodevila, E., & Varon, J. (2005). Purple urine bag syndrome. *American Journal of Emergency Medicine, 23,* 521–524.

van den Eijkel, E., & Griffiths, P. (2006). Catheter valves for indwelling urinary catheters: A systematic review. *British Journal of Community Nursing, 11,* 111–112, 114.

Vapnek, J.M., Maynard, F.M., & Kim, J. (2003). A prospective randomized trial of the LoFric hydrophilic coated catheter versus conventional plastic catheter for clean intermittent catheterization. *Journal of Urology, 169,* 994–998.

Verleyen, P., De Ridder, D., Van Poppel, H., & Baert, L. (1999). Clinical application of the Bardex IC Foley catheter. *European Urology, 36,* 240–246.

Vickerman, J. (2006). Selecting urinals for male patients. *Nursing Times, 102*(19), 47–48.

Wald, H., Epstein, A., & Kramer, A. (2005). Extended use of indwelling urinary catheters in postoperative hip fracture patients. *Medical Care, 43,* 1009–1017.

Wald, H., & Kramer, A.M. (2007). Nonpayment for harms resulting from medical care catheter-associated urinary tract infections. *JAMA, 298,* 2782–2784.

Warren, J.W. (2005). Nosocomial urinary tract infections. In G.L. Mandell, J.E. Bennett, & R. Dolin (Eds.), *Mandell, Douglas, and Bennett's principles and practice of infectious diseases* (6th ed., pp. 3370–3381). Philadelphia: Elsevier Saunders.

Warshaw, E., Nix, D., Kula, J., & Markon, E.E. (2002). Clinical and cost effectiveness of a cleanser protectant lotion for treatment of perineal skin breakdown in low-risk patients with incontinence. *Ostomy Wound Management, 48*(6), 44–51.

Watson, N.M., Brink, C.A., Zimmer, J.G., & Mayer, R.D. (2003). Use of the Agency for Health Care Policy and Research Urinary Incontinence Guideline in nursing homes. *Journal of the American Geriatrics Society, 51,* 1779–1786.

Webb, R.J., Lawson, A.L., & Neal, D.E. (1990). Clean intermittent self-catheterisation in 172 adults. *British Journal of Urology, 65,* 20–23.

Webster, J., Hood, R.H., Burridge, C.A., Doidge, M.L., Phillips, K.M., & George, N. (2001). Water or antiseptic for periurethral cleaning before urinary catheterization: A randomized controlled trial. *American Journal of Infection Control, 29,* 389–394.

Wein, A.J. (2002). Neuromuscular dysfunction of the lower urinary tract and its management. In P.C. Walsh, A.B. Retik, E.D. Vaughn, & A.J. Wein, (Eds.), *Campbell's Urology* (8th edition) (pp. 931–966). Philadelphia: Saunders.

Weld, K.J., & Dmochowski, R.R. (2000). Effect of bladder management on urological complications in spinal cord injured patients. *Journal of Urology, 163,* 768–772.

West, D.A., Cummings, J.M., Longo, W.E., Virgo, K.S., Johnson, F.E., & Parra, R.O. (1999). Role of chronic catheterization in the development of bladder cancer in patients with spinal cord injury. *Urology, 53*(2), 292–297.

Wilcox, M.H., Fawley, W.N., Wigglesworth, N., Parnell, P., Verity, P., & Freeman, J. (2003). Comparison of the effect of detergent versus hypochlorite on environmental contamination and incidence of *Clostridium difficile* infection. *Journal of Hospital Infection, 54,* 109–114.

Williams, M.E. (2005). How do we teach clean intermittent self-catheterization using touch technique? *Rehabilitation Nursing, 30,* 171–172.

Wong, E.S., & Hooten, T.M. (1981). Guidelines for the prevention of catheter-associated urinary tract infections. In *Guidelines for the prevention and control of nosocomial infections* (pp. 1–5). Atlanta: Centers for Disease Control and Prevention. Retrieved December 27, 2007, from http://www.cdc.gov/ncidod/dhqp/gl_catheter_assoc.html

Woodbury, M.G., Hayes, K.C., & Askes, H.K. (2008). Intermittent catheterization practices following spinal cord injury: A national survey. *Canadian Journal of Urology, 15*(3), 4065–4071.

Wyndaele, J.J., & Maes, D. (1990). Clean intermittent self-catheterization: A 12-year followup. *Journal of Urology, 143,* 906–908.

Zehrer, C.L., Newman, D.K., Grove, G.L., & Lutz, J.B. (2005). Assessment of diaper clogging potential of petrolatum moisture barriers. *Ostomy/Wound Management, 51*(2), 54–58.

11

Evaluation and Management
of Pelvic Organ Prolapse

Pelvic organ prolapse (POP) is a condition unique to women in which the pelvic organs (bladder, uterus, and/or rectum) descend downward within the pelvis, herniate ("drop") through the vaginal wall, and in some cases pass outside the vagina, bulging through the introitus. Prolapse is considered a type of herniation.

POP has been noted throughout civilization, and approaches to its management have at times been bizarre. Ancient Greek physicians characterized the uterus as erratic (i.e., the *Corpus Hippocraticum*) and believed that, when it suffered from an "imbalance of moisture" (i.e., when it was diseased), it would "wander" throughout the body in search of relief. Thus they believed a prolapsed uterus wandered outside the abdomen because it was searching for moisture, or urine. They also believed that the uterus was a tainted organ full of evil spirits that should be left alone to heal itself. However, if it did not, they suggested bleeding or cupping the prolapsed area; applying sponges and hard objects (initial type of pessary) dipped in hot water, honey, wine, or oil; or fumigating the external genitalia in an effort to purge the sinister uterus, and coax it back to its normal location (Shah, Sultan, & Thakar, 2006). As medicine evolved, approaches to prolapsed pelvic organs have also changed and evolved.

At least 50% of women who have had children will develop some type of POP (Marinkovic & Stanton, 2004; Olsen, Smith, Bergstrom, Colling, & Clark, 1997), but most women are asymptomatic. Treatment should be reserved for symptomatic women with few exceptions. Hendrix and colleagues (2002) reported the results of the Women's Health Initiative, noting that 41% of women ($n = 27,342$) with an intact uterus had some form of prolapse, and 38% of women who had undergone a hysterectomy had some form of POP. However, symptoms were not assessed in these women, so the degree to which POP is bothersome has not been well documented. In a population-based study of 2,001 randomly selected women in a Kaiser Permanente Medical Care Program in Northern California, symptomatic prolapse (self-report of a feeling of bulge, pressure, or protrusion or a visible bulge from the vagina) was identified in 6% of women; of these women, 50% reported moderate or great distress and 35%

reported that the symptoms affected at least one physical, social, or sexual activity (Rortveit et al., 2007). POP is the leading indication for hysterectomy in postmenopausal women (Kesharvarz, Hillis, Kieke, & Marchbanks, 2002).

Women have a lifetime risk of 11% of undergoing an invasive surgical procedure for treatment of POP (Olsen et al., 1997). The prevalence of uterine prolapse has been reported to be 14.2%, that of cystocele 34.3%, and that of rectocele 18.6% (Hendrix et al., 2002). POP is an important condition in women with pelvic floor dysfunction because treatment and comorbidities cost more than $1 billion (Subak et al., 2001; Weber & Richter, 2005), with POP noted in 1998 as one of the three most common diagnoses associated with hysterectomy (Popovic & Kozak, 2000).

A general lack of understanding about the natural history and causes of POP continues to exist, but certain factors may increase the risk of prolapse (Jelovsek, Maher, & Barber, 2007):

- Neuromuscular damage (injuries to or deterioration of the nerves, muscles, and connective tissue) secondary to vaginal childbirth. The more children a woman has, the more chances she has of developing POP. Cesarean section seems to protect against prolapse development, whereas forceps delivery increases risk (Lukacz, Lawrence, Contreras, Nager, & Luber, 2006; Moalli, Jones Ivy, Meyn, & Zyczynski, 2003).

- Effects of menopause (a decrease in the hormone estrogen)

- Increasing age

- Prior pelvic surgery (e.g., hysterectomy) or trauma

- Chronic increases in intra-abdominal pressure resulting from chronic cough, chronic constipation and straining for stool evacuation, obesity, or chronic lifting (e.g., occupational)

- Intrinsic factors such as race (Caucasian women have a higher prevalence), genetics (family history of POP), anatomy, connective tissue, and neurological conditions

CLINICAL EVALUATION

POP, depending on the degree, is often asymptomatic and is usually found incidentally (e.g., during workup for a recurrent urinary tract infection) because early stages do not cause any symptoms. Women usually will seek treatment when they see or feel a bulge of tissue that protrudes out of the vagina. Most women may experience little or no symptoms early in the day but will notice changes as the day goes on, especially if they are working in jobs that require long periods of standing (e.g., teaching) or lifting. As many as 32%–98% of women are reported to have some degree of POP on physical examination (Handa, Garrett, Hendrix, Gold, & Robbins, 2004; Hendrix et al., 2002; Nygaard, Bradley, & Brandt, 2004), but only 4%–10% of women report symptoms

---

Box 11.1   Common complaints of women with POP

Urinary

- Incontinence
- Overactive bladder symptoms of urgency and frequency
- Weak or prolonged urinary stream
- Hesitancy
- Feeling of incomplete emptying (especially with grades 3 and 4)
- Need for manual reduction of prolapse to start or complete voiding
- Need for position change to start or complete voiding

Vaginal

- Sensation of a bulge or protrusion
- Seeing or feeling a bulge or protrusion
- Pressure
- Heaviness

Bowel

- Fecal incontinence (flatus, or liquid or solid stool)
- Feeling of incomplete emptying
- Straining during defecation
- Urgency to defecate
- Need for digital evacuation to complete defecation
- Need for splinting, or pushing on or around the vagina or perineum, to start or complete defecation
- Feeling of blockage or obstruction during defecation

Sexual

- Dyspareunia
- Decreased sensation during intercourse

---

of POP (Ghetti, Gregory, Edwards, Otto, & Clark, 2005; Swift, Tate, & Nicholas, 2003). Symptoms may arise from all affected organs in the pelvis (Box 11.1). Once it becomes bothersome, women will report pelvic, sexual, urinary, and bowel symptoms. At least one third of women will report fecal incontinence or defecation problems. Questionnaires useful in assessing for POP are available, such as the Pelvic Organ Prolapse Distress Inventory 6 (POPDI-6) (Barber, Kuchibhatla, Pieper, & Bump, 2001; Barber, Walters, Bump, 2005). Helpful questions include:

- Usually experience *pressure* in the lower abdomen?

- Usually experience *heaviness* or *dullness* in the pelvic area?

- Usually have a bulge or something falling out that you can see or feel in your vaginal area?

- Usually experience a feeling of incomplete bladder emptying?

- Ever have to push up on a bulge in the vaginal area with your fingers to start or complete urination?

- Ever have to push on the vagina or around the rectum to have or complete a bowel movement?

Mechanical breakdown in the system of pelvic supports and organs can lead to urinary incontinence (UI). If the woman has anterior vaginal wall prolapse or if the prolapse extends beyond the hymen, causing compression or kinking of the urethra, she is more likely to have obstructive symptoms such as urinary hesitancy, intermittent flow, or weak, prolonged urinary stream and incomplete bladder emptying.

Types of POP

POP occurs with descent of one or more pelvic structures: the cervix and vaginal apex, the anterior vagina (usually with the bladder), the posterior vagina (usually with the rectum), and the peritoneum (small intestine) (ACOG Committee on Practice Bulletins—Gynecology, 2007). Prolapse is categorized as urethrocele, cystocele, uterine prolapse, vaginal vault prolapse, rectocele, rectal prolapse, and enterocele. The signs and symptoms of each are defined as follows:

- *Urethrocele*—descent of the lower part of the urethra into the vagina.

- *Cystocele*—descent or prolapse of the anterior vaginal wall with the bladder behind it (Figure 11.1A). This is the most typical segment of the vagina to prolapse. Symptoms may include vaginal discomfort or pain, UI, and difficulty with voiding. Some women may need to manually push the prolapse back toward the bladder in order to urinate. As a cystocele worsens, it can cause kinking of the urethra, producing symptoms that suggest bladder outlet obstruction. It can also mask stress UI (SUI).

- *Uterine prolapse*—descent of the neck of the uterus and cervix into the vagina. Symptoms may include urinary urgency and frequency, UI, feeling of incomplete bladder emptying (especially with grade 3 or 4 prolapse), discomfort, pressure or a bulging feeling in the vagina or perineum, a feeling as though one is sitting on a tennis ball, vaginal dryness or irritation, dyspareunia, anorgasmia, UI during intercourse, and in some cases blood-stained vaginal discharge. Some women may also report lower back pain/discomfort that worsens during the day and is relieved by lying down.

- *Vaginal vault prolapse*—a weakening at the top of the vagina (apex or apical) that causes the vagina to start to fold onto itself, moving toward the external opening of the vagina (Figure 11.2). If the vaginal tissue is left

A

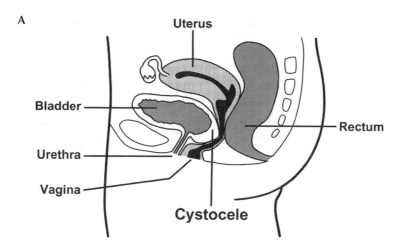

B

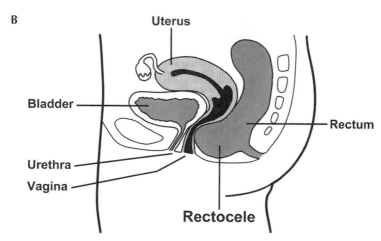

C

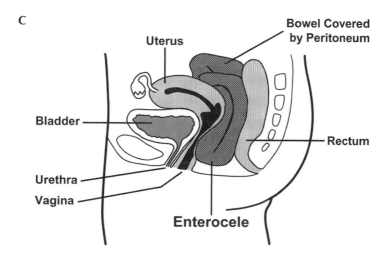

Figure 11.1.   Categories of prolapse. *A,* Cystocele. *B,* Rectocele. *C,* Enterocele. (Courtesy of Robin Noel.)

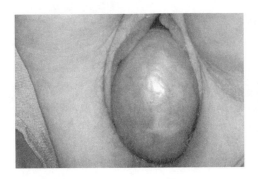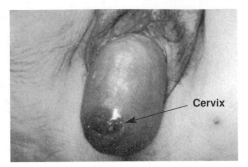

Figure 11.2.   Examples of vaginal vault prolapse.

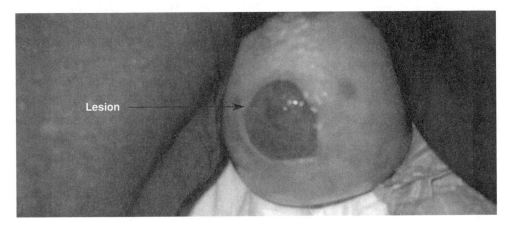

Figure 11.3.   Vaginal vault prolapse with open mucosal lesion.

exposed or rubs against a perineal pad, lesions can occur (Figure 11.3). Vaginal vault prolapse is more common in women who have had a hysterectomy. Symptoms may include pelvic or vaginal pressure or both, low back pain, bleeding, difficulty voiding and defecating, vaginal ulceration, and erosions of the exteriorized cervix that has been rubbing on clothing or perineal pads. These women may also have pain or discomfort when standing for prolonged periods. This discomfort is relieved by lying down.

- *Rectocele*—protrusion of the posterior vaginal wall with the rectum behind it (Figure 11.1B). Symptoms may include pelvic and vaginal pressure, vaginal bulge or mass, laxity with intercourse, difficulty with bowel movements necessitating digital evacuation, constipation, and fecal incontinence. Women may report vaginal splinting (placing the fingers in the vagina and pushing the prolapse back into the rectal space) to aid in defecation.

- *Rectal prolapse*—complete eversion of the rectum through the anal canal. The prolapsed tissue has a target-like appearance with circular folds of tissue protruding from the anus, often up to 10–15 cm. Symptoms mostly involve difficulty with defecation.

- *Enterocele*—bulging and herniation of the top of the vagina and part of the small intestine against the back wall of the vagina (Figure 11.1C). Symptoms may include pelvic pressure and lower backache that worsens throughout the day and is relieved by lying down. Some women may need to press down on the bulge in order to have a bowel movement.

Assessment of the extent of prolapse should be made during a Valsalva maneuver (having the women cough or bear down as though she is having a bowel movement). Although a bivalve speculum should be used to observe the cervix, a split-speculum examination with the posterior blade alone is used for the remainder of the speculum examination. This allows for analysis of each compartment—anterior, posterior, and apical—for evidence of prolapse or other abnormalities. To assess for anterior vaginal wall and apex prolapse, the bottom half of a Sims speculum is inserted into the vagina, pressure is applied to the posterior wall of the vagina, and the woman is asked to strain while the clinician notes the descent of the anterior wall (indicating that the bladder and uterus have lost support) and records the maximal descent. The woman is then asked to strain while the clinician withdraws the speculum until the apex/cervix does not descend further. If the bulge is emanating from the anterior vaginal wall, indicating that the bladder is herniating through, it is described as a cystocele. To assess posterior wall descent, the half-speculum is flipped to retract the anterior wall, the woman is asked to strain, and the clinician records the maximal descent of the posterior wall. Posterior "descent" or "protrusion" may indicate uterine prolapse or a rectocele or enterocele. If the prolapse can be pushed back inside the vagina, and does not appear to be arising from either the anterior or posterior wall, then a uterine prolapse or vaginal vault prolapse has been detected.

Decrease of normal levator ani muscle tone—by denervation or direct muscle trauma—results in an open urogenital hiatus (see Chapter 3). An open urogenital hiatus can be determined by the width of the introitus or vaginal opening. A wide opening indicates pelvic floor muscle weakness, which allows the introitus to distend and makes retention of a pessary less likely. Anal sphincter tone at rest and while squeezing should be evaluated to assess damage from chronic rectal prolapse. The clinician should also assess for vaginal and vulvar atrophy because some believe its presence precludes the use of a pessary. Most clinicians who fit women for pessary use, including one of the authors (DKN), use local topical estrogen to improve atrophy.

Measurement Systems for POP

In order to properly evaluate and record POP, some type of grading scale should be employed. For a basic evaluation of prolapse, some clinicians will

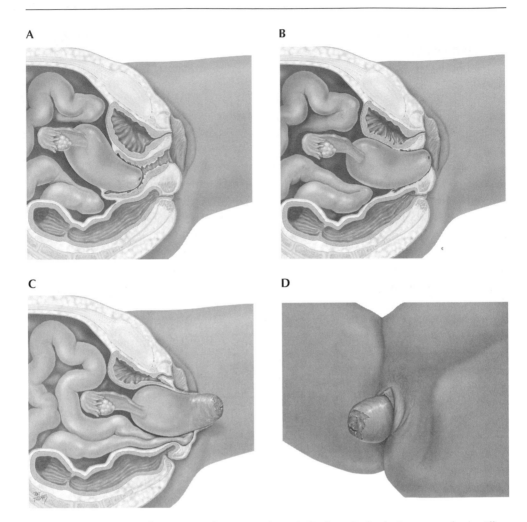

Figure 11.4.   Uterine prolapse. *A,* Grade 1. *B,* Grade 2. *C,* Grade 3. *D,* Grade 4 or procendentia. (Illustrations courtesy of Coloplast.)

refer to the prolapse as mild (prolapse with a leading edge that does not protrude to the level of the hymenal ring), moderate (prolapse that extends to, or slightly beyond, the hymen), or severe (prolapse that extends well beyond the vaginal opening). Several systems have been developed to classify POP. The Baden-Walker system (Baden & Walker, 1992) is a 5-point grading system for POP that is in widespread clinical use:

Grade 0—no prolapse

Grade 1—the prolapse descends or bulges halfway down to the hymen (opening of the vagina) (Figure 11.4A)

Grade 2—descent of the prolapse to the hymen (Figure 11.4B)

Grade 3—the prolapse protrudes halfway from the hymen (Figure 11.4C)

Grade 4—maximum descent; the vagina, with the vaginal vault and uterus, protrudes completely outside the body without a Valsalva maneuver (also known as *procidentia,* the most severe form of prolapse) (Figure 11.4D)

The Pelvic Organ Prolapse Quantification (POPQ) grading system is a tool used to quantitatively describe prolapse (Bump et al., 1996). Introduced for use in clinical practice and research, the POPQ not only identifies the area of involvement, but also renders an exact measurement. It is particularly useful to follow a patient for progression of prolapse because measurements that are discrete and reproducible are taken at specific sites on the external genitalia and along the vaginal wall. Alternative methods are not as useful. Using qualitative descriptors referencing the tissue that is prolapsed (such as cystocele, rectocele, and uterine prolapse) does not describe the degree of the problem, and staging (e.g., 0–4) uses ranges rather than specific measurements.

The POPQ measures the position of fixed vaginal points in relation to the hymenal ring. Measures are taken in centimeters while the patient is straining (bearing down or Valsalva maneuver); negative numbers refer to structures above or proximal to the hymen and positive numbers refer to structures below or distal to the hymen. Box 11.2 describes how to perform the POPQ measurements, and Figure 11.5 shows the quantification of these measurements. The measuring process takes approximately 1 minute and requires only a speculum and a cotton-tipped swab (Q-Tip) marked off with 1-cm hash marks (using a Magic Marker, with double hash marks at 5 and 10 cm for ease of reading). Diokno and Borodulin (2005) reported on a simple adjustable speculum that can accomplish POPQ. Although these measurements are taken with the patient recumbent, it is a good idea to have the patient stand and cough to see if the prolapse is more severe. Degree of increased severity must be approximated with this maneuver.

Because 38%–72% of women with POP will have some evidence of bladder outlet obstruction caused by the prolapse compressing or "kinking" the urethra, a postvoid residual (PVR) measurement should be performed. Most cases of increased PVR will resolve after active treatment. Urodynamic studies in this population can reveal over- or underactivity.

MANAGEMENT

Initially, observation is appropriate management when medically safe (i.e., no erosion or obstruction), and when preferred by the patient. Such patients are generally asymptomatic, with little or no bother. There is some evidence that pelvic floor muscle training may improve symptoms and prevent or stabilize anterior prolapse.

Primary treatment for POP is generally the use of an intravaginal mechanical support device called a pessary, a device that is approved by the U.S. Food and Drug Administration. Seventy percent of pelvic floor dysfunction

Box 11.2   Pelvic Organ Prolapse Quantification (POPQ) Measurement[a]

Prolapse should be evaluated relative to a fixed anatomic landmark that can be consistently and precisely identified. The hymen is a fixed point of reference used throughout the POPQ system. The anatomic position of the six defined points for measurements should be expressed in centimeters above or proximal to the hymen (negative number) or centimeters below or distal to the hymen (positive numbers), with the plane of the hymen defined as zero. Stages are assigned according to the most severe portion of the prolapse when the full extent of the protrusion has been demonstrated. Stages are subgrouped according to which portion of the lower reproductive tract is the most distal part of the prolapse by use of letter qualifiers.

- The first measurement is the **genital hiatus (gh)**—measure from the middle of the external urethral meatus to the posterior midline of the hymenal ring. This measurement is particularly useful in predicting the ability to fit the woman with a pessary, because this measurement should optimally be smaller than the width of the apex.

- The second measurement is the **perineal body (pb)**—measure from the posterior margin of the genital hiatus to the middle of the anal opening.

- The third measurement is the **total vaginal length (tvl)**—measure by inserting a speculum into the vagina, and placing a cotton-tipped swab into the posterior fornix (or at the cuff) with the vagina reduced to normal position.

- Move the swab to the front of the cervix (or leave at the cuff in a hysterectomized patient). The speculum is removed with the swab in place, and the woman is asked to cough or bear down, to reproduce her prolapse. Watch the swab for descent toward the hymenal ring. The mark on the swab equal to the hymenal ring is the measurement of **point "C"** (also called the apex with strain). For example, if the cervix or cuff comes to the hymenal ring, that measurement would equal 0. If the cervix or cuff descends to 1 cm inside the hymenal ring, the "C" measurement would be –1. If the cervix or cuff protrudes 2 cm outside the hymenal ring, that measurement would be +2. (Measurements above the hymen are recorded as negative numbers, whereas measurements past the hymenal ring are recorded as positive numbers. This is true for all measurements taken along the vaginal walls as well.)

- Anterior wall position measurements

  - Take the speculum apart and insert the posterior blade to support the posterior wall of the vagina. The swab is placed midline along the anterior wall, with the cotton tip 3 cm from the hymenal ring. This is **point Aa**.

  - The woman is asked to cough again, and this point is now observed for movement toward/out of the introitus. The amount of movement is recorded as none (measurement remains at –3) to fully extended outside the hymen (+3), or anywhere in between.

  - Measure the point along the anterior wall that prolapses the *most*. This is **point Ba**. The amount of movement is recorded as anywhere from –3 (no movement) to the full length of the vagina (if this is outside of the introitus, it will be recorded as a positive number).

- Posterior wall position measurements

  - Remove the speculum blade, flip it over to support the anterior wall, and reproduce along the posterior wall the measurements taken along the anterior wall to determine **point Ap** and **point Bp**.

- Remove the speculum and perform a bimanual pelvic exam. At this time, the last POPQ measurement—the length of the cervix—is estimated. The estimated length of the cervix is added to the point "C" measurement, to measure **point "D,"** which is the posterior fornix or cul-de-sac (with strain). (It is not applicable in the hysterectomized patient.) For example, if point "C" is at –5, and the cervical length is estimated at 1 cm, point "D" would be –6.

Adapted from material developed by Mary Ann Geary, RN, MSN, Partners for Continence, Morristown, NJ, 2006.
[a]Figure 11.6 presents a graphic illustration of these measurements and information for staging POP based on the measurements.

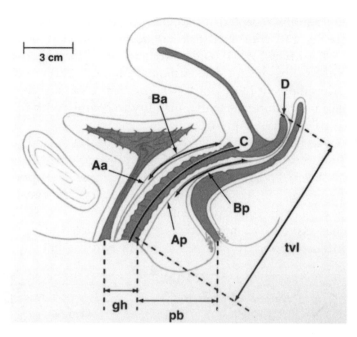

Figure 11.5.   Pelvic organ prolapse quantification (see Box 11.2 for abbreviations.) (From Bump, R.C., Mattiasson, A., Bo, K., Brubaker, L.P., DeLancey, J.O., Karskov, P., et al. [1996]. The standardization of terminology of female pelvic organ prolapse and pelvic floor dysfunction. *American Journal of Obstetrics and Gynecology, 175,* 10–17; reprinted by permission.)

specialists use a pessary as first-line therapy (Cundiff, Weidner, Visco, Bump, & Addison, 2000). It can be used temporarily while the woman is waiting for surgery, or can be used as a permanent device to support prolapse in women who have failed POP surgery or are poor candidates for surgery. It is also used diagnostically, inserted during urodynamic studies to try and predict which women will be helped by surgical correction, to assess whether symptom relief will be obtained with prolapse repair, and to unmask UI (particularly SUI). Although not a cure, as a medical treatment the use of a pessary has many potential benefits for the patient: it is low cost, it provides quick and effective relief of symptoms, it is not a permanent treatment, and it does not preclude the woman from opting for surgery. Some pessaries (e.g., incontinence pessary) may improve SUI. It has low risk because it is a noninvasive treatment (Trowbridge & Fenner, 2007).

A vaginal pessary is an effective and simple method of alleviating symptoms of POP and associated pelvic floor dysfunction (Fernando, Thakar, Sultan, Shah, & Jones, 2006). Two Cochrane Database Systematic Reviews (Adams, Thomson, Maher, & Hagen, 2004; Hagen, Stark, Maher, & Adams, 2004) have noted the lack of randomized controls in studies on the use of mechanical devices for POP. However, since the first edition of this book was published in 2002, there has been an increase in documented use of a pessary in women of all ages, so information on these devices is readily available. Pessaries have also been readily accepted by women as providing medium-term (1–2 years) satisfaction, and continued use has been reported (Clemons, Aguilar, Sokol, Jackson, & Myers, 2004). Older women (>65 years) tend to be longer term pessary users. Reasons for discontinuation include severe posterior vaginal prolapse, development of de novo SUI, and desire for surgery. Contraindications for their use include dementia, inability to comply with follow-up, and persistent vaginal infections or erosions.

A pessary is the oldest form of treatment for prolapse, and the word *pessary* can be found in both Greek and Latin literature. Some type of mechanical device has been reported since 400 B.C., the time of Hippocrates, who mentioned the use of fruit (a pomegranate) soaked in wine and placed in the vagina to support a POP. Homemade remedies continue, because one of the authors (DKN) has assessed women with POP who reported using a "sweet potato" and a kitchen sponge. Figure 11.6B shows two vaginal support devices

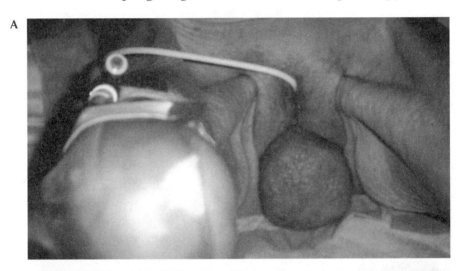

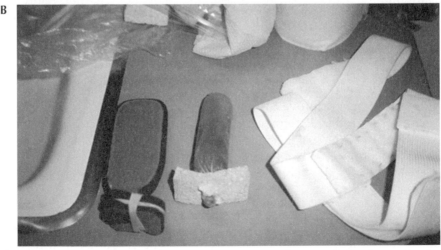

Figure 11.6. *A,* Vaginal vault prolapse causing urinary retention necessitating the use of an indwelling catheter. *B,* Homemade vaginal support devices made by husband of the woman in photo 11.6A.

with straps that were made by the spouse of a woman one of the authors (DKN) visited in the home several years ago. The woman had a vaginal vault prolapse (see Figure 11.6A) that was causing incomplete bladder emptying, necessitating an indwelling catheter. She had worn these devices for 2 years before discontinuing use because of discomfort.

Pessaries are very effective for premenopausal women with grades 1-4 prolapse. Posterior vaginal wall defects are not as adequately managed with pessaries as other defects. Women report improved lower urinary tract symptoms of urgency, frequency, and incontinence, as well as improved ambulation, with the use of a pessary. Most symptoms of prolapse (bulge and pressure) improve in 71%–90% of women (Clemons, Aguilar, Sokol, et al., 2004; Fernando et al., 2006). In addition, personal care is made easier and perineal hygiene is improved. A pessary may prevent further progression of the prolapse because this device may provide support and prevent constant strain on the connective tissue that supports the pelvic organs (Handa & Jones, 2002). Frail older women with large vaginal vaults and grade 4 prolapse are frequently not good surgical candidates. A well-fitting pessary is often the preferred alternative; however, these women usually have a difficult time retaining the pessaries currently on the market.

Types of Pessaries

A pessary comes in several sizes and shapes and is made of nonallergic silicone material with internal moldable steel reinforcement. The material is soft and pliable, does not absorb odors or secretions, and is resistant to breakdown with repeated cleaning or if autoclaved. Rigid pessaries are no longer used. Figure 11.7 shows the different types of pessaries and Appendix Table 11.1 provides a comprehensive review of available pessary types, indications, and fitting instructions. Pessary manufacturers are listed in Appendix B (Resources). The color of the pessary is either white (Coloplast, Bioteque) or pink (CooperSurgical [formerly distributed by Milex]). Some feel that the material and firmness of the pessary differ according to the manufacturer (Bioteque products are firmer, CooperSurgical and Coloplast products are softer). The best pessary is the one that supports the prolapse and stays in place when the woman walks and does her daily routine. It should not be painful; rather, the woman should not know it is there.

The manufacturers usually recommend a certain pessary for different types and degrees of prolapse. However, selection depends on a number of factors:

- Location and severity of prolapse
- Woman's weight and physical capacity
- Whether the woman is sexually active (ring, oval, or dish types are preferred)
- Previous pelvic surgery (e.g., hysterectomy). A pessary will work best if the uterus is present.

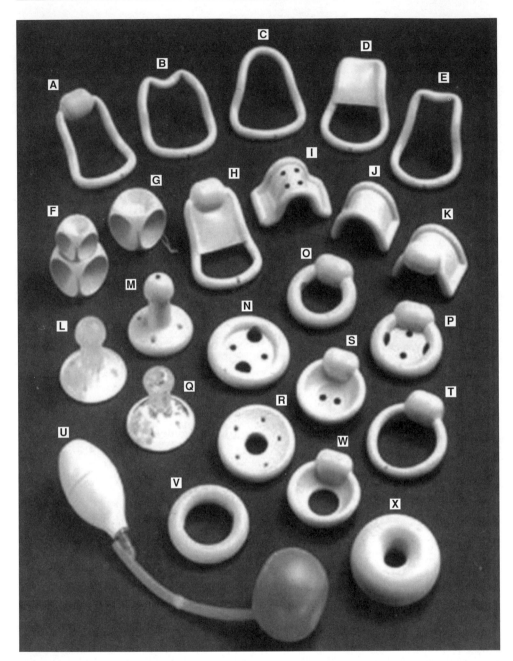

Figure 11.7. Various types of pessaries*. (A) Hodge with knob (folding). (B) Risser (folding). (C) Smith (folding). (D) Hodge with support (folding). (E) Hodge (folding). (F) Tandem-Cube. (G) Cube. (H) Hodge with support (knob/folding). (I) Regula (folding). (J) Gehrung (folding). (K) Gehrung with knob (folding). (L) Gellhorn 95% rigid (clear). (M) Gellhorn (flexible). (N) Ring with support (folding). (O) Ring with knob (folding). (P) Ring with support and knob (folding). (Q) Gellhorn (clear, short stem). (R) Shaatz (folding). (S) Incontinence Dish with support (folding). (T) Incontinence Ring (flexible). (U) Inflatoball 100% latex. (V) Ring (folding). (W) Incontinence Dish (folding). (X) Donut (autoclavable). (Courtesy of CooperSurgical.)

*Pessaries with a "knob" are primarily used in women who have stress UI to add support or compression at the vesicourethral junction.

- Length of the vagina (a shortened vagina, 6 cm or less, may be seen following hysterectomy)

- Size of the introitus (the larger the introitus—4 fingerbreadths or more—the greater the chance that the pessary will be expelled)

The pessary can be either supportive (e.g., ring, Gehrung) or space filling or "occupying" (e.g., cube, Inflatoball). A support pessary uses a spring mechanism that rests in the posterior fornix against the cervix. A space-filling pessary creates suction between the device and vaginal walls or just fills (occupies) the vaginal vault (Trowbridge & Fenner, 2007). A space-occupying pessary can be attempted for the relief of symptoms of a rectocele. Clinicians have noted that the ring pessary and incontinence dish are the most commonly used pessaries and the Gehrung and cube the least used (Komesu et al., 2007). The ring pessary, with or without support, is easily managed and allows for intercourse. Over two thirds of women with POP can be successfully fitted with a ring pessary (Clemons, Aguilar, Sokol, et al., 2004). The oval ring pessary, with or without support, may be useful in women with vaginal narrowing secondary to vaginal surgery or vaginal stenosis from aging and atrophy. A Gellhorn pessary is a space-occupying (completely fills the vaginal vault) pessary and is the second most common choice of pessary. The top of the Gellhorn pessary is a wide, flat disk that suctions against the vaginal wall. It can cause ulcerations. It has either a short or long stem depending on the length of the vagina. Because the cube pessary fills the entire vaginal vault, there is no area for drainage, which can lead to vaginal discharge and infection. Also, a cube prohibits vaginal intercourse if the woman is unable to remove it herself. In cases of severe prolapse, in which the vagina cannot retain a single pessary, the use of a tandem-cube pessary or double pessaries (e.g., a donut with a Gellhorn) may be recommended. Both the donut and Inflatoball pessaries should be removed and cleaned at least every 2–3 days and need special care.

There are also incontinence pessaries (ring, dish, or Marland) that are used to prevent SUI (Farrell, Singh, & Aldakhil, 2004). As opposed to a regular pessary, which is placed against the cervix in the posterior fornix, the incontinence pessary is placed at the base of the bladder to occlude, compress, or support the urethra and support the bladder neck (Dierich & Froe, 2000). This type of pessary restores continence by stabilizing the bladder base, decreasing bladder neck descent, allowing proper pressure transmission to the urethra, and by enhancing urethral resistance through significantly increased functional length and closure pressure (Noblett, McKinney, & Lane, 2008). If properly fitted, an incontinence pessary prevents urine loss during coughing, laughing, and other physical exertion activities when standing (Culligan & Heit, 2000). A study of 38 women with SUI showed that an incontinence ring pessary was an effective long-term device for 16% (6) of them (Robert & Mainprize, 2002).

Fitting a Pessary

Helen is an example of a woman who has successfully used a pessary. She is 69 years old and has managed her uterine prolapse with a pessary for the past 6 years. She was diagnosed with stage III anterior vaginal wall prolaspe with minimal descent of her cervix and stage II posterior wall prolapse. Her only urinary symptoms were occasional urinary urgency with no incontinence. Helen's gynecologist suggested prolaspe surgery, but she was reluctant to undergo the procedure because of a history of DVT and her current use of Coumadin. She was referred to one of the authors (DKN) for pessary fitting. Helen was successfully fitted with a ring with support pessary (size 6). She performs self-care of the pessary, removing and cleaning it at least 2 to 3 times per week. She uses VagiFem estradiol tablets intravaginally twice a week and will occasionally use TrimoSan vaginal jelly. She continues to be free of urinary and/or pelvic symptoms, has normal PVRs, and, surprisingly, has never experienced a urinary tract and/or vaginal infection or other pessary-related complications. Helen is very pleased with her current management and returns for follow-up pessary visits with DKN every 6 months.

Fitting the most appropriate pessary takes skill, experience, and trial and error but is essential for effectiveness (Carcio, 2004; Fritzinger, Newman, & Dinkin, 1997; Hanson, Schulz, Flood, Cooley, & Tam, 2006). It takes time and patience to fit pessaries, particularly in older women. Clemens et al. (2004) found that a mean of 2.2 pessaries per patient must be tried to achieve the best fit. Women with anterior vaginal wall prolapse should be counseled about unmasking or worsening UI. Most women have never seen a pessary and fear the "unknown." For this reason, women should be shown the different pessaries prior to insertion. Medical models or pictures should be used to explain their use and exactly where each provides support. Allowing the woman to hold and feel the pessary should alleviate some of her fear. Many women note the similarities between the contraceptive diaphragm and a pessary.

Prior to insertion of a pessary for fitting, the patient is asked to void. It is helpful if the bowels are also empty. A pelvic exam should always be performed before the introduction and fitting of a pessary because it helps to determine the appropriate pessary diameter. In general, the largest pessary the woman can comfortably accommodate should be fitted. The pessary rim's outside diameter is measured in inches. The clinician can use the fingers for approximation of size by determining the width and length (from the posterior fornix to under the symphysis pubis) of the vaginal vault. Manufacturers of pessaries will provide a fitting set, which may be a valuable aid in selecting the correct pessary. To measure, the clinician should insert the middle finger behind the cervix in the posterior fornix and place the index finger against the pubic notch. The distance between the two fingers is used as a starting point in pessary sizing. The pessary with the diameter that best approximates this distance is determined. This is similar to fitting a diaphragm, aiming for the largest size that fits comfortably.

The use of a local or topical estrogen cream or a water-soluble gel lubricant applied to the pessary aids in the success of pessary fitting. The entering end of the pessary is lubricated lightly and inserted so that part of the ring is behind the cervix and the opposite side is behind the pubic notch. Applying the lubricant to the vaginal opening instead of to the pessary will prevent the examiner's gloves from sliding off the pessary. Carcio (2004) suggested mixing lubricant with lidocaine 2% gel to decrease discomfort.

Like a diaphragm, the pessary is put into the vagina. Most are advanced to the posterior fornix behind the symphysis pubis and rest against the cervix, lifting or supporting the prolapsed pelvic organs. Once in place, the pessary is allowed to expand to its normal shape. It is recommended that the clinician rotate the pessary a quarter turn to prevent it from folding or being pushed out. The clinician should sweep a finger around the perimeter of the ring to check for pressure points. To avoid risk of pressure necrosis, the clinician should be able to insert a finger between the rim of the pessary and the vaginal walls. Urinary retention can result if the pessary compresses the urethra against the pubic bone. A well-supported pessary should not be visible. If the pessary does not fit properly, a smaller or larger size is tried. The pessary should be fitted for comfort and support.

Once the pessary is inserted, postfitting maneuvers are recommended. The woman should be examined in the standing position to determine proper positioning of the pessary, as well as possible discomfort. The woman should not be uncomfortable with the pessary in place because she should not be able to feel a properly fitted pessary. Once in place, the pessary should not dislodge when she is standing, sitting, squatting, or bearing down. The clinician should ask the woman to bear down while standing to determine

- if the pessary has descended to the introitus (if so, it will eventually fall out)
- if a cystocele or rectocele is bulging around the pessary
- if the pessary is becoming dislodged.

The woman should then spend about an hour walking and standing, and should also void with the pessary in place prior to leaving the medical facility to determine the risk of dislodgment. Dislodgment occurs most commonly during voiding or defecation. If the pessary becomes dislodged, the clinician should increase the pessary size or change to a different type (e.g., a space-occupying pessary).

Proper fitting may require several tries. Once fitted, most women are satisfied with the use of their pessary, and nearly all prolapse symptoms and approximately 50% of urinary symptoms (UI and voiding dysfunction) usually resolve within 2 months (Clemons, Aguilar, Tillinghast, Jackson, & Myers, 2004). Signs that a pessary size or shape may need to be changed include

- If the woman reports a slow urine stream when voiding, the pessary size should be decreased.

- If the woman feels the pessary move or shift, the size should be increased.

- If the woman complains of difficulty with bowel movements, the size should be decreased because the pessary may be pushing into the rectum, causing stool to get "stuck."

Unfortunately, many primary care physicians, geriatricians, and urologists are not familiar with pessary use (Cundiff et al., 2000). Pessaries are usually fitted by gynecologists, nurse practitioners, and nurse midwives (Carcio, 2004; Fitzinger, Newman, & Dinkin, 1997; Hanson et al., 2006; Luft, 2006; Maito Quam, Craig, Danner, & Rogers, 2006; McIntosh, 2005; Newman, 2007; Pott-Grinstein & Newcomer, 2001). Hanson et al. (2006) reported on 1,216 women who presented to a nurse-managed (continence nurse advisor) continence clinic in Canada. In this population, 1,043 women (86%) could be fitted with a pessary and 74% were successful with its use. Women with a cystocele (82%) or uterine prolapse (83%) were most successfully fitted. In this study, the ring, ring with support, and Gellhorn pessaries were more successful than the incontinence dish or ring and the Shaatz pessaries. As to complications in this study group, 88.5% ($n = 1,092$) did not have any reported complications, 8.9% developed erosions, 2.5% developed some type of vaginal infection, and 0.1% stopped using their pessary. Failure to retain a pessary is associated with increasing parity, previous pelvic surgery, and previous hysterectomy (Fernando et al., 2006; Maito et al., 2006).

Pessary Care

A new pessary should be washed with soap and water prior to insertion to remove the thin layer of powder coating the surface. Pessaries can be autoclaved using pre–vacuum sterilization parameters of 132°C ± 3°C for 4 minutes and gravity displacement sterilization parameters of 121°C ± 3°C for 30 minutes (CooperSurgical, personal communication, January 2007). A donut pessary should not be autoclaved. All pessaries can also be boiled for 15 minutes or cold sterilized with Cidex (Johnson & Johnson) or chlorophenyl (Bard-Parker), then thoroughly rinsed with water.

The method of care and the frequency of pessary removal differ from one type of pessary to another. A recommended follow-up visit protocol includes checking the pessary for size and support at 7–10 days after insertion, then 1 month later. If the woman cannot care for the pessary herself but is otherwise doing well with its use, then pessary care or follow-up with the clinician should occur at a minimum of every 2–3 months. If the woman performs self-care, then routine visits may be scheduled once or twice a year.

At the first follow-up visit, women should be questioned concerning pessary comfort, voiding, defecation, dislodgment, and self-care. At that visit, the woman is taught how to perform self-care, and demonstrates removal and insertion of the pessary. The visit should include a speculum vaginal examination to determine evidence of pressure, vaginal wall lesions, discharge, and allergic reactions. The pessary should be removed and washed with anti-bacterial cleanser and water, and a vaginal wash performed consisting of the insertion of 15 mL of povidone-iodine (Betadine) followed by rinsing with sterile water to remove excess discharge and secretions. (Pessary fitting and insertion can be billed under CPT code 57160, and vaginal irrigation under CPT code 57150; the actual device, which is Medicare reimbursable, can be billed under HCPCS A4562.)

The optimal pessary regimen is for the patient to perform self-care, re-moving and cleaning the pessary nightly with reinsertion in the morning. Many women prefer to remove the pessary at night in anticipation of sexual activity. Some patients remove and clean the pessary weekly. Some elderly women are unable to grasp the pessary for removal, and, for those, another option would be for their spouse or partner to remove the device. The use of a "pessary hook" (see Table 11.1) can assist the woman with removal of pes-saries that have holes because the hook can be inserted through the hole. Trowbridge and Fenner (2005) recommended tying either dental floss or monofilament suture to the pessary before insertion to aid in removal.

Although the materials used to make currently available pessaries are nontoxic, they will trap vaginal secretions, causing odor and discharge. A pessary can increase normal vaginal secretions (usually creamy). The use of TRIMO-SAN, an acidic vaginal jelly, is recommended because it is purported to help restore and maintain vaginal acidity and reduce odor-causing bacte-ria. Frequent use of this product may lead to bacterial vaginosis (BV) in cer-tain women, so we recommend its use only weekly. If the vaginal secretions are green or brown in color and have a foul odor, then a culture should be ob-tained because BV may be present. BV typically manifests with an increased thin, milky vaginal discharge and a foul or fishy odor. Douching should be discouraged because it has been shown to increase the prevalence of BV (Schwebke, Desmond, & Oh, 2004; Zhang et al., 2004).

Clinicians must emphasize the importance of follow-up pessary care. Re-gardless of whether a woman performs self-care, all should receive written in-structions about the use of a pessary. (For helpful information, see the patient education tool "Using a Pessary for Pelvic Organ Prolapse" on the companion CD.) Also, clinicians should consider having the patient routinely perform pelvic floor muscle exercises because these exercises have been shown to limit the progression of mild prolapse (Handa et al., 2004). Finally, the useful life of a pessary is limited, and it may need to be replaced as often as every 6 months. It may also be necessary to fit the woman with a different size or type of pes-sary after a period of time.

Pessary-Related Complications

The most common pessary-related complaints are pessary dislodgment—"it fell out"—UI, and rectal pain. Other complaints include perineal itching; foul odor; localized pain; inability to urinate, empty the bladder, or have bowel movements; and back pain. Disadvantages of a pessary include the requirement for ongoing care, risk of vaginal infection, and irritation. Vaginal mucosa ulceration, erosion, or both more commonly occur in postmenopausal women, and can be treated with a low-dose vaginal estrogen cream, $\frac{1}{4}$ to $\frac{1}{2}$ applicatorful twice a week (discussed in Chapter 9). Estrogen will thicken the vaginal wall, thus preventing erosion. Some clinicians use the Estring vaginal ring, placing it in the ring pessary with support or inserting it in the vagina before inserting the pessary.

A poorly fitted or neglected pessary can cause erosion through the vagina into the bladder or rectum. Uninterrupted pessary use can lead to chronic bacterial colonization and subsequent urosepsis (Roberge, McCandlish, & Dorfsman, 1999). Contraindications to the use of a pessary include persistent vaginal erosions or infections, endometriosis, and inability to comply with follow-up care (e.g., a woman with dementia who does not have a reliable caregiver). Chronic irritation, erosion, ulceration of the vagina, and vaginal fistula can occur in women who do not care for the pessary properly or who do not comply with regular follow-up (Luft, 2006). Adverse effects include back pain, BV, and bleeding (Alnaif & Drutz, 2000). If vaginal spotting or bleeding occurs, a pelvic examination should be performed to determine the presence of ulcers. If found, the pessary should be removed for 2–3 weeks to allow the ulcer to heal.

Chronic irritation, erosion, and ulceration of the vagina, as well as vaginal fistula (rare), can occur in women who do not properly care for their pessary or who do not go for regular follow-up visits with their doctor or nurse (Kankam & Geraghty, 2002). If ulceration and abrasion of the vaginal wall occur, the pessary should be removed until the lesions heal, and pessary size should be reduced. These women should be prescribed transvaginal estrogen to heal vaginal erosion and lacerations. Women who have not experienced UI should be warned that they have a risk of "potential" UI, which may have been previously masked by the prolapse. If SUI occurs, the clinician should suggest an incontinence pessary. A pessary left in place for prolonged periods of time or one that is "forgotten" can become embedded in the vaginal mucosa and cause harmful complications, and may be difficult to remove. Vaginal cancers have been reported in two women who were lost to follow-up (Jain, Majoko, & Freites, 2006). The authors postulated that a vaginal pessary may predispose to cancer through recurrent ulceration or erosions. Chronic inflammation due to the presence of a foreign body occurs, and poor hygiene may play a role.

Leukorrhea (a white watery discharge from the vagina) is probably the most common problem associated with pessary use. The vaginal environment alters with insertion of the pessary because the pessary is viewed as a foreign body; anaerobic bacteria and yeast may overgrow in relation to their normal balance with lactobacilli and other aerobic bacilli. This condition causes BV and has been reported to be prevalent in 32% of pessary users (Alnaif & Drutz, 2000). Cultures are not recommended. If symptomatic, according to the

Centers for Disease Control and Prevention (CDC) guidelines (CDC, Workowski, & Berman, 2006), women with BV should be treated with one of the following

- metronidazole 500 mg orally twice daily for 7 days
- metronidazole gel 0.75% intravaginally for 5 days
- clindamycin cream 2% intravaginally once a day for 7 days.

Other drugs, such as oral metronidazole 2 g orally in a single dose, are effective but have higher relapse rates after 2 weeks. If significant and offensive discharge persists, the pessary should be removed for 1 month. If vaginal discharge occurs frequently, the pessary should be removed and cleansed on a more frequent basis.

Reasons for Pessary Discontinuation

Not all women opt to use a pessary. Many do not want a foreign object inserted in their vagina. Many older patients have never used a contraceptive diaphragm or a tampon, so they are uncomfortable with a vaginal device. Once inserted, continuation is not always guaranteed. Women discontinue pessary use for multiple reasons, which include "not staying in well," and "it was uncomfortable" (Komesu et al., 2007, p. 620e3). Others discontinue because of the inconvenience or new-onset incontinence (Nguyen & Jones, 2005). New SUI can occur after pessary insertion, which can be a cause of dissatisfaction and is one of the primary reasons for discontinuation of a pessary. Urinary retention can result if the pessary compresses the urethra into the symphysis. A concern is when the woman is lost to follow-up, forgets she has a pessary, and goes for a long period of time without pessary care. The following case illustrates this concern.

> Several years ago, one of the authors (DKN) was asked by the charge nurse of a long-term care facility in a suburban Philadelphia nursing home to assess a female resident whose daughter had asked if her mother's pessary had been removed. The resident had been in the facility for 2 years and had dementia. The staff had been unaware that the resident had a pessary. The author asked the resident's certified nurse assistant (CNA) for assistance with pessary removal because the resident's dementia might make her uncooperative, and she might not be amenable to a pelvic examination.
>
> On opening the resident's door, the odor was overwhelming; when the CNA was questioned, she noted that the woman seemed to always have a bladder infection with very foul-smelling, brown-colored urine. The resident was then asked if she had a pessary. The "demented" resident replied "Yes, that blue thing [older models were colored blue], my doctor usually takes care of it." The resident was asked if she would like to have it removed. The response was "Yes, it hurts." The CNA confirmed that the

resident had been complaining of back pain, which staff had thought was another sign of a urinary tract infection.

When removing the resident's adult brief, brown-colored discharge was noted in the perineal area of the pad. The drainage was vaginal discharge, not urine, and the odor was probably not from the resident's urine but from the vagina. The pessary, which was a ring with support, was grasped and turned for removal. A large amount of brown vaginal drainage was noted. The odor was so strong that the CNA almost fainted. Betadine vaginal douches were prescribed once a day for 7 days. At a 1-month return visit, the resident had been infection free, in both the bladder and vagina, was without vaginal drainage, and her back pain had resolved.

Other Vaginal Support Devices

Some clinicians have found that the use of a tampon in the vagina will reduce SUI during exercising. Several disposable intravaginal devices have been introduced (e.g., Conveen Continence Guard, Contiform) that have been used to elevate the bladder neck. These devices resemble tampons and may be available in several sizes (Contiform) (Morris & Moore, 2003; Mouritsen, 2001). They are currently not available in the United States. One vaginal support device that is available is the Colpexin Sphere (Adamed, Frisco, Texas). This device elevates and supports the pelvic organs and can also be used with pelvic floor muscle training (PFMT) to treat POP (Lukban, Aguirre, Davila, & Sand, 2006). The Colpexin Sphere is made of medical-grade plastic and comes in six sizes. It is inserted into the vagina using the provided applicator or by hand (Figure 11.8). Unlike a pessary, its use is recommended as part of a program that includes PFMT (Sasso, 2006). Adverse events reported include vaginal irritation or burning, discomfort or spotting, yeast infection, and urinary tract infection.

Another product available for POP is the V-Brace by Fembrace (http:// www.fembrace.com/) (Figure 11.9). This is an external support garment for women that applies pressure upward in the perineum and may be helpful in reducing the discomfort from POP. It resembles a corset, and is adjustable and machine washable. It may be appropriate for women who do not want to try or have failed with a pessary and are not candidates for surgery.

SURGERY FOR POP

At least 1 in every 10 women will have POP so severe it will require surgery. Candidates for surgery include women with symptomatic and severe POP or who have failed or declined a pessary. Over 225,000 women in the United States have surgery each year for POP, but this represents a small fraction of women with this disorder (DeLancey, 2005; Weber, 2007). Surgery for POP should correct the specific pelvic floor defects that are present; in other words,

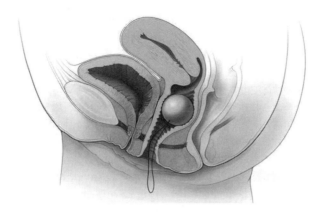

Figure 11.8.   Colpexin Sphere. (Courtesy of Adamed.)

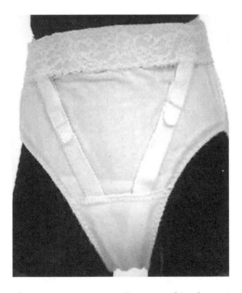

Figure 11.9.   V-Brace. (Courtesy of Fembrace.)

it should correct the specific prolapse and restore anatomy and function. Surgery has a reported success rate of 65%–90%, but repeat operations occur in 30% of women (Brubaker et al., 2003).

Surgical treatment for POP can be categorized broadly into reconstructive and obliterative techniques. Reconstructive surgery can be via the abdomen (open or laparoscopic abdominal sacrocolpopexy) or through the vagina using fascia, mesh tape, or sutures that suspend the prolapsed organs. The preferred method is via the vagina and involves repair with some combination of resuspension of the anterior, apical, or posterior vaginal wall. The current philosophy for a primary surgical approach to POP is to perform a vaginal procedure (e.g., vaginal sacrospinous colpopexy), virtually always with hysterectomy and occasionally with some form of vaginal cuff suspension and a variety of concomitant procedures (including colporrhaphy or continence procedures such as a Burch colposuspension) (discussed in Chapter 12). These procedures have varied success rates and can have multiple complications, including new incontinence, hemorrhage, hematoma, nerve damage, voiding difficulties, dyspareunia, recurrence of prolapse, and mesh erosion. Brubaker et al. (2006) found that postoperative SUI was significantly reduced in women who underwent abdominal sacrocolpopexy surgery for prolapse in combination with Burch colposuspension. A Cochrane Database review noted that abdominal sacrocolpopexy surgery was associated with a lower rate of prolapse recurrence and dyspareunia than vaginal surgery, but there was longer operating time, longer return to normal daily activities, and increased cost (Maher, Baessler, Glazener, Adams, & Hagen, 2008). Laparoscopic and robotic technologies are available. Success is dependent on the expertise and experience of the individual surgeon.

Obliterative surgery, such as total colpocleisis, corrects POP by moving pelvic viscera back into the pelvis and closing off the vagina either partly or totally. This procedure is usually reserved for women who are elderly, medically compromised, at increased surgical risk, and no longer sexually active and agree to permanent vaginal closure.

Appendix Table 11.1   Review of pessary types

Support
Ring (with and without support)   Oval ring (with or without support)

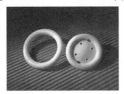   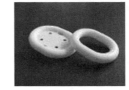

Picture courtesy of Coloplast   *Picture courtesy of Bioteque*

Description

- A "folding pessary" that uses a spring mechanism.
- The ring with support folds along one axis only. It has 2 small and 2 large holes; when folded, the 2 small holes touch each other.
- Most commonly used sizes are 3, 4, or 5.
- Sizes 11, 12, and 13 contain a wire coil that must be removed before MRI or x-ray studies.
- One of the most commonly used pessaries, and simplest to use and fit because the ring mimics that of a contraceptive diaphragm.
- Fit client with largest comfortable size.

Indications

- Ring without support—grades 1 and 2 uterine prolapse (anterior wall prolapse) only.
- Both types—grades 2 and 4 uterine prolapse complicated by a mild cystocele, anterior vaginal wall prolapse, and apical prolapse.
- Requires good perineal body or levator tone.
- The uterus and cervix can herniate (drop) through hole in center of the ring and oval ring without support pessaries.
- The oval-shaped ring pessary may be useful for women with some degree of vaginal narrowing (result of vaginal stenosis from aging and atrophy).

Fitting instructions

- Fold the pessary by bringing the small holes together and insert it downward.

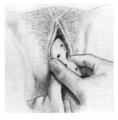

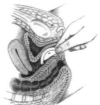

Pictures courtesy of CooperSurgical

(continued)

- After passing the introitus, allow the pessary to open again into a ring shape.
- Advance past the cervix until the leading edge reaches the posterior fornix, behind the symphysis pubis.
- Once inserted, rotate the pessary 90° so that one small hole is anterior (and the other small hole is posterior) to decrease risk of expulsion.

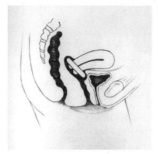

Picture courtesy of CooperSurgical

- To remove, insert a finger under the rim and turn the pessary 90° to facilitate bending; the notches will face the introitus.

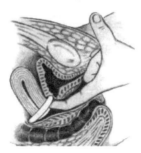

Picture Courtesy CooperSurgical

- Avoid putting a finger in the hole during removal.
- Women who have difficulty with self-removal can use a pessary hook that is inserted through the hole and "hooked" around the rim to remove the pessary.

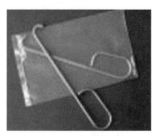

Picture courtesy of Bioteque

Gehrung without a knob	Gehrung with a knob
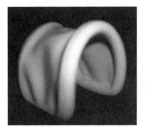	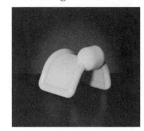
Picture courtesy of CooperSurgical	*Picture courtesy of CooperSurgical*

Description

- Arch-like moldable "U" shape provides broad support under the bladder and prevents the descent of the uterus.
- Derives its support from the remnants of the levator ani sling laterally.
- Can be molded and manually shaped to fit the individual patient.
- Common sizes: 3–5.
- Contains a wire coil that must be removed before x-ray or MRI studies.

Indications

- Designed to support uterine anterior and posterior vaginal wall prolapse. It is used with second- to fourth-degree cystocele and to thin out a rectocele.
- Is more adaptable in cases in which a cystocele tends to slip out when other pessaries are used.
- Gehrung with a knob is used for SUI.

Fitting instructions

- Fold the pessary by squeezing the two arches together.
- Insert with concavity downward for anterior vaginal wall prolapse, or with concavity upward for posterior vaginal wall prolapse.
- Insert it past the cervix and into the posterior fornix.
- Once it is in the vagina, allow the arch to open to its normal shape and rotate the pessary into position.
- The base of the arch should rest on the posterior vaginal wall, and the curve supports the anterior wall.
- Lateral bars should straddle the rectum for uterine and anterior wall prolapse, and should straddle the bladder for posterior wall prolapse.
- A correctly placed pessary should have both heels resting on the pelvic floor with the arches and cross support forming a bridge to raise the bladder.

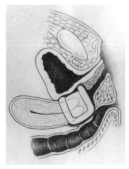

Picture courtesy of CooperSurgical

(continued)

- Remove the pessary by gradually pushing the arch of the pessary off the cervix while turning it so that the heels or supports of the pessary are turned 90°.

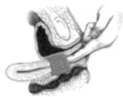

- Then fold the pessary, forming an arch that is in the up position and gently pulling the pessary with one heel first through the introitus.

Space-Filling or Space-Occupying

Gellhorn—"soft" silicone with standard or short stem	Gellhorn—95% "rigid" acrylic, with standard or short stem
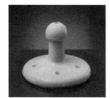	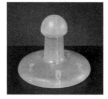
Picture courtesy of CooperSurgical	*Picture courtesy of CooperSurgical*

Description

- Common sizes: 2¼ to 3½ inches.
- Rigid Gellhorn pessary not recommended because of high rate of erosions and ulcerations.
- Difficult removal and insertion for patient.
- Prohibits vaginal intercourse if patient is unable to self-remove.

Indications

- Used for grades 3 and 4 prolapse, including procidentia (apical prolapse). This pessary relies on the integrity of the pelvic floor muscle and intact perineum for its retention.
- It must be removed for sexual intercourse.
- Most difficult-to-remove pessary.

Fitting instructions

- If a small size is used, fold disk (concave side), then gently push pessary into the upper vagina.
- If unable to fold, insert it edgewise almost parallel to the introitus.

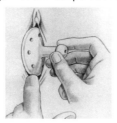

Picture courtesy of CooperSurgical

- Use a corkscrew motion while introducing the pessary into the vagina.
- The wide, flat surface (disk) should be toward the anterior vaginal wall. It should rest against the cervix or be suctioned against the upper vagina if the cervix is absent.

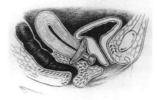

Picture courtesy of CooperSurgical

- The stem of the pessary may be seen at the introitus with a Valsalva maneuver, but ideally should rest against the posterior vaginal wall as indicated in the picture below.

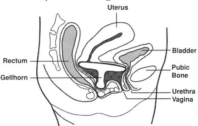

Picture courtesy of Robin Noel

- To remove, work the stem of the Gelhorn to the introitus and grasp it.

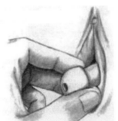

Picture courtesy of CooperSurgical

- It may be necessary to "break the seal" of the disk first by inserting a finger behind the disk, then grasping the stem with fingers or an instrument (tenaculum or ring forceps).
- Gently rock the stem side to side and pull downward and out.
- If this does not break the suction, then inject water through the hole in the stem as depicted in the illustration below. This will usually break the seal.

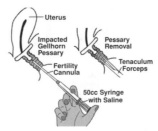

Picture courtesy of Robin Noel

(continued)

Donut

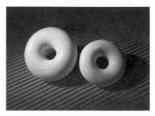

Picture courtesy of Coloplast

Description

- Space-filling device that functions by occupying a space larger than the genital hiatus.
- Common sizes: 2–4.
- Difficult insertion and removal for patient.

Indications

- Thicker than the ring, it is useful for grade 3 or 4 uterine prolapse, vaginal vault prolapse, or both (posterior and procidentia prolapse).

Fitting instructions

- The donut pessary can be compressed to simplify insertion and removal. Squeeze the sides to reduce the diameter of the donut pessary.
- Insert the compressed pessary past the cervix and into the posterior fornix.
- Once the pessary has passed the introitus, allow it to expand to its normal shape.

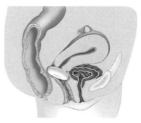

Picture courtesy of Coloplast

- Remove by placing your index finger into the center hole of the pessary and, with the thumb, compress the pessary.
- Then angle the compressed pessary downward and pull gently through the introitus.

Inflatoball

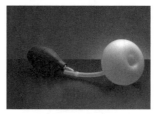

Picture courtesy of CooperSurgical

Description
• Space-occupying Inflatoball provides general support to prolapsing vaginal structures. It has a filling port that allows for inflation with air and deflation for removal. It is made of latex rubber, which absorbs odors, so should be removed and cleansed every 2 to 3 days. • Common sizes: medium to large. • Difficult to retain.

Indications
• Adequate integrity of the introital opening is necessary for this pessary to remain in place, but the patient does not need an intact perineum or competent levator ani muscle.

Fitting instructions
• Inflate Inflatoball once in the vagina using a small handheld pump. 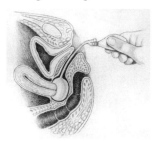 *Picture courtesy of CooperSurgical* • The inflation port may be able to be tucked into the vagina. • When removing the pessary, deflate by releasing the stopcock and allowing the air to escape.

Cube

Available with and without drains
(holes that allow for drainage)

Tandem-cube

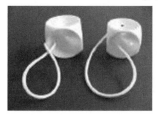

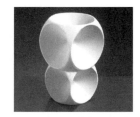

Picture courtesy of Bioteque   *Picture courtesy of CooperSurgical*

Description
• Space-filling device that functions by creating suction between the device's six sides and the vaginal walls. • Common sizes: 2–4. • Some designs include a string attached to the body of the cube. • Tandem-cube is used when a single cube provides inadequate support.

Indications
• Effective in some older patients in whom there is markedly decreased vaginal tone (rarely used), or grade 3 or 4 uterine and vaginal vault prolapse.

(continued)

- Tandem cube is used for grade 3 prolapse or procidentia when a single cube is inadequate.
- Can cause vaginal ulceration and discharge.
- Using a cube with holes may decrease ulcerations and discharge.
- This is the pessary of "last resort."

Fitting instructions

- Compress the two sides of the cube and advance it to the most posterior and apical portion of the vagina.

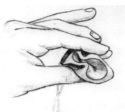

Picture courtesy of CooperSurgical

- Once the pessary has passed the introitus, allow the cube to expand to its normal shape.
- The attached silicone tie is an aid in removing the cube pessary.

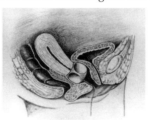

Cube
Picture courtesy of CooperSurgical

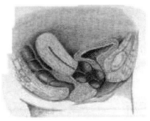

Tandem-cube
Picture courtesy of CooperSurgical

- Remove the cube by breaking the suction or seal and gently pulling down on the silicone tie until the pessary can be reached and compressed with the thumb and index finger. Once the walls are collapsed, they are easy to remove.
- Then angle the compressed cube downward and pull gently through the introitus.

Shaatz

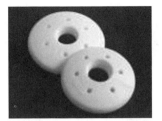

Picture courtesy of Bioteque

Description

- Was the original hard black rubber pessary.

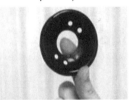

- Resembles the Gellhorn without the stem.

Indications

- Used in uterine or vaginal vault prolapse.

Fitting instructions

- Fold the Shaatz pessary so that the leading edge of the formed crescent points in a downward direction.
- Then insert the Shaatz past the cervix and into the posterior fornix.
- Once the pessary has passed the introitus, allow it to expand to its normal shape.

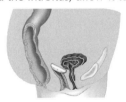

Picture courtesy of Coloplast

- To remove the pessary, try to fold it into a crescent shape and carefully withdraw.

Incontinence Pessary

Incontinence ring with or without support	Marland (with or without support)

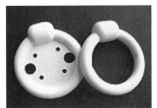

Picture courtesy of Bioteque

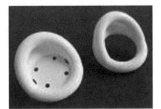

Picture courtesy of Bioteque

(continued)

Incontinence dish with support

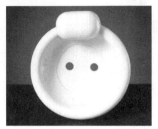

Picture courtesy of CooperSurgical

Incontinence dish without support

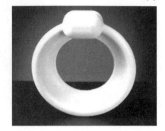

Picture courtesy of CooperSurgical

Description

- Has a midline knob or paraurethral prong to stabilize the urethrovesical junction when increases in intra-abdominal pressure occur.
- Common sizes: 2–7 (for incontinence ring with or without support).
- Common sizes: 3–5 (for incontinence dish with support).

Indications

- Supports the urethra in a more retropubic position, which prevents SUI in women with or without advanced prolapse.
- Incontinence ring is the initial pessary of choice for SUI.

Fitting instructions

- All incontinence pessaries are inserted, folded, and removed similar to the ring pessary. The knob of the pessary should rest at the level of the urethrovesical junction.

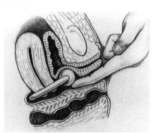

Incontinence ring
Picture courtesy of CooperSurgical

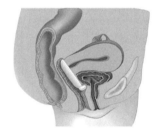

Incontinence dish
Picture courtesy of Coloplast

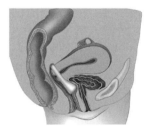

Marland
Picture courtesy of Coloplast

Key: MRI = magnetic resonance imaging; SUI = stress urinary incontinence.

REFERENCES

ACOG Committee on Practice Bulletins—Gynecology. (2007). ACOG Practice Bulletin No. 85: Pelvic organ prolapse. *Obstetrics and Gynecology, 110,* 717–729.

Adams, E., Thomson, A., Maher, C., & Hagen, S. (2004). Mechanical devices for pelvic organ prolapse. *Cochrane Database of Systematic Reviews,* (2), CD004010.

Alnaif, B., & Drutz, H.P. (2000). Bacterial vaginosis increased in pessary users. *International Urogynecology Journal and Pelvic Floor Dysfunction, 11,* 219–222.

Baden, W.F., & Walker, T. (1992). Fundamentals, symptoms and classification. In W.F. Baden & T. Walker (Eds.), *Surgical repair of vaginal defects* (p. 14). Philadelphia: J.B. Lippincott.

Barber, M.D., Kuchibhatla, M.N., Pieper, C.F., & Bump, R.C. (2001). Psychometric evaluation of 2 comprehensive condition-specific quality of life instruments for women with pelvic floor disorders. *American Journal of Obstetrics and Gynecology, 185,* 1388–1395.

Barber, M.D., Walters, M.D., & Bump, R.C. (2005). Short forms of two condition-specific quality-of-life questionnaires for women with pelvic floor disorders (PFDI-20 and PFIQ-7). *American Journal of Obstetrics and Gynecology, 193,* 103–113.

Brubaker, L., Cundiff, G., Fine, P., Nygaard, I., Richter, H., Visco, A., et al. for the Pelvic Floor Disorders Network. (2003). A randomized trial of colpopexy and urinary reduction efforts (CARE): Design and methods. *Controlled Clinical Trials, 24,* 629–642.

Brubaker, L., Cundiff, G.W., Fine, P., Nygaard, I., Richter, H.E., Visco, A.G., et al., for the Pelvic Floor Disorders Network. (2006) Abdominal sacrocolpopexy with Burch colposuspension to reduce urinary stress incontinence. *New England Journal of Medicine, 354,* 1557–1566.

Bump, R.C., Mattiasson, A., Bo, K., Brubaker, L.P., DeLancey, J.O., Klarskov, P., et al. (1996). The standardization of terminology of female pelvic organ prolapse and pelvic floor dysfunction. *American Journal of Obstetrics and Gynecology, 175,* 10–17.

Carcio, H. (2004). The vaginal pessary: An effective yet underused tool for incontinence and prolapse. *ADVANCE for Nurse Practitioners, 12*(10), 47–56.

Centers for Disease Control and Prevention, Workowski, K.A., & Berman, S.M. (2006). Sexually transmitted diseases treatment guidelines, 2006. *MMWR Recommendations and Reports, 55*(RR-11), 1–95.

Clemons, J.L., Aguilar, V.C., Sokol, E.R., Jackson, N.D., & Myers, D.L. (2004). Patient characteristics that are associated with continued pessary use versus surgery after 1 year. *American Journal of Obstetrics and Gynecology, 191,* 159–164.

Clemons, J.L., Aguilar, V.C., Tillinghast, T.A., Jackson, N.D., & Myers, D.L. (2004). Patient satisfaction and changes in prolapse and urinary symptoms in women who were fitted successfully with a pessary for pelvic organ prolapse. *American Journal of Obstetrics and Gynecology, 190,* 1025–1029.

Culligan, P.J., & Heit, M. (2000). Urinary incontinence in women: Evaluation and management. *American Family Physician, 62,* 2433–2444, 2447, 2452.

Cundiff, G.W., Weidner, A.C., Visco, A.G., Bump, R.C., & Addison, W.A. (2000). A survey of pessary use by members of the American Urogynecologic Society. *Obstetrics and Gynecology, 95,* 931–935.

DeLancey, J.O. (2005). The hidden epidemic of pelvic floor dysfunction: Achievable goals for improved prevention and treatment. *American Journal of Obstetrics and Gynecology, 192,* 1488–1495.

Dierich, M., & Froe, F. (2000). *Overcoming incontinence.* New York: John Wiley & Sons.

Diokno, A.C., & Borodulin, G. (2005). A new vaginal speculum for pelvic organ prolapse quantification (POPQ). *International Urogynecology Journal and Pelvic Floor Dysfunction, 16,* 384–388.

Farrell, S.A., Singh, B., & Aldakhil, L. (2004). Continence pessaries in the management of urinary incontinence in women. *Journal of Obstetrics and Gynaecology Canada, 26,* 113–117.

Fernando, R.J., Thakar, R., Sultan, A.H., Shah, S.M., & Jones, P.W. (2006). Effect of vaginal pessaries on symptoms associated with pelvic organ prolapse. *Obstetrics and Gynecology, 108,* 93–99.

Fritzinger, K.G., Newman, D.K., & Dinkin, E. (1997). Use of a pessary for the management of pelvic organ prolapse. *Lippincott's Primary Care Practice, 1,* 431–436.

Ghetti, C., Gregory, W.T., Edwards, S.R., Otto, L.N., & Clark, A.L. (2005). Pelvic organ descent and symptoms of pelvic floor disorders. *American Journal of Obstetrics and Gynecology, 193,* 53–57.

Hagen, S., Stark, D., Maher, C., & Adams, E. (2004). Conservative management of pelvic organ prolapse. *Cochrane Database of Systematic Reviews,* (2), CD003882.

Handa, V.L., Garrett, E., Hendrix, S., Gold, E., & Robbins, J. (2004). Progression and remission of pelvic organ prolapse: A longitudinal study of menopausal women. *American Journal of Obstetrics and Gynecology, 190,* 27–32.

Handa, V.L., & Jones, M. (2002). Do pessaries prevent the progression of pelvic organ prolapse? *International Urogynecology Journal and Pelvic Floor Dysfunction, 13,* 349–352.

Hanson, L.M., Schulz, J.A., Flood, C.G., Cooley, B., & Tam, F. (2006). Success of pessary use in the conservative management of incontinence and pelvic organ prolapse. *International Urogynecology Journal and Pelvic Floor Dysfunction, 14,* 142.

Hendrix, S.L., Clark, A., Nygaard, I., Aragaki, A., Barnabei, V., & McTiernan, A. (2002). Pelvic organ prolapse in the Women's Health Initiative: Gravity and gravidity. *American Journal of Obstetrics and Gynecology, 186,* 1160–1166.

Jain, A., Majoko, F., & Freites, O. (2006). How innocent is the vaginal pessary? Two cases of vaginal cancer associated with pessary use. *Journal of Obstetrics and Gynaecology, 26,* 829–830.

Jelovsek, J.E., Maher, C., & Barber, M.D. (2007). Pelvic organ prolapse. *Lancet, 369,* 1027–1038.

Kankam, O.K., & Geraghty, R. (2002). An erosive pessary. *Journal of the Royal Society of Medicine, 95,* 507.

Kesharvarz, H., Hillis, S.D., Kieke, B.A., & Marchbanks, P.A. (2002). Hysterectomy surveillance—United States, 1994–1999. *MMWR Surveillance Summary, 51*(SS05), 1–8.

Komesu, Y.M., Rogers, R.G., Rode, M.A., Craig, E.C., Gallegos, K.A., Montoya, A.R., et al. (2007). Pelvic floor symptom changes in pessary users. *American Journal of Obstetrics and Gynecology, 197,* 620.e1–620.e6.

Luft, J. (2006, March). Pelvic organ prolapse. *Nurse Practitioner,* pp. 170–185.

Lukacz, E.S., Lawrence, J.M., Contreras, R., Nager, C.W., & Luber, K.M. (2006). Parity, mode of delivery, and pelvic floor disorders. *Obstetrics and Gynecology, 107,* 1253–1260.

Lukban, J.C., Aguirre, O.A., Davila, G.W., & Sand, P.K. (2006). Safety and effectiveness of Colpexin Sphere in the treatment of pelvic organ prolapse. *International Urogynecology Journal and Pelvic Floor Dysfunction, 17,* 449–454.

Maher, C., Baessler, K., Glazener, C.M., Adams, E.J., & Hagen, S. (2008). Surgical management of pelvic organ prolapse in women: A short version Cochrane review. *Neurourology and Urodynamics, 27,* 3–12.

Maito, J.M., Quam, Z.A., Craig, E., Danner, K.A., & Rogers, R.G. (2006). Predictors of successful pessary fitting and continued use in a nurse-midwifery pessary clinic. *Journal of Midwifery and Women's Health, 51,* 78–84.

Marinkovic, S.P., & Stanton, S.L. (2004). Incontinence and voiding difficulties associated with prolapse. *Journal of Urology, 171,* 1021–1028.

McIntosh, L. (2005). The role of the nurse in the use of vaginal pessaries to treat pelvic organ prolapse and/or urinary incontinence: A literature review. *Urologic Nursing, 25,* 41–48.

Moalli, P.A., Jones Ivy, S., Meyn, L.A., & Zyczynski, H.M. (2003). Risk factors associated with pelvic floor disorders in women undergoing surgical repair. *Obstetrics and Gynecology, 101,* 869–874.

Morris, A.R., & Moore, K.H. (2003). The Contiform incontinence device—efficacy and patient acceptability. *International Urogynecology Journal and Pelvic Floor Dysfunction, 14,* 412–417.

Mouritsen, L. (2001). Effect of vaginal devices on bladder neck mobility in stress incontinent women. *Acta Obstetricia et Gynecologica Scandinavica, 80,* 428–431.

Newman, D.K. (2007, January). Nonsurgical solutions for POP. *Nursing Spectrum,* pp. 12–13.

Nguyen, J.N., & Jones, C.R. (2005). Pessary treatment of pelvic relaxation: Factors affecting successful fitting and continued use. *Wound, Ostomy, and Continence Nursing, 32,* 255–261.

Noblett, K.L., McKinney, A., & Lane, F.L. (2008). Effects of the incontinence dish pessary on urethral support and urodynamic parameters. *American Journal of Obstetrics and Gynecology, 198*(5), 592.e1-5.

Nygaard, I., Bradley, C., & Brandt, D., for the Women's Health Initiative. (2004). Pelvic organ prolapse in older women: Prevalence and risk factors. *Obstetrics and Gynecology, 104,* 489–497.

Olsen, A.L., Smith, V.J., Bergstrom, J.O., Colling, J.C., & Clark, A.L. (1997). Epidemiology of surgically managed pelvic organ prolapse and urinary incontinence. *Obstetrics and Gynecology, 89,* 501–506.

Popovic, J.R., & Kozak, L.J. (2000). National hospital discharge survey: Annual summary, 1998. *Vital and Health Statistics, Series 13: Data from the National Health Survey, 148,* 1–194.

Pott-Grinstein, E., & Newcomer, J.R. (2001). Gynecologists' patterns of prescribing pessaries. *Journal of Reproductive Medicine, 46,* 205.

Roberge, R.J., McCandlish, M.M., & Dorfsman, M.L. (1999). Case reports: Urosepsis associated with vaginal pessary use. *Annals of Emergency Medicine, 33,* 581–583.

Robert, M., & Mainprize, T.C. (2002). Long-term assessment of the incontinence ring pessary for the treatment of stress incontinence. *International Urogynecology Journal and Pelvic Floor Dysfunction, 13,* 326–329.

Rortveit, G., Brown, J.S., Thom, D.H., Van Den Eeden, S.K., Creasman, J.M., & Subak, L.L. (2007). Symptomatic pelvic organ prolapse: Prevalence and risk factors in a population-based, racially diverse cohort. *Obstetrics and Gynecology, 109,* 1396–1403.

Sasso, K.M. (2006). The Colpexin Sphere: A new conservative management option for pelvic organ prolapse. *Urologic Nursing, 26,* 433–441.

Schwebke, J.R., Desmond, R.A., & Oh, M.K. (2004). Predictors of bacterial vaginosis in adolescent women who douche. *Sexually Transmitted Diseases, 31,* 433–436.

Shah, S.M., Sultan, A.H., & Thakar, R. (2006). The history and evolution of pessaries for pelvic organ prolapse. *International Urogynecology Journal and Pelvic Floor Dysfunction, 17,* 170–175.

Subak, L.L., Waetjen, L.E., van den Eeden, S., Thom, D.H., Vittinghoff, E., & Brown, J.S. (2001). Cost of pelvic organ prolapse in the United States. *Obstetrics and Gynecology, 98,* 646–651.

Swift, S.E., Tate, S.B., & Nicholas, J. (2003). Correlation of symptoms with degree of pelvic organ support in a general population of women: What is pelvic organ prolapse? *American Journal of Obstetrics and Gynecology, 189,* 372–377.

Trowbridge, R.E., & Fenner, D.E. (2005). Conservative management of pelvic organ prolapse. *Clinical Obstetrics and Gynecology, 48,* 668–681.

Trowbridge, E.R., & Fenner, D.E. (2007). Practicalities and pitfalls of pessaries in older women. *Clinical Obstetrics and Gynecology, 50,* 709–719.

Weber, A.M. (2007). Elective cesarean delivery: The pelvic perspective. *Clinical Obstetrics and Gynecology, 50,* 510–517.

Weber, A.M., & Richter, H.E. (2005). Pelvic organ prolapse. *Obstetrics and Gynecology, 106,* 615–634.

Zhang, J., Hatch, M., Zhang, D., Shulman, J., Harville, E., & Thomas, A.G. (2004). Frequency of douching and risk of bacterial vaginosis in African American women. *Obstetrics and Gynecology, 104,* 756–760.

12

Overview of Surgical Intervention for Incontinence

Stress urinary incontinence (UI) is the leakage of urine with effort or physical exertion, such as coughing, sneezing, and straining. It can be caused by changes in the support (musculature, ligaments) or innervation of the bladder, bladder outlet, sphincter, and urethra. Conservative therapy such as pelvic floor muscle training may be effective, especially in mild cases. However, many patients with stress UI may choose to discontinue an initial trial of conservative therapy or may eventually become dissatisfied or disenchanted with these therapies because of cost, discomfort, inconvenience, lack of motivation, or lack of efficacy. For these individuals, numerous surgical methods have been described and in many cases may be the best and only option. The goal of surgical treatment of stress UI is to provide sufficient urethral closure to prevent urine from leaking from the urethra during increases in intra-abdominal pressure, while preserving voluntary, low-pressure, and complete bladder emptying.

Urgency UI, usually attributed to bladder dysfunction, involves overactive bladder symptoms of urgency and frequency that can be successfully managed with behavorial modification and drug therapy in many cases. Refractory urgency UI may improve with injections of botulinum toxin and with sacral neuromodulation.

Numerous surgical and invasive methods have been described for treatment of UI. The following methods are reviewed in this chapter:

- Retropubic colposuspension—open and laparoscopic

- Sling procedures, including bladder neck and midurethral tape procedures

- Periurethral injections

- Detrusor or suburothelial botulinum toxin (Botox) injections

- Artificial urinary sphincter

- Sacral neuromodulation

SURGICAL OPTIONS FOR STRESS UI IN WOMEN

If conservative therapy fails and better resolution is still desired, stress UI in women is typically treated with surgery, and more than 200 different operations have been designed. These procedures generally aim to improve the support to the proximal urethra and/or bladder neck and to correct deficient urethral closure during increases in intra-abdominal pressure. There is disagreement, however, regarding the precise mechanism by which continence is achieved with surgical manipulation. The surgeon's preference and expertise, coexisting problems, and the anatomic features and general health condition of the individual often influence the choice of procedure. In general, surgical correction of stress UI, urethral hypermobility, or intrinsic (urethral) sphincter dysfunction (ISD) (see Chapter 4) is directed primarily toward one or both of the following two goals:

1. Providing a "backboard" of support against which the urethra is compressed during increases in intra-abdominal pressure.

2. Creating coaptation, compression, or both, or otherwise augmenting the urethral resistance provided by the intrinsic sphincter unit, with (e.g., sling) or without (e.g., periurethral injectables) affecting urethral and bladder neck support.

Choice of Operation

The number of surgical procedures for stress UI doubled in the mid-1990s (Boyles, Weber, & Meyn, 2004), and from this large number, it is obvious that no "perfect" procedure exists (Rovner & Wein, 2004). Yet, the quest for the ideal procedure with the highest effectiveness, least morbidity, and greatest cost-effectiveness is still ongoing. As with most surgeries, the best stress UI operation, in terms of results, is the first procedure. All experts agree that surgery for recurrent incontinence may have a poorer outcome because scarring is usually present and complications are more likely to occur.

Surgeries directed toward repositioning or stabilizing the bladder neck and proximal urethra are often classified according to the operative approach: retropubic (transabdominal) or transvaginal (Smith & Moy, 2004). Traditional routes of surgery for stress UI include the abdominal route (retropubic urethropexy) and the combined technique used in sling procedures (abdominal and vaginal). Retropubic suspension procedures include the Burch colposuspension and the Marshall-Marchetti-Krantz (MMK) bladder neck suspension. The abdominal and combined abdominal-vaginal routes have drawbacks, including the risks of incisional hernia, incisional pain, and delayed recovery. Because of these drawbacks, laparoscopic suspension surgery for stress UI has become an alternative to other traditional abdominal approaches, but it may not be as successful. When the vaginal approach is being considered, additional procedures may be performed at the same time, such as anterior and posterior colporrhaphy and vaginal hysterectomy, in symptomatic women with pelvic organ prolapse (see Chapter 11). The newer midurethral "tension-free" vaginal tape procedures provide a backboard against which the urethra is compressed during increases in intra-abdominal pressure. Coaptation (joining together or fitting of two surfaces) of the proximal urethra/bladder neck can also be achieved by these or by the classic pubovaginal sling procedure. Some degree of coaptation is generally necessary when a significant degree of ISD is present.

It is important to understand that the outcome definition of improvement/ cure is not standardized for any incontinence procedure (Kobashi & Govier, 2005). Rapp and Kobashi (2008) noted that "completely dry" represents the strictest criteria for success and it is achieved in the minority of patients. "Cure" is not the same outcome, as it may denote "rare" UI episodes or "pad-free." The stricter the definition, the poorer the results. Long-term reports indicate "success" (improvement/ cure) rates of 60%–90% for sling tape and suspension procedures. In a follow-up study of women who had undergone a midurethral tension-free tape procedure, Ulmsten, Johnson, and Rezapour (1999) found 86% success at 3 years; however, the definition of success was less than 10 g of UI on a 24-hour pad test, not really a "dry" outcome. Unfortunately, the success rate for surgery may not be as high for older women, especially if the woman has detrusor overactivity, urgency, and frequency present in addition to stress UI.

Preoperative Preparation

If a surgical procedure is to be performed, the woman should be properly informed of its risks and benefits, including the expected postoperative course. Informed consent should include a discussion of potential postoperative complications and their treatments, which should be considered as part of the decision making. Prevailing expert opinion suggests that surgery should be delayed until childbearing is complete.

One complication is the possibility of postoperative urinary retention (1%–15%) that occurs immediately after the procedure but usually resolves either quickly or within 4–6 weeks postoperatively. It is important to discuss the method of urine drainage (suprapubic or urethral catheter) during the immediate postoperative period. An intermittent catheterization program may be necessary if spontaneous voiding does not occur immediately after a voiding trial. Another important adverse event that needs discussion preoperatively is the potential for aggravating preexisting or creating de novo (new) urgency and UI symptoms. Self-reported new symptoms or worsening of urgency or incontinence can occur in up to 25% of women after surgery. This can be a very bothersome symptom to women, but there also is a good chance that, if preexisting, such symptoms may subside spontaneously. Older women (>75 years) are more likely to experience postoperative urinary retention, urgency UI, and treatment failure following sling surgery (Anger, Litwin, Wang, Pashos, & Rodríguez, 2007).

Experiencing overactive bladder symptoms during the postsurgical period significantly diminishes patient satisfaction, regardless of personal goal achievement (Hullfish, Bovbjerg, & Steers, 2004). Therefore, patient-centered surgical outcomes have been shown to be important when discussing this intervention for women with UI. Mahajan, Elkadry, Kenton, Shott, and Brubaker (2006) reported on patient satisfaction 1 year after surgery for stress UI (slings and Burch colposuspension) and pelvic organ prolapse, and noted that those women with any urgency UI reported reduced satisfaction rates compared with the overall group (69% of subjects with < 80% satisfaction vs. 77% in the group as a whole). They also showed that incomplete resolution of symptoms (20%) was the second most common reason for less than 100% satisfaction with surgical outcomes. Patient satisfaction with surgical outcomes after surgery is highly subjective and is determined by the achievement of personal goals for surgery.

Types of Procedures

As previously mentioned, several different surgical procedures and many different approaches (e.g., passing needles from above or below, through the vagina) are used for stress UI. This section provides a synopsis of the current procedures.

Retropubic Suspensions (MMK, Burch)

Retropubic suspension involves raising the vesicourethral junction and the anterior vagina by suturing surrounding tissues to the underside of the pubis or to tissue on the pelvic sidewalls. The current mode of action hypothesis proposes that the bladder neck and proximal urethra are then in a position where increases in intra-abdominal pressure are transmitted at least equally to the outlet as to the bladder, and the Burch colposuspension (and variations) also strengthens the suburethral supporting layer, theoretically allowing better proximal urethral compression during effort (Brubaker, 2004). When it is "open," the approach is through an incision in the lower abdomen, usually a transverse incision above the symphysis pubis.

Complications   Postoperative complications specific to retropubic suspensions include voiding dysfunction such as urinary retention, de novo urgency, and vaginal prolapse, especially apical and posterior wall prolapse. There is a greater risk for postoperative pelvic organ prolapse after Burch colposuspension, when compared with anterior colporrhaphy and sling procedures. There is also a potential problem with osteitis pubis and osteomyelitis with the MMK procedure as sutures are placed through the periosteum of the pubis (Kammer-Doak, Cornella, Magrina, Stanhope, & Smilack, 1998).

Outcomes   Research has shown that the retropubic suspension is an effective surgical technique for women with stress and mixed UI, resulting in long-term cure for most women. The Burch procedure has shown good short-term and long-term success, with overall cure rates of 68.9%–88.0% for open retropubic colposuspension (Lapitan, Cody, & Grant, 2005). After 5 years, up to 70%–80% of women have reported themselves to be "dry" (Lapitan et al., 2005). There is a higher efficacy following the Burch colposuspension when compared to the MMK. Some surgeons still use Burch colposuspension as the primary surgery in women with stress UI.

Laparoscopic Burch Colposuspension

A laparoscopic approach may also be used to perform the Burch colposuspension. Advantages of the laparoscopic approach include smaller skin incisions and quicker postoperative recovery and return to work. Disadvantages may include longer operative times, especially during the surgeon training period, and technical difficulty. A Cochrane review indicated that the cure rate for laparoscopic colposuspension trended lower compared to the open approach, but more well-designed randomized trials are needed (Dean, Ellis, Wilson, & Herbison, 2006). The "success" probably depends more on the experience of the surgeon than anything else.

Bladder Neck Sling Procedures

The sling is designed to support the bladder neck and urethra. The most commonly performed bladder neck sling is the autologous pubovaginal fascial sling. This technique restores periurethral support and, in cases of ISD, improves coaptation (closing) of the urethral seal using the woman's own tissue. The sling forms a backboard to support the urethra while providing a mild component of urethral compression. The sling should generally be placed under minimal tension (Figure 12.1), but more compression may be required depending on the degree of ISD. This procedure is typically performed primarily through a vaginal approach, with an abdominal incision needed for some techniques requiring access to the rectus fascia (fibrous tissue of the rectum). Whether the sling should be placed at the bladder neck/proximal urethra or midurethra is debatable. Typically, a material is brought from underneath the urethra to a superior fixation point above using fascia, bone anchors (Figure 12.2), or no fixation at all (Brubaker, 2004). Methods for anchoring the sling also have varied widely, including use of sutures tied above the rectus abdominis muscle (central muscle that runs down the front of the abdomen). The advent of newer, minimally invasive modifications of the sling surgery has increased its popularity.

Sling Material   Slings use a variety of materials to provide a backstop to the urethra. Sling material is biocompatible, meaning the material does not incite a hostile reaction (Table 12.1) (Gomelski & Dmochowski, 2007), although some synthetic materials have been found to be associated with higher rates of erosion and sinus formation. Many other types of materials have been tried, including xenografts. The "gold standard," the autologous pubovaginal fascial

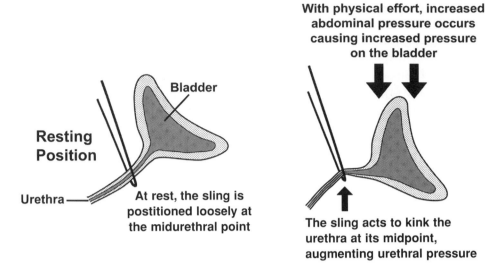

Figure 12.1. Positions of midurethral slings. (Courtesy of Robin Noel.)

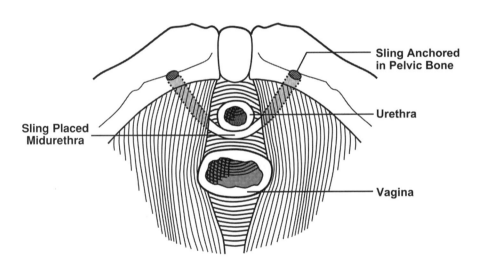

Figure 12.2. Bone anchor sling. (Courtesy of Robin Noel.)

sling, is commonly harvested from the rectus abdominis (Brubaker et al., 2006). The advantages of autologous fascial slings include the use of the woman's own tissues, thus minimizing the risk of infection and erosion and improving long-term results. However, disadvantages include longer operative times, increased hospitalization, and increased pain and time to recover because of the abdominal incision and necessary dissection.

Table 12.1 Types of sling material

Material	Description
Autologous tissue	Derived or transplanted from the same individual's body so biocompatibility is good. Rectus fascia (suprapubic area) or fasia lata (from the greater trochanter) are the material of choice. Urethral erosion is rare.
Allografts	Nonautologous material taken from an organism of the same species, cadaveric tissue, or acellular dermis. Potential for disease transmission.
Xenografts	Material originating from an organism of a different species (nonhuman). Porcine and bovine tissues are common sources. May lose tensile strength.
Synthetic mesh	Material, such as mesh, that is engineered in a laboratory. Synthetic meshes are either absorbable or nonabsorbable, of which the latter is preferred.

Complications   Similar to retropubic colposuspensions, bladder neck slings have an approximate risk of voiding dysfunction of 5%–15%, prolonged urinary retention of 2%–10%, and de novo urge symptoms of 5%–15%. If voiding dysfunction secondary to obstruction occurs, an additional operation may be required to release (lysis) or remove the sling. The lysis technique involves blunt and sharp dissection of periurethral and retropubic scar tissue to free the urethra. Evidence-based treatment recommendations for post-sling voiding dysfunction are lacking, but only a small minority of women are permanently unable to urinate and require intermittent self-catheterization indefinitely.

Efficacy   It appears as though slings have improved continence outcomes when compared to the Burch suspension (Novara et al., 2007). Albo et al. (2007) reported on a multicenter, randomized clinical trial sponsored by the National Institutes of Health comparing two procedures—the pubovaginal sling, using autologous rectus fascia, and the Burch colposuspension—among women with urethral hypermobility and pure or stress-predominant incontinence. Just over half the women underwent concomitant surgery for pelvic organ prolapse. A total of 655 women underwent either the sling procedure (326) or the Burch procedure (329), with 520 women (79%) completing the outcome assessment. The researchers had two primary outcomes to measure success in terms of overall UI and SUI. Treatment success was defined as: 1) no self-reported symptoms of urinary incontinence; 2) an increase of less than 15 g in pad weight during a 24-hour pad test; 3) no incontinence episodes recorded in a 3-day diary; 4) a negative urinary stress test; and 5) no re-treatment for urinary incontinence (including behavioral, pharmacologic, and surgical therapies). At 24 months, success rates were higher for women who underwent the sling procedure than for those who underwent the Burch procedure, for both the overall category of success (47% vs. 38%) and the category specific to stress incontinence (66% vs. 49%). However, more women who underwent the sling procedure had uri-

nary tract infections, difficulty voiding, and postoperative urgency incontinence. However, new-onset urgency UI (3%) was low in both groups, much less
than reported in previous studies. It may be that this symptom was underesti-
mated because the definition was restricted to patients who received treatment.
It should be noted that the criteria for "success" were quite rigid, hence the
lower numbers than seen in other series in which the outcome was more loosely
defined. The definition of success specific to stress UI was limited to no self-
reported symptoms of stress UI, a negative stress test, and no re-treatment for
stress incontinence. The authors concluded that the autologous fascial sling resulted in a higher rate of successful treatment of stress UI, but also greater morbidity, than the Burch suspension. Success rates declined steadily over the
2-year follow-up period, so there is a need for long-term follow-up in these
women.

In women without stress UI who are undergoing abdominal sacrocolpopexy (a procedure that involves providing support of the vaginal vault by af-
fixing it to the periosteum of the sacrum following a hysterectomy) for pelvic
organ prolapse, the addition of a Burch colposuspension at the time of the abdominal sacrocolpopexy has been shown to significantly reduce postoperative
symptoms of stress UI without increasing other lower urinary tract symptoms
(Brubaker et al., 2006).

Midurethral Slings—Newer Procedures

The most recent variations of the sling procedure include the popular and minimally invasive midurethral slings—tension-free vaginal tape (TVT), suprapubic arch sling (SPARC), and transobturator tape (TOT)—that aim to maintain
or improve continence results and decrease morbidity. This approach involves
the placement of a strip (referred to as "tape") of some type of sling material
under the midurethra and behind the pubic symphysis in a tension-free manner (see Figure 12.1). The tape is believed to reinforce the suburethral ligaments
and suburethral vaginal wall to provide a backboard against which the urethra
is compressed during increases in intra-abdominal pressure. This procedure is
significantly different from the classical pubovaginal procedure because the
sling mesh is placed at the midurethra rather than at the urethrovesical junction (bladder neck). In addition, because it requires less dissection around the
urethra, it is less likely to disrupt the blood and nerve supply to the urethra.

Although synthetic midurethral slings placed via the retropubic or abdominal and transobturator routes have proven to be efficacious and are generally safe, complications can cause substantial morbidity and patient dissatisfaction. These complications are usually related to the technique of sling
placement or to the type of material used. Many of these techniques are performed blindly with instruments such as trocars (French for "three side"; a
hollow cylinder with a sharply pointed end that is used to introduce the mesh)
and without finger guidance, which can lead to bladder perforation and other
rare and more severe complications (e.g., bowel or major vessel injuries).

Tension-Free Vaginal Tape (TVT) *(Gynecare, Sommerville, NJ)*   TVT was the first new sling described, wherein a thin mesh made of monofilament polypropylene threads is placed without superior fixation, other than the tissue resistance against the material itself. TVT aims to restore continence by providing a firm backboard for the urethra to close against during episodes of increased intra-abdominal pressure. The TVT sling differs from traditional bladder neck slings that have a potential obstructive component. Because the TVT sling is not anchored to the pubic bone, ligaments, or rectus fascia, it is considered "free of tension." The result is a midurethral support that limits urethral descent, improves the stabilization mechanism generated by pubourethral ligaments and levator ani muscles, and reinforces support of the backboard vaginal hammock. It is held in place by friction, not sutures. The ends of the tape are cut just below the skin's surface. TVT may re-create the pubourethral ligament or cause a "kinking" at the midurethra during increased pressure without compressing the urethra at rest, so it is not obstructive.

Procedure   The TVT procedure is most often done under general anesthesia, but in some individuals it may be performed under local or minimal regional anesthesia. It is most often performed on an outpatient basis. Operative time is short and, in general, postoperative pain and recovery are less severe than with pubovaginal slings and retropubic colposuspensions. A retropubic "bottom to top" approach is used. Two small suprapubic skin incisions are made, and one small incision is made in the vagina over the midurethra. A thin mesh tape is then passed vaginally up through the suprapubic incision on either side with needles, and the mesh is situated at the midurethra, tension free (Figure 12.3).

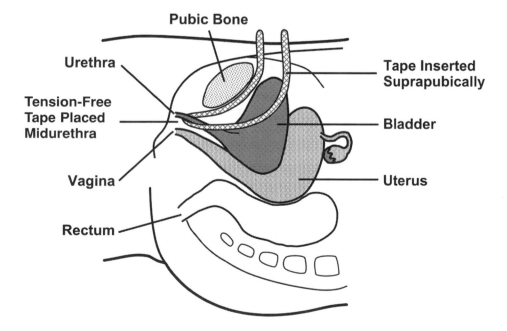

Figure 12.3.   Intraoperative placement of a tension-free vaginal tape sling. (Courtesy of Robin Noel.)

Two midurethral slings have been introduced that include the MiniArc (American Medical Systems) and the TVT Secure (Gynecare/Ethicon). These are shortened slings that allow for sling fixation at the pubic ramus.

Complications   TVT is considered a safe and successful procedure. Because the tape is placed loosely beneath the urethra, it provides support without repositioning the bladder neck or proximal urethra and should result in less postoperative voiding dysfunction than with open procedures. The most common complications related to the TVT procedure are voiding difficulties and obstructive symptoms (8%–17%), bladder perforations (2.7%–17%), and symptoms of urgency (5%–15%), all of which are complications normally associated with stress UI surgery (Novara et al., 2007). The urgency may be permanent. Urinary retention requires reoperation in 1%–2.8% of patients. Another complication of concern is mesh or tape erosion and infection. Although rare, serious complications have been reported with this technique, including vascular and bowel injuries related to the passage of the sling through the retropubic space (Karram, Segal, Vassallo, & Kleeman, 2003).

Efficacy   Ulmsten et al. (1999) reported that, at 2–3 years following the TVT procedure, 86% of women were dry, an additional 13% were improved, and 3% had no improvement. Nilsson, Kuuva, Falconer, Rezapour, and Ulmsten (2001) reported 5-year subjective and objective cure rates as 84.7% cure rate, 10.6% improvement rate, and a low 4.5% failure rate. In 2004, Ward and Hilton published results from a large, multicenter randomized trial comparing the TVT procedure to the open Burch colposuspension. At 2 years, the authors found no difference in success rates between the two procedures. Depending on how missing data were treated, objective cure ranged from 63% to 85% for the TVT group and from 51% to 87% for the colposuspension group. Women in the TVT group were less likely to have voiding dysfunction requiring self-catheterization and had shorter recovery times.

Transobturator Tape (TOT).   *Varieties include Monarc (American Medical Systems, Minneapolis, MN), Uratape (Mentor Corp, Santa Barbara, CA), and Obtryx Transobturator (Boston Scientific, Natick, MA).* TOT is also a midurethral sling with principles and mechanisms of action similar to those of TVT. However, rather than passing through the retropubic space, it is passed through the medial portion of the obturator foramen to the suburethral location, creating a hammock that should support the urethra, as occurs with TVT (Delorme, 2001). Some advantages may be a decreased chance of vascular, bowel, and bladder injury, as well as decreased de novo urgency (Giberti, Gallo, Cortese, & Schenone, 2007). Other advantages are similar to those for the TVT procedure in that the TOT procedure is minimally invasive, and sometimes performed under local or light regional anesthesia on an outpatient basis. The TOT procedure also has a short operative time and patients recover quickly. A proposed advantage of the TOT procedure is a decreased risk of bleeding because no needles are passed through the retropubic space and the great ves-

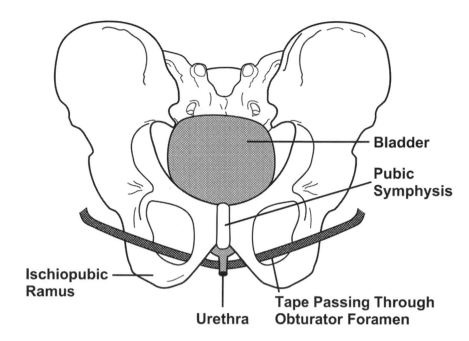

Figure 12.4.   Transobturator sling. (Courtesy of Robin Noel.)

sels are at less risk (Delorme, Droupy, de Tayrac, & Delmas, 2004). This also theoretically decreases the risk of bowel and bladder injury (Barber et al. 2008). Another proposed advantage is lower risk of urinary retention, urinary tract infection, and voiding dysfunction because of less risk of overcorrection (Morey et al., 2006). Longer follow-up will be necessary to determine if the results are durable and the purported advantages are true.

Procedure   A small incision is made in each groin where the thigh meets the abdomen near the vagina, and a vaginal incision is made in the anterior vagina over the midurethra. A thin strip of Prolene mesh tape is placed under the midurethra that passes behind the ischiopubic ramus, punctures the obturator membrane, and passes through each corresponding groin incision (Figure 12.4). The ends of the tape are cut at the incision. It does not enter the retropubic space and was designed to decrease morbidity associated with the TVT procedure.

Complications   The greatest risk with the TOT sling may be injury to the obturator nerve and vessels, as both are close to placement of the mesh. Postoperative leg pain is usually transient and is reported in less than 10% of women (Mahajan, Kenton, Bova, & Brubaker, 2006). The TOT sling can also have mesh erosion/extrusion. Botros et al. (2007) compared 276 subjects with stress or mixed UI who underwent retropubic midurethral sling procedures (TVT, $n = 99$; SPARC, $n = 52$) or TOT sling procedures (Monarc, $n = 125$). Those who underwent the TOT procedure had a significantly lower rate of de novo urgency UI than those who underwent the other midurethral sling procedures. In this study, rates of resolution of detrusor overactivity, urgency UI, and de novo urgency did not differ between the groups.

Efficacy   Two published meta-analyses evaluating TOT and retropubic midurethral slings for the treatment of SUI identified a total of 13 randomized trials comparing these two techniques (Latthe, Foon, Toozs-Hobson, 2007; Sung, Schleinitz, Rardin, Ward, Myers, 2007). In each of the 13 trials, no significant difference was found in the subjective continence rates between the two procedures. Barber et al. (2008) found that the TOT was not inferior to TVT for the treatment of SUI and results in fewer bladder perforations.

Suprapubic Arch Sling (SPARC™) *(American Medical Systems, Minnetonka, MN)*   The SPARC™ was the first commercially available midurethral sling system that allowed the surgeon to place a midurethral synthetic sling from an abdominal (suprapubic) approach using two small incisions above the pubic bone rather than a vaginal approach (Staskin & Tyagi, 2006). It uses a loosely woven monofilament polypropylene mesh.

Procedure   The major difference between the SPARC™ and the TVT procedures is trocar size and the route of delivery. TVT trocars are passed via a vaginal-to-suprapubic route or "top to bottom" approach. In contrast, the smaller SPARC™ trocars, which are two thin, curved stainless steel needles, are passed from a suprapubic approach to the vagina (Figure 12.5). They both involve a vaginal incision. Some urologists prefer this procedure to the TVT because they are more familiar with the suprapubic method of needle insertion.

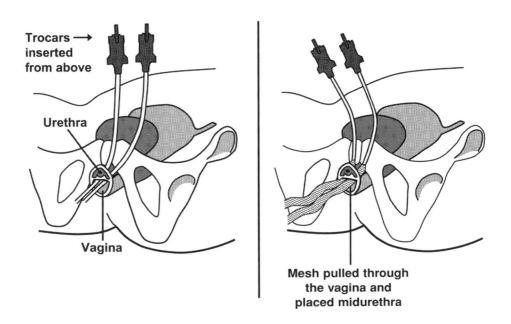

Figure 12.5.   SPARC midurethral sling. (Courtesy of Robin Noel.)

Complications   As with the other surgical procedures, postoperative complications can occur. Hodroff, Sutherland, Kesha, and Siegel (2005) reported the need to do a sling release in 4.3% of their SPARC™ patients. Others have noted an incidence of vaginal erosions (1.2%), urethral erosions (0.6%), and urinary retention (6.5%) (Hammad, Kennedy-Smith, & Robinson, 2005).

Efficacy   Subsequent comparative studies have shown the SPARC™ procedure to have success rates similar to those of the TVT procedure in the short term (Andonian, Chen, St-Denis, & Corcos 2005; Dalpiaz, Primus, & Schips, 2006).

Rapp and Kobashi (2008) conducted a retrospective review of patients undergoing SPARC™ (314 patients) and autologous pubovaginal sling (127 patients) placement. Questionnaire surveillance (Urogenital Distress Inventory and Incontinence Impact Questionnaire) and additional items addressing satisfaction were completed on 204 patients with the SPARC™ and 67 with a pubovaginal sling. Success rates were compared using alternate definitions of success across all outcomes measures (e.g., dry rate, pad rate, percent improvement, and degree of satisfaction). Rapp and Kobashi found wide variations in outcomes depending on the definition used for success. The SPARC™ success range was 33% to 87%, whereas the pubovaginal sling range was 40% to 79%. Total absence of leakage was the strictest definition of success while continued use of one to three panti-liners was associated with the highest success rates. In addition, 74% of patients with SPARC™ placement and 66% with the pubovaginal sling reported willingness to undergo sling surgery again despite the treatment failing to meet the criteria for success under multiple definitions.

INJECTION THERAPY FOR STRESS INCONTINENCE

As more women and men seek treatment of stress UI, the demand for minimally invasive therapies has increased. One minimally invasive treatment is injection therapy of "bulking" agents, referred to as "periurethral injection." Although no one claims to know exactly how they work, they probably improve the "seal" of the urethra so it can withstand increased intra-abdominal pressure and maintain closure as the bladder fills with urine. Materials are implanted via a periurethral (alongside the urethra) or, in most cases, a transurethral (through the urethra) route, under cystoscopic guidance. This procedure is performed in the office or in an ambulatory or hospital surgery setting.

This therapy, although originally advocated and approved for women for the treatment of stress UI with ISD and a low abdominal leak point pressure but not hypermobility alone, has been more recently used in stress UI with or without hypermobility (see Chapter 4). It is also used but without marked success in men with stress UI. This therapy can be performed on almost any individual as long as he or she is infection free, has a pliable urethra into which the material can be injected, and lacks hypersensitivity to the agent. Urethral bulking agents offer a less invasive augmentation of the urethra than sling procedures and artificial urinary sphincters and are popular with patients who wish to avoid surgery of any kind, especially elderly women (Dmochowski, 2005). However, compared with slings and urethropexy, treatment with injectable agents has a markedly lower improvement/cure rate and significantly diminished longevity (Appell, Dmochowski, & Herschorn, 2006). Such therapy has a low complication rate and a variable "success" rate, as shown in mainly short-term studies, and improves quality of life. Overall "success" rates for periurethral injections in women are reported by some to be as high as 80%, with 40% cured and 40% improved (Keegan, Atiemo, Cody, McClinton, & Pickard, 2007). The efficacy generally decreases over time.

These injections are usually reimbursable under almost all insurance carriers as long as ISD and low Valsalva leak point pressures have been determined to exist (McGuire, 2006). Therefore, injection therapy may be considered as a first-line treatment option for patients who have failed conservative therapy such as pelvic floor muscle training and who decline or have a contraindication for surgical intervention.

Injection Procedure

Prior to injection therapy, individuals should have a thorough evaluation of symptoms, including complex urodynamic studies (see Chapter 6). The procedure can be performed either transurethrally or periurethrally. In the transurethral approach, a spinal or special angled needle is placed through a urethroscope or cystoscope and the instrument is advanced into the proximal urethra. The needle penetrates the urethral mucosa, and the bulking material is injected (Figure 12.6). Careful needle placement is necessary to minimize extravasation of the bulking agent. This is done by creating a long tunnel while preventing the needle from moving too superficially, which may cause rupture of the urethral mucosa. It is thought that the implant should be positioned at the bladder neck or proximal urethra. Different sites can be chosen, such as the 3 o'clock and 9 o'clock or the 4 o'clock and 8 o'clock positions, or until good coaptation (urethral closure) is achieved (see Figure 12.6). The procedure is completed when the urethral mucosa moves together with occlusion of the urethral lumen. After injecting, the cystoscope should not be advanced past injected areas, and only small in-and-out catheters (8–12 Fr) should be inserted if necessary, because larger catheters may result in compression or extrusion of the bulking agent.

Perioperative antibiotic coverage is recommended for 2–3 days. If urinary retention occurs, an indwelling catheter should be avoided; instead, the individual should be instructed to perform clean intermittent catheterization using a small (10- to 14-Fr) catheter. In addition, during the procedure the second and third injections must be positioned correctly with respect to the first injection, because there is a risk of puncturing the previous implant. Immediate repeat injections as well as future injections may be necessary.

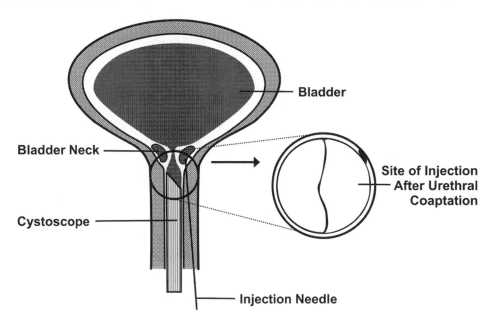

Figure 12.6. Periurethral injection procedure. (Courtesy of Robin Noel.)

Types of Injection Material

The ideal material should be biocompatible and nonallergic. It should also retain its bulking ability for a long period of time and not biodegrade or migrate. It is also important that the material is easy to prepare and implant. Ease of introduction, using a relatively simple technique, and satisfactory long-term continence after insertion are other prerequisites for the ideal material (Chapple et al., 2005). Materials used include collagen, carbon-coated beads, and synthetic bone components (e.g., Coaptite Injectable Implant; Boston Scientific). Autologous fat (the fat used is harvested from the abdominal wall) is biocompatible and has been used in smaller numbers of procedures, but success was considerably lower than that with other injectables. The following is a short review of the most commonly used injection materials.

Collagen/Bovine Collagen *(Contigen; C.R. Bard, Covington, GA)*

Several materials have been used over the years to enhance bladder outlet resistance and to correct ISD, the most common of which is collagen. Contigen is a glutaraldehyde cross-linked (GAX) bovine collagen. Used since 1993, its advantage is its long history of use, ease of administration, and lack of migration. Shortcomings such as lack of stability in the body have hampered its ability to achieve long-term durable success. Disadvantages include the need to undergo a skin test before use, because up to 4% of patients may have an allergic reaction as a result of its bovine origin. The need for repeat injections and degradation are also considerations.

Efficacy of periurethral Contigen injections has been studied mostly in women. Reported success rates vary widely and range from 86% of patients remaining dry at 3 months to 20% remaining dry at 48 months (Lightner, 2002; Madjar, Covington-Nichols, & Secrest, 2003; Schulz, Hager, Stanton, & Baessler, 2004). Collagen has been shown to be equally effective in individuals with hypermobility or ISD (Herschorn & Radomski, 1997; Herschorn, Steele, & Radomski, 1996). Reported cure rates for transurethral retrograde collagen injection in men for stress UI after radical prostatectomy range from 5% to 20% (Keegan et al., 2007). Maintenance of good results in the long term may occur with durability of the initial procedure itself or with reinjections with additional collagen. Because GAX collagen has the potential for eliciting an allergic reaction, is expensive, and requires more treatment sessions to attain continence, the search has continued for a better injectable.

Carbon-Coated Zirconium Beads *(Durasphere; Boston Scientific)*

Durasphere is composed of pyrolytic carbon-coated zirconium beads in a carrier gel. It is not degraded, and the large size of the beads theoretically prevents their migration from the injection site, a problem with previously tested substances such as polytetrafluoroethylene (Teflon). Durasphere is thicker (more viscous) than collagen and initially was more difficult to administer than Contigen. A newer agent, Durasphere EXP, has lessened this problem. Because of the synthetic nature of this product, it is not reactive; therefore, no skin testing needs to be performed. It has been shown to be comparable in efficacy to Contigen (Lightner et al., 2001). Also, the initial and repeated injection volumes of Durasphere were significantly less than those of collagen. When compared to collagen, the adverse events are similar, but Durasphere seems to have an increased short-term risk of urgency and urinary retention. Pelvic radiographs obtained at 1 and 2 years after injection show stability of the bulking agents at the injection site. This suggests potential improved durability, but the beads can migrate (Pannek, Brands, & Senge, 2001).

Silicone Polymers *(Macroplastique; Uroplasty, Inc., Minneapolis, MN)*

Silicone polymers are soft, flexible, highly textured, irregularly shaped implants within a carrier of hydrogel in which the solid particle content is 33% of the total volume. However, the agent must be injected with a high-pressure injection gun because of its viscous nature. The Macroplastique Implantation System allows consistent placement of the implants at predefined depths and angles at the 6, 10, and 2 o'clock positions of the midurethra within the same circumferential plane. In order to identify the site of implantation correctly, the ruler/measuring scale on the top side of the device is used. The standard implantation position is defined by withdrawing the device from the urethra to the appropriate location of the midurethra (i.e., a 10- to 15-mm distance from the level of the bladder neck). Outcomes are similar to other injection material, but long-term data are limited (Tamanini, D'Ancona, & Netto, 2006).

The risks of biodegradation and migration of this bulking agent are uncertain. No definitive evidence has been reported that silicone elastomers are associated with acquired connective tissue disease.

Calcium Hydroxyapatite *(Coaptite; BioForm Medical, Inc., Franksville, WI)*

Calcium hydroxyapatite is a synthetic version of material found naturally in bone and teeth. It is a nonantigenic bulking agent consisting of hydroxyapatite spheres in an aqueous gel composed of sodium carboxylmethylcellulose. Calcium hydroxyapatite is formulated to prevent distant migration. Radiographs and ultrasound scans will identify calcium hydroxyapatite at the injection site. Because this is a relatively new agent, very few data are available on efficacy and complications. This agent has injection characteristics similar to those of collagen.

Complications of Periurethral Injections

The potential complications of all periurethral injections include de novo urgency and urinary retention, which may last a few days (Dmochowski, 2005). Urinary retention ranges from 1% to 21% and can be managed with intermittent catheterization or short-term indwelling catheterization. Urinary tract infection occurs in 1%–25% of individuals, and hematuria occurs in 2%. Other rare complications include periurethral abscess formation. With injection of Contigen, a delayed skin reaction is associated with arthralgia in 0.9% of cases. A concern with some bulking agents is migration because smaller size particles (e.g., as with Teflon injections) can migrate to distant locations.

OTHER URETHRAL TREATMENTS

A new therapy (Renessa; Novasys Medical, Newark, CA) uses radiofrequency energy to heat urethral tissue to low temperatures, causing local denaturation of collagen. Shrinkage occurs and the treated tissue is firmer, resulting in increased resistance to involuntary leakage with increased intra-abdominal pressure. Outcome data are very limited.

SURGERY FOR MALE STRESS UI

Male stress UI is the result of de novo sphincter insufficiency or trauma and is a potential complication of prostate surgery (radical prostatectomy, resection of the prostate). It is estimated that, in the United States, 7% of men older than 60 years—or approximately 3.4 million men—have daily incontinence (Penson et al., 2005). It is estimated that 6%–20% of men have persistent (from 12 to >60 months) and significant postprostatectomy stress UI (Penson et al., 2005; Steineck et al., 2002). However, only 6%–7% of men undergo subsequent surgical treatment. In these men, except for pelvic floor muscle training, additional treatment is not recommended for at least 6 months to 1 year after surgery (Klingler & Marberger, 2006).

Periurethral injections can be used in men with slight stress UI but, in contrast to women, in men their outcomes are often suboptimal and transitory. The artificial urinary sphincter (AUS) is currently the preferred treatment in men with moderate to severe UI. However, this involves a very experienced surgeon and an open operation. Men receiving an AUS may also experience a degree of residual UI (Dalkin, Wessells, & Cui, 2003). New techniques include the insertion of periurethral balloons and bulbourethral slings. This section discusses the bulbourethral sling and the AUS.

Sling Procedure

Compression of the bulbar urethra in men with stress UI is an old technique that was abandoned primarily because of poor long-term results and many complications. The original techniques consisted of compressing the bulbar urethra by means of an acrylic cylinder and then a silicone pad. The current version uses a perineal approach to compress the bulbar urethra by means of a sling attached to the pubic bone (Figure 12.7). This bone-anchored male sling system is a synthetic mesh that exerts pressure on the urethra.

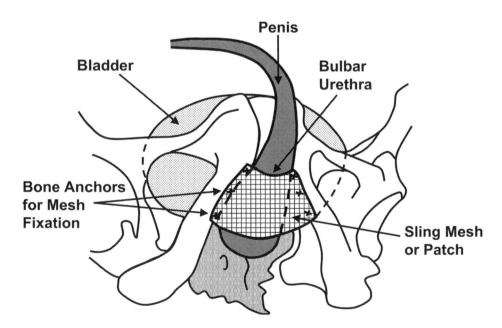

Figure 12.7.   InVance male sling. (Courtesy of Robin Noel.)

Procedure

This is a minimally invasive procedure that can be performed on an outpatient basis. In this procedure, six bone screws are used for mesh fixation, obviating the abdominal incision and offering a reliable point of fixation.

Complications

Postoperative perineal pain and transient urinary retention can occur, as can infection. In addition, there is a potential risk of pubic osteitis, given the fact that the screws are attached to the bone.

Efficacy

The best and most consistent results will be achieved in men who have mild to moderate incontinence (using fewer than three perineal pads per day). With an average follow-up of 12 months, Comiter (2002) reported a "success rate" of 76%. Outcomes are inferior in men who have undergone pelvic radiation and in those with severe UI. As the time from placement progresses, the "success" rates, in the hands of many, seem to decline.

Artificial Urinary Sphincter

The AUS is considered the gold standard for surgical treatment of persistent or severe sphincteric UI in men. It is a prosthetic device that can substitute for the individual's sphincteric mechanism and prevent or reduce urine leakage during increases in intra-abdominal pressure (Quallich & Ohl, 2003a). This prosthesis is used primarily in men and only rarely in women. Candidates include men with severe stress UI following prostate surgery, especially radical prostatectomy. Other candidates for the AUS include men with congenital disorders of the bladder, those who have had unsuccessful reconstructive surgery to the urethra or bladder, some individuals with neurological injury, and selected women with stress UI (Quallich & Ohl, 2003a; Staskin & Comiter, 2007). These individuals have usually failed other treatment (e.g., pelvic floor muscle training). Potential downsides include infection, mechanical failure, and erosion into the urethral lumen.

AUS Device

The current model (AMS 800; American Medical Systems), with some improvements, has been available for more than 20 years. It is made of silicone elastomer and has several cuff sizes. The device consists of three components: a cuff that encircles the urethra, a fluid-filled reservoir (balloon) in the retropubic space, and a pump for activation/deactivation placed in the scrotum (or labia in women) (Figure 12.8). Fluid transfer from the cuff to the reservoir is accomplished by active "pumping" while refilling of the cuff occurs by the

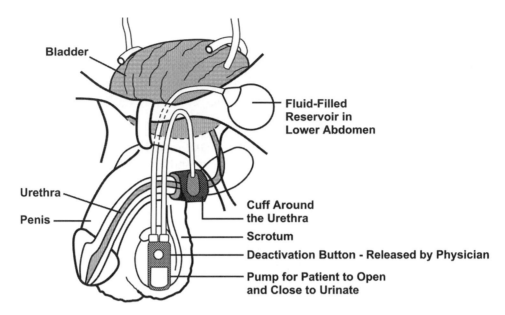

Figure 12.8. Artificial urinary sphincter (AUS). (Courtesy of Robin Noel.)

pressure gradient from the reservoir that traverses a resistor implanted in the pump mechanism.

AUS Procedure and Activation

Prior to AUS implantation, individuals should undergo urodynamic testing to document ISD or some other sphincteric malfunction (see Chapter 4). Patients who are found to have refractory detrusor overactivity, decreased detrusor compliance, or small bladder capacity are not good candidates for surgery. Cystoscopy is also usually indicated preoperatively. To be a good candidate for the AUS, the individual must have adequate understanding of the device, as well as the dexterity to use the pump, normal bladder compliance, and, ideally, normal detrusor function to completely empty the bladder. Patients should be informed about all aspects of this procedure prior to implantation.

The cuff is generally placed around the bulbar urethra (in women, the AUS cuff is placed around the bladder neck). The reservoir is placed in the lower abdomen next to the bladder. The fluid in the cuff gently compresses the urethra and occludes it. The device is typically in the "activated" state—that is, the cuff is inflated, compressing the urethra. Once activated, a few pumps of the bulb in the scrotum by the patient transfers fluid from the cuff (around the urethra) to the reservoir in the lower abdomen, opening the urethra and allowing voiding to occur (Figure 12.9). The reservoir will hold the fluid so urine may pass from the bladder. In 3–4 minutes, the fluid will return (via a one-way valve) from the balloon down to the cuff to close off the ure-

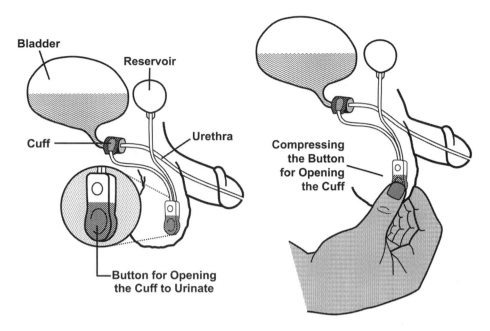

Bladder

Reservoir

Cuff

Urethra

Compressing the Button for Opening the Cuff

Button for Opening the Cuff to Urinate

Figure 12.9.   Artificial urinary sphincter (AUS). Compression of the pump to move fluid from the cuff to the reservoir allows urine to pass from the bladder. (Courtesy of Robin Noel.)

thra again and stop urinary leakage. After voiding, the pressure in the cuff returns to its normal level. After surgery, the device is temporarily deactivated. This is to allow complete urethral healing before active compression. The patient remains incontinent (Quallich & Ohl, 2003b). This deactivation of the device can also be used when the patient needs to be catheterized or to have other urinary tract instrumentation. If the individual achieves satisfactory continence with the device deactivated, then it is never activated. If required, device activation is usually done 6–8 weeks postoperatively.

Device Complications

AUS implantation is a surgical procedure that can have significant adverse complications. Postoperatively, hematoma can occur in the scrotum or present as a fluid collection (Staskin & Comiter, 2007). Men may temporarily need to apply a pressure dressing, and men may need to wear a scrotal support. The greatest risks are AUS infection and urethral erosion, often reported together, which are usually seen within the first 3 months after surgery (Petrou, Elliott, & Barrett, 2000; Venn, Greenwell, & Mundy, 2000). The infection rate with first implant has been reported as 1%–3% and is higher in men who have undergone pelvic radiation. Signs of an infection include erythema, tenderness, and swelling in the scrotum or any site that has a component of the device. One of the initial symptoms of infection is scrotal pain.

Pain in the perineum, irritative voiding symptoms, bloody urethral discharge, swelling around the cuff, and hematuria may indicate cuff erosion into the urethra. AUS urethral cuff erosion occurs in up to 5.0% of cases, usually within 3–4 months after implantation (Raj, Peterson, & Webster, 2006). Traumatic or prolonged urinary catheterization can cause cuff erosion into the urethra or device malfunction. To decrease the risk of cuff erosion, the cuff should be deactivated before a urethral catheter is inserted, and in women during pregnancy and labor. Treatment of an infected or eroded AUS is removal of the device. A second system can be implanted within 3–6 months with good success rates (Staskin & Comiter, 2007).

Other complications include mechanical failures as well as fluid leak from rupture or perforation of any of the parts, tube kinking, pump malfunction, and connector separations. Nonmechanical failure includes cuff erosion into the urethra, pain, and insufficient cuff pressure or reservoir migration.

Efficacy

When performed by an experienced urologist, implantation of the AUS is effective for a highly selected group of patients with moderate to severe stress UI. Almost all outcomes have been reported in men. Total continence following AUS insertion in men after prostatectomy has been reported to be approximately 75% (Petrou et al., 2000), and significant improvement in continence has been achieved in more than 90% (Litwiller, Kim, Fone, DeVere White, & Stone, 1996). Even when not completely dry, men uniformly report greater than 90% satisfaction rates with its use. Expert urologists compared 108 men ($n = 53$) and women ($n = 55$) who underwent an AUS implantation and found that the device performed well in women but was better in men in terms of dryness and longer device duration before failure (Petero & Diokno, 2006). Overall satisfactory continence rates were similar between men (81%) and women (84%). However, the AUS placed in women had a durability twice that in men (5 vs. 11 years), with some using the device in a deactivated mode. Despite good outcomes, only a small percentage of potential candidates receive an AUS (Reynolds, Patel, Msezane, Luciono, & Rapp, 2007).

Patient Education

Thorough understanding of AUS care is essential for long-term success with this device. Individuals must have adequate cognition and be motivated to care for their AUS. They need detailed, complete instructions on the use of the device, awareness of the fact that there may be some degree of incontinence following AUS implantation, and understanding that the complications include cuff erosion or device malfunction. Medic Alert bracelets (provided free by American Medical Systems) should be routinely worn after AUS placement. Individuals will need to inform other health care providers prior to urinary tract instrumentation because catheterization of a patient with a closed

AUS can cause serious complications (cuff erosion, infection). If the patient needs catheterization, the device should be deactivated by pressing the deactivation button. A 14- or 16-Fr catheter can then easily slide through the urethra without difficulty. If the individual requires an indwelling catheter, then the AUS should remain deactivated (Mulholland & Diokno, 2004).

BOTULINUM TOXIN INJECTION THERAPY FOR NEUROGENIC AND NON-NEUROGENIC BLADDER OVERACTIVITY

Botulinum toxin (BTX) is a neurotoxin produced by the gram-negative anaerobic bacterium *Clostridium botulinum*. Botulism, the disease, results from toxin exposure and includes limb paralysis, dysarthria, facial muscle weakness, dyspnea, constipation, urinary retention, and ophthalmoplegia. Toxin exposure commonly occurs from lower gastrointestinal tract exposure to the bacteria resulting from the ingestion of contaminated food, especially after poor canning practices. Today, BTX has moved from a cause of life-threatening disease to a medical therapy. There are seven serological forms of BTX: A, B, C, D, E, F, and G. Currently, botulinum toxin serotype A (BTX-A) (Botox; Allergan, Inc., Irvine, CA) is the most commonly used form of BTX for medical applications (Mucksavage, Smith, & Moy, 2006).

Botulinum Toxin A

BTX-A injections have been used for many years to treat conditions such as facial muscle paralysis and for aesthetics (e.g., wrinkles). BTX-A is becoming an increasingly used injection material for patients with certain urological conditions. Injection sites include the detrusor muscle or suburothelium, the striated sphincter, and the prostate, depending on the condition being treated. Although it is currently not approved by the U.S. Food and Drug Administration (FDA) or the European regulatory agencies for urological conditions, its use in investigational protocols and "off-label" use continue to grow. Specific situations in which Botox injections have been used include patients with neurogenic and non-neurogenic detrusor overactivity (DO), interstitial cystitis, and prostate disorders (Kim, Thomas, Smith, & Chancellor, 2006). BTX-A injection into the striated sphincter is also being used to treat patients with spinal cord injury with outlet obstruction due to detrusor–sphincter dyssynergia. BTX-A striated sphincter injection can be an alternative to self-catheterization in some individuals with urinary retention related to detrusor hypocontractility from neurological disease because it leads to urethral sphincter relaxation. This may improve bladder emptying but may also result in stress UI. Before receiving Botox injections for a urological purpose, patients need to be informed of indications, side effects, and postinjection complications.

Mechanism of Action (Bladder Usage)

BTX-A is a highly potent neurotoxin that acts on peripheral nerve endings to inhibit the release of acetylcholine and probably other neurotransmitter vesicles at the presynaptic neuromuscular junction. When this occurs, contractile receptors in the detrusor muscle are not stimulated, and voluntary and involuntary bladder contractions are suppressed (Chancellor & Chartier-Kastler, 2000). It is likely that a similar inhibitory action occurs in the sensory response as well. The majority of studies have shown no muscle fibrosis, and the drug is as effective in reinjection as it was at first usage. Patients with preexisting neurological disorders affecting transmission at the neuromuscular junction are advised not to undergo any form of treatment with BTX (Mahajan & Brubaker, 2007).

Botox Injection Procedure

BTX-A is injected into the bladder with a flexible cystoscope in an outpatient setting, generally using local anesthesia (intraurethral lidocaine jelly). Children and more anxious patients are injected under general anesthesia. Usually a total of 300 units of BTX-A is injected for neurogenic individuals, although dosage schedules have not been firmly established for neurogenic or nonneurogenic voiding dysfunction. Care must be taken in preparation of the toxin suspension because suspension strength is determined by the amount of saline used to reconstitute the purified crystalline form of the toxin. Each vial contains 100 units of toxin, and it is diluted in 1 mL of injectable saline. For a 300-unit total, three vials must be used to yield a total of three 1-mL syringes, each filled with 100 units of BTX-A at a concentration of 10 units per 0.1 mL. A fourth 1-mL syringe of injectable saline is used to flush any residual toxin contained in the needle sheath. The medication is injected using a 23-gauge needle tip that has a 5 mm-long sheath, allowing the physician to control the depth of the injection into the bladder muscle. Each injection site receives 0.1 mL of the BTX solution, so a total of 20–30 sites are generally injected (Figure 12.10). But there is no consensus on injection sites within the bladder. Patients with overactive bladder and poor bladder contractility may receive less (e.g., 100 units total) to try to avoid urinary retention.

Safety and Side Effects

BTX-A injections in the lower urinary tract have been reported to be safe because BTX typically affects only the local tissue into which it is injected. Adverse effects related to BTX-A detrusor muscle injections can be divided into local and systemic effects (Nitti, 2006). Local effects include pain, infection, and hematuria. These are due to the procedure and not the toxin. In addition,

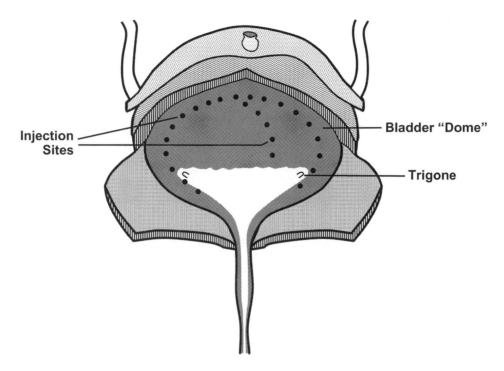

Figure 12.10.   Botulinum A toxin injection sites. (Courtesy of Robin Noel.)

intradetrusor injections can be associated with excessive detrusor relaxation, resulting in detrusor underactivity and subsequent transient elevation of postvoid residual volume or urinary retention. Therefore, after injection, post-void residual volumes should be monitored. Patients who are treated long term with BTX may develop antibodies, which appear to cause no side effects other than rendering subsequent BTX treatments less effective or ineffective. If this occurs with BTX-A treatments of the bladder, some evidence suggests that switching to a different formulation of BTX may be effective. To prevent antibody development, the FDA recommends dosing intervals of no less than 8 weeks between treatments for BTX at other sites in the body. Other recommendations include 1) using the minimum effective dose and 2) avoiding booster injections. Generally, the effects last for 4–6 months.

The authors would like to note that the FDA has received reports of systemic adverse reactions, including respiratory compromise and death, following the use of botulinum toxins types A and B for both FDA-approved and unapproved uses. The reactions reported are suggestive of botulism, which occurs when botulinum toxin spreads in the body beyond the site where it was injected. The most serious cases had outcomes that included hospitalization and death and occurred mostly in children treated for cerebral palsy–associated limb spasticity. More information is available at the FDA's Web site (http://www.fda.gov/cder/drug/early_comm/botulinium_toxins.htm).

Contraindications

Contraindications include pregnancy, breast feeding, myasthenia gravis, Eaton-Lambert syndrome, amyotrophic lateral sclerosis, and the concomitant use of aminoglycosides. It also should be noted that some BTX-A preparations use stabilizers such as albumin derived from human blood, which may be a cultural or religious issue with some individuals.

Efficacy

Many studies have documented the positive outcomes of BTX-A bladder injections; only a few are discussed here. Schmid et al. (2006) studied 23 men and 77 women with a mean age of 63 years (range, 24–89) with non-neurogenic overactive bladder, including urgency–frequency syndrome, and incontinence. Urgency disappeared in 82% of these individuals, and incontinence resolved in 86%, within 1–2 weeks after BTX-A injections. Mean frequency decreased from 14 to 7 micturitions daily (50% decrease), and nocturia decreased from 4 to 1.5 micturitions. Urodynamic findings indicated a 56% increase in maximal bladder capacity (increased from 246 to 381 mL); mean volume at first urge to void increased from 126 to 212 mL and mean urge volume increased from 214 to 309 mL. There were no severe side effects except temporary urinary retention in four cases. The mean duration of effect was at least 6–12 months.

Schurch et al. (2005) conducted a placebo-controlled, prospective, randomized study in patients who had neurogenic DO (e.g., resulting from spinal cord injury, multiple sclerosis, or myelomeningocele). BTX-A injections of 200 and 300 units reduced UI by an average of 50%, an effect that lasted for the duration of the 24-week study. Reitz et al. (2004) reported on a 200-subject (131 males and 69 females), multicenter, European open-label study of BTX-A in neurogenic DO. All subjects presented with neurogenic DO, and in 92 cases this was accompanied by detrusor–sphincter dyssynergia. Clean intermittent self-catheterization was performed by 188 subjects to empty their bladder, and 12 subjects relied on indwelling catheters because of severe incontinence. Before injection, 163 subjects were on anticholinergic drugs. The subjects on antimuscarinic agents were allowed to continue the drugs, even though the response was less than adequate. These investigators, too, showed significant improvements in urinary symptoms, with 73% of incontinent subjects becoming continent at 12 weeks; in 72% of these, complete continence persisted at 36 weeks. Also of interest was the fact that, at 12 weeks, antimuscarinic agents were discontinued in 28% and reduced in 72% of subjects.

At this time, BTX-A has not been approved by the FDA for any urological therapy.

NEUROMODULATION: SACRAL NERVE STIMULATION

Neuromodulation through sacral nerve stimulation (SNS) involves the use of mild electrical pulses to stimulate the sacral nerve roots associated with voiding function (see Chapter 3). SNS modulates the abnormal involuntary reflexes of the lower urinary tract and restores voluntary control. Medtronic (Minneapolis, MN) received approval to market an SNS therapy called InterStim as a treatment option for patients with refractory voiding dysfunction.

Mechanism of Action

The mechanism of action of SNS is unknown. It is hypothesized that the effects depend on electrical stimulation of somatic afferent axons in the spinal roots, which in turn modulate voiding and continence reflex pathways in the central nervous system. It is believed that the close contact between the nerve root and the electrical stimulation source offers the distinct advantage of more durable, consistent control of lower urinary tract dysfunction. The afferent system is the most likely target because beneficial effects can be elicited at intensities of stimulation that do not activate movements of striated muscles (Leng & Chancellor, 2005; Leng & Morrisroe, 2006). SNS paradoxically has been successful in managing both DO and idiopathic non-obstructive urinary retention. For urgency UI, SNS is thought to promote more normal detrusor muscle activity and behavior by 1) stimulating the striated muscle of the external urethral sphincter and increasing inhibitory reflex neural feedback to the sacral cord centers controlling detrusor activity, and 2) activating other inhibiting peripheral and central afferent pathways involved in the micturition reflex. In patients with incomplete bladder emptying or urinary retention symptoms, SNS is believed to suppress overactivity of the guarding reflex, stabilizing the pelvic floor and improving the voiding pattern (Leng & Chancellor, 2005; Leng & Morrisroe, 2006). "Awareness of the pelvic floor" allows for voluntary relaxation of these muscles, in turn permitting initiation of the voiding reflex (Chancellor & Chartier-Kastler, 2000; DasGupta & Fowler, 2003). However, Goh and Diokno (2007) found that those individuals who are able to void some amount of urine, despite having urinary retention, are more likely to have treatment success.

Indications for InterStim Therapy

Michelle was 33 years old when she was referred to a urologist for voiding symptoms of urinary urgency and frequency. She had been diagnosed with fibromyalgia 12 months earlier. At that time, she was successfully treated by one of the authors (DKN) with behavioral interventions to in-clude bladder training with urge suppression techniques and biofeed-back-assisted pelvic floor muscle exercises. Two years later, she started noticing an increase of urgency and frequency that did not appear to im-prove with the behavioral therapies. Michelle's primary care physician prescribed an antimuscarinic medication that decreased these symptoms. One year later, after an episode of generalized muscle weakness and fa-tigue, she started noticing urinary hesitancy and the feeling that she was not completely emptying her bladder. Her urologist noted an elevated postvoid residual of 475 cc, and urodynamic studies indicated poor blad-der contraction with no apparent obstruction. Michelle was prescribed self-catheterization 4 to 5 times per day. Six months of vaginal pelvic floor electrical stimulation did not improve her symptoms. When Michelle was 39, her urologist suggested that she consider neuromodulation with an implantable stimulator as she continued with nonobstructive urinary re-tention. After stage I, Michelle started to void in small amounts, and by three weeks she was able to decrease catheterizations to twice a day. She opted to undergo stage II, and within six months she was voiding sponta-neously and could discontinue cathing. In 2008, Michelle is 4 years post-implant, continues to void completely, and has no other urinary symp-toms. She turned off the stimulator prior to undergoing a hysterectomy in 2007 and experienced post-operative urinary retention. She saw DKN who turned the stimulation back on and reprogrammed the unit. Michelle continues to void normally and is free of any other urinary symptoms.

In 1997 InterStim® therapy was approved by the FDA for refractory ur-gency UI and for urgency–frequency syndrome and nonobstructive chronic urinary retention (incomplete or complete urinary retention) in 1999. "Refrac-tory" means the patient must have failed conservative therapy, including drug therapy with two different medications and behavioral interventions (biofeed-back-assisted pelvic floor muscle training, bladder training) (see Chapters 8 and 9). They also may have failed external pelvic floor muscle electrical stimulation. Patients with other pathological conditions, including chronic pelvic pain, constipation/obstipation, irritable bowel syndrome, and fecal incontinence may also benefit from SNS therapy, but these conditions have not received FDA approval for Interstim therapy. Symptoms must be present for at least 2 months, be documented on a 3-day/3-night voiding diary, and have resulted in significant difficulty with activities of daily living. Prior to SNS, patients should undergo a thorough evaluation, including urodynamics (see Chapter 6).

InterStim System

The InterStim® Therapy System is considered minimally invasive technology and is often referred to as a "bladder pacemaker." The InterStim® Therapy System has the following components: 1) implantable neurostimulator (INS or

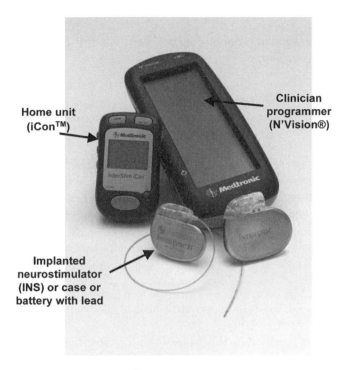

Figure 12.11.   InterStim® devices. (Courtesy of Medtronic.)

IPG), 2) implanted lead (tined) with four stimulating electrodes, 3) physician programmer, and 4) patient programmer (the iCon) (Figure 12.11). These implanted components (InterStim Tined Lead Model 3093, InterStim INS Model 3023, or InterStim II INS Model 3058) form the electrical circuit that delivers therapeutic electrical stimulation to the sacral nerve roots.

InterStim Implantation Technique

SNS is a minimally invasive procedure that is completed in two stages: Stage 1 is a clinical trial of a temporary or permanent lead for external stimulation and stage 2 is implantation of a subcutaneous implantable pulse generator, the INS or battery (Vasavada & Rackley, 2007). The specifics of the two stages are outlined in Box 12.1 and shown in Figure 12.12. Stage 1 is a completely reversible diagnostic procedure that can be performed with a percutaneous needle electrode or as a staged implant using the surgically implantable lead as the test lead. The purpose of the stimulation test is to locate and identify the sacral nerves, verify the neural integrity of these nerves, allow the patient to feel the stimulation, and assess the response. A successful response to stimulation is defined in Box 12.2. The external test stimulator unit or the INS emits an electrical pulse that travels through a conducting wire to the site of nerve stimulation, then back to the INS through another conducting wire (all within

Box 12.1   Interstim implantation procedure

Stage 1 (Testing Stage)

- Lead placement for needle test stimulation can be performed in a surgery center or office or as an outpatient surgical procedure.

- One method involves percutaneous lead insertion. The second method requires a minimal surgical incision, inserting a tined lead in a sutureless anchoring system.

- The procedure can be performed under a combination of intravenous short-acting sedation and supplemental local anesthesia so as to allow for intraoperative patient response to stimulation.

- The tined lead, with four electrodes at the distal tip, is inserted in a sacral foramen, most commonly the S3 foramen (alternatively, the S4 foramen) (see Figure 12.12).

- Mild electrical pulses stimulate the sacral nerves, and adequate electrode placement is confirmed by obtaining appropriate motor and sensory responses (see Table 12.2).

- The proximal end of the tined lead is tunneled laterally to a small (1-inch) incision in the upper gluteal tissue, creating a pocket for placement of the INS in stage II. It is then connected to a percutaneous extension that is then tunneled contralaterally and then connected to a cable (gray) that is connected to the external stimulator device (with adjustable settings) for 3–4 weeks (see Figure 12.12).

- Anteroposterior and lateral radiographs are used to determine the final lead placement.

Stage 2

- The percutaneous extension with cable is discarded and the proximal end of the tined lead is attached to an INS (case or battery).

- The INS is positioned in a pocket in the upper buttock region (see Figure 12.12).

- The patient should feel a comfortable sensation (vibrating, pulsating, tingling, and tickling) in an appropriate sensory location (e.g., perineum, vagina, and rectum).

Key: INS = implantable neurostimulator.

the lead or extension) to complete an electrical circuit and deliver therapy (see Figure 12.13).

This trial period of stage 1 allows patients to try the therapy and assess not only its efficacy but also its tolerability and sensation so that they can determine whether they want to proceed to stage 2, implantation. All sensations depend on lead location, amplitude, electrode configuration, and patient-specific anatomy. The programming of each electrode may produce different sensations: distal electrodes produce more anterior sensations (vaginal and scrotal) and proximal electrodes produce more posterior sensations (gluteal). If a satisfactory sacral motor and sensory response to stimulation is achieved with stage 1 testing (Table 12.2), then the same successful lead or electrode becomes part of the definitive implantation device. If the patient's symptoms decrease by at least 50% within a 3- to 4-week period of time as recorded in a voiding diary, the patient returns for the implantation, which is a short procedure that involves attachment of the tined lead to the INS, placed in an upper gluteal pocket. If the patient does not achieve any benefit from SNS, then the tined lead or electrode and its temporary percutaneous wires can be easily disconnected and removed.

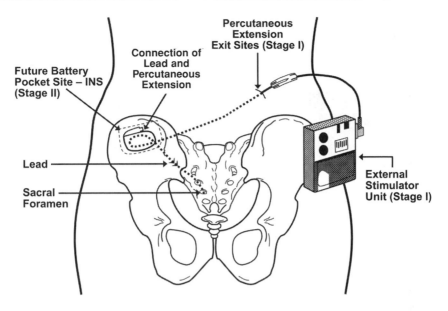

Figure 12.12.   Placement of InterStim® with implantable neurostimulator (INS) internal case (battery) in upper buttock, with lead placement. (Courtesy of Robin Noel.)

Box 12.2   Determining InterStim stage 1 outcomes based on 4-day voiding diary

Refractory Urge Incontinence: > 50% improvement in

- Number of leaking episodes per day
- Severity of leaking episodes per day
- Number of incontinence absorbent products used per day

Urgency–Frequency Syndrome (overactive bladder without incontinence): > 50% improvement in

- Number of voids per day
- Volume of voids per day
- Degree of urgency

Chronic Urinary Retention

- Catheterized volume versus voided volume
- Number of catheterizations per day versus number of voids per day
- >50% decrease in the number of catheterizations
- >50% increase of voided volumes

SNS Programming

Programming, accomplished with the use of a remote electronic programming device called the "N'Vision Clinician Programmer," (Figure 12.11) is important to achieve the best possible outcomes for the individual user, to confirm the integrity of the implanted system, to analyze implant settings, and to troubleshoot

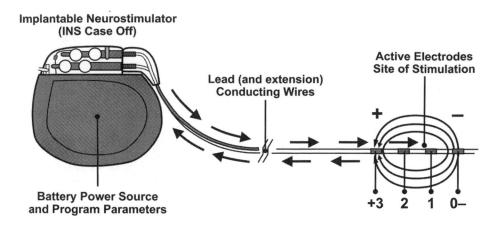

Figure 12.13.   InterStim "electric current."

Table 12.2   Sacral motor and sensory response

	Innervation	Response		Sensation
S2	Primary somatic contributor to pudendal nerve for external sphincter, leg, and foot.	Pelvic floor—clamp[a] of anal sphincter	Foot/calf/leg: plantar flexion of entire foot, contraction of calf, leg/hip rotation	"Pulling in" sensation in the cocyxx, vagina, or base of the penis.
S3	All pelvic autonomic functions and striated muscle (levator ani).	Bellows[b]	Plantar flexion of great toe, occasionally other toes (sciatic nerve stimulation)	"Pulling in" sensation in rectum, extending to the labia or scrotum. Tingling sensation in the external genitalia.
S4	Pelvic autonomic and somatic functions. No lower extremity (leg or foot) response.	Bellows[b]	No lower extremity motor stimulation	"Pulling in" sensation in rectum only (activation of the posterior levator ani muscles).

Adapted from material by Medtronic (Minneapolis, MN), 2007.

[a]Clamp: Contraction of the anal sphincter and, in men, retraction of the base of the penis. By moving the buttocks aside, one can see anterior-posterior shortening of the perineal structures.

[b]Bellows: Contraction of the levator ani muscles, causing a "bellows" contraction of the perineum (deepening and flattening of the intergluteal fold) and a pulling inward of the anus.

Table 12.3   Primary parameters of electrical stimulation pulse

Parameter	Definition	Components
Amplitude (A)	Strength or intensity of the stimulation, measured in volts (V).	• Increased amplitude equates to greater intensity. Decreased amplitude equates to less intensity. • Typical settings are between 1.0 and 4.0 V and are determined by user comfort. • Adjusted until "sensation" is felt comfortably; should *not* be painful. • May need to be increased to maintain urinary control.
Pulse Width (PW)	Time or duration of the stimulation pulse, measured in microseconds (µsec).	• A typical PW setting is between 180 and 270 µsec. • An increase in PW may widen the area of the stimulation, increasing the pulse duration. • Decreasing the PW decreases the pulse duration. • As the PW is increased, IPG battery longevity is decreased.
Rate (R)	Speed of the perceived sensation; represents the number of times a pulse is delivered, which is measured in pulses per second (pps) or Hertz (Hz).	• Increased rate feels more like a "flutter." • Decreased rate feels more like a "tapping." • A typical rate setting is between 10 and 19 Hz. • As rate is increased, IPG battery longevity decreases.
Mode	Mode of stimulation, which can either be continuous or can cycle (on/off). A common setting is 20 seconds "on" and 8 seconds "off."	• Cycling mode may have the benefit of maintaining the person's sense of awareness of the pelvic floor. • Cycling is preferred over continuous to save the life of the battery.
Electrode Polarity	Can be unipolar or bipolar, but bipolar is recommended over unipolar to save the life of the battery	• Must have at least one positive and one negative electrode. • A change in active electrodes changes the location of the stimulation pattern. • Unipolar: any combination of electrodes (0, 1, 2, 3) with at least one *negative* electrode and the case (INS battery) *positive*, as shown below 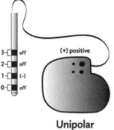 **Unipolar** • Bipolar: system with current flowing between one or more negative electrodes. The INS battery or case is "off" and a *positive* and *negative* charge on the electrodes (0, 1, 2, 3). Example would be 1 is "negative" and 2 is "positive." 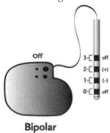 **Bipolar**

Key: INS = implantable neurostimulator; IPG = implantable pulse generator.

any problems. Clinicians are provided this unit by the manufacturer to establish and adjust settings for the patient's INS, following stage 2. The entry of these clinician-determined parameters and settings is called "programming." Primary parameters of this stimulation pulse are amplitude, pulse width, rate, mode, and electrode polarity and are defined in Table 12.3. Programming parameters may have to be changed in the first weeks and months after the system is implanted to optimize therapy, user comfort, and battery longevity (Rittenmeyer, 2008a, 2008b). Programming is usually performed at each patient visit to determine remaining battery life, patient's use since last visit, and the continuity of the electric circuit through electrode impedance measurements. A very high impedance (>4,000 ohms) in more than four electrodes may indicate an open circuit. Very low impedance measurements (<50 ohms) indicate a short circuit. Anteroposterior and lateral radiographs will show any coiling or break in the wire (Diokno, Burgess, & Mulholland, 2003).

Patient Programmer

Patients are able to adjust certain settings using a unit called the iCon Patient Programmer. This unit allows the patient to turn the stimulation on and off, as well as increase or decrease amplitude of the stimulation, and to move between preset programs created by the clinician (Figure 12.14).

Side Effects and Adverse Events

Before considering InterStim therapy, patients should be made aware of both the advantages and potential adverse events associated with this therapy. If problems occur, they may relate to the therapy, the device, or the procedure and include adverse changes in voiding function (bowel, bladder, or both). Common adverse events are pain at the implant or lead site (up to 25% of patients), lead-related problems such as lead migration (16%), replacement and repositioning of the INS (15%), wound problems (7%), adverse effects on bowel function (6%), infection (5%), and generator problems (5%) (Leng & Morrisroe, 2006). Permanent removal of the electrode has been reported in 9% of individuals. Overall, reoperation can be necessary in one third of implanted individuals. The most common reason for surgical revision was relocation of the generator because of pain and infection (Brazzelli, Murray, & Fraser 2006). Change in sensation of stimulation can occur and is described as uncomfortable (jolting or shocking) by some patients.

Malfunctioning SNS devices may result from lead disruption after a traumatic event, implant migration, or a dead battery (battery life is commonly 7–10 years) (Gaynor-Krupnick, Dwyer, Rittenmeyer, & Kreder, 2006). Other problems that may cause a malfunctioning InterStim® device are suboptimal programming settings (impedance levels, pulse width, pulse rate, frequency, and energy level), sensory discomfort, motor changes (lower extremity or great toe spasm), overly tight lead connection, a broken fiber, poor nerve conduction, lead migration (trauma, fall, hematoma), infection, generator site pain, and sensory discomfort.

A

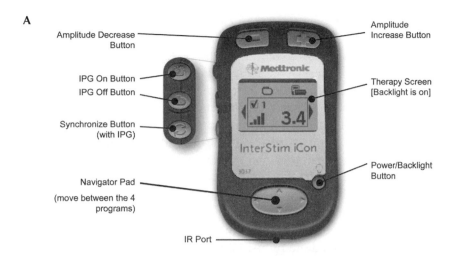

Amplitude Decrease Button

Amplitude Increase Button

IPG On Button

IPG Off Button

Synchronize Button (with IPG)

Therapy Screen [Backlight is on]

Power/Backlight Button

Navigator Pad (move between the 4 programs)

IR Port

B

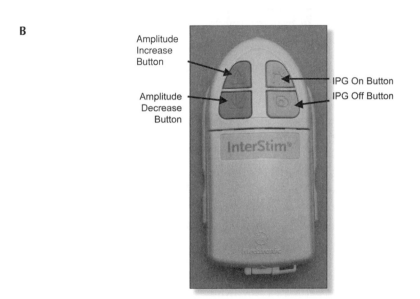

Amplitude Increase Button

Amplitude Decrease Button

IPG On Button

IPG Off Button

Figure 12.14. InterStim iCon home patient programmer. (IPG = implantable pulse generator; IR = infra red). *A,* Current model (3037). *B,* Older model (3031A). (Courtesy of Medtronic.)

Device Discomfort

Discomfort at the site of the INS device can occur as a result of pocket-related or output-related causes. Pocket-related causes of discomfort include infection, pocket location (waistline), pocket dimension (too tight, too loose), seroma, and erosion. Output-related causes include sensitivity to unipolar stimulation (if this mode is used) or current leak. To troubleshoot this problem, the clinician should turn off the device and ask the patient if the discomfort is still present to differentiate pocket-related from output-related causes. If the discomfort is persistent, the cause is not related to the device output. In the absence of clinical signs of infection, pocket-related causes such as pocket size, seroma, and erosion must be considered.

If the discomfort disappears when the device is turned off, device output is likely causing discomfort. If the stimulation program used was unipolar, switching to bipolar stimulation may eliminate discomfort. Some patients are sensitive to the unipolar mode of stimulation because the positive pole is the neurostimulator itself. Another possibility is leakage of fluid into the connector, which creates a short circuit whereby the current from the device follows this fluid pathway out to the patient's tissues. Most patients report this as a burning sensation. Although current is following this fluid to the tissues, because some current also may be getting to the electrodes, some patients feel burning in the implant pocket as well as stimulation in the perineum. Reprogramming around this can be done by using different electrode combinations. If reprogramming is unsuccessful, the "burning" sensation may nonetheless be tolerable (it will not harm the individual's tissues); if not, a revision surgery may be necessary to dry out the connection sites.

Precautions and Contraindications

InterStim® therapy is not intended for patients with mechanical outlet obstruction. The safety and effectiveness of magnetic resonance imaging (MRI) for patients using the InterStim device has not been established, so undergoing MRI is not recommended. If an individual with an InterStim device has an electrocardiogram done, INS activity may be recorded as part of the electrocardiogram. The INS should be turned off before the test. Continuous cardiac monitoring and pacemaker interrogation are recommended during lead wire placement, with testing to maximal SNS to assure that no inhibition or interference occurs. In addition, the InterStim unit should be turned off during pregnancy. Diathermy is contraindicated because it generates heat that is transferred to the lead and may result in tissue damage. InterStim users may also want to avoid prolonged stays in hot tubs.

Efficacy

The safety and efficacy of SNS with respect to refractory urgency UI, urgency–frequency syndrome, and nonobstructive urinary retention has been demonstrated in several long-term clinical studies. A major limitation to the efficacy of InterStim® is that information is not available or not reported pertaining to the number of patients who fail initial PNE or stage I trials or those who do not opt to move to stage II implant. So it is *not* known what percentage of patients who fail stage I or the number who do not advance to permanent implant but rather have the tined lead removed. This should be reported to determine the true "cure" or "improvement." A systematic review by Brazzelli and colleagues (2006) listed cure and improvement rates at 6 months in patients with urgency incontinence randomized to a stimulation or a delayed group. Overall, 50% of patients in the stimulation group achieved complete continence or greater than 90% improvement in the main incontinence symptoms compared with 1.6% of patients in the delay group. A 50% improvement in main incontinence symptoms was observed in approximately 37% and 3% of patients in the stimulation and delay groups, respectively. Case series have shown that 67% of patients become dry or achieve a greater than 50% improvement in symptoms after implantation. Incontinence episodes, leakage severity, voiding frequency, and pad use were significantly lower after implantation. Benefits were reported to persist 3–5 years after implantation (Brazzelli et al., 2006).

Jonas and colleagues (2001) reported on subjects with idiopathic urinary retention, comparing subjects ($n = 37$) who received early implantation to a control group ($n = 31$). The primary end point of residual volume was significantly higher in the control group at 6 months' follow-up. Significantly more subjects continued to require catheterization in the control group (81% vs. 40%). Clinical improvement was maintained throughout the 18-month period after implantation. With inactivation of the neuromodulator, the voiding diary parameters returned to baseline values, indicating that the underlying cause of retention was not cured by treatment.

Wallace, Lane, and Noblett (2007) reported good results in 28 of 33 subjects (85%) with underlying neurological disease (13 of 16 subjects [81%] with multiple sclerosis, 4 of 6 subjects [67%] with Parkinson's disease, and 11 of 11 subjects [100%] with other neurological disorders) who underwent InterStim implantation. Incontinence episodes per 24 hours decreased by 68%, number of voids per 24 hours decreased by 43%, nocturia decreased by 70%, and there was a 58% reduction in intermittent self-catheterization per 24 hours. Ninety-three percent of subjects reported overall satisfaction.

Comiter (2003) performed a prospective study that evaluated SNS for the treatment of refractory interstitial cystitis. Interstitial cystitis is not an approved indication for SNS, but the technique can be used to treat the urgency and frequency seen in these individuals. At a mean of 14 months' follow-up, urinary frequency had decreased from 17.1 to 8.7 voids per day, mean voided volume had increased from 111 to 264 mL, and pain had decreased from 5.8 to 1.6 on a scale of 1 to 10. Ninety-four percent of subjects with implants demonstrated a sustained improvement in symptoms. These results await confirmation.

CONCLUSIONS

Surgical treatment for UI includes sling surgery and injections for stress UI, an artificial sphincter for stress UI, botulinum toxin injections, and neuromodulation with a "bladder pacemaker" for urgency and frequency. The decision to perform surgery for the treatment of UI should be made only after a precise, focused assessment. This assessment should include a comprehensive clinical evaluation with an objective confirmation of the pathophysiological diagnosis and severity of urinary loss, a correlation of the anatomic and physiological findings with the surgical plan, an estimation of surgical risk, an estimation of the impact of the proposed surgery on the patient's quality of life, and a determination of patient expectations of this treatment.

REFERENCES

Albo, M.E., Richter, H.E., Brubaker, L., Norton, P., Kraus, S.R., Zimmern, P.E., et al. for the Urinary Incontinence Treatment Network. (2007). Burch colposuspension versus fascial sling to reduce urinary stress incontinence. *New England Journal of Medicine, 356,* 2143–2200.

Andonian, S., Chen, T., St-Denis, B., & Corcos, J. (2005). Randomized clinical trial comparing suprapubic arch sling (SPARC) and tension-free vaginal tape (TVT): One-year results. *European Urology, 47,* 537–541.

Anger, J.T., Litwin, M.S., Wang, Q., Pashos, C.L., & Rodríguez, L.V. (2007). The effect of age on outcomes of sling surgery for urinary incontinence. *Journal of the American Geriatrics Society, 55,* 1927–1931.

Appell, R.A., Dmochowski, R.R., & Herschorn, S. (2006). Urethral injections for female stress incontinence. *BJU International, 98*(Suppl. 1), 27–30.

Barber, M.D., Kleeman, S., Karram, M.M., Paraiso, M.F., Walters, M.D., Vasavada, S., & Ellerkmann, M. (2008). Transobturator tape compared with tension-free vaginal tape for the treatment of stress urinary incontinence: A randomized controlled trial. *Obstetrics & Gynecology, 111*(3), 611–621.

Botros, S.M., Miller, J.J., Goldberg, R.P., Gandhi, S., Akl, M., Beaumont, J.L., et al. (2007). Detrusor overactivity and urge urinary incontinence following trans obturator versus midurethral slings. *Neurourology and Urodynamics, 26,* 42–45.

Boyles, S.H., Weber, A.M., & Meyn, L. (2004). Ambulatory procedures for urinary incontinence in the United States, 1994–1996. *American Journal of Obstetrics and Gynecology, 190,* 33–36.

Brazelli, M., Murray, A., & Fraser, C. (2006). Efficacy and safety of sacral nerve stimulation for urinary urge incontinence: A systematic review. *Journal of Urology, 175,* 835–841.

Brubaker, L. (2004). Surgical treatment of urinary incontinence in women. *Gastroenterology, 126*(1 Suppl. 1), S71–S76.

Brubaker, L., Cundiff, G.W., Fine, P., Nygaard, I., Richter, H., Visco, A., et al. for the Pelvic Floor Disorders Network. (2006). Abdominal sacrocolpopexy with Burch colposuspension to reduce urinary stress incontinence. *New England Journal of Medicine, 354,* 1557–1566.

Chancellor, M.B., & Chartier-Kastler, E.J. (2000). Principles of sacral nerve stimulation (SNS) for the treatment of bladder and urethral sphincter dysfunctions. *Neuromodulation, 3,* 15–26.

Chapple, C.R., Wein, A.J., Brubaker, L., Dmochowski, R., Pons, M.E., Haab, F., et al. (2005). Stress incontinence injection therapy: What is best for our patients? *European Urology, 48,* 552–565.

Comiter, C.V. (2002). The male sling for stress urinary incontinence: A prospective study. *Journal of Urology, 167,* 597–601.

Comiter, C.V. (2003). Sacral neuromodulation for the symptomatic treatment of refractory interstitial cystitis: A prospective study. *Journal of Urology, 169,* 1369–1373.

Dalkin, B.L., Wessells, H., & Cui, H. (2003). A national survey of urinary and health related quality of life outcomes in men with an artificial urinary sphincter for post-radical prostatectomy incontinence. *Journal of Urology, 169,* 237–239.

Dalpiaz, O., Primus, G., & Schips, L. (2006). SPARC sling system for treatment of female stress urinary incontinence in the elderly. *European Urology, 50,* 826–830.

DasGupta, R., & Fowler, C.J. (2003). The management of female voiding dysfunction: Fowler's syndrome—a contemporary update. *Current Opinion in Urology, 13,* 293-299.

Dean, N.M., Ellis, G., Wilson, P.D., & Herbison, G.P. (2006). Laparoscopic colposuspension for urinary incontinence in women. *Cochrane Database of Systematic Reviews,* (3), CD002239.

Delorme, E. (2001). Trans-obturator urethral suspension: A minimally invasive procedure to treat female stress urinary incontinence. *Progress in Urology, 11,* 1306–1313.

Delorme, E., Droupy, S., de Tayrac, R., & Delmas, V. (2004). Transobturator tape (Uratape): A new minimally-invasive procedure to treat female urinary incontinence. *European Urology, 45,* 203–207.

Diokno, A.C., Burgess, S., & Mulholland, T. (2003). Complication of the sacral neuromodulator: Lead avulsion and wire disruption. *Journal of Urology, 169,* 283–284.

Dmochowski, R.R. (2005). Current use of injectables for female stress urinary incontinence. *Reviews in Urology, 7*(Suppl. 1), S12–S21.

Gaynor-Krupnick, D.M., Dwyer, N.T., Rittenmeyer, H., & Kreder, K.J. (2006). Evaluation and management of malfunctioning sacral neuromodulator. *Urology, 67,* 246–249.

Giberti, C., Gallo, F., Cortese, P., & Schenone, M. (2007). Transobturator tape for treatment of female stress urinary incontinence: Objective and subjective results after a mean follow-up of two years. *Urology, 69,* 703–707.

Goh, M. & Diokno, AC. (2007). Sacral neuromodulation for nonobstructive urinary retention—is success predictable? *Urology, 178,* 197–199.

Gomelski, A., & Dmochowski, R.R. (2007). Biocompatibility assessment of synthetic sling materials for female stress urinary incontinence. *Journal of Urology, 178*(4 Pt 1), 1171–1181.

Hammad, F.T., Kennedy-Smith, A., & Robinson, R.G. (2005). Erosions and urinary retention following polypropylene synthetic sling: Australasian survey. *European Urology, 47,* 641–646.

Herschorn, S., & Radomski, S.B. (1997). Collagen injections for genuine stress urinary incontinence: Patient selection and durability. *International Urogynecology Journal, 8,* 18–24.

Herschorn, S., Steele, D.J., & Radomski, S.B. (1996). Followup of intraurethral collagen for female stress urinary incontinence. *Journal of Urology, 156,* 1305–1309.

Hodroff, M.A., Sutherland, S.E., Kesha, J.B., & Siegel, S.W. (2005). Treatment of stress incontinence with the Sparc sling: Intraoperative and early complications of 445 patients. *Urology, 66,* 760–762.

Hullfish, K., Bovbjerg, V., & Steers, W. (2004). Patient-centered goals for pelvic floor dysfunction surgery: Long-term follow-up. *American Journal of Obstetrics and Gynecology, 191,* 201–205.

Jonas, U., Fowler, C.J., Chancellor, M.B., Elhilali, M.M., Fall, M., Gajewski, J.B., et al. (2001). Efficacy of sacral nerve stimulation for urinary retention: Results 18 months after implantation. *Journal of Urology, 165,* 15–19.

Kammer-Doak, D.N., Cornella, J.L., Magrina, J.F., Stanhope, C.R., & Smilack, J. (1998). Osteitis pubis after Marshall-Marchetti-Krantz urethropexy: A pubic osteomyelitis. *American Journal of Obstetrics and Gynecology, 179,* 586–590.

Karram, M.M., Segal, J.L., Vassallo, B.J., & Kleeman, S.D. (2003). Complications and untoward effects of the tension free vaginal tape procedure. *Obstetrics and Gynecology, 101,* 929–932.

Keegan, P., Atiemo, K., Cody, J., McClinton, S., & Pickard, R. (2007). Periurethral injection therapy for urinary incontinence in women. *Cochrane Database of Systematic Reviews,* (3), CD003881.

Kim, D.K., Thomas, C.A., Smith, C., & Chancellor, M.B. (2006). The case for bladder botulinum toxin application. *Urologic Clinics of North America, 33,* 503–510.

Klingler, H.C., & Marberger, M. (2006). Incontinence after radical prostatectomy: Surgical treatment options. *Current Opinion in Urology, 16,* 60–64.

Kobashi, K.C., & Govier, F. (2005). The completely dry rate: A critical re-evaluation of the outcomes of slings. *Neurourology & Urodynamics, 24*(7), 602–605.

Lapitan, M.C., Cody, D.J., & Grant, A.M. (2005). Open retropubic colposuspension for urinary incontinence in women. *Cochrane Database of Systematic Reviews,* (3), CD002912.

Latthe, P.M., Foon, R., & Toozs-Hobson, P. (2007). Transobturator and retropubic tape procedures in stress urinary incontinence: A systematic review and meta-analysis of effectiveness and complications. *BJOG, 114,* 522–531.

Leng, W.W., & Chancellor, M.B. (2005). How sacral nerve stimulation neuromodulation works. *Urologic Clinics of North America, 32,* 11–18.

Leng, W.W., & Morrisroe, S.N. (2006). Sacral nerve stimulation for the overactive bladder. *Urologic Clinics of North America, 33,* 491–501.

Lightner, D., Calvosa, C., Andersen, R., Klimberg, I., Brito, G., Snyder, J., et al. (2001). A new injectable bulking agent for treatment of stress urinary incontinence: Results of a multicenter, randomized, controlled, double-blind study of Durasphere. *Urology, 58,* 12–15.

Lightner, D.J. (2002). Review of the available urethral bulking agents. *Current Opinion in Urology, 12,* 333–338.

Litwiller, S.E., Kim, K.B., Fone, P.D., DeVere White, R.W., & Stone, A.R. (1996). Postprostatectomy incontinence and the artificial urinary sphincter: A long-term study of patient satisfaction and criteria for success. *Journal of Urology, 156,* 1975.

Madjar, S., Covington-Nichols, C., & Secrest, C.L. (2003). New periurethral bulking agent for stress urinary incontinence: Modified technique and early results. *Journal of Urology, 170*(6 Pt. 1), 2327–2329.

Mahajan, S.T., & Brubaker, L. (2007). Botulinum toxin: From life-threatening disease to novel medical therapy. *American Journal of Obstetrics and Gynecology, 196,* 7–15.

Mahajan, S.T., Elkadry, E.A., Kenton, K.S., Shott, S., & Brubaker, L. (2006). Patient-centered surgical outcomes: The impact of goal achievement and urge incontinence on patient satisfaction one year after surgery. *American Journal of Obstetrics and Gynecology, 194,* 722–728.

Mahajan, S.T., Kenton, K., Bova, D.A., & Brubaker, L. (2006). Transobturator tape erosion associated with leg pain. *International Urogynecology Journal and Pelvic Floor Dysfunction, 17,* 66–68.

McGuire, E.J. (2006). Urethral bulking agents. *Nature Clinical Practice: Urology, 3,* 234–235.

Morey, A.F., Medendorp, A.R., Noller, M.W., Mora, R.V., Shandera, K.C., Foley, J.P., et al. (2006). Transobturator versus transabdominal midurethral slings: A multi-institutional comparison of obstructive voiding complications. *Journal of Urology, 175*(3 Pt. 1), 1014–1017.

Mucksavage, P., Smith, A.L., & Moy, M.L. (2006). The use of botulinum toxin in the treatment of refractory overactive bladder. *Ostomy/Wound Management, 52*(12), 28, 30, 32–33.

Mulholland, T.L., & Diokno, A.C. (2004). The artificial urinary sphincter and urinary catheterization: What every physician should know and do to avoid serious complications. *International Urology and Nephrology, 36,* 197–201.

Nilsson, C.G., Kuuva, N., Falconer, C., Rezapour, M., & Ulmsten, U. (2001). Long-term results of the tension-free vaginal tape (TVT) procedure for surgical treatment of female stress urinary incontinence. *International Urogynecology Journal, 2*(Suppl.), 5–8.

Nitti, V.W. (2006). Botulinum toxin for the treatment of idiopathic and neurogenic overactive bladder: State of the art. *Reviews in Urology, 8,* 198–208.

Novara, G., Ficarra, V., Boscolo-Berto, R., Secco, S., Cavalleri, S., & Artibani, W. (2007). Tension-free midurethral slings in the treatment of female stress urinary incontinence:

A systematic review and meta-analysis of randomized controlled trials of effectiveness. *European Urology, 52,* 663–679.

Pannek, J., Brands, F.H., & Senge, T. (2001). Particle migration after transurethral injection of carbon coated beads for stress urinary incontinence. *Journal of Urology, 166,* 1350–1353.

Penson, DF, McLerran, D, Feng, Z, Li, L, Albertsen, PC, Gilliland FD, et al. (2005). 5-Year urinary and sexual outcomes after radical prostatectomy: Results from the Prostate Cancer Outcomes Study. *Journal of Urology, 173,* 1701–1705.

Petero, V.G., & Diokno, A.C. (2006). Comparison of the long-term outcomes between incontinent men and women treated with artificial urinary sphincter. *Journal of Urology, 175,* 605–609.

Petrou, S.P., Elliott, D.S., & Barrett, D.M. (2000). Artificial urethral sphincter for incontinence. *Urology, 56,* 353.

Quallich, S.A., & Ohl, D.A. (2003a). Artificial urinary sphincter: Part I. *Urologic Nursing, 23,* 259–263, 268.

Quallich, S.A., & Ohl, D.A. (2003b). Artificial urinary sphincter: Part II: Patient teaching and perioperative care. *Urologic Nursing, 23,* 269–273.

Raj, G.V., Peterson, A.C., & Webster, G.D. (2006). Outcomes following erosions of the artificial urinary sphincter. *Journal of Urology, 175,* 2186–2190.

Rapp, D.E., & Kobashi, K.C. (2008). Outcomes following sling surgery: Importance of definition of success. *Journal of Urology, 180,* 998–1002.

Reitz, A., Stohrer, M., Kramer, G., Del Popolo, G., Chartier-Kastler, E., Pannek, J., et al. (2004). European experience of 200 cases treated with botulinum-A toxin injections into the detrusor muscle for urinary incontinence due to neurogenic detrusor overactivity. *European Urology, 45,* 510–515.

Reynolds, W.S., Patel, R., Msezane, L., Luciono, A., & Rapp, D.E. (2007). Current use of artificial urinary sphincters in the United States. *Journal of Urology, 178,* 578–583.

Rittenmeyer, H. (2008a). Sacral nerve neuromodulation (InterStim). Part I: Review of the InterStim system. *Urologic Nursing, 28,* 15–20.

Rittenmeyer, H. (2008b). Sacral nerve neuromodulation (InterStim). Part II: Review of programming. *Urologic Nursing, 28,* 21–25.

Rovner, E.S., & Wein, A.J. (2004). Treatment options for stress urinary incontinence. *Reviews in Urology, 6*(Suppl. 3), S29–S47.

Schmid, D.M., Sauermann, P., Werner, M., Schuessler, B., Blick, N., Muentener, M., et al. (2006). Experience with 100 cases treated with botulinum-A toxin injections in the detrusor muscle for idiopathic overactive bladder syndrome refractory to anticholinergics. *Journal of Urology, 176,* 177–185.

Schulz, J.A., Hager, C.W., Stanton, S.L., & Baessler, K. (2004). Bulking agents for stress incontinence: Short-term results and complications in a randomized comparison of periurethral and transurethral injections. *International Urogynecology Journal and Pelvic Floor Dysfunction, 15,* 261–265.

Schurch, B., de Seze, M., Denys, P., Chartier-Kastler, E., Haab, F., Everaert, K., et al. for the Botox Detrusor Hyperreflexia Study Team. (2005). Botulinum toxin type A is a safe and effective treatment for neurogenic incontinence: Results of a single treatment, randomized, placebo controlled 6-month study. *Journal of Urology, 174,* 196–200.

Smith, A.L., & Moy, M.L. (2004). Modern management of women with stress urinary incontinence. *Ostomy/Wound Management, 50*(12), 32–39.

Staskin, D.R., & Comiter, C.V. (2007). Surgical treatment of male sphincteric urinary incontinence: The male perineal sling and artificial urinary sphincter. In A.J. Wein, L.R. Kavoussi, A.C. Novick, A.W. Partin, & C.A. Peters (Eds.), *Campbell's urology* (9th ed., pp. 2391–2403). Philadelphia: Elsevier Saunders.

Staskin, D.R., & Tyagi, R. (2006). SPARC-midurethral sling suspension system. In L. Cardozo & D. Staskin (Eds.), Textbook of female urology and urogynecology (2nd ed., pp. 925–934). United Kingdom: Isis Medical Media, LTD.

Steineck, G., Helgesen, F., Adolfsson, J., Dickman, P.W., Johansson, J.E., Norlén, B.J., et al. for the Scandinavian Prostatic Cancer Group Study Number 4. (2002). Quality of life after radical prostatectomy or watchful waiting. *New England Journal of Medicine, 347,* 790.

Sung, V.W., Schleinitz, M.D., Rardin, C.R., Ward, R.M., & Myers, D.L. (2007). Comparison of retropubic vs transobturator approach to midurethral slings: A systematic review and meta-analysis. *American Journal of Obstetrics & Gynecology, 197,* 3–11.

Tamanini, J.T., D'Ancona, C.A., & Netto, N.R. (2006). Macroplastique implantation system for female stress urinary incontinence: Long-term follow-up. *Journal of Endourology, 20,* 1082–1086.

Ulmsten, U., Johnson, P., & Rezapour, M. (1999). A three-year follow up of tension free vaginal tape for surgical treatment of female stress urinary incontinence. *British Journal of Obstetrics and Gynaecology, 106,* 345–350.

Vasavada, S.P., & Rackley, R.R. (2007). Electrical stimulation for storage and emptying disorders. In A.J. Wein, L.R. Kavoussi, A.C. Novick, A.W. Partin, & C.A. Peters (Eds.), *Campbell's urology* (9th ed., pp. 2147–2167). Philadelphia: Elsevier Saunders.

Venn, S.N., Greenwell, T.J., & Mundy, A.R. (2000). The long-term outcome of artificial urinary sphincters. *Journal of Urology, 164*(3 Pt. 1), 702–706.

Wallace, P.A., Lane, F.L., & Noblett, K.L. (2007). Sacral nerve neuromodulation in patients with underlying neurologic disease. *American Journal of Obstetrics and Gynecology, 197,* 96.e1–96.e5.

Ward, K.L., & Hilton, P. (2004). A prospective multicenter randomized trial of tension-free vaginal tape and colposuspension for primary urodynamic stress incontinence: Two-year follow-up. *American Journal of Obstetrics and Gynecology, 190,* 324–331.

13

Continence Nurse
Specialists and Service Models

Evaluation and treatment of urinary incontinence (UI), overactive bladder, and related pelvic floor disorders is a changing and expanding area of practice for physicians, allied health professionals such as physical therapists, and nurses—especially advanced practice nurses (APNs). Almost every day, health care providers encounter people with incontinence, despite the fact that UI is not always the reason for the initial contact. Surprisingly, physicians and nurses inquire about UI in only a minority of their at-risk patients (see Chapter 2), even though primary care providers can be effective in treating incontinence by conservative measures when educated and motivated (Newman et al., 2005).

It is thought that screening for UI and related disorders will occur only if those responsible for primary health care are educated about these conditions, learn to ask people about the problem, and know how to refer appropriately. One of the barriers is that most doctors, nurses, and allied health professionals receive little if any basic training in UI. Organizations such as the Agency for Healthcare Research and Quality (AHRQ), the American Urological Association, the American College of Obstetrics and Gynecology, and the American Medical Directors Association have established guidelines for medical practitioners concerning UI in adults, but these measures are largely ignored by the medical community.

Nurses are the core of UI care because management of urine and feces has been a part of nursing practice since Florence Nightingale's time. Nurses have appropriate interpersonal and technical skills, and they use an informal approach that is attractive to patients (Du Moulin, Hamers, Paulus, Berendsen, & Halfens, 2005). Many nurses have great expertise in caring for incontinent patients because they have dealt with people with socially embarrassing conditions. Many have developed advanced skills for UI assessment and treatment, and these nurses are the ideal professionals to provide specialized continence services (Matharu et al., 2004). Their numbers are increasing, but there are no academic or clinical proficiency requirements in the United States in order to be considered a "continence nurse practitioner" or "continence nurse specialist." Those nurses who do specialize in continence care have obtained their knowledge and skills through self-motivated activities. This chapter discusses the role of the nurse as a continence expert and reviews some existing models for delivery of continence care.

GROWTH OF CONTINENCE CARE NURSE SPECIALISTS

The scope and extent of nursing services for UI differ throughout the world. Appendix Table 13.1 reviews the categories of nurse specialists who provide continence services throughout the world. These services have primarily targeted UI, and few nurse specialists provide bowel services (Norton, 2004). Two models that have been comprehensively used in countries such as Australia, New Zealand, and the United Kingdom are the *continence nurse advisor* (CNA) and the *nurse continence advisor* (NCA), both of whom are registered (generalist) nurses with specialized training in UI (Wells, 2000). In the past several years, particularly in the United Kingdom, the United States, and Australia, nurses with additional nursing education (graduate or doctorate level) have evolved into *continence nurse practitioners* (CNP). These three roles are overlapping in duties.

Advanced Practice Nurse Continence Specialists

Despite the lack of formal training, CNPs in the United States are a growing group of nurses—APNs—who have taken up the AHRQ's recommendations, incorporating them into evidence-based clinical practice and care pathways (Newman, 2006; Newman & Palumbo, 1994; Newman, Parente, & Yuan, 1997; Sampselle et al., 2000; Watson, Brink, Zimmer, & Mayer, 2003). APNs are clinical nurse specialists, nurse practitioners, nurse midwives, and nurse anesthetists who have completed a Master of Science degree in nursing. Starting in 2015, nurse practitioner entry level into advanced practice will be at the doctorate level (e.g., Doctorate in Nursing Practice [DNP]). These health care providers are knowledgeable about a wide range of medical health conditions and practice with a physician collaborator to maximize patient outcomes in acute, primary, home care, outpatient, and long-term care (LTC) settings. APN competencies include, but are not limited to,

1. Ability to conduct comprehensive assessment based on advanced knowledge of human sciences and extended skills in diagnostic decision making

2. Ability to differentiate between normal and abnormal findings

3. Knowledge of pharmacokinetics and phamacodynamics and ability to prescribe appropriate drug therapy

4. Ability to make informed and autonomous decisions about all aspects of a person's assessment and treatment

The Wound, Ostomy, and Continence Nurses Society has a postgraduate course that includes a curriculum for UI. Appendix Table 13.2 provides a sample of a curriculum for a continence nurse specialist compiled by one of the authors (DKN) (Jirovec, Wyman, & Wells, 1998; Newman, 2006; Rogalski, 2005).

Studies have shown that people are satisfied with the care given by APNs, particularly nurse practitioners, who have been shown to spend more time with patients (Wong & Chung, 2006). APNs' quality of care is comparable with that of physicians, and prescriptive authority (e.g., diagnostic tests, medications) is part of their practice (Horrocks, Anderson, & Salisbury, 2002). Jha, Moran, Blackwell, and Greenham (2007) noted that 35% of women attending gynecology outpatient departments with incontinence problems could be effectively managed by urogynecology specialist nurses.

In the United States, APNs have become increasingly interested in and knowledgeable about the assessment, diagnosis, and treatment of people suffering with UI. Like nurses in other countries, these nurses are developing a nursing subspecialty in the care of individuals with UI. These APNs provide comprehensive assessment and noninvasive treatment and act as educators and researchers. Nurses are often successful at engaging their patients to share personal information related to their health, and thus should take the leadership role in providing health promotion information. To successfully promote healthy lifestyles in old age, bladder control educational information must be included. Nurses can be the change agent in providing a public health population-based approach to continence promotion (Palmer & Newman, 2006). However, because the United States does not have well-developed external funding of continence nurse services, growth in this area is nurse dependent.

These APNs practice either independently in solo practices or as part of a multidisciplinary team (Cacchione & Decker, 2004; Carcio, 2003; Klay & Marfyak, 2005; Mason, Newman & Palmer, 2003; McDowell, Burgio, Dombrowski, Loches, & Rodrequez, 1992). Appendix Box 13.1 reviews various continence practice models that are managed by APNs. The development of continence practices has been aided by the broadening of authority for APNs, including 1) the ability to receive direct reimbursement from insurers such as Medicare, Medicaid, health maintenance organizations, and other private insurers; 2) the implementation of prescriptive authority; and 3) the removal of barriers to independent practice (Newman, 1996). These changes have given APNs the opportunity to expand services for the management of UI. They usually serve as clinical support for nurses who have incontinent patients, and they are catalysts for improved care and coordination of services (Ostaszkiewicz, 2006).

A more recent growth of these services is among geriatric APN specialists practicing in home care and LTC settings, providing expert consultation in UI and related disorders (Jacobs, Wyman, Rowell, & Smith, 1998; Newman et al., 1997; Thompson & Smith, 2002; Wells, 2000; Zarowitz & Ouslander, 2007).

Many have developed innovative approaches to management of UI in nursing homes. Ryden et al. (2000) demonstrated significantly improved outcomes for three clinical problems—UI, depression, and pressure ulcers—when gerontology APNs worked with nursing facility staff to implement scientifically based protocols. This study also showed that consistent educational efforts with staff and residents produced interventions that improved or stabilized the level of UI in many people.

One of the authors (DKN) has provided UI consultation in both of these settings and has developed setting-specific materials for this care. For example, Appendix Box 13.2 outlines a protocol for LTC settings for a bladder and bowel program, and Appendix Box 13.3 outlines steps used for implementing such a program, in the LTC setting. Bucci (2007) developed the CHAMMP (Continence, History, Assessment, Medications, Mobility, Plan) tool to educate staff on a comprehensive continence assessment and to assist in implementation of individualized plans of care. The CHAMMP program improved one facility's Quality Measure Indicator Report.

Some APNs have also been active in developing health promotion programs (e.g., Dry Anticipations by the Oklahoma State Health Department; Dry Expectations and Bladder Health by one of the authors [DKN] with Rutgers University School of Nursing and Philadelphia Corporation For Aging in Philadelphia) for community centers (McFall, Yerkes, Belzer, & Cowan, 1994; Newman, Wallace, & Blackwood, 1996; Palmer & Newman, 2006). One of the authors (DKN) also maintains an online searchable database of professional continence providers for use by consumers, health care professionals, and industry leaders called SEPHIA's Choice (http://www.sephiaschoice.com). The web site also offers health professionals, group medical practices, and medical institutions the opportunity to perform unlimited searches on an ongoing basis. One of the authors (DKN) also maintains a web site specifically for continence nurses and other pelvic health professionals that provides continuing education programs and downloadable patient education tools and records (http:// www.ContinenceNurse.net).

Educational Preparation

A survey of nurses attending a national nursing conference on UI asked about educational preparation related to this condition (Jacobs et al., 1998). Fewer than half (40%) of respondents reported receiving an academic education, including course work in accredited postbaccalaureate or graduate programs, related to UI. Most nurses (76%) obtained instruction at professional conferences, at continence clinics supervised by nurse practitioners or physicians, through on-the-job training, by self-study, and in in-service programs. Information was also obtained from courses on the application of equipment and modalities sponsored by companies who provide urodynamic or biofeedback equipment or both. There have not been more recent surveys of this group.

Nurses have undertaken certain activities to further their expertise in this area, including reading medical and nursing journals, attending professional meetings, observing clinical findings of other health care professionals (urologists, urogynecologists, or gynecologists), and joining professional organizations to discuss topics related to the care of incontinent patients. One of the authors (DKN) and colleagues (Newman et al., 1994) reported on a clinical and didactic training program held from 1987 to 1994 that trained 82 health care professionals on the identification, assessment, and evaluation of UI. The professionals attending this program completed "hands-on" training in the application of behavioral interventions, including biofeedback and pelvic floor electrical stimulation. These individuals were able to observe clinical practice in all settings, including hospital-based clinics, private practice, LTC, and home care. Participants included 76 nurses (6 nurses with Ph.D.s in nursing, 45 APNs, and 25 registered nurses), 2 physical therapists, 1 physician assistant, and 3 physicians. Time spent in training averaged 5 days but ranged from 3 to 21 days. Many of these professionals were able to expand a continence practice in their geographic area. One such practitioner, Cindy Maloney Monaghan, is profiled in Appendix Box 13.1.

Outcomes of Nurse Continence Services

By providing patient-tailored and holistic care and using evidence-based treatment options, nurses can adequately diagnose and treat individuals suffering from incontinence. Urological nurses have been trained as "teachers" to successfully implement behavior modification in group programs (Lajiness, Wolfert, Hall, Sampselle, & Diokno, 2007). Although nurses can provide effective interventions in the area of UI, there is limited research on effective interventions for bowel incontinence.

Specialized continence nurses are readily accepted by people with urinary symptoms. Also, there is wide acceptance of nurse-directed continence services, particularly nurse-run clinics (Wong & Chung, 2006). Shaw, Williams, and Assassa (2000) conducted a postal survey of people receiving services for UI by CNPs. Participants expressed satisfaction with nurse-led services because of the interpersonal skills, technical skills, and communication and information-giving abilities of the nurses. This is in line with previous studies that have consistently identified these attributes as important predictors of patient satisfaction with nursing, despite variation in context and methodology (L.H. Thomas & Bond, 1996). There is now some evidence that treatment of incontinent community-dwelling individuals by a nurse is beneficial in terms of clinical outcomes (Du Moulin, Hamers, Paulus, Berendsen, & Halfens, 2007). Important aspects for a successful nurse continence service are the educational preparation of nurses, use of evidence-based protocols, frequent nurse–patient interaction that serves to reinforce treatments, nurse-led urodynamic investigations, and nurse contact with a specialist medical team (e.g., urology).

Kate Williams, a continence nurse researcher in the United Kingdom, has reported in several publications on positive outcomes of interventions delivered by nurses trained in UI management using a comprehensive approach (Williams, 2000; Williams, Assassa, Smith, Shaw, & Carter, 1999; Williams et al., 2000, 2005). She reported on a randomized, controlled study of 3,746 community-dwelling individuals greater than 40 years of age (61% women) who had incontinence, frequency, urgency, and nocturia all impacting quality of life (Williams et al., 2005). Twenty-one generalist nurses who were trained as CNPs delivered evidence-based behavioral interventions using predetermined care pathways in four visits over an 8-week period to 2,958 individuals. Standard care consisting of access to existing continence services, including CNAs, was provided to 788 individuals. At 3 months, more subjects in the CNP group than the standard care group had improvement in more than one symptom or reported no symptoms (cure).

Incontinence interventions provided by nurses may also result in reduced costs. An Australian study by Moore et al. (2003) compared outcomes in 145 women presenting with stress UI, with or without urge UI, randomly allocated to a standardized regimen with an NCA or treatment by a urogynecologist. The treatment by the NCA took a median of 160 minutes, but cost $59.20 (Australian) compared with 90 minutes of gynecologist time at a cost of $189.70. At 2.5 years, 29% of the NCA group and 41% of the gynecologist group were dry. The authors concluded that similar results were achieved at lower cost using the NCA.

INCONTINENCE PRACTICE MODELS

The organization of incontinence services depends on the organization and structure of health services generally (Newman et al., 2005). Few studies exist that directly compare the effectiveness of specific health care delivery systems on continence care. Enthusiasts have conducted research, but the results may not generalize to the wider setting. Most models have combined the expertise of multidisciplinary providers to maximize service delivery (Cheater et al., 2006). Although some might argue that a multidisciplinary approach is ideal, the reality is not always smooth. In some situations, rivalries and competition between medical specialties surface. This may be caused by competition for patients and income or by disputes over the demarcation of the scope of different disciplines (e.g., the boundary between urology and gynecology or between nursing and physical therapy).

UI is so widespread and affects so many different types of people that those experiencing UI may seek help from any type of health care provider. It is impractical, therefore, to expect individuals to be treated only by specialized continence programs. Mode of service delivery is an important factor that affects patient outcomes, but there have been few systematic evaluations of service interventions for urinary symptoms. Primary care providers will remain the professionals who will first screen for, identify, and evaluate people for these conditions. However, the need for more complex and specialized evaluation and treatment through specific services or practices (e.g., "continence centers") is growing.

The goals of specialized continence centers include providing high-quality, cost-effective care; promoting access to health care for an underserved population; and acting as a source of referral to other providers, particularly primary care providers. These centers are an attractive addition to a hospital or urology practice because they provide secure revenue-generating services. A continence center usually offers the combined knowledge of experts in the field of UI and voiding and pelvic floor dysfunction. Hospital-based continence centers provide increased referrals to urology and gynecology departments for more comprehensive urodynamic studies and surgical procedures. Many have hospital-based video-urodynamic radiology suites. Urologists specialize in treating problems of the urinary tract in both men and women. In fact, a growing number of urologists, collaborating with APNs, are focusing solely on treating the genitourinary problems of women and men, particularly UI, overactive bladder, interstitial cystitis, and related conditions (see Appendix Box 13.1). Changes in reimbursement for nonsurgical treatments such as biofeedback therapy, pelvic muscle electrical stimulation, and neuromodulation have allowed urologists, urogynecologists, and other professionals to consider the expansion of current treatments (pharmacological and surgical) to alternative treatments such as pelvic muscle rehabilitation.

Identifying a management approach for UI that decreases patient dependency or caregiver burden can be a daunting task and requires a professional who has expertise in assessment of complex situations and environments. Management also includes the identification of the appropriate product or device, so professionals need to be knowledgeable about all products available. The challenge is to plan a service that ensures a systematic care pathway (i.e., a stepwise progression of investigation and treatment that each patient follows without overlaps or omissions) and the best use of limited resources (Newman, in press). Models for continence services take several different forms, ranging from comprehensive treatment centers to a program within an established practice (see Appendix Box 13.1).

There are multidisciplinary models that target incontinence or pelvic floor disorders and combine the expertise of APNs and registered nurses working with urologists, geriatricians, gynecologists, and urogynecologists. These nurses may receive on-the-job training from a practicing physician whose background and interests lie in the care of women with urinary dysfunction, or may receive training in preceptorships available from these physicians, or during attendance at instructional seminars or conferences on continence care, or from a combination of these sources. These collaborators will incorporate UI evaluation within an existing private practice, open a clinic within an outpatient hospital setting, or establish a freestanding practice separate from existing medical services.

A trend for hospital systems is to establish "women's centers," which typically include continence services. Usually, these centers are given names that identify the specifics of the services provided. Names such as Bladder Control Center, Pelvic Floor Dysfunction Center, Incontinence Treatment Center, Continence Center, Center for Continence and Pelvic Health, Bladder Wellness Center, Continence Management Program, Urofitness, Urology Wellness Center, and Urohealth are just a few examples. These centers provide all-inclusive evaluation and treatment services, and frequently serve as sites for research and professional training. Such a center should have three main components: 1) clinical and direct patient care, 2) research, and 3) education of health care professionals (Appendix Box 13.4).

The Internet is growing as a useful health education and outreach tool for people with a stigmatized illness such as UI (Berger, Wagner, & Baker, 2005, Boyington, Dougherty, & Yuan-Mei, 2003; Diering & Palmer, 2001; Sandvik, 1999). One of the authors (DKN) has maintained an Internet web site (http://www.seekwellness.com/incontinence) since 1994 that has provided health information on all aspects of UI.

CONCLUSION

The trend seen in health care practice today is for a more comprehensive medical approach to bladder and pelvic floor disorders. The most urgent educational need is being seen at the undergraduate medical and nursing levels. Given these two changes, more professionals will be prepared to detect the problem of UI and make appropriate treatment or referral decisions. Also, the increasing number of continence nurse specialists practicing in "Centers of Excellence" will help to fill the ever-increasing need for health care providers with detailed knowledge of UI and related disorders.

REFERENCES

Berger, M., Wagner, T.H., & Baker, L.C. (2005). Internet use and stigmatized illness. *Social Science and Medicine, 61,* 1821–1827.

Borrie, M.J., Bawden, M., Speechley, M., & Kloseck, M. (2002). Interventions led by nurse continence advisers in the management of urinary incontinence: A randomized controlled trial. *CMAJ, 166,* 1267–1273.

Boyington, A.R., Dougherty, M.C., & Yuan-Mei, L. (2003). Analysis of interactive continence health information on the web. *Journal of Wound, Ostomy, and Continence Nursing, 30,* 280–286.

Bucci, A.T. (2007). Be a continence champion: Use the CHAMMP Tool to individualize the plan of care. *Geriatric Nursing, 28,* 120–124.

Cacchione, P.Z., & Decker, S.A. (2004). Caring for the incontinent elder: Advanced practice nursing concepts. *Clinics in Geriatric Medicine, 20,* 489–497.

Carcio, H. (2003). Comprehensive continence care: The nurse practitioner's role. *ADVANCE for Nurse Practitioners, 11*(10), 26–36.

Cheater, F.M., Baker, R., Reddish, S., Spiers, N., Wailoo, A., Gillies, C., et al. (2006). Cluster randomized controlled trial of the effectiveness of audit and feedback and educational outreach on improving nursing practice and patient outcomes. *Medical Care, 44*, 542–551.

Diering, C., & Palmer, M.H. (2001). Professional information about urinary incontinence on the World Wide Web: Is it timely? Is it accurate? *Journal of Wound, Ostomy, and Continence Nursing, 27*, 1–9.

Du Moulin, M.F., Hamers, J.P., Paulus, A., Berendsen, C., & Halfens, R. (2005). The role of the nurse in community continence care: A systematic review. *International Journal of Nursing Studies, 42*, 479–492.

Du Moulin, M.F., Hamers, J.P., Paulus, A., Berendsen, C., & Halfens, R. (2007). Effects of introducing a specialized nurse in the care of community-dwelling women suffering from urinary incontinence. *Journal of Wound, Ostomy, and Continence Nursing, 34*, 631–640.

Horrocks, S., Anderson, E., & Salisbury, C. (2002). Systematic review of whether nurse practitioners working in primary care can provide equivalent care to doctors. *BMJ, 324*, 819–823.

Jacobs, M., Wyman, J.F., Rowell, P., & Smith, D. (1998). Continence nurses: A survey of who they are and what they do. *Urologic Nursing, 18*, 13–20.

Jha, S., Moran, P., Blackwell, A., & Greenham, H. (2007). Integrated care pathways: The way forward for continence services? *European Journal of Obstetrics, Gynecology, and Reproductive Biology, 134*, 120–125.

Jirovec, M.M., Wyman, J.F., & Wells, T.J. (1998). Addressing urinary incontinence with educational continence-care competencies. *Image: Journal of Nursing Scholarship, 30*, 375–378.

Klay, M., & Marfyak, K. (2005). Use of a continence nurse specialist in an extended care facility. *Urologic Nursing, 20*, 1–4.

Lajiness, M.J., Wolfert, C., Hall, S., Sampselle, C., & Diokno, A.C. (2007). Group session teaching of behavioral modification program for urinary incontinence: Establishing the teachers. *Urologic Nursing, 27*, 124–127.

Mason, D., Newman, D., & Palmer, M. (2003, March). State of the science on urinary incontinence. *American Journal of Nursing, Supplement, 7*.

Matharu, G.S., Assassa, R.P., Williams, K.S., Donaldson, M.K., Matthews, R.J., Tincello, D.G., et al. for the Leicestershire MRC Incontinence Study Team. (2004). Continence nurse treatment of women's urinary symptoms. *British Journal of Nursing, 13*, 140–143.

McDowell, B.J., Burgio, K.L., Dombrowski, M., Loches, J.L., & Rodrequez, E. (1992). An interdisciplinary approach to the assessment and behavioral treatment of urinary incontinence in geriatric outpatients. *Journal of Applied Gerontology, 40*, 370–374.

McFall, S.L., Yerkes, A.M., Belzer, J.A., & Cowan, L.D. (1994). Urinary incontinence and quality of life in older women: A community demonstration in Oklahoma. *Family and Community Health, 17*, 64–75.

Moore, K.H., O'Sullivan, R.J., Simons, A., Prashar, S., Anderson, P., & Louey, M. (2003). Randomised controlled trial of nurse continence advisor therapy compared with standard urogynaecology regimen for conservative incontinence treatment: Efficacy costs and two year follow-up. *British Journal of Obstetrics and Gynaecology, 10*, 649–657.

Newman, D., Smith, D., Blackwood, N., Wallace, J., Gerhard, C., & Manning, M. (1994, January). Educating health care professionals about continence services [Poster Presentation]. In *Abstracts of the Multi-Specialty Nursing Conference on Urinary Incontinence*, Phoenix, AZ, pp. 148–149.

Newman, D.K. (1996). Program and practice management for the advanced practice nurse. In A.B. Hamric, J.A. Spross, & C.M. Hanson (Eds.), *Advanced nursing practice* (pp. 545–568). Philadelphia: W.B. Saunders.

Newman, D.K. (2006). Role of continence nurse specialists. In L. Cardozo & D. Staskin (Eds.), *Textbook of female urology and urogynaecology* (2nd ed., pp. 65–80). Abingdon, UK: Informa Healthcare.

Newman, D.K. (in press). Community awareness and education. In G.H. Badlani, G.W. Davila, M.C. Michel, & J.M.C.H. de la Rosette (Eds.), *Continence in males and females: Current treatment concepts and treatment strategies*. London: Springer-Verlag Ltd.

Newman, D.K., Denis, L., Gruenwald, I., Ee, C.H., Millard, R., Roberts, R., et al. (2005). Promotion, education and organization for continence care. In P. Abrams, L. Cardozo, S. Khoury, & A. Wein (Eds.), *Incontinence: Proceedings from the Third International Consultation on Incontinence* (pp. 35–72). Plymouth, UK: Health Publications, Ltd.

Newman, D.K., & Palumbo, M.V. (1994). Planning an independent nursing practice for continence services. *Nurse Practitioner Forum, 5*, 190–193.

Newman, D.K., Parente, C.A., & Yuan, J.R. (1997). Implementing the Agency for Health Care Policy and Research urinary incontinence guidelines in a home health agency. In M.D. Harris (Ed.), *Handbook of home health care administration* (2nd ed., pp. 394–403). Gaithersburg, MD: Aspen Publishers.

Newman, D.K., Wallace, J., & Blackwood, N. (1996). Promoting healthy bladder habits for seniors. *Ostomy/Wound Management, 42*, 18–28.

Norton, C. (2004). Nurses, bowel continence, stigma and taboos. *Journal of Wound, Ostomy, and Continence Nursing, 31*, 85–94.

Ostaszkiewicz, J. (2006). A clinical nursing leadership model for enhancing continence care for older adults in a subacute inpatient care setting. *Journal of Wound, Ostomy, and Continence Nursing, Nov-Dec;33*(6):624-629.

Palmer M.H., & Newman, D.K. (2006). Bladder control educational needs of older adults. *Journal of Gerontological Nursing, 32*(1), 28–32.

Rogalski, N.M. (2005). A graduate nursing curriculum for the evaluation and management of urinary incontinence. *Educational Gerontology, 31*, 139–159.

Ryden, M.B., Snyder, M., Gross, C.R., Savik, K., Pearson, V., Krichbaum, K., et al. (2000). Value-added outcomes: The use of advanced practice nurses in long-term facilities. *The Gerontologist, 40*, 654–662.

Sampselle, C.M., Wyman, J.F., Thomas, K.K., Newman, D.K., Gray, M., Dougherty, M., et al. (2000). Continence for women: A test of AWHONN's evidence-based protocol in clinical practice. *Journal of Obstetric, Gynecologic, and Neonatal Nursing, 29*, 18–26.

Sandvik, H. (1999). Health information and interaction on the Internet: A survey of female urinary incontinence. *BMJ, 319*, 29–32.

Shaw, C., Williams, K.S., & Assassa, R.P. (2000). Patients' views of a new nurse-led continence service. *Journal of Clinical Nursing, 9*, 574–582.

Thomas, L.H., & Bond, S. (1996). Measuring patients' satisfaction with nursing: 1990–1994. *Journal of Advanced Nursing, 23*, 747–756.

Thomas, S., Billington, A., & Getliffe, K. (2004). Improving continence services—a case study in policy influence. *Journal of Nursing Management, 12*, 252–257.

Thompson, D.L., & Smith, D.A. (2002). Continence nursing: A whole person approach. *Holistic Nursing Practice, 16*(2), 14–31.

Watson, N.M., Brink, C.A., Zimmer, J.G., & Mayer, R.D. (2003). Use of the Agency for Health Care Policy and Research urinary incontinence guideline in nursing homes. *Journal of the American Geriatrics Society, 51*, 1779–1786.

Wells, M. (2000). The role of the nurse in urinary incontinence. *Baillière's Best Practice and Research: Clinical Obstetrics and Gynaecology, 14*, 335–354.

Williams, K. (2000). Good practice guidance for continence services. *British Journal of Nursing, 9*, 530.

Williams, K.S., Assassa, R.P., Cooper, N.J., Turner, D.A., Shaw, C., Abrams, K.R., et al. for the Leicestershire MRC Incontinence Study Team. (2005). Clinical and cost-effectiveness of a new nurse-led continence service: A randomised controlled trial. *British Journal of General Practice, 55*, 696–703.

Williams, K.S., Assassa, R.P., Smith, N.K., Jagger, C., Perry, S., Shaw, C., et al. (2000). Development, implementation and evaluation of a new nurse-led continence service: A pilot study. *Journal of Clinical Nursing, 9,* 566–573.

Williams, K.S., Assassa, R.P., Smith, N.K., Shaw, C., & Carter, E. (1999). Educational preparation: Specialist practice in continence care. *British Journal of Nursing, 8,* 1198–1207, 1202, 1204.

Wong, F.K., & Chung, L.C. (2006). Establishing a definition for a nurse-led clinic: Structure, process, and outcome. *Journal of Advanced Nursing, 53,* 358–369.

Wyman, J.F., Bliss, D.Z., Dougherty, M.C., Gray, M., Kass, M., Newman, D.K., et al. (2004). Shaping future directions for incontinence research in aging adults. *Nursing Research, 53*(6 Suppl.), S1–S10.

Zarowitz, B.J., & Ouslander, J.G. (2007). The application of evidence-based principles of care in older persons (issue 6): Urinary incontinence. *Journal of the American Medical Directors Association, 8,* 35–45.

Appendix Table 13.1 Categories of Continence Nurse Specialists

Model	Description	Background
Continence nurse advisor (CNA)	Acts as a liaison for continence services, and guides patients through the referral route most appropriate to their particular needs. Currently, the CNA has four main areas of responsibility: • clinical—involving patient assessment, management, and treatment • administrative—including monitoring supplies, protocols, and the budget for incontinence care in his or her specific health district • educational—for patients, consumers, and other nurses • research	This model originated in the United Kingdom with the goal to use a nurse as the reference point for the medical care of incontinence, both urinary and fecal. Physicians developed specialty continence assessment clinics and promoted the role of the CNA as a major contributor in the British health care system. Initially, the growth was slow; however, as manufacturing companies developed disposable incontinence products, many government health authorities saw the need for an advisor to assist with their use. Multiple branches of the government fund these nurse specialists and assign them to a geographic location, usually a district health authority, and determine the scope of practice (S. Thomas, Billington, & Getliffe, 2004). In the United Kingdom, this specialty of incontinence nurses has evolved into a national professional organization—the Association for Continence Advice (ACA)—that includes both nurses and physical therapists ("physios" in the United Kingdom) who deal with individuals with incontinence (Borrie, Bawden, Speechley, & Kloseck, 2002). Many other countries have developed this role (e.g., Australia, Canada, other European countries).

Role	Description	Evolution
Nurse continence advisor (NCA)	More independent nurse role that is usually associated with community/area health centers, where NCAs may have variable professional support from general or primary care physicians and family practice physicians. NCAs often work in both hospitals and the community, and the service is focused on primary care assessment of individuals and organization of free incontinence product delivery to the home.	This role has evolved in Canada and Australia, and a number of studies support the efficacy of the NCA in the delivery of community continence care (Borrie et al., 2002).
Continence nurse practitioner (CNP)	Nurses who have developed expertise (mostly through "hands-on" and didactic training) caring for incontinent patients. There are no academic or clinical proficiency requirements to be considered a "continence nurse practitioner" or "continence nurse specialist." In the United States, most of these nurses have graduate-level nursing degrees and are certified to independently assess, diagnose, treat (including prescribing medications), and provide management options. These services are provided in fully equipped "continence clinics" with a collaborating physician or through independent practice (e.g., long-term care consultation).	This role has evolved into an informal nursing subspecialty, especially in the United States, where APNs have the ability and training to provide care at the primary care level independently or in collaboration with physicians. APN responsibilities are similar to those identified in countries where "Continence Nurses" are organized. The United Kingdom and Australia have this model also. Research in the United Kingdom has shown that CNP assessment has the potential to assign individuals to the correct conservative treatment, thereby shortening waiting times for urodynamics and specialist assessment (Matharu et al., 2004). In a series of studies performed in Leicestershire, UK, the short- and long-term outcomes of a new CNP-led service for urinary symptoms were examined and evaluated (Williams, 2000; Williams, Assassa, Smith, Shaw, & Carter, 1999). The need for CNPs for care of older adults has been identified as a growing need (Wyman et al., 2004).

Adapted from Newman (2006) and Newman et al. (2005).

Appendix Table 13.2   Sample curriculum outline for continence nurse specialist

Topic	Content
Urinary incontinence	Overview • History • Current state of prevalence, impact, risk factors • Management guidelines (AHRQ, AMDA, AUA, CMS Tag F315 guidance)
Genitourinary system	Anatomy and physiology • Kidneys, bladder, urethra, pelvic floor, prostate • Voiding physiology • Structure, function, age-related changes • Pathophysiology • Transient versus established causes of UI • Neurological causes
Assessment	History • Identification of UI • Mental, functional, environmental status • Physical examination: general, neurological, abdominal, pelvic/genital (including prolapse assessment), rectal • Provocative stress/urge testing • Analysis of voiding records, pad tests • Diagnostics: Q-Tip test, U/A, PVR, blood studies, radiology • Urodynamics: simple, office based; advanced/video • Indications for referral to specialist
Management	Behavior modification • Instruction on lifestyle changes, bladder training, and timed voiding programs • Implementation of pelvic floor muscle training and rehabilitation: use of adjuncts (biofeedback, pelvic floor stimulation) • Prescribing drug therapy • Surgical intervention (pre- and postoperative care, neuromodulation programming) • Use of containment devices, catheters, and other products
Clinical skills	Cognitive (identification of need for counseling on behavior modification, to include information on diet irritants and other lifestyle changes) Psychomotor (e.g., external catheter application, pelvic floor muscle exercise teaching)
Documentation	Documentation (setting appropriate reimbursement/coding requirements)
Goals of management	• Patient expectations • Provider/employer management

Adapted from Jirovec et al. (1998), Newman (2006), and Rogalski (2005).

Key: AHRQ = Agency for Healthcare Research and Quality; AMDA = American Medical Directors Association; AUA = American Urological Association; CMS = Centers for Medicare & Medicaid Services; PVR = postvoid residual; U/A = urinalysis; UI = urge incontinence.

Appendix Box 13.1   Continence practice models

Urologic Center of Excellence for Continence Care

Diane Newman, RNC, M.S.N., CRNP, FAAN; Alan J. Wein, M.D., Ph.D. (hon); M. Louis Moy, M.D.; Philip Hanno, M.D.

The Penn Center for Continence and Pelvic Health, a collaboration between the authors of this book and two of their colleagues, is part of the Division of Urology at the University of Pennsylvania in Philadelphia. The center is considered a regional Center of Excellence for the evaluation, diagnosis, and treatment of all nonmalignant disorders of the pelvis. Appendix Box 13.4 is an outline of the specific services offered by this center. Through the combined experience and cooperation of three urologists and an APN, the center offers complex diagnostic testing, all surgical treatments, and the latest advances in nonsurgical treatments such as behavioral modification and pelvic floor muscle training using biofeedback and electrical stimulation. The center also handles management for those individuals with chronic incontinence through use of products and devices.

Multi-Setting Practice for Continence

Cindy Maloney Monaghan, RNC, M.S., FNP (Director)

Seton Health Incontinence and Wound Services (SHIWS) was established in 1993 at the Seton Health Incontinence Treatment Center, and is primarily a nurse practitioner practice that is part of a community hospital in Troy, New York. Services include evaluation and treatment of individuals with urinary incontinence. Patients include all ages and both sexes. SHIWS's focus over the years has been to evaluate, diagnose, and treat incontinence utilizing the least invasive approach possible. Nurse practitioner (NP) staff evaluate patients in an office setting and in 12 skilled nursing facilities. During the summer of 2005, wound care services were added to the program, providing services in both the nursing home and office setting. Two of the NPs are certified in wound management. Because many people with wounds have incontinence, SHIWS is able to address both conditions. SHIWS's outpatient setting offers free community bladder screening days every couple of months. These screenings attract 20–30 people, the majority of whom request treatment. Consultation in skilled nursing facilities involves evaluation of residents, with special attention to possible functional components of incontinence. SHIWS's approach includes both formal and informal in-service training for the staff and residents.

Another component in the practice is participation in several research, including pharmaceutical investigational trials. Staff have published continuing medical education articles describing clinical experience and analyzing outcomes of the effects of local estrogen on urinary tract infections in elderly nursing home residents.

Multispecialty Continence Services for Women

Leslie Saltzstein Wooldridge, CNP (Gerontological Nurse Practitioner)

The Bladder Control Clinic (BCC) is part of Hackley Health at the Lakes Women's Center in Muskegon, Michigan. It is a place for women to come for comprehensive management of continence care. The BCC staff comprise a multidisciplinary team, including a geriatric nurse practitioner, a urologist, a physical therapist, and a psychologist. Complete assessments include a full range of urodynamics to guide proper treatment and referral. The role of the

(continued)

Appendix Box 13.1 *(continued)*

physical therapist is to treat pelvic pain with exercises, vaginal stretching, and other therapeutic techniques that treat hypertonicity and disorders that contribute to pain. The psychologist counsels women with interstitial cystitis and weight management issues. In addition, the BCC includes obstetrics and gynecology services, internal medicine, and bone density and mammography screening. There is also a separate, daily service for invited specialists (e.g., dermatologists, plastic surgeons, infertility specialists, orthopedic doctors, ophthalmologists), including a menopause clinic. The focus of the BCC is the treatment of incontinence problems with techniques such as behavioral interventions, including fluid management, control of constipation, and bladder emptying and storage conditions. Pessary fitting and management, as well as pelvic floor rehabilitation (including biofeedback and pelvic floor stimulation), round out the scope of the practice. Multiple meetings are held in the evenings in the Community Room, including interstitial cystitis and weight management support groups that are directed toward maintaining bladder health. "Lunch and Learn" educational sessions are conducted twice monthly by specialists who speak to the public on the latest care and treatment for women's health. A discussion on prevention of incontinence through the life span is a quarterly event that also coincides with a bladder screening program. Women feel comfortable and less threatened in this environment because they are free to discuss their problems with the nurse practitioner.

Leslie Saltzstein Wooldridge, a recognized expert continence nurse specialist, also serves the community by providing continence services at a continuum-of-care facility that includes apartments for older adults, assisted living facilites, and a skilled nursing facility where residents have the opportunity to be seen at an on-site "clinic" for all their urinary incontinence needs.

Urology Continence Center

Cheryl LeCroy, M.S.N., RN (Clinical Coordinator)

The Virginia Women's Continence Center (VWCC) at the Virginia Women's Center in Richmond, Virginia, is a Center of Excellence for women. This unique private practice incorporates a urologist as an integrated member of a large obstetrics and gynecology group practice. The VWCC was established in 2006 and is staffed with an advanced practice nurse (APN) who is the clinical coordinator and with nurses trained in continence care. The VWCC utilizes various comprehensive diagnostic procedures and testing and medical evaluation. Nonsurgical treatments of behavioral modification, dietary modification, pelvic floor muscle training, incontinence containment devices and pads, and medications are all utilized and valued. Collaboration with local physical therapists for biofeedback and pelvic floor muscle evaluation and rehabilitation also plays an important role. A full range of state-of-the-art surgical techniques for incontinence is available. A multidisciplinary approach is utilized to provide the highest possible care to patients.

VWCC offers one-stop, comprehensive health care for women of all ages. This includes routine health maintenance and promotion, mammography services, pregnancy and delivery, menopause management, osteoporosis detection and treatment, and assessment and treatment of urinary incontinence, voiding dysfunction, and pelvic pain. A registered dietitian and clinical psychologist are on staff at the center as well. The role of the APN at the VWCC is to perform all complex urodynamics, assist in pre- and postoperative education and care, assist in adjustment of medications, provide counseling for incontinence products and skin care, coordinate and provide treatments for indwelling catheter patients, and provide staff and patient education. In addition, the APN develops patient and staff educational materials and works in conjunction with local nursing and outreach agencies in the area. The urologist and the APN lecture locally and nationally and are recognized as experts in the field of continence care.

Urogynecology Continence Practice

Mary Ann Geary, M.S.N., APN-C (Women's Health Nurse Practitioner)

Urogynecology is an optimal model for providing continence services for women. A hospital-owned urogynecology practice at the Atlantic Health System branches in Morristown, New Jersey (Morristown Memorial Hospital) and Summit, New Jersey (Overlook Hospital) combines the expertise of a women's health nurse practitioner and a urogynecologist to treat pelvic organ prolapse, urinary frequency/urgency and incontinence, painful bladder syndrome, pelvic pain, and dyspareunia. The nurse practitioner's role within this practice is to address the medical management of pelvic organ prolapse, urinary frequency/urgency, and incontinence as well as other pelvic floor disorders. This role includes performing pessary fitting, biofeedback-assisted pelvic floor muscle training, bladder instillations, and medication management, as well as teaching behavioral methods such as bladder retraining, urge suppression, fluid management, and elimination of bladder irritants to address lower urinary tract symptoms. Ms. Geary sees new patients in the practice and does urodynamic testing. She also consults in long-term care facilities to address issues related to urinary incontinence through her own private practice, Partners for Continence.

University-Based School of Nursing Continence Practice

Jean Wyman, RN-C, Ph.D.

Minnesota Continence Associates (MCA) is a clinical practice of the University of Minnesota (Minneapolis) School of Nursing that provides comprehensive, coordinated care for adolescents and adults with pelvic health and continence issues. MCA offers many options in developing a nonsurgical treatment plan that is tailored to each patient's needs and preferences. Staffed by three expert and experienced nurse practitioners who are faculty members of the University of Minnesota School of Nursing, MCA provides continence care to patients in their clinic-based practices in the Women's Health Center and the Department of Urology, and at the University of Minnesota Medical Center, Fairview, as well as at various assisted living facilities and nursing homes throughout the Twin Cities metropolitan area. As part of the University of Minnesota physicians group, MCA nurse practitioners are able to work in multidisciplinary teams offering individuals a full spectrum of diagnostic and medical options.

Appendix Box 13.2   Bladder and bowel protocol for long-term care (LTC)

The overall goal is for the continence nurse consultant to assist the LTC staff in

- Assessing the resident's medical, cognitive, and functional status to determine impact on the resident's risk of becoming or remaining incontinent or developing a related bladder problem (e.g., urinary tract infection [UTI])

- Planning and implementing continuous individualized interventions to prevent urinary incontinence (UI) and UTIs and determining medical necessity for indwelling urinary catheters

- Maintaining normal bladder function or achieving restored or improved bladder function in appropriately identified residents

- Recognizing and addressing changes in the individual resident's status that may increase the resident's risk for incontinence or UTI or may signal attainment of the established goal regarding bladder function

- Reassessment of residents who have a change in bladder or bowel function

The continence nurse consultant will

- Evaluate and assess residents with UI and related problems, to include comprehensive medical history, modified physical examination, determination of bladder function, and urinalysis

- Review bladder and bowel records obtained by staff

- Conduct environmental, functional, and mental status evaluations to determine deterrents to continence

- Identify, with staff assistance, daily habits, frequency, and circumstances of bladder or bowel dysfunction

- Establish a diagnosis of the type of incontinence and contributing factors

- Provide assistance to LTC staff by participating in rounds or care plan conferences on identified residents

- Assess bowel function, with implementation of a bowel regimen

- Develop a behavior program to include toileting assistance or prompted voiding

- Develop retraining programs, to include bladder training and pelvic floor muscle training, for appropriately motivated and cognitively intact residents with appropriate biofeedback training, pelvic floor electrical stimulation, or both

- Assess all residents with indwelling urinary catheters for catheter removal and implement a voiding or intermittent catheterization program as needed

- Implement the use of appropriate collection or containment devices (or both) or management strategies for individuals with chronic, long-term UI who cannot be otherwise managed

- Design an ongoing care plan, in partnership with the LTC staff, to implement revisions as needed

Appendix Box 13.3   Steps to Implementing a Continence Program in Long-Term Care

First Step

The keys to success of a bladder and bowel continence program include a commitment by the key decision makers, including the nursing home owner (individual or corporate), administrator, and director of nursing. To meet the implementation goal, a staff education (in-service) program on the bladder and bowel retraining program should be scheduled to include nursing staff on all three shifts. All employees should be expected to participate in the education program. There must be ongoing continuing education to inform and educate new staff as to the techniques and principles of continence management.

Second Step

A meeting is scheduled with the medical director to discuss the bladder and bowel retraining program's assessment techniques, treatment, and management strategies. It is important that the medical director understands the concepts of this program and supports its implementation. A chart order for a bladder and bowel evaluation of a resident should be obtained from the medical director or the resident's family physician by the nursing home nursing staff. If appropriate, a letter explaining the program is sent to the resident's family physician to inform him or her of implementation of the program. Residents with urinary incontinence (UI) and a variety of bladder-related problems are assessed. Appropriate referrals are residents with UI and who have an indwelling urinary catheter (see Chapter 2), including residents who

- Have complaints of urinary frequency, urgency, and "always running to the bathroom"

- Have new onset of episodic UI or have a change in urinary function

- May benefit from a prompted voiding program

- Are using absorbent products, other toileting aids (e.g., bedpans), or intermittent or external catheters

- Have indwelling catheters and need assessment for alternative management and evaluation of catheter-related problems

- Have related problems such as pelvic organ prolapse, fecal incontinence, constipation, and other bowel problems

Third Step

It is the responsibility of the nursing home staff to notify residents and families about initiation of the program, citing goals and benefits of the program. Many residents and families are unaware of federal and state regulations (e.g., Tag F315) that govern the development and implementation of programs for bladder and bowel retraining in nursing homes (see Chapter 2). It is important that residents and families are notified of the program prior to implementation to allow for informed consent. It will definitely be considered an asset, by both the public and regulatory agencies, for a nursing home to have in place an established and organized program for the treatment of incontinence. It is recommended that notification be given to the residents, families, or both in the form of a letter or public announcement. This letter should be part of the facility's admission packet so all newly admitted residents and families are aware of the program. Convening a public meeting or speaking with family members at a scheduled evening gathering to explain the program may be appropriate.

Appendix Box 13.4   Outline of Continence Services

A. Clinical Services

1. Evaluation and assessment of incontinence and pelvic disorders:

    –   Urodynamics: simple, complex, and video

    –   Anal manometry

    –   Pelvic ultrasonography

    –   Cystoscopy

    –   Pudendal nerve motor latency testing

2. Surgical treatments for urinary and fecal incontinence and pelvic organ prolapse.

3. Behavioral and medical interventions:

    –   Behavior modification/lifestyle changes and coping skills to maximize bladder control and related medical problems.

    –   Ensuring long-term transference of skills learned to the patient's daily life.

    –   Bladder retraining.

    –   Pelvic floor muscle rehabilitation to include biofeedback therapy.

    –   Pelvic floor electrical stimulation to increase strength, coordination, and control of bladder and pelvic muscles.

    –   Pessary fitting for women with pelvic organ prolapse.

    –   Management of long-term chronic incontinence that has not been amenable to medical treatments. This may involve working with families and caregivers.

    –   Implementation of the use of appropriate collection and containment devices, catheters, or other products that will include management strategies where appropriate.

B. Research

1. Identify and investigate new and promising alternatives to current therapies.

2. Use current relationship with industry to identify appropriate funding opportunities.

3. Explore other possible funding (e.g., National Institutes of Health, Robert Wood Johnson Foundation) and professional relationships for inclusion in research.

C. Professional Training

1. Educate medical students, residents, and fellows in urology, gynecology, and surgery, and allied health personnel.

2. Provide courses and continuing medical education initiatives both nationally and regionally.

3. Offer fee-based on-site mentoring and clinical training in the evaluation and management of incontinence and pelvic disorders to physicians, nurses, and other allied health personnel.

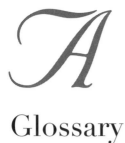

Glossary

Absorbent products Pads and garments, either disposable or reusable, worn to contain urinary incontinence or uncontrolled urine leakage. Absorbent products include shields, guards, undergarment pads, combination pad-and-pant systems, diaper-like garments, and bed pads.

Acetylcholine (Ach) Substance (neurotransmitter) that plays an important part in the transmission of nerve impulses in the nervous system. Ach causes some smooth muscles to contract, including the bladder smooth muscle.

Acontractile detrusor Detrusor muscle that cannot be demonstrated to contract during testing (urodynamic studies).

Activities of daily living Activities necessary to meet essential human needs, such as bathing, grooming, toileting, and social interactions.

Acute incontinence Incontinence that comes on suddenly, usually caused by a new illness or condition, and is often easily reversed with appropriate treatment of the condition that caused it.

Allergic vulvitis Itching (pruritus), irritation, and burning of the vulva with a history consistent with allergen exposure; lack of infectious cause.

Anal fissure A small tear or cut in the skin around the anus that can cause pain, bleeding, or both.

Anal fistula A hollow tract connecting a primary opening inside the anal canal to a secondary opening in the perianal skin.

Anal sphincters Two rings of muscles surrounding the rectum and anus, which help control passage of bowel movements and prevent leakage of stool between bowel movements.

Anorectal Pertaining to the anus and rectum considered together.

Antibiotics Substances that inhibit the growth of or kill microorganisms (bacteria and viruses); used to treat infections.

Anticholinergic drugs A class of drugs that block the effects of acetylcholine, a chemical that causes the bladder to contract. An antimuscarinic drug will facilitate storage of urine in a patient with overactive bladder and involuntary bladder contractions by increasing bladder capacity and decreasing bladder overactivity. Side effects may include dry mouth and constipation.

Anus   Final 2 inches of the rectum, surrounded by the internal anal sphincter and the external sphincter.

Areflexia   Absence of reflexes.

Artificial urinary sphincter   Mechanical device surgically implanted into the patient that consists of a cuff placed around the bulbar urethra or bladder neck, a pressure-regulating balloon, and a pump. The device is used to control opening and closing of the urethra manually, and the procedure is the most commonly used surgical procedure for the treatment of severe male urethral sphincter deficiency.

Atonic or hypotonic bladder   A bladder lacking normal tone or strength, often caused by peripheral neuropathies, such as diabetes mellitus or chronic overdistention from any cause. The bladder is flaccid and overdistended with urine. Overflow incontinence may occur.

Autoimmune   Condition in which the body produces antibodies to its own tissue.

Autologous   Refers to cells, tissues, or even proteins that are reimplanted in the same individual they came from. Often used when describing material for stress urinary incontinence surgery.

Bacteria   Microscopic organisms that can cause infection and are usually treated with antibiotics.

Bacteriuria   Bacteria present in the urine at a sufficient level of colony-forming units (cfu).

Bedside commode   Portable toilet used by individuals who have difficulty ambulating to standard facilities.

Behavioral techniques   Specific interventions designed to alter the relationship between the patient's symptoms and his or her behavior, environment, or both for the treatment of maladaptive urinary voiding patterns. This may be achieved by modification of the behavior or the environment of the patient, or both.

Benign prostatic hyperplasia (BPH)   A benign (noncancerous) common disorder of men older than 50 years; generally characterized by enlargement of the prostate, which may press against the urethra and interfere with the flow of urine. BPH is the most common cause of anatomic bladder outlet obstruction in elderly men.

Biofeedback therapy   Behavioral technique that uses specialized instruments to help individuals learn how to consciously control involuntary (not under conscious control) responses such as muscle contractions. The person receives a visual, auditory, or tactile signal (the feedback) that indicates how well the person's muscles are responding to the commands of his or her nervous system. The signal is derived from a measurable physiological parameter, which is subsequently used in an educational process to accomplish a specific therapeutic result. The signal is displayed in a quantitative way, and the person is taught how to alter it and thus control the physiological process. An example is using electromyography or pressure recordings to teach pelvic floor muscle exercises.

Bladder   Hollow, muscular organ lying in the lower abdomen and pelvis that stores and empties urine. The bladder has only two functions: to expand to allow the storage of urine at low pressure and to contract to enable the expulsion of urine. The term *detrusor* is often used to refer to the smooth muscle of the bladder.

Bladder cancer   Carcinoma originating in the epithelium that lines the bladder. Tumors in the bladder may be benign or cancerous. Bladder cancers account for 2%-6% of all cancers in the United States and are 3 times more prevalent in men than in women. Bladder cancer can spread throughout the body, so early detection is critical. After prostate cancer, bladder cancer is the most common urinary tract cancer.

Bladder catheterization   Procedure in which a catheter is passed through the urethra and into the bladder for the purpose of draining urine and/or to perform diagnostic tests of bladder or urethral function.

Bladder Diary or bladder record   Daily record of bladder habits documenting urination and episodes of incontinence.

Bladder neck   The portion of the bladder where it narrows to join the urethra, like the neck of a funnel.

Bladder reflex arc   The transmission of nerve impulses from stretch receptors in the bladder to the spinal cord and back to the bladder, which causes the bladder to contract.

Bladder training   Behavioral technique that requires the patient to resist or inhibit the sensation of urgency (the strong desire to urinate), to postpone voiding, and to urinate according to a timetable rather than with each urge to void.

Bowel movement   Act of passing feces through the rectum and anus.

Bowels   Another word for "intestines."

Candidiasis   Characteristic patch of erythema (redness) containing macules or papules with satellite lesions, caused by infection with the fungus *Candida*. Frequently associated with itching.

Caregiver burden   The strain or load borne by an individual caring for an older family member or other person with chronic illness or disability. Can develop in either an informal caregiver providing unpaid assistance to a family member or friend who needs help with one or more activities of daily living or in formal caregivers who are paid to provide assistance to a person who needs help with one or more activities of daily living.

Caruncle (urethral caruncle)   Small, red, benign swelling that is visible at the posterior part of the urethral meatus. Occurs chiefly in postmenopausal women and usually causes no symptoms.

Cathartics   Medications that increase the clearing of intestinal contents. Also known as laxatives.

Catheter   Narrow, flexible rubber, latex, or Silastic tube that is passed through the urethra or inserted through the lower abdomen and into the bladder for the purpose of draining urine or performing diagnostic tests of bladder or urethral function.

Catheterization   Techniques for bladder emptying employing the use of a thin tube (catheter) inserted through the urethra or through the anterior abdominal wall into the bladder to drain the bladder.

Cervix   Lower portion of the uterus that connects with the vagina.

Cholinergic   Relating to fibers in the nervous system that release acetylcholine.

Chronic candidal vulvovaginitis   Variable erythema, edema, or thick white discharge of the vulva and vagina, caused by infection with the fungus *Candida*; pruritus is common. Potassium hydroxide microscopy or culture positive.

Clinical practice guidelines   Set of systematically developed statements or recommendations designed to assist the practitioner and patient in making decisions about appropriate health care for specific clinical circumstances. Such guidelines are designed to assist health care practitioners in the prevention, diagnosis, treatment, and management of specific clinical conditions.

Compression device   Device used to put direct pressure on the urethra, causing it to remain closed until the device is removed and the bladder is allowed to drain. Also known as a penile clamp.

Condom catheters   Condom-like device placed over the penis to allow bladder drainage and collection of urine. *See* External (condom) catheters.

Continence   Ability to exercise voluntary control over the urge to urinate (urinary continence) or defecate (fecal continence) until an appropriate time and place can be found.

Continuous urinary incontinence   Leakage of urine without a precipitating factor such as exertion or effort or urgency. Generally associated with a nonfunctional bladder neck and proximal urethra.

Coudé catheter   Curved-tipped catheter that allows for the passage of the catheter beyond certain urethral, prostatic, or bladder neck impediments that may pose problems for a straight catheter.

Credé maneuver   Method of applying direct pressure with one or two hands to the abdomen over the bladder in order to empty or help empty the bladder.

Cystitis   Irritation or inflammation of the bladder, usually caused by an infection.

Cystocele   Intrusion, bulging, or herniation of the bladder into the vagina, usually caused when the pelvic muscles that support the bladder and urethra are stretched or damaged.

Cystometry   Test used to assess the function of the bladder by measuring the pressure or volume as the bladder is slowly being filled. Cystometry is used to assess detrusor activity, sensation, capacity, and compliance. There are different variations of the test depending on the problem being investigated, but regardless of the technique, cystometry involves insertion of a catheter into the bladder.

Cystoscopy   Procedure used to diagnose urinary tract disorders and provide a direct view of the urethra and bladder by inserting a thin, flexible, lighted telescope-like instrument into the bladder through the urethral meatus under anesthesia (local or general); provides visualization of the urethra and bladder for diagnostic or treatment purposes.

Daytime frequency Number of voids recorded during waking hours, including the last void before sleep but excluding the first void after waking and rising in the morning.

Decreased bladder compliance Failure to store urine in the bladder at low pressure caused by the loss of bladder wall elasticity and of bladder accommodation. This condition may result from fibrosis in the bladder wall due to obstruction or a neurological disease or injury, radiation cystitis, or inflammatory bladder conditions such as chemical cystitis. Compliance refers to the change in pressure with respect to the volume contained.

Decubitus ulcer Area of local tissue necrosis (death or damage) that usually develops where soft tissues are compressed between bony prominences and any external surface for prolonged periods.

Defecation Act of having a bowel movement.

Dehydration State that occurs when not enough fluid is present to fulfill the body's fluid needs.

Dementia General loss of short- and long-term memory and mental deterioration. It may affect emotions, abstract thinking, judgment, impulse control, and learning and can cause functional incontinence.

De novo New, as in "de novo (new) symptoms."

Detrusor Used to describe the smooth muscle of the bladder wall.

Detrusor hyperactivity with impaired bladder contractility (DHIC) Condition characterized by involuntary detrusor contractions during bladder filling and urine storage, causing urgency and perhaps urgency incontinence, but unable to empty the bladder completely during voiding because of poor/decreased bladder contractility.

Detrusor overactivity Urodynamic observation characterized by involuntary detrusor contractions during bladder filling, which may be spontaneous or provoked.

Detrusor overactivity incontinence Incontinence caused by an involuntary detrusor contraction.

Detrusor-sphincter dyssynergia (DSD) Inappropriate contraction of the striated muscle surrounding and in the urethra, or both, concurrent with an involuntary contraction of the detrusor. Occasionally voiding may be prevented altogether.

Detrusor underactivity Contraction of reduced strength, duration, or both generally resulting in prolonged bladder emptying, failure to achieve complete bladder emptying within a normal time span, or both.

Diabetic neuropathy Condition in which portions of the nerves have degenerated as a result of diabetes.

Disimpaction   Act of removing stool from the rectum that could not be eliminated normally.

Diuresis   Production of excessive amounts of urine that may precipitate urinary incontinence or overactive bladder. Can be caused by medical problems such as diabetes mellitus and edema.

Diuretic   Agent (e.g., drug, alcohol, caffeine) that increases the excretion of water from the body (referred to as diuresis) by causing the kidneys to produce more urine.

Diverticula   Outpouches in the walls of organs that, if found in the bladder or urethra, can hold excess urine and become infected or inflamed.

Dysuria   Painful or difficult urination.

Eczema   Pruritic (causing itching) dermatitis that occurs as a reaction to a drug or some other skin contact. Characterized in the acute state by an erythema; edema (swelling) associated with serious exudates between the cells of the epidermis; and an inflammatory infiltrate in the dermis, causing oozing, vesiculation, crusting, and scaling of the epidermis.

Electrical stimulation   Application of electric current to stimulate or inhibit the pelvic floor muscles or their nerve supply in order to induce a direct therapeutic response.

Electromyography (EMG)   Diagnostic test used to measure the electrical activity of striated muscles. Can be done with needle electrodes inserted into the muscle or with "patch" electrodes on the skin over the muscle(s).

Enterocele   Prolapse or falling down of the intestines into the vagina.

Enuresis   Involuntary loss of urine during sleep (bed-wetting).

Epididymitis   Inflammation of the epididymis, the structure at the back area of the testicle through which the sperm pass after being produced in the testicle. Generally results in pain, and may be accompanied by dysuria, urinary frequency, and occasional fever.

Episiotomy   Surgical cut made, just before delivery of a baby, into the muscular area between the vagina and anus (perineum) to enlarge the vaginal opening so as to ease childbirth through the vagina.

Erythema   Redness of the top layer of the skin.

Established (chronic) incontinence   Pattern of incontinence that is chronic or longstanding in nature.

Estrogen   Hormone produced primarily by the ovaries. Estrogen is believed to play a major role in maintaining the strength and tone of the pelvic floor and the mucosal surface of the vagina.

Evacuation   Another word for "bowel movement."

External (condom) catheters   Devices made from latex, rubber, polyvinyl chloride, or silicone that are used for externally draining the bladder. They are secured on the shaft of the penis by some form of adhesive and connected to urine collecting bags by a tube. Also called penile sheaths.

External sphincter   Band of striated muscle innervated through the pudendal nerve and found below the internal sphincter. It is under voluntary control and helps to maintain urinary and fecal continence. Location is around the proximal urethra. This is the muscle that a person contracts when given the command to "stop voiding."

Fecal impaction   Large amount of hardened stool in the rectum that an individual is unable to pass. A fecal impaction may present as small amounts of watery and incontinent stool.

Fecal incontinence   Accidental and involuntary loss of liquid or solid stool or gas from the anus.

Feces   Waste material from the intestines. Feces are composed of bacteria, undigested food, and material sloughed from the intestines.

Fistula   Abnormal passage or connection between two organs. Examples are vesicovaginal (bladder and vagina), ureterovaginal (urethra and vagina) and enterovesical (bowel and bladder) fistulae.

Flatulence   Release of gas through the anus.

Fracture pan   Specially designed bedpan for individuals who are unfit to lift their hips to position themselves on the bedpan. A handle allows the caregiver to remove the pan gently, without turning or lifting the user.

Frequency   Voiding more than 8 times in a 24-hour period.

Frequency-volume chart   Records the volumes voided as well as the time of each micturition, day and night, for at least 24 hours.

Gas   Material that results from swallowed air or that is created when bacteria in the colon break down waste material. Gas that is released from the rectum is called flatulence.

Habit training   Behavioral technique that calls for scheduled toileting at regular intervals on a planned basis to prevent incontinence.

Hematuria   Blood in the urine, which may be gross (seen with the naked eye) or miscrosopic (seen under the microscope).

Hesitancy   Difficulty or delay in initiating voiding, resulting in delay in the onset of voiding after the person is ready to pass urine.

Hormone   A substance that stimulates the function of a gland. Hormones circulate in the bloodstream and control the actions of certain cells and organs.

Hydronephrosis   Dilation of the renal pelvis and calices and sometimes the collecting ducts. Hydronephrosis is secondary to obstruction of urine flow by calculi, tumors, neurological disorders, or any of various congenital anomalies.

Hydrophilic-coated catheter   One-time-use tube devices that are coated with a substance that absorbs water and binds it to the device's surface.

Hyperreflexia   Overactivity of reflexes generally as a result of loss of central nervous system control.

Iatrogenic   Due to the action of a health care provider or a prescribed therapy.

Idiopathic   A disease or process occurring without a known cause.

Impaction   Blockage in the rectum composed of a large amount of dried stool that is difficult to evacuate. *See also* Fecal impaction.

Incontinence   Accidental or involuntary loss of urine or feces (stool). A person may have urinary or fecal incontinence or both (sometimes called double incontinence).

Indwelling catheter   Tube device inserted into the bladder to drain the urine continuously. Sometimes called a Foley catheter.

Indwelling urethral catheterization   Process of inserting a tube device into the bladder through the urethra to drain urine continuously.

Inflammatory bowel disease (IBD)   A chronic inflammatory condition of the digestive tract. Ulcerative colitis and Crohn's disease are the most common.

Intermittency   Term used when the individual describes urine flow that stops and starts on one or more occasions during voiding. Also called intermittent stream.

Intermittent (in-and-out) catheterization   The use of catheters inserted through the urethra into the bladder every 3-6 hours for bladder drainage in people with urinary retention. Intermittent catheterization performed by the person at home is called clean intermittent catheterization (CIC).

Internal sphincter   Smooth muscle at the base of the bladder (or rectum) that functions as an involuntary sphincter. In the bladder, this is at the bladder neck and proximal urethra.

Intravenous pyelogram or urogram (IVP or IVU)   Serial radiographs of the urinary tract taken after intravenous injection of radiopaque dye.

Intravesical   Within the bladder.

Intravesical pressure   Pressure within the bladder.

Intrinsic sphincter deficiency (ISD)   Cause of stress urinary incontinence in which the urethral sphincter mechanisms are unable to contract and generate sufficient resistance to prevent urinary leakage, especially during stress maneuvers. ISD may be due to congenital sphincter weakness, such as myelomeningocele or epispadias, or it may be acquired subsequent to prostatectomy, trauma, radiation therapy, or sacral spinal cord injury or disease. Individuals affected by the most severe ISD generally have gravitational incontinence (they leak when they stand up).

Introitus   External vaginal opening.

Irritable bowel syndrome (IBS)   Recurrent abdominal pain and diarrhea (often alternating with constipation); often associated with emotional stress.

Kegel exercises   Exercises named after Dr. Arnold Kegel, a gynecologist who first prescribed a specific set of pelvic floor muscle exercises to women for the treatment of urinary stress incontinence in the 1940s. *See* Pelvic muscle exercises.

Kidney   One of two paired urine-making organs that lie behind the rib cage against the posterior body wall musculature. Their principal function is to filter the blood to separate out waste products, which are combined with excess water to form urine.

Lichen planus   White reticulate lesions often accompanied by vaginal discharge, pruritus, burning, dyspareunia, and bleeding with intercourse; may have erosions, erythema, buccal lesions, or papulosquamous plaques.

Lichen sclerosis   Vulvar thinning, whitening, and wrinkling; agglutination of labia. Pruritus may be severe.

Lower urinary tract   Consists of the bladder, prostate gland (in men), urethra, and urinary sphincters.

Lower urinary tract symptoms (LUTS)   A group of symptoms including 1) incontinence, 2) weak stream, 3) hesitancy, 4) urgency of urination, 5) nocturia, 6) post-void dribbling, and 7) intermittency, or an interrupted urinary stream.

Maceration   Softening of the skin by soaking in fluids; skin appears white and waterlogged.

Meatus   Opening to the urethra.

Micturition   Passing of urine; another term for urination or voiding.

Minimum Data Set (MDS)   Federally mandated screening and assessment form for Medicare- and Medicaid-certified long-term care facilities in the United States. This form is completed for each resident within 14 days of admission to the facility, quarterly, and when there is a significant change in the resident's status. An annual update is also required. The information collected in the MDS is used in planning the care of the individual.

Mixed urinary incontinence   Combination of involuntary leakage associated with urgency and also with stress (e.g., exertion, effort, sneezing, and coughing). The person has both urge and stress urinary incontinence.

Mucosa   Innermost lining of the bladder and gastrointestinal tract; mucous membrane.

Nervous system   Voluntary nervous system and involuntary nervous system, which are composed of the brain, the spinal cord, sensory nerves, which provide messages to the brain from the body, and motor nerves, which provide messages from the brain to various parts of the body, particularly the muscle component.

Neural   Referring to the nerves.

Neurogenic bladder dysfunction   Condition in which there is an abnormality of the nerve supply to and from the lower urinary tract that results in an inability to properly store or empty urine. It is usually caused by neurological conditions, such as diabetes, stroke, or spinal cord injury.

Nighttime frequency   Needing to void one or more times per night between the time the person goes to bed with the intention of sleeping and the time the person wakes with the intention of rising.

Nocturia   Complaint by the individual of being awakened at night one or more times because of the need or urge to urinate.

Nocturnal enuresis   Complaint of loss of urine during sleep. In children it is called bed-wetting.

Nocturnal polyuria   Present when more than one third of the 24-hour output occurs at night (normally the 8 hours while the person is in bed). The nighttime urine output excludes the last void before sleep but includes the first void of the morning.

Obstruction   Blockage.

Overactive bladder   Condition characterized by urgency, with or without urgency incontinence, usually with frequency and nocturia.

Overflow incontinence   Involuntary loss of urine associated with overdistention of the bladder. Overflow incontinence results from urinary retention that causes the capacity of the bladder to be overwhelmed. Continuous or intermittent leakage of a small amount of urine results.

Painful bladder syndrome (bladder pain syndrome)   Complaint of suprapubic pain related to bladder filling, accompanied by other symptoms such as increased daytime and nighttime frequency, in the absence of proven urinary tract infection or other obvious pathology. This term is now generally used in place of "interstitial cystitis."

Palpate/palpation   To feel with the palmar surface of the hands and fingers to delineate organs, masses, and tenderness during a physical examination.

Parasympathetic nerves   A component of the autonomic nervous system. Stimulation of the parasympathetic nervous system that innervates the bladder promotes voiding by stimulating the bladder muscle (detrusor) to contract, causing the urge sensation, and by indirectly relaxing the internal urethral sphincter, which allows urine to enter the urethra. Stimulation of the parasympathetic nervous system that innervates the intestinal tract will increase motility and secretion.

Pelvic diaphragm   The musculature of the pelvic floor.

Pelvic muscle exercises (PMEs)   Repetitive active exercise of the pelvic floor muscles to improve urethral resistance and urinary control. Also called Kegel exercises, pelvic floor muscle exercises, or pelvic floor muscle training.

Pelvic muscles   General term referring to the muscles of the pelvic diaphragm and urogenital diaphragm as one unit. These muscles form a "hammock" slung from the front of the pelvis to the back. They support the organs of the pelvis: the bladder, uterus, and rectum. Also referred to as pelvic floor muscles.

Pelvis   Ring of bones at the lower end of the trunk in which the pelvic organs lie.

Perineum (perineal body)   Area between the vagina and anus in women and between the scrotum and anus in men.

Pessary   Device for women that is placed in the vagina (intravaginal) to treat prolapse of pelvic organs by supporting or lifting these organs.

Pharmacological treatment   Treatment by the use of medications.

Phimosis   When the orifice of the foreskin is constricted, preventing retraction of the foreskin over the glans of the penis.

Polyuria   Increase in the volume of urine excreted on a daily basis (usually > 2.8 L in 24 hours). Can be a result of uncontrolled diabetes mellitus or the administration of a diuretic.

Postmicturition dribble   Involuntary loss of urine after a person has finished voiding.

Postvoid residual (PVR) volume   Amount of fluid remaining in the bladder immediately following the completion of urination. Estimation of PVR volume can sometimes be made by abdominal palpation and percussion or bimanual examination. Specific measurement of PVR volume can be accomplished by catheterization, pelvic ultrasound, radiography, or radioisotope studies. Ultrasound is commonly used and is noninvasive.

Pressure sore   Lesion resulting from prolonged pressure and involving loss of integrity of skin or damage to underlying tissue. *See also* Decubitus ulcer.

Prevalence   Number of cases of a disease existing in a population at a given time.

Prolapse   To slide forward or downward, usually referring to the pelvic organs herniating into an adjacent structure, such as the prolapse of the bladder, uterus, or rectum through the vagina. Prolapses are staged, using objective criteria, by the severity of the maximum protrusion of the prolapse during examination.

Prompted voiding   Behavioral technique for use primarily with dependent people or those with cognitive impairment. Prompted voiding attempts to teach the incontinent person to be aware of his or her incontinence status and to request toileting assistance, either independently or after being prompted by a caregiver.

Prostate   Walnut-shaped gland in men that surrounds the urethra between the base of the bladder and the pelvic floor.

Prostatitis   Irritation or inflammation of the prostate. May or may not be associated with a bacterial infection.

Proximal urethra   Portion of the urethra closest to the bladder.

Pubic symphysis   The center front portion of the pelvic bone.

Pubococcygeus muscle   Another name for the levator ani muscle, one of the pelvic muscles that holds the pelvic organs in place.

Pudendal canal syndrome   Unilateral genital pain, often increased with sitting.

Pudendal nerve   Main nerve that innervates all of the muscles of the pelvic floor, including the external urinary sphincter. The pudendal nerve originates from spinal nerves S_2–S_4 (the sacral micturition center) and causes the external urinary sphincter to contract, aiding urinary continence.

Pyuria   White blood or "pus" cells present in the urine, which is a hallmark of an inflammatory response.

Rectocele   Bulging of the rectum into the space normally occupied by the vagina, suggesting weakness of the pelvic floor.

Rectum   Last segment of the colon, or large intestine; the lowest part of the bowel, found right before the anus.

Reflux   Backward flow, as in reflux from the bladder through the ureters, vesico-uretero reflux.

Rehab urinals   Portable receptacles for collecting urine, usually made of plastic or metal, that are specifically designed to aid individuals who have decreased dexterity or functional ability.

Resident Assessment Protocol (RAP)   Part of the Minimum Data Set that assists the nurse to assess the cause of various disruptions or conditions. The RAP provides a systematic method of assessment and is used in the development of the care plan for the individual residing in a nursing home.

Residual urine   Urine retained in the bladder after voiding as a result of incomplete emptying. Also, known as postvoid residual or "PVR."

Restraints   Medications or devices (e.g., belts, straps, jackets, and chairs) used to immobilize a person.

Retracted penis   Penis with a penile shaft of decreased length. The penis retracts into the pelvic area and can resemble an uncircumcised penis.

Risk factor   Quality that makes a person more susceptible to a specific disease.

Scheduled toileting   Assistance to toilet or use of a bedpan or urinal offered on a fixed schedule, for example, every 2–4 hours.

Scrotal abscess   Bacterial infection of the scrotum, causing a localized collection of pus, swelling, and pain.

Sepsis   Presence of bacterial or viral organisms in the blood. Sepsis in the genitourinary tract is referred to as urosepsis.

Skin sealant   Compound that provides a clear copolymer layer to the skin that assists in removal of adhesive on the skin.

Sphincter   Muscular structure that opens and closes.

Stenosis   Narrowing; decrease in diameter.

Straining to void   Muscular effort used to initiate, maintain, or improve the urinary stream.

Stress maneuvers   Activities that increase pressure in the bladder, such as coughing and laughing. They are used as a diagnostic test to check for stress urinary incontinence.

Stress urinary incontinence   Involuntary loss of urine from the urethra as a result of effort or physical exertion (e.g., during coughing and laughing).

Stricture   Narrowing usually caused by scarring; decrease in diameter (e.g., urethral stricture).

Suppositories   Medications adapted for introduction into the rectum, vagina, or urethra. Suppository bases are solid at room temperature but melt or dissolve at body temperature.

Suprapubic   Above the pubic bone.

Suprapubic catheterization   A surgical procedure involving insertion of a tube or similar instrument through the anterior abdominal wall above the symphysis pubis into the bladder to permit urine drainage from the bladder.

Sympathetic nerves   "Fight or flight" component of the autonomic nervous system. They originate in the thoracic and lumbar region of the spinal cord. Stimulation of the sympathetic nervous system that innervates the bladder is thought to promote bladder filling by relaxing the bladder (detrusor) muscle and contracting the internal proximal portion of the urethral sphincter to prevent urine from entering the urethra. Stimulation of sympathetic fibers that innervate the intestine will cause reduced motility and reduced secretions.

Tenesmus   An urgent need to have a bowel movement.

Topical   Application of a medication (e.g., cream, ointment) to a specific site or location, usually on the skin or external mucosa.

Transient (acute) urinary incontinence   Temporary episodes of urinary incontinence that are generally reversible once the cause or causes of the episodes are identified and treated. An example would be transient incontinence due to a severe bladder infection causing severe urgency.

Trigone   Triangle-shaped area on the posterior surface of the bladder between the bladder neck and the two ureteral orifices. The trigone is a very sensitive area of the bladder muscle because of its high concentration of nerves.

Ureters   Two very thin muscular tubes about 8 or 9 inches long that transport urine from the kidneys to the bladder.

Urethra   Narrow tube through which urine flows from the bladder to the outside of the body; the external opening of the urethra is at the end of the penis in men and just above the vaginal opening in women.

Urethral dilation   Procedure in which a blunt metal instrument, called a dilator, is passed through the urethra for the purpose of opening scar tissue (i.e., stricture).

Urethral incompetence   A failure of the urethral sphincter (closure) mechanism that allows for urine leakage.

Urethral obstruction   Blockage of the urethra causing difficulty with urination, usually caused by a stricture or, in men, by an enlarged prostate.

Urethral pressure profilometry (UPP)   Test used to measure pressures in the urethra.

Urethral sphincter mechanism   Segment of the proximal urethra that influences storage and emptying of urine in the bladder. It aids bladder voiding by relaxing, which opens the outlet from the bladder, allowing urine to flow from the bladder to the outside of the body. A deficiency of the urethral sphincter mechanism may allow leakage of urine in the absence of a detrusor contraction. *See* Intrinsic sphincter deficiency.

Urethral stricture   Narrowing of the urethra.

Urethrocele   Prolapse or herniation of the urethra into the vaginal wall.

Urge   Sensation from the bladder producing the desire to void.

Urge incontinence or urgency incontinence   Involuntary and accidental loss of urine when the person is aware of the need to get to the bathroom but is not able to hold the urine long enough to get there. Usually, it is accompanied by or immediately preceded by urgency.

Urgency   Strong, intense, and often sudden desire to void that is difficult to postpone. Urgency, with or without urgency incontinence and usually with frequency and nocturia, can be described as overactive bladder syndrome, urge syndrome, or urgency-frequency syndrome.

Urinalysis   Chemical or microscopic analysis of the urine.

Urinary incontinence (UI)   Involuntary or accidental loss (leakage) of urine.

Urinary meatus   External opening of the urethra.

Urinary retention   Inability to empty urine from the bladder, which can be caused by atonic bladder or obstruction of the urethra.

Urinary system   Part of the body (kidneys, ureters, bladder, and urethra) that produces, stores, and eliminates urine.

Urinary tract   Refers to the entire urine passageway from the pelvis of the kidney to the urinary orifice through the ureters, bladder, and urethra.

Urinary tract infection (UTI)   Infection in the urinary tract caused by the invasion of disease-causing microorganisms that proceed to establish themselves, multiply, and produce various symptoms in their host. UTI in women is known as cystitis. In men, infection is usually associated with obstruction to the flow of urine, such as prostate gland enlargement.

Urinate   To void or to pass urine.

Urination   Act of passing urine.

Urine   Liquid waste products filtered from the blood and combined with excess water by the kidneys; usually has an amber color. Average amount of urine excreted in 24 hours is 40–60 ounces (1,200–1,800 mL).

Urine culture   Test to determine whether bacteria are present in the urine. It is generally performed by placing a drop of urine on a culture plate containing agar, a jelly-like substance full of nutrients that promote the growth and multiplication of bacteria. If there are bacteria in the urine, they will start to grow and form colonies on the agar and, within a few days, they will be visible to the naked eye. The type of bacteria can be determined by the color and appearance of the colonies. The number of bacteria are determined by estimating the number of colonies per milliliter.

Urodynamic tests   Tests designed to measure the function of the bladder and the urethra during bladder filling and storage, and during emptying. *See* Cystometry, Electromyography, Urethral pressure profilometry, and Uroflowmetry.

Uroflowmetry   Urodynamic test that measures urine flow either visually, electronically, or with the use of a disposable flowmeter unit.

Urosepsis Infection of the urinary tract that causes bacteria to enter the bloodstream, generally causing fever, drop in blood pressure, increased heart rate, and dysfunction of various vital organs.

Uterine prolapse Dropping of the uterus from its normal position, with the cervix closer to or protruding outside the vagina.

Vagina Collapsible cylinder of smooth muscle with its opening located between the urethral orifice and the anal sphincter of women and its origin at the cervix. Also known as the birth canal.

Vaginismus Pelvic floor muscle spasm present at and accentuated by examination.

Valsalva maneuver Action of closing the airways and straining down on the abdominal muscles (such as when straining to have a bowel movement).

Void Another word for "urinate."

Voiding or Bladder Diary (bladder record) Record maintained by the individual or caregiver that is used to record the frequency, timing, amount of voiding, and/or other factors associated with the patient's urinary incontinence.

Voiding reflex Reflex in which the bladder indicates to the brain that it is full of urine, and the brain signals the bladder to contract and empty.

Vulvar atrophy Pale, thinning mucosa in the vulvar area of the vagina, possible tears or petechiae. White blood cells and parabasal cells are present in vaginal discharge.

Vulvar intraepithelial neoplasia White or multicolored, elevated lesions, possibly warty. Patient may be asymptomatic or have pruritus.

Warning time The time from the first sensation of urgency to the time of voiding or incontinence.

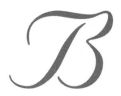

Resources

MANUFACTURERS OF DRUGS AND PRODUCTS

This is a list of the major manufacturers of products and devices for urinary incontinence (UI) management. Included are their Internet Web site and toll-free customer service line. Most of these products are mentioned throughout the book. These manufacturers have additional educational material on UI and their products.

3M Health Care
3M Center, Building 275 4W 02
St. Paul, MN 55144-1000
(888) 364-3577
http://www.3M.com/healthcare/
Skin care and perineal cleanser products: Cavilon no-sting barrier film; Cavilon One-Step Skin Care Lotion and Skin Cleanser; Emollient Cream; Moisturizing, Durable Barrier Cream; No Sting Barrier Film

A+ Medical Products, Inc.
442 Mitchell Hollow Road
Windham, NY 12496
(888) 843-3334
http://www.aplusmedical.com/
Female catheter guide, urinal

AdaMed
3101 Gaylord Parkway
Frisco, TX 75034
(866) 871-9654
http://www.colpexin.com/
Intravaginal device (Colpexin Sphere)

AdaMed
5385 Five Forks Trickum Road, Suite 200K
Stone Mountain, GA 30087
(866) 306-5263
http://www.adamedinc.com/
Bedside commodes, raised toilet seats, and other bathroom products

Allergan Medical Affairs
2525 Dupont Drive
Irvine, CA 92612
(800) 433-8871
http://www.botox.com/
http://www.sancturaxr.com/
Manufacturer of Botox botulinum toxin type A and Sanctura (trospium chloride)

AlphaDry Medical LLC
1211 Edgewater NW, Suite 2
Salem, OR 97304
(877) 235-9379
http://www.alphadry.com/
Reusable external collection system

American Biffy Company
674 Wells Road
Boulder City, NV 89005
(877) 422-4339
http://www.biffy.com/
Bidet attachment that can be
mounted on toilet, providing
complete perineal care

American Medical Systems
10700 Bren Road West
Minnetonka, MN 55343
(800) 328-3881
http://www.americanmedical
systems.com/
Artificial urinary sphincters,
AdVance male sling, midurethral
slings for women

Arcus Medical, LLC
900 Tulip Drive, Suite B
Gastonia, NC 28052
(877) 272-8763
http://www.arcusmedical.com/
Afex incontinence management
system, urinary collection bags,
underpads

Astellas Pharma US, Inc.
Three Parkway North
Deerfield, IL 60015-02537
(800) 888-7704
http://www.us.astellas.com/
Overactive bladder drug VESIcare
(solifenacin succinate) and benign
prostatic hypertrophy alpha blocker
Flomax (tamsulosin)

Astra Tech, Inc.
21535 Hawthorne Boulevard, Suite 525
Torrance, CA 90503
(877) 456-3742
http://www.astratechusa.com/

Manufactures LoFric Primo, a
hydrophilic urinary catheter, and
other catheter products

**A-T Surgical Manufacturing Co.,
Inc.**
115 Clemente Street
Holyoke, MA 01040
(800) 225-2023
http://www.a-tsurgical.com/
Reusable pads, catheter straps, and
holders

Augusta Medical Systems
1025 Broad Street
Augusta, GA 30903
(800) 827-8382
http://www.augustams.com/
New products for the treatment of
mildly incontinent to fully
incontinent individuals

Aventis Pharmaceuticals
399 Interpace Parkway
Parsippany, NJ 07054
(800) 207-8049
http://www.aventispharma-us.com/
Nasal spray/tablets for nocturnal
enuresis

Bard Medical Division
C.R. Bard, Inc.
8195 Industrial Blvd
Covington, GA 30014
(800) 526-4455
http://www.bardmedical.com/
products/urology.aspx
Large variety of indwelling, intermittent, and external catheter and
drainage bag products; also carries
skin care and perineal cleanser
products called "Special Care" and
periurethral bulking agent (Contigen)

Bedwetting Store
17737 New Hampshire Avenue
Ashton, MD 20861
(800) 214-9605
http://www.bedwettingstore.com/
Bedwetting items and waterproof
bedding

BioDerm, Inc.
12320 73rd Court, North
Largo, FL 33773
(800) 373-7006
http://www.libertypouch.us/
External collection system (Liberty
Pouch)

Bioteque America, Inc.
3631 Yale Way
Fremont, CA 94538
(800) 889-9008
http://www.bioteque.com/
Large selection of vaginal pessaries

Boston Scientific Corporation
One Boston Scientific Place
Natick, MA 01760-1537
(888) 272-1001
http://www.bostonscientific.com/
Midurethral sling material and
Coaptite injectable implant

Calmoseptine, Inc.
16602 Burke Lane
Huntington Beach, CA 92647
(800) 800-3405
http://www.calmoseptine
ointment.com/
Skin care ointment (Calmoseptine
Ointment)

Carbon Medical Technologies, Inc.
1290 Hammond Road
St. Paul, MN 55110-5867
(888) 207-0262

info@carbonmed.com
Injectible periurethral bulking agent
(Durasphere)

Care-Tech® Laboratories, Inc.
3224 South Kingshighway Boulevard
St. Louis, MO 63139
(800) 325-9681
http://www.caretechlabs.com/
Skin care and perineal cleanser
products (Barri-Care)

Carrington Laboratories, Inc.
2001 Walnut Hill Lane
Irving, TX 75038
(800) 358-5205
http://www.carringtonlabs.com/
Skin care, perineal cleanser, and
deodorizer products (Carrington)

Chester Labs, Inc.
1900 Section Road, Suite A
Cincinnati, OH 45237
(800) 354-9709
http://www.chester-labs.com/
Skin care products, perineal
cleansers, and odor eliminators
(April Fresh)

Coloplast Corporation (now home
to Mentor Urology)
200 South 6th Street, Suite 900
Minneapolis, MN 55402
(800) 525-8161
http://www.coloplast.com/
Large variety of indwelling,
intermittent, and external catheters
(including the McGuire reusable
external catheter/urinal) and
drainage bags (Conveen), pessary
product line and skin care and
perineal cleanser products (Sween
Cream, Xtra-Care Lotion, Critic Aid

Clear Moisture Barrier) and other products (Baza Clear Moisture Barrier Ointment and Protect Cream)

Convatec
100 Headquarters Park Drive
Skillman, NJ
(800) 422-8811
http://www.convatec.com/
Skin care and perineal cleanser products (Sensi-Care Perineal/Skin Cleanser, Aloe Vesta skin care products, 2-n-1 Body Wash & Shampoo, Bathing Cloths, 3-n-1 Cleansing Foam); Flexi-strap anchor, Flexi-Seal fecal incontinence management system

Cook Urological Inc.
1100 West Morgan Street
P.O. Box 227
Spencer, IN 47460
(800) 457-4448
http://www.cookurological.com/
Urodynamic catheters, inflatable penile compression device, external catheters

Cook Wound/Ostomy/Continence
1100 West Morgan Street
Spencer, IN 47460
(800) 454-5400
http://www.cookwoc.com/
Penile compression device (penile clamp), pessaries, and catheters

CooperSurgical
95 Corporate Drive
Trumbull, CT 06611
(800) 621-1278
http://www.milexproducts.com/
Large selection of vaginal pessaries (Milex)

Cure Medical
2113 Seville Ave.
Newport Beach, CA 92661
(800) 570-1778
http://www.curemedical.com
Intermittent catheters that are latex and DEHP free and have smooth, polished eyelets

Dale Medical Products, Inc.
P.O. Box 1556
7 Cross Street
Plainville, MA 02762-0556
(800) 343-3980
http://www.dalemed.com/
Anchor straps for catheters (leg and abdominal)

DesChutes Medical Products, Inc.
1011 SW Emkay Drive, Suite 104
Bend, OR 97702
(800) 383-2588
http://www.deschutesmed.com/
Pelvic muscle strengthening device (Myself)

Dumex Medical
825 Franklin Court, Unit G
Marrietta, GA 30067
(877) 796-8637
http://www.woundcaredirect.com/
Skin care and perineal cleanser and deodorizer products (PrimaDerm); reusable absorbent pads and products

E.K. Johnson
4869 "G" Street
Springfield, OR 97478
(541) 746-6126
Spill-proof Rehab Urinal

Empi, Inc.
599 Cardigan Rd

St. Paul, MN 55126-4099
(800) 328-2536
http://www.empi.com/
Portable pelvic floor muscle exerciser and electrical stimulators for home use (Minnova, Innova, InnoSense)

Ethicon Women's Health & Urology (Gynecare)
Route 22 West
Somerville, NJ 08876
(888) 493-2673
http://www.gynecare.com/
Material for midurethral sling

Fembrace, Inc.
P.O. Box 951
Honsey, NY 10952
(877) 535-6800
http://www.fembrace.com/
V-Brace product for pelvic organ prolapse

First Quality Products, Inc.
80 Cuttermill Rd, Suite 500
Great Neck, NY 11021
(800) 227-3551
http://www.firstquality.com/
Disposable absorbent incontinence products (Prevail)

GOJO Industries Inc.
P.O. Box 991
Akron, OH 44309-0991
(800) 321-9647
http://www.GOJO.com/
Skin care and perineal cleanser products (Provon)

Greenwald Surgical Co., Inc.
2688 DeKalb Street
Lake Station, IN 46405
(888) 962-1829
http://www.greenwaldsurgical.com/
Cunningham and Baumrucker penile clamp

GT Urological, LLC
1313 5th Street Southeast
Minneapolis, MN 55414
(877) 488-4379
http://www.gturological.com/
Disposable pouch for male stress UI

Gyrus/ACMI
300 Stillwater Ave
Stamford, CT 06902
(800) 852-9361
http://www.circoncorp.com/
Urodynamic UI evaluation system and biofeedback system

Healthpoint
3909 Hulen Street
Fort Worth, TX 76107
(800) 441-8227
http://www.healthpoint.com/
Skin care and perineal cleanser and deodorizer products (Proshield, Proshield Foam & Spray Incontinent & Total Body Cleanser, Proshield Plus Skin Protectant)

Hollister, Inc.
2000 Hollister Drive
Libertyville, IL 60048
(888) 740-8999
http://www.hollister.com/
Wide variety of external male catheters and pouches (e.g., for retracted penis), external female pouches, intermittent catheters, catheter drainage bags, odor eliminator products, and skin care (Restore) and perineal cleansers products; electromyography/ biofeedback equipment

Humanicare International, Inc.
9 Elkins Road
North Brunswick, NJ 08816
(888) 232-7000
http://www.humanicare.com/
Disposable and reusable absorbent
products (Dignity)

Hygienics Industries
3968 194th Trail
Miami, FL 33160
(800) 498-7051
http://www.hygienics.com/
Reusable absorbent products
(Safe & Dry)

Incontinent Control Devices
2727 Bens Branch Drive #1302
Kingwood, TX 77339
(281) 360-4638
http://www.procon2.com/
Rectal catheter with inflatable cuff
used for fecal incontinence

J.T. Posey Company
5635 Peck Road
Arcadia, CA 91006-0020
(800) 447-6739
http://www.posey.com/
Reusable catheter supplies, catheter
tube holder and drainage bag straps,
sheath holder for external catheter,
and urine drainage bag holder/
cover

Kendall Company
Tyco Healthcare
15 Hampshire Street
Mansfield, MA 02048
(800) 962-9888
http://www.kendallhq.com/
Indwelling catheter (Curity) and
external collection bags, skin care
products (Vaseline)

Kendall Confab Retail Group
601 Allendale Road
King of Prussia, PA 19406
(610) 265-5000
http://www.confab.com/
Disposable absorbent products

Kimberly Clark Corporation
Adult Care Division
P.O. Box 2020
Neenah, WI 54956-9002
(888) 525-8388
http://www.depend.com/
http://www.poise.com/
Retail supplier of absorbent products
(Depend); first to introduce
protective underwear and
pantiliners for incontinence

Laborie Medical
400 Avenue D, Suite 10
Williston, VT 05495-7828
(800) 522-6743
http://www.laborie.com/
Catheter straps, home wetness
monitor, and complex urodynamic
and biofeedback equipment

Lantiseptic
P.O. Box 7329
Marietta, GA 30065
(800) 241-6996
http://www.lantiseptic.com/
Skin protection products

Life-Tech, Inc.
4235 Greenbriar Drive
Stafford, TX 77477-3995
(800) 231-9841
http://www.life-tech.com/
Urodynamics equipment

Maddak, Inc.
661 Route 23 South
Wayne, NJ 07470

(973) 628-7600
http://www.maddak.com/
Bathroom toileting aids

M.C. Johnson Co., Inc.
Suite 201
8801 Business Park Drive
Ft. Myers, FL 33912-6007
(800) 553-8483
http://www.mcjohnson.com
Cath-Secure catheter holder

MedGyn Products, Inc.
328 North Eisenhower Lane
Lombard, IL 60148
(800) 451-9667
http://medgyn.com/pessaries.htm
Distributors of pessary devices

Medical Technologies of Georgia
15151 Prater Drive
Covington, GA 30014
(888) 511-4239
www.medtechga.com
Distributors of closed system
intermittent catheters

Mediwatch
1501 Northpoint Parkway, Suite 103
West Palm Beach, FL 33407
(888) 471-2611
http://mediwatch.com
Manufacturer of urodynamic
equipment and portable ultrasound
equipment

Medline Industries, Inc.
One Medline Place
Mundelein, IL 60060
(800) MEDLINE
http://www.medline.com/
Indwelling and intermittent
catheters, drainage bags, disposable
absorbent products, skin creams
and cleansers (Aloetouch Premium
Cleansing Cloths, ReadyBath cleans-
ing systems, Sooth & Cool No-Rinse
Perineal Wash w/Aloe and Moistur-
izing Lotion, Remedy Calazime
Protectant Paste, Dimethicone
Moisture Barrier, Skin Repair Cream,
Soothe & Cool Moisture Barrier
Ointment, Zinc Oxide Barrier)

Medtronic Corp
710 Medtronic Parkway
Minneapolis, MN 55432-5604
(800) 328-0810
http://www.interstim.com/
Implantable electrical stimulator
(Interstim)

Nature Plus, Inc.
555 Lordship Boulevard
Stratford, CT 06615
(203) 380-0316
http://www.nature-plus.com/
Odor eliminator

Neotonus
30 South Park Square, Suite 201
Marietta, GA 30060-8613
(800) 895-4298
http://www.neotonus.com/
Noninvasive and painless treatment
for UI, pelvic pain, and other
conditions (NeoControl)

Neurodyne Medical Corp
52 New Street
Cambridge, MA 02138
(800) 963-8633
http://www.neumed.com/
Electromyography/biofeedback
equipment

**Novartis Pharmaceuticals
Corporation**
One Health Plaza
East Hanover, NJ 07936
(888) 669-6682
http://www.enablex.com/

In partnership with Procter & Gamble, distributes overactive bladder drug Enablex (darifenacin)

Opticon Medical
7001 Post Road, Suite 100
Dublin, OH 43016
(614) 336-2000
http://www.opticonmedical.com/
OPTICON-*vf* urethral insert

Ortho Women's Health and Urology
OrthoUrology
1000 Route 202, Box 300
Raritan, NJ 08869
(800) 526-7736
http://www.ortho-mcneil
pharmaceutical.com/
http://www.ditropanxl.com/
http://www.orthoelmiron.com/
Ditropan XL (oxybutynin chloride) drug treatment for overactive bladder; Elmiron (pentosan polysulfate sodium) for interstitial cystitis and painful bladder syndrome

Paper-Pak Products, Inc.
1029 Old Creek Road
Greenville, NC
(800) 428-8363
http://www.attends.com/
Disposable absorbent incontinence products (Attends)

Pfizer Corporation
235 East 42nd Street
New York, NY 10017
(866) 776-3700
http://www.detrolla.com/
Detrol (tolterodine tartrate) for overactive bladder; Vagifem (estradiol hemihydrate) vaginal tablets for atrophic vaginitis

Preferred Medical Devices, Inc.
6400 Congress Avenue, Suite #1700
Boca Raton, FL 33487
(866) 381-4134
http://www.urassist.com/
UrAssist collection system

Principle Business Enterprises
P.O. Box 129
Dunbridge, OH 43414-0129
(800) 467-3224
http://www.tranquilityproducts.com/
Disposable absorbent products (Tranquility)

Prometheus Group
1 Washington Street, Suite 303
Dover, NH 03820
(800) 442-2325
http://www.theprogrp.com/
Manufacturers of the Pathway CTS 2000 Pelvic Muscle Rehabilitation System, which has electromyography, biofeedback, and stimulation

Rochester Medical Corporation
One Rochester Medical Drive
Stewartville, MN 55976
(800) 243-3315
http://www.rocm.com/
Specially coated intermittent catheters, indwelling and external catheters, antibacterial catheters, and FemSoft urethral insert

Rusch, Inc.
(866) 246-6990
http://www.teleflexmedical.com/
http://www.originalbellybag.com/
Indwelling and intermittent catheters, collection bags, pessary, Cunningham penile clamp, abdominal leg bag for indwelling or suprapubic catheters (Belly Bag)

Salk, Inc.
320 Washington St.
Brookline, MA 02445
(800) 343-4497
http://www.healthdri.com/
Reusable absorbent products

SCA Personal Care
2929 Arch Street
Suite 600
Philadelphia, PA 19104
(800) 992-9939
http://www.tena.com/
Disposable absorbent products
(Tena, Serenity) and skin cleansers
(TENA Wash Cream and Wash
Cloths)

Smith & Nephew, Inc.
11775 Starkey Road
Largo, FL 33779
(800) 876-1261
http://www.securacare.com/
http:///www.snwmd.com/
Skin care products (Triple Care),
including cream and perineal
cleansers, protectants, and
moisturizers (Secura)

SRS Medical Corp.
8672 154th Avenue, NE
Redmond, WA 98052
(800) 345-5642
http://www.srsmedical.com/
Uodynamics, biofeedback, vaginal
cones, and penile clamp

Standard Textile Company
1 Knollcrest Drive
P.O. Box 371805
Cincinnati, OH 45222-1805
(800) 999-0400
http://www.standardtextile.com/
Reusable absorbent products

Summitt Industries
P.O. Box 7329
Marrietta, GA 30065
(800) 241-6996
http://www.lantiseptic.net/
Skin care products (Lantiseptic)

Sunrise Medical, Inc.
7477 East Dry Creek Parkway
Longmont, CO 80503
(800) 333-4000
http://www.sunrisemedical.com/
Raised toilet seats

Swiss-American Products, Inc.
4641 Nall Road
Dallas, TX 75244
(800) 633-8872
http://www.elta.net/
Skin care products (Elta Lite
Moisturizer)

T-DOC Company, LLC
5 Edgemoor Road, Suite 212
Wilmington, DE 19809
(800) 520-8362
www.tdocllc.com
Manufacturer of air-charged
urodynamic catheters

Thought Technology Ltd.
2180 Belgrave Ave
Montreal, QC, Canada
(800) 361-3651
http://www.thoughttechnology.com/
Electromyography/biofeedback
equipment, neuromuscular
stimulators

Timm Medical Technologies
6585 City West Parkway
Eden Prairie, MN 55344
(800) 438-8592
http://www.timmmedical.com/
Penile compression device, vaginal
weights

TransAqua
1860 South York Road
Gastonia, NC 28031
(800) 769-1899
http://www.trans-aqua.com/
Reusable absorbent products
(HealthDri)

TYCO Healthcare Kendall
15 Hampshire Street
Mansfield, MA 02048
(800) 962-9888
http://www.kendallhq.com/
http://www.tycohealthcare.com/
Urine collection systems;
incontinence absorbent products,
including WINGS brand

Urocare Products, Inc.
2735 Melbourne Ave
Pomona, CA 91767
(800) 423-4441
http://www.urocare.com/
External catheter (reusable latex bag)
and supplies (Uro-Cath and
Uro-Bond IV, a brush-on silicone
adhesive used for securing male
external catheters)

Uro Concepts, Inc.
P.O. Box 6635
Malibu, CA 90264
(310) 457-8350
http://www.betterpant.com
Undergarment for securing catheters

Uroplasty, Inc.
5420 Feltl Road
Minnetonka, MN 55343
(866) 258-2182
http://www.uroplasty.com/
Urgent PC Neuromodulation System
for percutaneous tibial nerve
stimulation (PTNS); Macroplastique
Implants for treatment of stress UI

Utah Medical Products, Inc.
7043 South 300 West
Midvale, UT 84047
(800) 533-4984
http://www.utahmed.com/
Pelvic floor electrical stimulator

Verathon Medical
(formerly Diagnostic Ultrasound)
21222 30th Drive, SE, Suite 120
Bothell, WA 98201
(800) 331-2313
http://www.dxu.com/
Portable ultrasound (BladderScan)

Warner Chilcott Company
Consumer Healthcare
201 Tabor Rd
Morris Plains, NJ 07950
(800) 521-8813
http://www.estrace.com/
Vaginal cream (Estrace)

Watson Pharma, Inc.
360 Mt. Kemble Avenue
P.O. Box 1953
Morristown, NJ 07962
(973) 355-8300
http://www.watsonpharm.com/
Overactive bladder transdermal drug
Oxytrol (oxybutynin)

Westons Internet Home Health
http://www.westons.ws/acatalog/
Westons_Health_Knee_Spreader_
W_ Mirror_17798.html#
Knee spreader with mirror for self-
catheterization

Wyeth-Ayerst Laboratories
Division of Home Products Corp.
P.O. Box 8299
Philadelphia, PA 19101
(800) 934-5556
http://www.premarin.com/
Conjugated equine estrogens
(Premarin oral, patch, vaginal cream)

MEDICAL SUPPLIERS OF INCONTINENCE PRODUCTS

This is a list of medical suppliers that provide direct-to-home distribution of specialty medical supplies, specifically urological supplies. They all have catalogs that can be obtained on request. This list is not all-inclusive but contains sources for products commonly used by clinicians and patients in the treatment of incontinence.

180 Medical
(877) 688-2729
http://www.180Medical.com/

A-Med Health Care
5302 Rancho Road
Huntington Beach, CA 92649
(800) 552-2633
http://www.a-med.com/

Bruce Medical Supply
411 Waverly Oaks Road, Suite 154
Waltham, MA 02452
(800) 225-8446
http://www.brucemedical.com/

Byram Healthcare Centers, Inc.–Home Health Supplies
440 Wheelers Farms Road, Suite 101-A
White Plains, NY 10605
(877) 902-9726
http://www.byramhealthcare.com/

CCS Medical and DS Medical
14255 49th Street North, Suite 301
Clearwater, FL 33762
(800) 726-9811
http://www.ccsmedical.com/
http://www.dsmedical.com/

Edgepark Surgical Inc.
1810 Summit Commerce Park
Twinsburg, OH 44087
(800) 321-0591
http://www.edgepark.com/

HDIS–Home Delivery Incontinent Supplies Co., Inc.
9385 Dielman Industrial Drive
Olivette, MO 63132
(800) 269-4663
http://www.hdis.com/

Liberty Medical
10045 South Federal Highway
Port St. Lucie, FL 34952
(800) 376-1599
http://www.libertymedical.com/

Medline Industries
One Medline Plaza
Mundelein, IL 60060
(800) 633-5463
http://www.medline.com/

Sterling Medical Services
2 Twosome Drive
Moorestown, NJ 08057
(800) 291-8500
http://www.sterlingmedical.com/

UroMed, Inc
1095 Windward Ridge Parkway, Suite 170
Alpharetta, GA 30005
(800) 403-9189
http://www.uromed.com/

RESOURCES

These professional organizations, consumer groups, and Internet sites provide education or information on incontinence, overactive bladder, and related disorders.

Agency for Healthcare Research and Quality (AHRQ)
(Formerly Agency for Health Care Policy and Research)
2101 East Jefferson Street, Suite 501
Rockville, MD 20852
(301) 427-1364
http://www.ahrq.gov/

American College of Obstetricians and Gynecologists (ACOG)
409 12th Street, SW
P.O. Box 96920
Washington, DC 20024
(800) 762-2264
http://www.acog.org/

American Physical Therapy Association (APTA)
Section on Women's Health
111 North Fairfax Street
Alexandria, VA 22314
(800) 999-2782
http://www.APTA.org/

American Urogynecologic Society (AUGS)
2025 M Street, NW, Suite 800
Washington, DC 20036
(202) 367-1167
http://www.augs.org/

American Urological Association (AUA)
1000 Corporate Boulevard
Linthicum, MD 21090
(866) 746-4282
http://www.auanet.org

American Urological Association Foundation
1000 Corporate Boulevard
Linthicum, MD 21090
(866) 746-4282
http://www.auafoundation.org/
http://www.urologyhealth.org/

Association of Women's Health, Obstetric and Neonatal Nurses (AWHONN)
2000 L Street, NW
Suite 740
Washington, DC 20036
(800) 673-8499
http://www.awhonn.org/

Centers for Medicare & Medicaid Services (CMS)
Survey & Certification Group
Division of Nursing Homes
http://www.cms.internetstreaming.com/
Guidance to Surveyors: Urinary Incontinence and Catheters—Tag F 315; webcast from October 2004 entitled "Urinary Incontinence, Volume II," which facilities have found helpful, can still be viewed under "Archived Webcasts."

FDA Office of Women's Health
(888) 463-6332
http://www.fda.gov/womens/pubs.html
Consumer publications on a variety of topics

International Continence Society
(ICS)
19 Portland Square, Bristol
Bristol BS2 8SJ United Kingdom
+44 117 9444881
http://www.icsoffice.org

International Foundation for
Functional Gastrointestinal
Disorders (IFFGD)
P.O. Box 170864
Milwaukee, WI 53217
(888) 964-2001
http://www.iffgd.org/

International Urogynecological
Association (IUGA)
2950 Cleveland Clinic Blvd
Weston, FL 33331
(954) 659-6209
http://www.iuga.org

Interstitial Cystitis Association (ICA)
110 North Washington Street,
Suite 340
Rockville, MD 20850
(800) 435-7422
http://www.ichelp.org

Kestrel Health Information, Inc.
206 Commerce Street
Hinesburg, VT 05461
(802) 482-4000
http://www.kestrelhealthinfo.com/

Krames
780 Township Line Road
Yardley, PA 19067-4200
(800) 333-3032
http://www.krames.com/
Patient education materials

Mayo Clinic Resources
http://www.mayoclinic.com/health/
urinary-incontinence/DS00404/

National Association for
Continence (NAFC)
P.O. Box 1019
Charleston, SC 29402
(800) 252-3337
http://www.nafc.org/

National Institute of Diabetes and
Digestive and Kidney Diseases
(NIDDK)
31 Center Drive, MSC 2560
Bethesda, MD 20892-2560
(301) 496-3583
http://www2.niddk.nih.gov/

National Institute on Aging (NIA)
National Institutes of Health
Building 31, Room 5C27
31 Center Drive, MSC 2292
Bethesda, MD 20892
(301) 496-1752
http://www.niapublications.org/

National Kidney and Urologic
Diseases Information Clearing
House
3 Information Way
Bethesda, MD 20892
(800) 891-5390
http://kidney.niddk.nih.gov/
kudiseases/pubs/uiwomen/index.htm

Simon Foundation for Continence
Box 835-F
Wilmette, IL 60091
(800) 237-4666
http://www.simonfoundation.org/

Society for Urodynamics
and Female Urology (SUFU)
1100 E. Woodfield Rd., Suite 520
Schaumburg, IL 60173
(847) 517-7225
http://www.sufuorg.com

Society of Urologic Nurses and Associates (SUNA)
East Holy Avenue, Box 56
Pitman, NJ 09071
(888) 827-7862
http://www.suna.org/

The Bathroom Diaries
http://www.thebathroomdiaries.com/
Clean restrooms around the world

Twin Rivers Stay-Dri Systems
1 Industrial Park Drive
P.O. Box 347
Livermore, KY 42352
(800) 248-5519
Fax: (270) 278-5202

US TOO! International Prostate Cancer Survivor Support Groups
5003 Fairview Avenue
Downers Grove, IL 60515
(800) 808-7866
http://www.ustoo.org/

Wellness Partners, LLC
237 Old Tilton Rd
Canterbury, NH 03224
(800) 840-9301
http://www.seekwellness.com/
Continence Center for consumers and professionals

Wound, Ostomy and Continence Nurses Society (WOCN)
4700 West Lake Ave
Glenview, IL 60025
(800) 224-9626
http://www.wocn.org/

Index

Page references followed by *f*, *t*, and *b* indicate figure, table, and box, respectively.

Abdomen bags, 440–441, 440*f*
Abdominal examinations, 180*b*, 201
Abdominal leak point pressure (ALPP), 223*t*–224*t*
Absorbent capacity, total, 371
Absorbent incontinence products, 368–377, 368*f*, 370*t*, 371*t*
Accessibility, toilets and, 392
ACE (angiotensin converting enzyme) inhibitors, 91*t*, 94
ACET study, 325
Acetylcholine, 76–78, 77*t*, 78*t*, 307, 312–313; *see also* Antimuscarinic medications
Acid mantle, 381
ACOVE-2 intervention, 29*t*
Acquisition rate, 371
Acupuncture, 20*t*, 299–300
Acute bacterial prostatitis, 19*t*
Acute care hospitals, 43–44, 103–104
Adenomas, 316
Adenosine triphosphate (ATP), 77*t*
Adrenergic receptors, 77
Adult briefs, 374, 375*f*
Advanced Practice Nurses
  advanced practice nurses as, 566–568
  categories of, 576–577
  control programs in LTC facilities and, 41
  educational preparation of, 568–569, 578
  outcomes of services of, 569–570, 582–584
  overview of, 565–566
Afex reusable ECC, 435*f*
Age
  antimuscarinic drugs and, 329–330
  changes in urinary tract and, 81–83
  financial aspects of incontinence and, 45
  misconceptions about, 28*t*
  pelvic floor muscle training and, 290–291
  prevalence and, 14–18, 16*f*
  prevention and, 48
  as risk factor, 108–109
Agency for Healthcare Research and Quality (AHRQ), 5, 175
AI, *see* Anal incontinence
AIDS, neurogenic bladder and, 104

Alcohol, 91*t*, 237
Alfuzosin, 114
Allodynia, 22*t*
Allografts, 529*t*
Allopurinol, 20*t*
Alpha blocker therapy, 20*t*, 114, 332
Alpha-adrenergic receptor agonists, 77, 91*t*, 340
Alpha-adrenergic stimulation, 67
AlphaDry Reservoir, 428, 434–435, 436*f*
ALPP, *see* Abdominal leak point pressure
Alzheimer's disease, 112
American Board of Obstetrics and Gynecology, 5
American Board of Urology, 5
American Medical Directors Association guidelines, 5
American Physical Therapy Association, 7
Amitriptyline, 21*t*
Amplitude, 296
Anal canal, 73–74
Anal (fecal) incontinence (AI), 2, 134–137
Anal plugs, 166
Anal sphincteroplasty, 168
Anal sphincters, 72, 74–76, 110–111, 132*f*, 133, 168
Anal "wink" reflex, 216, 216*f*
Analgesics, 145
Anchoring, 414–415, 415*f*, 416*f*
Angiotensin, 77*t*, 316
Anismus, 138
Anorectal angle, 72, 73*f*, 132*f*
Anorectal examinations, 214–215
Anorectal pathology, 135*t*
ANP, *see* Atrial natriuretic peptide
Antacids, 145
Anthraquinones, 162*t*
Antibiotic-coated catheters, 409–410, 409*f*
Antibiotics, 19*t*, 145, 418–419, 421
Anticholinergic load, 329–330
Anticholinergic medications, *see* Antimuscarinic medications
Antidepressants, 23*t*, 91*t*, 103, 309*b*, 340–342; *see also* Tricyclic antidepressants

Antidiuretic hormones, 81, 237
Antifungal agents, 386
Antimuscarinic Clinical Effectiveness Trial
    (ACET), 325
Antimuscarinic medications
    benign prostatic hyperplasia and, 332–333
    bladder function and, 91t, 92
    bowel dysfunction and, 145
    children and, 333–334
    community-based studies of, 325–326
    comparisons of efficacy and tolerability of,
        324–325
    considerations when selecting, 326–328
    contraindications, side effects of, 334–337
    dementia and, 330–331
    long-term care facilities and, 331–332
    mechanism of action of, 312
    muscarinic receptors and, 312–316, 313t,
        314f, 315f
    neurological diseases and, 333
    overview of, 308–311, 309b
    review of available, 316–324, 317t
    use of in older adults, 329–330
Apex with strain, 494b
Applicator catheters, 430, 431f
Arcus tendineus fasciae pelvis, 70
Arginine vasopressin (AVP), 81
Arthritis, 114
Artificial anal sphincters, 168
Artificial urinary sphincters (AUS), 541–545,
    542f, 543f
Ascorbic acid, 419, 446
Assessment; see also Evaluation
    clinical, 177–182
    cognitive, 182
    environmental barriers and, 180b, 183–185
    functional, 180b, 182–183
    overview of, 175–177, 226f
Association for Continence Advice (ACA), 576
Asymptomatic inflammatory prostatitis, 19t
Atenolol, 91t
Atrial natriuretic peptide (ANP), 114
Atrophic urethritis, 90t, 92–93
Atrophic vaginitis, 205–206, 343
AUS, see Artificial urinary sphincters
Autologous tissue, 529t
Autonomic nervous system, 74–75
AVP, see Arginine vasopressin

Bacteremia, 399
Bacterial infections, 19t, 380t
Bacterial vaginosis, 503–505
Bacteriuria, 93, 217–218, 400–401, 401f, 442,
    446
Balloon expulsion test, 153
Balloon size, 407, 407f
Bathroomdiaries.com, 102

Baumrucker clamps, 465, 466f
Baxter diagnostic tape, 206
BCC, see Bladder Control Clinic
Beck Geriatric Depression Scale Short Form,
    182
Bedding, 377
Bedpans, 391
Bedside bags, 437, 437f, 438
Bee pollen extract, 20t
Beers Criteria, 331
Behavior modification, 245–247, 246f, 247f,
    284–293; see also Pelvic floor muscle
    training (PFMT); Toileting programs
Belly Bags, 415, 440, 440f
Benign prostatic enlargement (BPE), 116b
Benign prostatic hyperplasia (BPH), 17, 68, 83,
    92, 116b, 332–333
Benign prostatic obstruction (BPO), 116b
Beta-adrenergic receptor antagonists, 91t, 314
Bethanechol, 339, 339t
Better Pant, 435f
Bifidobacterium spp., 164
Billing codes, 366, 468
Biofeedback therapy
    equipment for, 277f, 278f, 279f, 280f
    pelvic floor muscle training (PFMT) and,
        21t, 165–166, 276–284, 277f, 278f,
        279f, 280f, 283f, 285f–287f
    vaginal weights and, 293–294, 294f
    vulvodynia and, 22t, 23t
Biofilms, 403, 410
Bioteque, 497, 509–510, 515, 517
Bisacodyl, 162t
Bladder and bowel diaries
    bladder training and, 261–262, 264
    evaluation and, 180b
    overview of, 196–199, 197f, 199f
    physician familiarity with, 5
    placebo effect and, 310
    scheduled voiding and, 252–253
Bladder and bowel records, 189b–190b,
    199–200
Bladder cancer, 405
Bladder Control Clinic (BCC), 579–580
Bladder drill, 261; see also Habit program
Bladder function tests, 191b
Bladder irrigation, 418
Bladder neck sling procedures, 527–530, 528f
Bladder outlet obstruction, 17
Bladder pacemakers, see InterStim Therapy
    System
Bladder retraining, 420–422
Bladder stones, 405, 447
Bladder stretching, 21t
Bladder training (BT), 245–246, 247f,
    249t–250t, 260–264, 275
"Bladder Training—Controlling Urgency and
    Frequency," 261

Bladders; *see also* Neurogenic bladder
  aging and, 83
  chronic incontinence and, 95
  common diagnoses and term definitions and,
    97*t*
  drug therapy for underactivity of, 339, 339*t*
  innervation of, 105*f*
  medications affecting, 91*t*
  nervous system and, 76–77, 76*t*
  neurotransmitters and, 117
  overflow urinary incontinence and, 103
  prolapse of, 189*b*
  self-care and, 236–237, 239–240
  structure and function of, 61–65, 64*f*
  urination cycle and, 79–81
BladderScan, 219*b*, 258–259, 265
Bleach, 442
Blockage, indwelling catheter and, 471
Blockers, 404, 417
Blocking devices, 463–464, 463*f*
Blood pressure, 119
Body-worn products, 368–377, 368*f*, 370*t*, 371*t*
Botulinum toxin (BTX-A) injections, 545–548,
  547*f*
Bovine collagen, 537–538
Bowel Continence Nursing (Norton and
  Chelvanayagam), 129
Bowel Disorders Profiles, 152–153
Bowel irrigation, 167*f*
Bowels
  anatomy and physiology of, 130–133
  constipation (chronic) and, 137–140
  defecation process and, 133–134
  diarrhea and, 142–143
  evaluation of function of, 147–153,
    148*b*–150*b*, 151*f*
  factors contributing to dysfunction of,
    143–147
  fecal (anal) incontinence and, 2, 134–137
  fecal impaction and, 140–142
  relationship of dysfunction of to UI,
    129–130
  stool collection devices and, 166–167, 166*f*,
    167*f*
  treatment of disorders of, 153–168
BPE, *see* Benign prostatic enlargement
BPH, *see* Benign prostatic hyperplasia
BPO, *see* Benign prostatic obstruction
Bradykinin, 77*t*, 316
Brain tumors, 106*t*
Brainstem, 75*f*, 78
Briefs, 368–377, 368*f*, 370*t*, 371*t*
Bristol Stool Form Scale, 147, 150, 151*f*, 153
BTX-A, *see* Botulinum toxin injections
Bulbocavernosus reflex (BCR), 216
Bulk formers, 159
Bulking agents, 535–539, 537*f*
Burch colposuspension, 508, 524, 526–527

Burgio, Kathy, 276
Bypassing, 471

Caffeine, 91*t*, 164, 234*b*, 236–237
"Caffeine Count," 236–237
Calcium channel blockers, 91*t*, 146
Calcium hydroxyapatite, 539
Candida spp., 22*t*, 23*t*
Candidiasis, 379*t*, 381, 381*b*, 382*f*
Candiduria, 402
Capsaicin, 316
CapSure, 463, 463*f*
Captopril, 91*t*
Carbon-coated zirconium beads, 538
Cardiac safety, 335–336
Caregiver burden, 32–33
Cascara sagrada, 162*t*
Catheter bypassing, 471
Catheter valves (CV), 443–444, 443*f*
Catheter-associated urinary tract infection
  (CAUTI); *see also* Bacteriuria
  acute care catheter use and, 397–398
  drainage bag care and, 442
  education and, 419–420
  indwelling urinary catheters and, 393, 399,
    402–403
  intermittent catheterization and, 446–447
Catheterization; *see also* Indwelling urinary
  catheters; Intermittent catheterization
  external catheter collection systems,
    425–437, 427*f*, 429*f*, 430*f*, 431*f*,
    432*f*–434*f*, 435*f*, 436*f*
  overview of, 392–393
  postvoid residual urine and, 218–219, 225*b*
  suprapubic, 422–425, 423*f*
  urinary drainage bags and, 437–442, 437*f*,
    438*f*, 439*f*, 440*f*, 441*f*
  valves and, 443–444, 443*f*
Cath-Secure catheter anchors, 416*f*
CAUTI, *see* Catheter-associated urinary tract
  infection
Centers for Medicare & Medicaid Services
  (CMS), 5, 6, 33–34, 36–37, 175, 328,
  331, 449*b*, 467, 503
Central nervous system, 78*t*
Cerebral cortex, 75*f*
Cerebral palsy, 104, 106*t*
Cerebrovascular accidents (CVA), 101, 106*t*,
  112–113
Certified nurse assistants, 42
Cesarean delivery, 47, 110, 111
CHAMMP tool, 568
Checking, 256
Childbirth
  anal sphincters and, 74, 76, 110–111
  bowel dysfunction and, 145
  pelvic floor muscle training and, 289–290

Childbirth *(continued)*
   pelvic organ prolapse and, 485, 486
   prevention and, 47–48
   as risk factor, 98–99, 100, 109–112
Children, 333–334
Chlamydia spp., 203
Chlorox, 442
Chlorpromazine, 91*t*
Cholinergic receptors, 76
Cholinergic stimulation, 67, 339, 339*t*
Cholinesterase inhibitors, 91*t*, 330–331
Chronic bacterial prostatitis, 19*t*
Chronic incontinence, 85, 95–104
Chronic pelvic pain (CPP), 21*t*, 299
Chronic pelvic pain syndrome (CPPS), 19*t*, 20*t*
CIC, *see* Clean intermittent catheterization
Circadian rhythms, 81–82
CISC, *see* Clean intermittent self-catheterization
Clamps, *see* Penile compression devices;
      Urethral inserts and clamps
Clean intermittent catheterization (CIC), 444,
   445, 446
Clean intermittent self-catheterization (CISC),
   444, 456–457
Clinical assessment, overview of, 177–182,
   178*b*–181*b*
Clock Drawing Test, 182
Clostridium difficile, 142, 419
CMS, *see* Centers for Medicare & Medicaid
      Services
Coagulase-negative staphylococci, 380*t*
Coagulase-positive staphylococci, 380*t*
Coaptation, 525, 527
Coaptite, 539
Coccygeus muscles, 69–70, 71
Cocoa, 236
Co-contraction, 72, 283–284
Cognition, 330
Cognitive assessment, 182, 187*b*
Collagen, 537–538
Collection products, *see* Management and
      collection products
Colon, structure and function of, 130–131,
   131*f*
Colonic inertia, 138
Coloplast, 497, 509, 514, 518
Colpexin Sphere, 506
Colpocleisis, 508
Colpopexy, 507–508
Colporrhaphy, 508
Colposuspension, 508, 524, 526–527
Commodes, 388–389, 389*f*
Comorbidity, 18, 23
Compression, spinal, 107*t*
Congestive heart failure, 90*t*, 94, 114
Constipation
   defined, 130
   DIAPPERS mnemonic and, 94

   medications for treatment of, 159, 160*t*–163*t*,
      164
   pelvic organ prolapse and, 192
   self-care and, 237
   as side effect of medication, 335
   types of, 137–140
Contained incontinence, 181, 247*f*
Containment, as current nursing focus, 7
Contigen, 537–538
Continence centers, 571
Continence champions, 259
Continence nurse advisors (CNA), 566, 576
Continence nurse practitioners (CNP), 566,
   569–570, 577
Contractibility, 281
Conveen SpeediCath, 453
Cook Continence Cuffs, 465, 466*f*
CooperSurgical, 497, 498*f*, 509–518
Corticosteroids, 20*t*, 23*t*
Coudé tips, 406, 406*f*, 449*b*, 451, 452*f*
Cough tests, 220
Coughing, 118, 211, 220, 240; *see also* Stress
     urinary incontinence (SUI)
CPPS, *see* Chronic pelvic pain syndrome
Cranberries, 93–94, 419
Credé maneuver, 240
Credentialing programs, 5
Cromolyn sodium, 23*t*
Cunningham compression devices, 465, 466*f*
CVA, *see* Cerebrovascular accidents
Cymbalta, *see* Duloxetine
CYP system, 322–323
Cystitis, 20*t*–21*t*
Cystocele, 189*b*, 488, 489*f*
Cystography, 221
Cystometrograms, 221, 222*t*–223*t*, 225–226,
   225*b*
Cystospaz, *see* Hyoscyamine

Darifenacin, 308, 311, 316–318, 317*t*, 336,
   347*t*, 350*t*, 351*t*, 353*t*
DDAVP, *see* Desmopressin acetate
Defecation, overview of, 133–134
Defecation schedules, 155*b*–156*b*, 158–159
Defecation urge, 144–145
Defecatory disorders, *see* Constipation
Defensive urination, 26, 96
Degenerative joint disease, 114
Dehydration, 94–95, 150, 235; *see also* Fluid
     intake
Delirium, 95
Delivery method, antimuscarinic drugs and,
   328
Dementia, 95, 106*t*, 112, 254*t*, 330–331
Demyelinating disease, 104
Dependent continence, 177, 247*f*
Depression, 18, 116–117, 146, 182

Dermatitis
  incontinence-associated (IAD), 377, 381
  perineal, 23, 378*t*, 427
  yeast-associated, 379*t*, 381, 381*b*, 382*f*
Desmopressin acetate (DDAVP), 338, 349*t*, 449
Detrol, *see* Tolterodine
Detrusor; *see also* Bladders
  acetylcholine and, 312–313
  aging and, 82
  bladder, urethral dysfunctions and, 97*t*
  caffeine and, 236–237
  normal bladder function and, 76*t*
  overview of, 61–63
  race and, 17
  urgency urinary incontinence and, 100–101
Detrusor hyperactivity with impaired bladder
      contractility (DHIC), 97*t*
Detrusor hyperreflexia, 97*t*, 101
Detrusor overactivity (DO), 101
Detrusor-sphincter dyssynergia (DSD), 97*t*,
      103, 450
DHEP, 452
DHIC, *see* Detrusor hyperactivity with
      impaired bladder contractility (DHIC)
Diabetes mellitus, 48, 103, 104, 107*t*, 113, 144,
      146
Diabetes mellitus autoantibody panel, 217–218
Diagnostic tests, 153, 190*b*–191*b*
Diapers, 368–377, 368*f*, 370*t*, 371*t*
DIAPPERS mnemonic, 88, 89*t*
Diaries, *see* Bladder and bowel diaries
Diarrhea, 135*t*, 142–143, 166, 383
Diet, 21*t*, 143–144, 154–158, 155*b*, 160*t*
  "What You Eat and Drink Can Affect Your
      Bladder," 234
Digestive tract, anatomy of, 131*f*
Digital stimulation, 164–165
Diltiazem, 91*t*
Dimethicone, 385, 470
Dimethylsulfoxide (DMSO), 21*t*–22*t*
Discoloration, purple, 442
Dislodgement, 471
Ditropan, *see* Oxybutynin
Diuretics, 81, 91*t*, 94, 237–238
DO, *see* Detrusor overactivity
Doctorate in Nursing Practice (DNP), 566
Documentation, indwelling urinary catheters
      and, 411–412, 412*b*
Docusate sodium, 160*t*
Donepezil, 330–331
Dopamine, 78*t*, 316
Double incontinence, 136–137
Double voiding, 239
Douches, 27
Down training, 284
Doxazosin, 91*t*
Drainage bags, 437–442, 437*f*, 438*f*, 439*f*, 440*f*,
      441*f*

Dribbling, 87*f*, 239
DRIP mnemonic, 88, 89*t*
Drip-collecting pouches, 373, 373*f*
Drug therapy, 307–309, 337–338, 349*t*–355*t*;
      see also Antimuscarinic medications
Dry mouth, 335
DSD, *see* Detrusor-sphincter dyssynergia
Duloxetine, 117, 293, 340–342
Durasphere, 538
Dutasteride, 116
Duty cycle, 297
Duvoid, *see* Bethanechol
Dyssynergic defecation, 138
Dysuria, 86*f*

Education, 3–8, 41–43, 419–420, 568–569,
      578
Effort-related urinary incontinence, *see* Stress
      urinary incontinence (SUI)
Elastomer latex, 396*t*
Elavi, *see* Amitriptyline
Electrical stimulation, *see* Pelvic floor electrical
      stimulation (PFES); Posterior tibial
      nerve stimulation
Electrolytes, 94–95
Electromyography (EMG), 207, 224*t*, 276–284,
      283*f*
EMG, *see* Electromyography
Emollients, 159, 160*t*, 469
Emptying/voiding symptoms, 87*f*, 104–105
Enablex, *see* Darifenacin
Enalapril, 91*t*
Encrustations, 403–404, 408, 471
Endopelvic fascia, 69, 70
Endothelin, 77*t*
Endurance, 281
Enemas, 140, 141–142, 162*t*
Enteral feedings, 142–143
Enterocele, 491
Enterococcus, 402
Environmental assessment, 180*b*, 183–185,
      187*b*–188*b*
Ephedrine, 91*t*, 340, 341*t*
Epididymitis, 405, 447
Episiotomy, 110
Erosions, urethral, 404, 404*f*
Erythema, 377, 378*t*
Escherichia coli, 19*t*, 93
Estrace, 345
Estradiol, 344*t*, 345
Estring, 345–346
Estrogen, 23*t*, 83, 92–93, 100, 205–206,
      342–346, 344*t*
Evadri Bladder Control System, 279*f*
Evaluation; *see also* Assessment; Physical
      examinations
  checklist for, 178*b*–181*b*

Evaluation *(continued)*
    histories and, 178*b*–180*b*, 185, 186*b*–191*b*,
        191–192
    overview of, 176*f*
    screening tools, voiding logs and, 193–200,
        193*b*, 194*b*, 194*t*, 197*f*, 199*f*
Excretion, antimuscarinic drugs and, 327
Exercise, 24, 119–120, 146–147, 154, 156*b*
"Exercising Your Pelvic Floor Muscles," 272
Ex-Lax, 162*t*
Extended-release drug formulations, 311,
        319–320
External anal sphincter, 73–74, 73*f*, 132*f*, 133
External catheter collection systems (EECS),
        425–437, 427*f*, 429*f*, 430*f*, 431*f*,
        432*f*–434*f*, 435*f*, 436*f*
External continence devices, 431, 432*f*–433*f*
External perianal pouches, 167, 168*f*
External pouches, 167, 168*f*, 431, 434, 434*f*
External stimulation, 164–165
External urethral devices, 463–464, 463*f*
External urethral sphincter, 67, 67*b*, 68, 71
Eyeball cystometrograms, 225–226, 225*b*

Fall alarms, 115*b*
Fallen uterus, 100
Falling, 115*b*
False passage creation, 447
Fatigue, 281
Fecal Collector, 167, 168*f*
Fecal containment devices, 166–167, 166*f*, 167*f*
Fecal impaction, 89*t*, 90*t*, 94, 140–142,
        214–215
Fecal incontinence, *see* Anal incontinence (AI)
Federal regulations, 36–38, 121, 331–332; *see
        also* Tag F315
FemAssist, 463
Fembrace, 506, 507*f*
FemSoft urethral insert, 460–461, 460*f*
Fesoterodine, 308, 323–324
Fiber, *see* Diet
Fibrous urogenital diaphragm muscles, 70–71
Filling symptoms, *see* Storage/filling symptoms
Financial aspects of incontinence, 44–46
Finasteride, 114
Fistulas, urethral, 405
FIT intervention, *see* Functional integrated
        graining intervention
Flavoxate, 337, 349*t*
FlexiSeal Fecal Collection Device, 166, 167*f*
Fluconazole, 23*t*
Fluid intake
    bowel dysfunction and, 144, 150, 154, 155*b*
    catheters and, 417, 448
    self-care and, 234–236, 234*b*
Foley, Frederick, 393
Foley catheters, *see* Indwelling urinary
        catheters

Folstein Mini-Mental State Examination, 182
Food and Drug Administration, 366, 367*b*
Fornix, posterior, 494*b*
Fracture pans, 391
Frequency, overview of, 86*f*
Frequency rate, 297
Friction, 381
Fulmer SPICES framework, 44
Functional assessment, 180*b*, 182–183, 187*b*
Functional capacity, 65
Functional constipation, *see* Normal-transit
        (functional) constipation
Functional integrated graining (FIT)
        intervention, 259
Functional urinary incontinence, 96*t*, 103–104
Furosemide, 91*t*

GABA, 78*t*
Gabapentin, 20*t*, 21*t*, 23*t*, 91*t*
Galantamine, 330–331
"Garage door" syndrome, 101–102
Gastroenteritis, 142
Geary, Mary Ann, 581
Gehrung, 511
Gellhorn, 512
Gellhorn pessaries, 498*f*, 499
Gender, 2, 13–18, 16*f*, 29*t*, 109
Genital hiatus, 202, 494*b*
Genitalia, 201–207, 202*f*, 203*f*
Genuine stress urinary incontinence, 97*t*; *see
        also* Stress urinary incontinence (SUI)
Glans penis, 66
Glutamate, 78*t*, 315
Glutaraldehyde cross-linked (GAX) bovine
        collagen, 537–538
Glycine, 78*t*
Glycosuria, 217–218
Gonococci, 203
Gram-negative bacteria, 380*t*
Gravitational urinary incontinence, 97*t*, 524
Guarding reflex, 68
Guillain-Barré syndrome, 104

Habit program, 249*t*
Hanno, Philip, 579
Head injuries, 106*t*
Heart rates, 335–336, 336
Help-seeking behavior, 26–27, 30
Hematuria, 217, 405, 447
Hemorrhoids, 135*t*, 144, 204, 282
Hesitancy, overview of, 87*f*
High-tone PFM dysfunction, 284
Hip fractures, 23
Hip protectors, 115*b*
Hiprex, 419
Histories, evaluation and, 121, 135*t*,
        178*b*–180*b*, 185, 186*b*–191*b*, 191–192

Home care setting, incontinence in, 30, 32–34
Hormone replacement therapy, 92–93
Huiyang, 299
Humectants, 469
Hydrogel, 397*t*, 408–409, 464
Hydrophilic-coated catheters, 452–454, 453*f*
Hygiene, misconceptions about, 29*t*
Hyoscyamine, *see* Propantheline
Hypercalcemia, 90*t*
Hyperglycemia, 90*t*, 94
Hyperpathia, 22*t*
Hypoactive bladder, 97*t*, 339, 339*t*
Hypocontractile bladder, 97*t*, 339, 339*t*
Hypoestrogenization, 83, 92, 205–206
Hypogastric nerves, 76*t*
Hyponatremia, 338
Hypothyroidism, 146
Hysterectomy, 90*t*, 100, 117–118, 485, 486

IAD, *see* Incontinence-associated dermatitis
ICIQ, *see* International Consultation on
    Incontinence Questionnaire
IC/PBS, *see* Interstitial cystitis/painful bladder
    syndrome
IIQ-7, 195
Iliococcygeus muscles, 69, 71, 207
Imipramine, 338–339, 350*t*
IMPACT study, 325–326
Impaction, 89*t*, 90*t*, 94, 140–142, 214–215
Impacts, women's statements about, 31*b*
Implementation, barriers to, 38–43
InCare Advance Plus, 453, 455*f*
Incomplete emptying, 87*f*, 339, 339*t*
Incontinence, 86*f*; *see also* Anal (fecal)
    incontinence; Double incontinence
Incontinence Impact Questionnaire 7 (IIQ-7),
    195
"Incontinence Patient Profile," 193
Incontinence pessaries, 499, 517–518
Incontinence practice models, *see* Practice
    models
Incontinence-associated dermatitis (IAD), 377,
    381
Independent continence, 177
Indigo, 442
Indwelling urinary catheters
    acute care use of, 397–399
    bacterial colonization prevention and,
        409–410, 409*f*
    bacteriuria and, 400–401, 401*f*
    balloon size and, 407, 407*f*
    best practices for care of, 410–422, 412*b*,
        415*f*, 416*f*
    biofilms and, 403
    changing schedule for, 410
    design of, 405–406
    encrustations and, 403–404
    home care use and, 400

indications for use of, 394–396, 398*b*
latex allergies and, 408–409
long-term care facilities and, 399
materials made of, 396*t*–397*t*, 408
overview of, 393–394, 394*f*, 395*f*
size and length of, 406
tips of, 406, 406*f*
troubleshooting of problems with, 471–472
types of, 396*t*–397*t*, 405
urethral damage and, 404–405, 404*f*
urinary tract infections and, 401*f*, 402–403
urosepsis and, 404
use and misuse of, 396–397
Inflatoball, 498*f*, 499, 514–515
InFlow intraurethral prosthesis, 461–462, 461*f*
Infrastructure, 40
Injection therapy, 535–536, 537–539, 537*f*, 539
Inpatient Prospective Payment System (IPPS),
    398
Inserts, *see* Urethral inserts and clamps
Insoluble dietary fiber, 156, 160*t*
Insurance, 366, 468
Interlabial sulci, 202
Intermittent catheterization (IC)
    bacteriuria and, 446
    cathether use and care and, 458
    closed or self-contained systems and, 454,
        455*f*, 456*f*
    complications from, 447
    materials made of, 451–454
    medicare and, 449*b*
    overview of, 444–445
    prevention of problems with, 448–450
    scheduling and, 454–455
    self-catheterization and, 456–458, 457*f*
    size and length of, 450–451, 451*f*
    sterile vs. clean, 445–446
    types of, 450, 452*f*, 453*f*
    urethral damage and, 447
    urinary tract infections and, 446–447
Intermittent stream, 87*f*
Internal anal sphincter, 73–74, 73*f*, 132*f*, 133
Internal obturator muscles, 73, 270–271
Internal urethral inserts, 459–463, 460*f*, 461*f*,
    462*f*
Internal urinary sphincter, 64, 67, 67*b*, 68
International Consultation on Incontinence,
    177, 310
International Consultation on Incontinence
    Questionnaire (ICIQ), 195
International Continence Society (ICS), 85, 102
InterStim Therapy System, 549–559, 551*f*,
    552*b*, 553*b*, 553*f*, 554*f*, 554*t*, 555*t*, 557*f*
Interstitial cystitis/painful bladder syndrome
    (IC/PBS), 20*t*–21*t*
Intertrigo, 378*t*
Intraurethral prostheses, *see* Internal urethral
    inserts
Intravesical therapy, 321

Intrinsic urethral (sphincter) deficiency (ISD), 97*t*, 524
InVance male slings, 540, 540*f*
IPPS, *see* Inpatient Prospective Payment System
Iron supplements, 146
Irrigation, 418
Irritable bowel syndrome, 146
Irritant dermatitis, 378*t*
ISD, *see* Intrinsic urethral (sphincter) deficiency

Kegel, Arnold, 266, 279, 280*f*
Kegel exercises, 266–267; *see also* Pelvic floor muscle training (PFMT)
"Key-in-the-lock" syndrome, 101–102
Kidneys, 61, 82
"The Knack," 269, 275–276

Lactobacilli, 164, 205–206, 343
Lactose intolerance, 143
Lactulose, 161*t*
Laparoscopic Burch colposuspension, 527
Lapides, Jack, 444
Large intestine, 130–132, 131*f*
Large-capacity bags, *see* Overnight bags
Latex, 396*t*, 397*t*
Latex allergies, 408–409
Laxatives, 94, 130, 140, 147
LeCroy, Cheryl, 580
Leg bags, 437*f*, 438–440, 438*f*, 441*f*
Leukorrhea, 504–505
Leukotrienes, 77*t*, 316
Levator ani muscles
   anatomy of, 69–70
   childbirth and, 110
   evaluation of, 207, 209–210
   pelvic floor muscle training and, 266, 267, 269, 272
   stress urinary incontinence and, 98
   structure and function of, 71–72
Levator prostatae muscles, 71
Levsin, *see* Hyoscyamine
Liberty Pouch, 431, 432*f*–433*f*
Lidocaine, vulvodynia and, 23*t*
Limbic system, 78
Limited mobility, 88–90, 90*t*, 104, 114
Lisinopril, 91*t*
Lithotomy position, 201, 204
LoFric catheter, 453
Long-term care facilities
   antimuscarinic medications and, 331–332
   bacteriuria and, 93
   bladder and bowel records in, 199–200
   causes of incontinence in, 35–36
   control programs in, 38–43, 39*b*
   dehydration and, 94

evaluation checklist for, 186*b*–191*b*
financial aspects of incontinence and, 45–46
functional urinary incontinence and, 103–104
incontinence in, 34–35
protocols for, 582–583
state and federal regulations and, 36–38, 39*b*
Lower extremity venous insufficiency, 114
Lower urinary tract, 61, 63*f*, 77*t*, 81–83
Lower urinary tract symptoms (LUTS), 85, 86*t*–87*t*, 114–116, 139
Low-tone PFM dysfunction, 284
Lubiprostone, 163*t*
Lubricants, 162*t*
Lupus erythematosus, 104

Maceration, 378*t*, 436
Macroplastique Implantation System, 538–539
Magnesium citrate, 161*t*
Management and collection products; *see also* Catheterization
   absorbent incontinence, 368–377, 368*f*, 370*t*, 372*f*, 373*f*, 374*f*, 375*f*
   classification and approval of, 367*b*
   overview of, 365–366
   perineal skin care and, 377–387, 378*t*–380*t*, 381*b*, 382*f*, 384*f*
   toileting substitutes and devices, 387–392, 389*f*, 390*f*, 392*f*
   "The Side Effects of Treatment for Overactive Bladder," 334
Manometry, 276, 279–280, 279*f*
Marland pessary, 517, 518
Marshall-Marchetti-Krantz (MMK) bladder neck suspension, 524, 526–527
MATRIX study, 326
Maximal voluntary contraction (MVC), 266
MCA, *see* Minnesota Continence Associates
McGuire reusable ECC, 435*f*
MDS, *see* Minimum Data Sets
Meatal plates, 459
Meatus urinarius, 65
Medicaid, *see* Centers for Medicare & Medicaid Services (CMS)
Medical directors, 40–41
Medicare, 6, 328, 449*b*, 467, 503
Medications; *see also* Drug therapy; Polypharmacy
   affecting bladder function, 91*t*
   bowel dysfunction and, 145–146, 150–152, 159, 160*t*–163*t*, 164
   caffeine and, 236
   dehydration and, 94
   toileting programs and, 259–260, 292–293
Men, 19*t*–20*t*; *see also* Gender
Menopause
   hypoestrogenization and, 83
   pelvic organ prolapse and, 485

prevalence and, 14
as risk factor, 98–99, 100, 112
urgency and, 1
Menstrual cycle, 22*t*
Menstrual pads, 376
Mental awareness, 103–104
Metabolic conditions, overview of, 90*t*
Methicillin-resistant *S. aureus, see* MRSA
Methylcellulose, 160*t*
Methylxanthines, 91*t*
Metoprolol, 91*t*
Micromotions, 312
Micturition (voiding), 78–81, 78*t*, 79*f*, 80*b*, 239–240
Midurethral slings, 528*f*, 530–535, 531*f*, 533*f*, 534*f*
Milex, *see* CooperSurgical
Milk of Magnesia, 161*t*
Mineral oil, 162*t*
Miniguard, 464, 464*f*
Minimum Data Sets (MDS), 35–36
Minnesota Continence Associates (MCA), 581
Minnova PFES device, 296*f*
Misconceptions, 2–3, 4, 27, 28*t*–29*t*
Misoprostol, 162*t*
Mixed urinary incontinence (MUI), 13–14, 14*f*, 96*t*, 102, 338–339, 349*t*–355*t*
Mnemonics, 88, 89*t*
Mobility, prevention and, 46
Moisturizers, 385, 469
Monaghan, Cindy Maloney, 579
Moniliasis, 379*t*, 381, 381*b*, 382*f*
Morbidity, 24
Moy, M. Louis, 579
MRSA, 399, 402
Mucosal lining, 65–66
Mucous glands, 65
MUI, *see* Mixed urinary incontinence
Multiple sclerosis, 101, 103, 104, 107*t*, 108, 113–114, 146
Multiple system atrophy, 106*t*
Multi-Setting Practice for Continence, 579
Multispecialty Continence Services for Women, 579–580
Muscarinic receptors, 312–316, 313*f*, 313*t*, 314*f*
Muscle relaxants, 20*t*
Myelitis, 107*t*
Myofascial release, 21*t*

Nabisco plant lawsuit, 121
Narcotic analgesics, 91*t*
National Institutes of Health (NIH), 19*t*, 20*t*, 46
N-DEO, 320
NDO, *see* Neurogenic detrusor overactivity
Nervous system
external sphincter and, 68

large intestine and, 132
neurogenic bladder and, 105*f*
obesity and, 119
pelvic floor muscles and, 207
rectum, anal canal and, 73
Neurogenic bladder, 104–108, 333–334, 337
Neurogenic detrusor overactivity (NDO), 97*t*, 101
Neurogenic lower urinary tract dysfunction, *see* Neurogenic bladder
Neuroleptics, 91*t*
Neurological examinations, 215–216, 216*f*
Neuromodulation therapy, 295, 549–559, 551*f*, 552*b*, 553*b*, 553*f*, 554*f*, 554*t*, 555*t*, 557*f*
Neuromuscular electrical stimulation, *see* Pelvic floor electrical stimulation (PFES)
Neurontin, *see* Gabapentin
Neurotransmitters, 63, 64, 76–77, 77*t*, 117, 315–316
NHQI, *see* Nursing Home Quality Initiative
NICHE project, 44
Nifedipine, 91*t*
Nighttime incontinence, 81, 86*f*
Nitric oxide, 77*t*, 316
Nitrite tests, 217
Nitrofurazone, 409–410, 409*f*
Nocturia, 23, 81–82, 86*f*, 100–101, 238–239
Nocturnal enuresis, 81, 86*f*
Nocturnal polyuria (NP), 81–82, 448–449
Nonadhesive catheters, 429, 430*f*
Non-blockers, 404
Norepinephrine, 77*t*, 78*t*, 315
Normal-transit (functional) constipation, 137
NP, *see* Nocturnal polyuria
NSAIDs, 91*t*, 145
Nurse continence advisors (NCA), 566, 570, 577
Nurses, 6–7, 28*t*–29*t*, 35, 41–43; *see also* Advanced Practice Nurses
Nurses' Health Study II, 118
Nurses Improving Care for Health System Elders, *see* NICHE project
Nursing Home Quality Initiative (NHQI), 36
Nursing homes, *see* Long-term care facilities

OAB, *see* Overactive bladder
OAB-q, 194*t*
Obesity, 46, 98–99, 118–119, 241; *see also* Weight gain
Obsessive toileting reduction, overview of, 264–266
Obstruction, indwelling catheter and, 471
Obstructive sleep apnea, 114
Occlusive devices, 459–463, 460*f*, 461*f*, 462*f*, 469
Occupational Safety and Health Administration (OSHA), 121

Odor, fear of, 27
Olive-tipped catheters, 451, 452f
On/off time, 297
Onuf's nucleus, 77, 78, 341
OPERA study, 324–325
Opioids, 91t, 145
OPTION-vf urethral inserts, 462–463
OSHA, see Occupational Safety and Health Administration
Osmotic agents, 159, 161t–162t
Osteoporosis, 114
Outcome and Assessment Information Set, 33–34
Outlet obstruction constipation, see Rectosigmoidal outlet delay
Out-of-pocket expenses, 46
Overactive bladder (OAB); see also Antimuscarinic medications
    defined, 13
    estrogen and, 342
    financial aspects of, 44–45
    gender and, 17
    prevalence of, 15
    prostatitis vs., 19t
    quality of life and, 25
    questionnaire for, 194t
    second-line medications for, 337–339, 349t–355t
    urgency urinary incontinence and, 100
Overflow anal (fecal) incontinence, 136
Overflow urinary incontinence, overview of, 96t, 102–103
Overnight bags, 437, 437f, 438
Oxybutynin
    biofeedback therapy and, 292–293
    blood-brain barrier and, 313
    neurogenic bladder and, 333–334
    older adults and, 329–330
    overview of, 308, 317t, 318–321, 347t–348t, 350t, 351t, 353t–354t
    problems associated with, 310–311
    tolterodine vs., 324
Oxytrol, 326, 350t

Pad tests, 220
Pad-and-pant systems, 374, 375f
Pads, 368–377, 368f, 370t, 371t
Paget's disease, 90t
Painful bladder syndrome, 20t–21t
Parachute jumping, 120
Paradoxical incontinence, 96t, 102–103
Paraphimosis, 206, 206f
Parasympathetic nervous system, 75, 76t
Parkinson's disease, 101, 106t, 113, 146, 333
Partial incontinence, 181
Patient Perception of Bladder Conditions (PPBC), 194, 194b, 325–326

Patterned Urge Response Toileting (PURT), 258–259
Payment, 328
Pelvic diaphragm muscles, 69–71, 70f
Pelvic examinations, 181b, 189b, 204–205
Pelvic Floor Clinical Assessment Group, 270
Pelvic floor disorders (PFDs), 1–2
Pelvic floor dyssynergia, 138
Pelvic floor electrical stimulation (PFES), 294–299, 296f
"Pelvic Floor Muscle Exercise Prescription," 274
Pelvic floor muscle training (PFMT)
    biofeedback and, 165–166, 276–284, 277f, 278f, 279f, 280f, 283f, 285f–287f
    childbirth and, 47
    evidence for effectiveness of, 288–290
    implementation of, 272–275
    mechanism of action of, 267–269
    muscle location and, 268f, 269–272
    overview of, 246, 266–267
Pelvic floor muscles
    aging and, 83, 108–109
    changes in with age, 81–83
    evaluation of, 207–213, 208b–209b, 210f, 213f
    exercises for, 189b
    fecal incontinence and, 135t
    location of, 268f, 269–272
    nervous system and, 76t, 105f
    overview of, 69–70, 69f, 70f, 72f, 267–269
    physical examination of, 207–213
    supportive structures of, 70–73
    weakness of as risk factor, 116
Pelvic nerves, 76, 76t
Pelvic organ prolapse (POP); see also Pessaries
    assessment of, 189b, 206, 486–488, 487b
    constipation and, 192
    estrogen and, 342
    management of, 493–497, 496f, 506, 507f
    measurement systems for, 491–493, 492f, 494b, 495f
    muscle weakness and, 116
    overflow urinary incontinence and, 103
    overview of, 485–486
    as pelvic floor disorder, 1–2
    pregnancy and childbirth and, 111
    stress urinary incontinence and, 100
    surgery for, 486, 506–508
    types of, 488–491, 489f, 490f
Pelvic Organ Prolapse Quantification (POPQ) grading system, 493, 494b, 495f
Pelvic pain assessment, 213–214, 214f
Pelvic surgery as risk factor, 98–99, 107t, 117–118
Penile compression devices, 464–467, 466f, 467f
Penis, urethra and, 66

Penn Center for Continence and Pelvic Health, 579
Performance on Timed Toileting Instrument (POTTI), 183
Perineal body, 494*b*
Perineal cleansers, 383–384, 384*f*, 469
Perineal dermatitis, 23, 378*t*, 427
Perineal membrane, 70–71
Perineal pads, 371–372, 373*f*
Perineal skin care, 377–387, 378*t*–380*t*, 381*b*, 382*f*, 384*f*, 469–470
Perineometers, 266, 279–280, 279*f*, 280*f*
Peripheral nervous system, 74
Periurethral injection, 535–539, 537*f*
Pessaries
    care of, 502–503
    complications with use of, 503–505
    fitting of, 500–502
    pelvic organ prolapse and, 493–497
    reasons for discontinuing use of, 505–506
    types of, 497–499, 498*f*, 509–518
Petrolatum-based skin protectants, 383, 385, 470
PFD, *see* Pelvic floor disorders
PFES, *see* Pelvic floor electrical stimulation
PFMT, *see* Pelvic floor muscle training
PH, 217, 381, 381*b*, 383, 403, 419
Pharmacological causes, 88
Phenylpropanolamine, 340, 341*t*
Phimosis, 436
Physical activity, *see* Exercise
Physical examinations
    abdominal, 180*b*–181*b*, 201
    anorectal examination and, 214–215
    bowel dysfunction and, 152
    general, 200–201
    genitalia (male) and, 180*b*, 204*b*, 206–207, 206*f*
    genitalia (female) and, 180*b*, 202*f*, 203*f*, 206
    neurological examination, 215–216, 216*f*
    pelvic floor muscle evaluation and, 207–213, 208*b*–209*b*, 210*f*, 212*f*
    pelvic pain assessment and, 181*b*, 205*f*, 213–214, 214*f*
    urological testing and, 181*b*, 216–227, 219*b*, 221*b*, 222*t*–224*t*, 225*b*
Physical therapists, education and, 7
Physician Voluntary Reporting Program (PVRP), 6
Physicians, misconceptions of, 28*t*–29*t*
Pill burden, 328
Placebo effects, 310
Polyacrylate, 371
Polycarbophil, 160*t*
Polymers, 371, 538–539
Polypharmacy, 88, 117, 329–330, 331
Polytetrafluoroethylene (PTFE), 396*t*, 408
Polyuria, 94, 114, 448–449

Polyvinyl pyrrolidone (PVP), 452–453
POP, *see* Pelvic organ prolapse
POPQ, *see* Pelvic Organ Prolapse Quantification grading system
Posterior fornix, 494*b*
Posterior tibial nerve stimulation (PTNS), 299, 300*f*
Postvoid dribbling, 87*f*, 239
Postvoid residual urine
    aging and, 82
    bladder retraining and, 421–422
    evaluation and, 181*b*, 191*b*
    intermittent catheterization and, 444–445
    overflow urinary incontinence and, 102
    overview of, 218–220
    pelvic organ prolapse and, 493
    physician familiarity with, 5
POTTI, *see* Performance on Timed Toileting Instrument
PPBC, *see* Patient Perception of Bladder Conditions
Practice models, 5, 566, 570–572, 579–581
PRAISED mnemonic, 88, 89*t*
Praising, 257–258
Prazosin, 91*t*
Predisposing conditions, 90*t*
Pregnancy, 98–99, 100, 109–112, 145, 289–290; *see also* Childbirth
Pressure, overview of, 86*f*
Pressure ulcers, 377, 380*t*, 382*f*, 399
Prevalence rates, 13–14, 14–18, 14*f*, 15*f*, 16*f*, 30, 137
Prevention of incontinence, overview of, 46–48
Pro-Banthine, *see* Propantheline
Probiotics, 164
Procidentia, 492*f*, 493
Products, *see* Management and collection products
Prokinetic agents, 161*t*
Prolapse, *see* Pelvic organ prolapse (POP)
Prometheus Feedback System, 277*f*, 284, 285*f*–287*f*
Prompted voiding (PV), 255–259; *see also* Bladder training (BT)
Propantheline, 337, 349*t*
Prophylaxis, 418–419, 421
Propranolol, 91*t*
Prostanoids, 77*t*, 316
Prostate cancer treatment, 90*t*, 100
Prostate disorders, 68, 114–116, 116*b*, 215; *see also* Benign prostatic hyperplasia (BPH)
Prostatectomies, 48, 100, 117–118, 290, 291*f*
Prostatic urethra, 66, 67
Prostatitis, 19*t*, 19*t*–20*t*, 93, 395
Protective acid mantle of the skin, 381
Protective underwear, 374, 374*f*
Proteus mirabilis, 93
Provocative stress tests, 220

Pruritus ani, 379t
Pseudoephedrine, 91t, 340, 341t
Psychological causes, 88
Psychotropic medications, 91t
Psyllium, 154
Pubic pressure urinals, 434–435, 435f
Pubococcygeus muscles, 69, 70, 71, 110, 207, 209–210
Puborectalis muscles, 69, 71–72, 74, 132, 132f, 207, 214–216
Pubovaginalis muscles, 71
PUBS, see Purple urine bag syndrome
Pudendal nerves, 68, 76, 76t, 110–111, 295, 298
Purple urine bag syndrome (PUBS), 442
PURT, see Patterned Urge Response Toileting
PVC catheters, 452
PVP, see Polyvinyl pyrrolidone
PVRP, see Physician Voluntary Reporting Program
Pyelonephritis, 446
Pyuria, 217

QT interval prolongation, 335–336
Q-Tip procedure, 203, 204b
Quality of life, 23–26, 325–326
Quercetin, 20t
Quick flicks, 269

Race, 14–18, 15f, 21t, 109
Radiofrequency thermal treatment, 539
Ramping, 296–297
RAP, see Resident Assessment Protocols
Recruitment, 72, 283–284
Rectal examinations, 181b
Rectal prolapse, 111, 490–491
Rectal surgery, 144
Rectoanal inhibitory reflex, 133
Rectocele, 489f, 490
Rectosigmoidal outlet delay, 138
Rectosphincteric anal (fecal) incontinence, 136
Rectum
    assessment of, 189b
    location of, 132f
    prolapse of, 189b
    structure and function of, 73–74, 73f, 131–132, 131f
    urogenital hiatus and, 71
Regulation 1910.141, 121
Rehabilitation centers, incontinence in, 43–44
Reliance, 459
Renessa, 539
Research projects, federal funding for, 3–4
Reservoir anal (fecal) incontinence, 136
Resident Assessment Protocols (RAP), 35, 36, 175
Rest breaks, 121

Restricted mobility, 88–90, 90t, 104, 114
Retropubic suspension, 526–527
Reusable ECCS, 434–435, 435f
Reusable incontinence products, 371, 372f
Re-wet value, 371
Rhabdosphincter, 65
Rhabdosphincter-skeletal muscle, 68
Risk factors
    age as, 108–109
    chronic, treatable conditions as, 112–114
    constipation and, 139
    depression as, 116–117
    family history and, 121
    fecal incontinence and, 134–136, 135t
    menopause as, 112
    obesity as, 118–119
    overview of, 90t
    pelvic floor muscle weakness as, 116
    pelvic surgery as, 98–99, 107t, 117–118
    physical activities as, 119–120
    polypharmacy as, 117
    pregnancy and childbirth and, 109–112
    prevention and, 46
    prostate disorders as, 114–116
    sex and race as, 109
    smoking as, 118
    work environment and, 120–121
Rivastigmine, 330–331

Sacral agenesis, 107t
Sacral nerve stimulation (SNS), 549–559, 551f, 552b, 553b, 553f, 554f, 554t, 555t, 557f
Sacrocolpexy, 507
Sampselle, Carolyn, 289
Sanctura, see Trospium
SANS protocol, 299
Saturation point, 371
Saw palmetto, 20t
Scheduled voiding/habit training, 247, 249t, 252–255, 261–263, 420–422
Schedules, see Defecation schedules
Screening tools, 193–196, 193b, 194b, 194t
Scrotal abscess, 447
Scrotal edema, 387
Scrotum, 207
Securement, 414–415, 415f, 416f
Self-adhesive catheters, 429, 429f, 432f–433f
Self-care
    bladder irritants and, 236–237
    fluid intake and, 234–236
    importance of, 3
    interstitial cystitis/painful bladder syndrome and, 21t
    irregularity, constipation and, 237
    nocturia management and, 238–239
    overview of, 26–27, 223–224, 234b
    smoking cessation and, 240–241

techniques to assist with, 239–240
weight reduction and, 241
Self-catheterization, 456–458, 457*f*
SEPHIA's Choice, 568
Serotonin, 77*t*, 117, 316, 340–342
Seton Health Incontinence and Wound
 Services (SHIWS), 579
Sexual intercourse, 25
Sexually transmitted diseases (STD), 22*t*
Shaatz pessaries, 517
SHIWS, *see* Seton Health Incontinence and
 Wound Services
Side effects
 alpha-adrenergic agonists and, 340
 anticholinergic-antimuscarinic agents and,
  334–337
 antidepressants and, 339, 341
 overview of, 350*t*
 transvaginal estrogen and, 344–345
Sigmoid colon, 131, 131*f*
Silicone, 396*t*, 397*t*, 408, 538–539
Silver alloy, 397*t*, 408, 409, 410
Skene's glands, 65
Skin, 336–337; *see also* Dermatitis; Perineal
 skin care
Skin care products, 383–387, 384*f*, 469–470
Skin patches, 311, 320–321, 328, 336–337
Sling procedures
 bladder neck sling procedures, 527–530
 male SUI and, 540–541, 540*f*
 materials used in, 529*t*
 midurethral slings, 528*f*, 530
 overview of, 524
 suprapubic arch sling (SPARC), 534–535,
  534*f*
Slow-transit constipation, 138
Smegma, 202, 206
Smoking, 46, 118, 240–241
Smooth sphincter, 64, 67, 67*b*, 68
Sneezing, *see* Stress urinary incontinence (SUI)
SNS, *see* Sacral nerve stimulation
Soaps, 383–384
Social incontinence, *see* Contained
 incontinence
Sodium biphosphate, 161*t*
Soldiers, 120
Solifenacin
 drug selection and, 311
 overactive bladder and, 308
 overview of, 317*t*, 321–322, 348*t*, 350*t*,
  351*t*–352*t*, 354*t*–355*t*
 safety and, 336
 tolterodine vs., 324–325
Soluble dietary fiber, 156, 160*t*
Somatic nervous system, 75–76, 76*t*
Sorbitol 60%, 161*t*
SPARC, *see* Suprapubic arch sling
Spastic pelvic floor syndrome, 138

Sphincter urethrae, 66*f*, 67
Sphincter vesicae, 66
Sphincteric urethra, 66, 67
Sphincteric urinary incontinence, *see* Stress
 urinary incontinence (SUI)
Sphincters; *see also* Artificial urinary
 sphincters; Internal anal sphincter
 anal canal and, 73–74, 73*f*
 childbirth and, 110–111
 fecal incontinence and, 135*t*
 location of, 132*f*
 stress urinary incontinence and, 98–99, 98*f*
 structure and function of, 67–68, 67*b*, 133
 urethra and, 65, 66*f*
SPICES framework, 44
Spina bifida, 104, 107*t*
Spinal cord, 75*f*
Spinal cord injuries
 catheters and, 444, 445
 CAUTI diagnosis and, 402–403
 neurogenic bladder and, 104–105,
  106*t*–107*t*, 108
 overflow urinary incontinence and, 103
 urgency urinary incontinence and, 101
Spinal lesions, 105, 106*t*–107*t*
State regulations, 36–38, 121
StatLock catheter anchors, 416*f*
STD, *see* Sexually transmitted diseases
Sterile catheterization technique, 444, 445–446
Stimulants, 159, 161*t*
Stimulation, external, *see* External stimulation
Stoller, Marshall, 299
Stool, devices for collection of, 166–167
Stool impaction, 89*t*, 90*t*, 94, 140–142,
  214–215
Stop-orders, 413
Storage/filling symptoms, 86*f*, 104–105, 308
Straight catheters, 451–452, 452*f*
Straining to void, overview of, 87*f*
Stress urinary incontinence (SUI); *see also*
 Surgery
 injection therapy and, 535–539, 537*f*
 medications for, 307, 340–342, 341*t*
 overview of, 13–14, 95–100, 96*t*, 523
 pelvic floor electrical stimulation and, 298
 pessaries and, 499, 505–506
 prevalence of, 14*f*
 prostatectomies and, 48
 sphincter muscles and, 98*f*
Stricture, urethral, 447
Strokes, *see* Cerebrovascular accidents (CVA)
Study of Women's Health Across the Nation
 (SWAN), 110
Suction devices, 464
SUI, *see* Stress urinary incontinence
Superabsorbent polymer (SAP), 371
Suppositories, 162*t*, 164
Suprapubic arch sling (SPARC), 534–535, 534*f*

Suprapubic catheters, 394*f*
Suprapubic tapping, 240
Surgery
  artificial urinary sphincters and, 541–545,
    542*f*, 543*f*
  bladder neck sling procedures, 527–530,
    528*f*
  bowel dysfunction and, 144, 167–168
  fecal incontinence and, 135*t*
  laparoscopic Burch colposuspension, 527
  midurethral slings, 528*f*, 530
  misconceptions about, 29*t*
  options for, 524–525
  overview of, 523
  overview of for female SUI, 524
  overview of for male SUI, 539–540
  for pelvic organ prolapse, 486, 506–508
  preoperative preparation and, 525–526
  retropubic suspension, 526–527
  as risk factor for incontinence, 98–99, 107*t*,
    117–118
  sling procedure for male SUI, 540–541,
    540*f*
  suprapubic arch sling (SPARC), 534–535,
    534*f*
  tension-free vaginal tape (TVT), 531–532,
    531*f*
  transobturator tape (TOT), 532–534, 533*f*
SWAN, *see* Study of Women's Health Across
  the Nation
Sympathetic nervous system, 75, 76*t*
Synthetic mesh, 529*t*

Tachykinins, 77*t*, 78*t*, 316
Tag F315, 39*b*, 175, 199–200, 248, 256
Tag F329, 331–332
Tampons, 506
Tamsulosin, 114
Teflon, 396*t*, 408
TENS, *see* Transcutaneous electrical nerve
  stimulation
Tension-free vaginal tape (TVT), 531–532, 531*f*
Terazosin, 91*t*
Terminal dribbling, 87*f*, 239
Testes, 207
Theophylline, 91*t*
Thioridazine, 91*t*
Tibial nerve stimulation, 299, 300*f*
Tiemann catheters, *see* Coudé tips
Timed toileting, *see* Scheduled voiding/habit
  training
"Tips for Keeping Your Bowels Moving," 158
Tofranil, *see* Imipramine
Toileting programs
  bladder training (retraining), 260–264
  drug therapy and, 259–260
  obsessive toileting reduction and, 264–266

overview of, 248–252, 250*t*–251*t*, 252*f*,
  259–260
prompted voiding, 255–259
scheduled voiding/habit training, 252–255
Toileting substitutes and devices, 387–392,
  389*f*, 390*f*, 392*f*
Toilet-mapping, 26, 102
Toilets, 388, 389*f*
Tokophobia, 111
Tolterodine
  bladder training and, 263
  cognition and, 330
  efficacy and tolerability of, 311
  overactive bladder and, 308
  overview of, 317*t*, 322, 348*t*–349*t*, 350*t*, 352*t*
  oxybutynin vs., 324
  solifenacin vs., 324–325
Topiramate, 21*t*
TOT, *see* Transobturator tape
Total vaginal length (tvl), 494*b*
Transcutaneous electrical nerve stimulation
  (TENS), 295
Transdermal delivery systems (TDS), 311,
  320–321, 328, 336–337
Transient incontinence, 85, 88–95, 89*t*
Transobturator tape (TOT), 532–534, 533*f*
Transurethral resection of the prostate, 118
Transvaginal estrogen, 343–346, 344*t*
Transverse abdominus (TrA) muscles, 270
Traumatic catheterization, 450
Traveling, 147
Treatments, misconceptions about, 29*t*
Tricyclic antidepressants, 23*t*, 91*t*, 308,
  338–339
Triggers, 101–102, 185, 240
Trigone, 61, 62, 63–64
TRIMO-SAN, 503
Trospium
  efficacy and tolerability of, 311
  overactive bladder and, 308
  overview of, 317*t*, 322–323, 349*t*, 350*t*, 352*t*,
    355*t*
  safety and, 336
TVT, *see* Tension-free vaginal tape
Two-piece catheters, 429, 429*f*
Type III stress urinary incontinence, 97*t*, 524

UDI-6, *see* Urogenital Distress Inventory 6
UDS, *see* Urodynamic studies
Ultrasonography, 218–219, 219*b*, 258–259, 265
Underactive bladder, 97*t*, 339, 339*t*
Undergarments, 374, 374*f*
Underpads, 377
Unnecessary Drugs (Tag F329), *see* Tag F329
"Up and Go" tests, 183
Up training, 284
Upper urinary tract, 61

Urease, 403
Urecholine, *see* Bethanechol
Urethral catheters, 394*f*
Urethral inserts and clamps
    external, 463–464, 463*f*, 464*f*
    internal, 459–463, 460*f*, 461*f*, 462*f*
    overview of, 458–459
    penile compression devices, 464–467, 466*f*, 467*f*
Urethral meatus, 66*f*
Urethral pressure profiles (UPP), 221, 223*t*
Urethral prolapse, 464
Urethral sphincters, 96–97, 100, 103, 204
Urethral stricture, 447
Urethras
    aging and, 82–83
    assessment of, 203, 203*f*
    control of in women, 66*f*
    damage to from indwelling urinary catheters, 404–405, 404*f*
    damage to from intermittent catheterization, 447
    innervation of, 105*f*
    stress urinary incontinence and, 96–98, 99*f*
    structure and function of, 64*f*, 65–67
Urethritis, 90*t*, 92–93, 404, 447
Urethrocele, 488
Urethrovaginal sphincter, 66*f*
Urge sensation perception, 82
Urge suppression/inhibition, *see* Bladder training (BT)
Urgency, overview of, 86*f*
Urgency urinary incontinence (UUI); *see also* Antimuscarinic medications
    overview of, 13–14, 96*t*, 100–102
    pelvic floor electrical stimulation and, 298–299
    prevalence of, 14*f*
    second-line medications for, 337–338, 349*t*–355*t*
Urgency wave, 261, 262*f*, 265
Urinals, 390–391, 390*f*, 392*f*
Urinalysis, 190*b*, 217–218
Urinary control inserts, *see* Internal urethral inserts
Urinary control pads, 464, 464*f*
Urinary drainage bags, 437–442, 437*f*, 438*f*, 439*f*, 440*f*, 441*f*
"Urinary Incontinence in Adults" (AHRQ), 5, 175
Urinary incontinence (UI), overview of, 13–14
Urinary meatus, 65, 203
Urinary retention, 82, 86*f*, 92, 461–462, 461*f*
Urinary sphincters, *see* Artificial urinary sphincters (AUS)
Urinary tract
    bladder structure and, 61–65, 64*f*
    micturition and, 78–81

nervous system and, 74–78, 75*f*, 76*t*, 77*t*, 78*t*
overview of, 61
pelvic floor muscle anatomy and, 69–73, 69*f*, 70*f*, 72*f*
prostate and, 68
rectum, anal canal and, 73–74
sphincters and, 67–68
structure and function of, 62*f*, 63*f*
urethra structure and, 64*f*, 65–67, 66*f*
vaginal structure and function and, 68–69
Urinary tract infections (UTI); *see also* Catheter-associated urinary tract infection (CAUTI)
    aging and, 82
    as cause of incontinence, 90*t*, 93
    correlation with, 18
    estrogen and, 92, 342
    intermittent catheterization and, 446, 448
    prostatitis and, 19*t*
    toilet accessibility and, 121
Urination cycle, 79–81, 79*f*
Urine, acidification of, 419
Urine culture and sensitivity (C&S), 190*b*–191*b*, 418
Urispas, *see* Flavoxate
Urodynamic studies (UDS), 220–221, 221*b*, 224*t*, 225–226
Uroflowmetry, 221, 224*t*
Urogenital atrophy, 205
Urogenital Distress Inventory 6 (UDI-6), 195
Urogenital hiatus, 71, 491
Urogynecology Continence Practice, 581
Urologic Center of Excellence for Continence Care, 579
Urologic Diseases in America Project, 108–109
Urological testing, 181*b*, 216–227, 219*b*, 221*b*, 222*t*–224*t*, 225*b*
Urosepsis, 404
Urothelium, 63
Uterine prolapse, 189*b*, 488, 489*f*, 492*f*
UUI, *see* Urgency urinary incontinence

Vagifem, 345–346
Vaginal tape procedures, 525, 530–532, 531*f*
Vaginal vault prolapse, 189*b*, 488–490, 490*f*
Vaginal weights (cones), 293–294, 294*f*
Vaginas, 68–69, 189*b*, 205–206
Vaginitis, 90*t*, 92–93, 205–206, 343
Valsalva maneuver, 133, 152, 204, 210, 240, 491
Valved urinary catheters, 462–463
Valves, *see* Catheter valves
Vancomycin-resistant *Enterococcus*, *see* VRE
Vasopressin, 338
V-Brace, 506, 507*f*
Venous insufficiency with edema, 90*t*, 94
Verapamil, 91*t*

VESIcare, *see* Solifenacin
Virginia Women's Continence Center (VWCC), 580
Voiding, *see* Micturition
Voiding diaries, *see* Bladder and bowel records
Voiding symptoms, *see* Emptying/voiding symptoms
VRE (vancomycin-resistant *Enterococcus*), 402
Vulvar vestibulitis (VVS), 22*t*
Vulvodynia, 22*t*–23*t*, 204
VWCC, *see* Virginia Women's Continence Center

Washable incontinence products, 371, 372*f*
Web sites, education and, 7
Weight gain, 24; *see also* Obesity
Wein, Alan J., 579
Wheat bran, 157–158

Whistle-tipped catheters, 406
Williams, Kate, 570
Women, *see* Gender
Women's centers, 572
Wooldridge, Leslie Saltzstein, 579–580
Workplace activities, 120–121
Wound, Ostomy, and Continence Nurses Society, 7, 567
Wyman, Jean, 261, 581

Xenografts, 529*t*

Yeast infections, 379*t*, 381, 381*b*, 382*f*

Zassi Bowel Management System, 166, 166*f*
Zinc oxide, 385, 470